RADIOLOGY OF THE PEDIATRIC CHEST
CLINICAL AND PATHOLOGICAL CORRELATIONS

Alvin H. Felman, M.D.

Professor, Departments of Radiology and Pediatrics
University of Florida College of Medicine,
  Jacksonville Campus
Radiologist, University Hospital
  and Nemours Children's Hospital
Jacksonville, Florida

Contributing Author

Mervyn D. Cohen, M.B., Ch.B.

Professor of Radiology
Indiana School of Medicine
Director of Radiology
James Whitcomb Riley Children's Hospital
Indianapolis, Indiana

McGraw-Hill Book Company

New York St. Louis San Francisco Auckland Bogotá Hamburg Johannesburg
Lisbon London Madrid Mexico Milan Montreal New Delhi Panama Paris
San Juan São Paulo Singapore Sydney Tokyo Toronto

Notice

Medicine is an ever-changing science. As new research and clinical experience broaden our knowledge, changes in treatment and drug therapy are required. The editors and the publisher of this work have checked with sources believed to be reliable in their efforts to provide drug dosage schedules that are complete and in accord with the standards accepted at the time of publication. However, readers are advised to check the product information sheet included in the package of each drug they plan to administer to be certain that the information contained in these schedules is accurate and that changes have not been made in the recommended dose or in the contraindications for administration. This recommendation is of particular importance in connection with new or infrequently used drugs.

This book was previously published under the title *The Pediatric Chest: Radiological, Clinical, and Pathological Observations* by Charles C Thomas, Publisher.

Radiology of the Pediatric Chest
Clinical and Pathological Correlations

1234567890 HAL HAL 89876

ISBN 0-07-020405-5

This book was set in Zapf Book Light by Compset, Inc.; the editor was T. Fiore Lavery; the production supervisor was Thomas J. LoPinto; the cover was designed by Edward R. Schultheis.
Arcata Graphics/Halliday was printer and binder.

Library of Congress Cataloging-in-Publication Data

Felman, Alvin H.
    Radiology of the pediatric chest.

    Includes bibliographies and index.
    1. Chest—Diseases—Diagnosis.   2. Pediatric respiratory diseases—Diagnosis.   3. Diagnosis, Radioscopic.   4. Pediatric diagnostic imaging.
    I. Cohen, Mervyn D.   II. Title. [DNLM: 1. Thoracic Radiography—in infancy & childhood. WS 280 F322r]
    RJ433.5.D5F45   1987   618.92′097540757   86-20911
    ISBN 0-07-020405-5

To my wife Lynne
my boys David, Robert, James—
this book is affectionately dedicated

Contents

Preface

The writer's only responsibility is to his art. He will be completely ruthless if he is a good one. He has a dream. It anguishes him so he must get rid of it. He has no peace until then. Everything goes by the board: honor, pride, decency, security, happiness, all, to get the book written. If a writer has to rob his mother, he will not hesitate; the "Ode on a Grecian Urn" is worth any number of old ladies.

William Faulkner, 1956

Of two things I am certain: (1) this book will never be confused with "Ode on a Grecian Urn," and (2) it could never have been written without the help of several, very reliable "ladies." Nevertheless, Faulkner's words have fueled my furnace for the last year, and I quote him with reverence, respect, and considerable tongue in check.

Physicians who care for children with respiratory tract illness must recognize the roentgenographic expression of a host of disorders. Radiologists, who wish to fulfill their role as consultants, must be familiar with the clinical manifestations of these diseases as well as their radiographic presentations. Rapid advances in our knowledge of pathophysiology and therapy, as well as the explosion of radiographic imaging technology, compound the task of each.

My major purpose is to bring together the clinical and radiologic features of pediatric chest diseases in a form that is comprehensible to the most uninitiated medical student, yet valuable to the sophisticated pediatric radiologist. The material is presented in a descriptive manner; structured algorithms and "cookbook" recipes are avoided since clinical presentations, available facilities, local customs, and individual expertise are rarely comparable. Well-informed clinicians, radiologists, and pathologists, trained to assess cases on their individual merits, should find the most logical path to the proper diagnosis and treatment regimen.

Section IV, "Roentgenographic Patterns in Pulmonary Disease," is devoted to four patterns that I have found reliable for pediatric chest interpretation. The "pattern" recognition and gamut list methodologies, so dear to medical students and residents, often suffer the danger of becoming the proverbial square pegs in round holes. This method should not be substituted for careful observation and description, logical analytical discussion, and reasonable differential diagnosis.

Discussions and illustrations of the associated pathologic processes are placed wherever needed to expand and clarify the behavior and nature of these abnormalities. My fascination with pathology reaches back to my monumental medical school chairman of pathology, Dr. Edward A. Gall, who continues to prod me from his grave in Cincinnati, Ohio. Time and distance offer no escape from him.

Without doubt, the most significant and rare stroke of genius was my decision to enlist the talents of Dr. Mervyn D. Cohen, of the James Whitcomb Riley Children's Hospital. With hardly a twitch of his whiskers, he accepted the challenge and, within several months, delivered three beautifully composed and illustrated chapters on chest imaging in children. His broad experience with computed tomography and his pioneering role in magnetic resonance imaging are unexcelled, and I value his contribution greatly.

As I close this prologue, my thoughts wander back to my roots in the Cincinnati College of Medicine, the Cincinnati Children's Hospital, and Dr. A. Ashley Weech, that marvelous pediatrician, educator, and humanitarian, whose legacy of inspiration lives within all of us who called him "Pappy." His words, his wisdom, his way with children, are entwined within these pages.

ALVIN H. FELMAN

Acknowledgments

Any attempt to acknowledge the many individuals who contributed to the production of this book is doomed to failure at the outset. Nevertheless, I cannot let the occasion pass without at least some effort.

The support of the photographic department of the University Hospital, headed by Stephen Englert, was willing and prompt, in spite of my many trying demands. Linda Laughton, a secretary of unexcelled skill, typed the original draft with a promptness and accuracy rarely found.

Many of the chapters were reviewed by Davey Volkhardt, editorial consultant for the University of Florida, Jacksonville campus. Davey is a writer and poet in her own right; a true woman of letters, the likes of whom I have not encountered since my days in high school English class. If any participles have been left dangling, or if my assault on the English language has at times exceeded the bounds of credulity, it is the result of my own stubborn ignorance and should cast no shadow on Davey's knowledge or the futile tenacity with which she so often tried to restrain me.

My wife, Lynne, was a constant source of support and inspiration; this book could never have been completed without her. She sat by my side in front of our word processor during the endless, tedious editing process and tried to keep me from writing foolishness. I would like to believe she was successful, but, in truth, her task was insurmountable.

Dr. Ronald Rhatigan, medical director and chairman of the Department of Pathology, was a willing and generous patron of this project, as were his associate pathologists, Drs. Jeffrey Goldstein and Carmela Monteira. Only a pathologist can experience the sheer terror and disruption of a radiologist in the pathology department. They suffered my bullish intrusions with patience and forbearance, even in the midst of their "frozen" sections.

Dr. William Donnelly of the University of Florida provided much of the pathologic material for the previous edition that has been carried over into this version. I again owe him my gratitude for his past contribution to this effort.

My thanks and appreciation are also expressed to the Department of Radiology chairman, Dr. Frederick Vines, and my colleagues and house officers, for their support and encouragement.

The unselfish willingness of so many of my colleagues in radiology to share their experiences is evident from the unique and beautifully documented cases that they contributed. Other authors whom I contacted were equally generous. I would like to recognize their contributions by listing their names below.

Eshan Afshani	Michael Hartenberg	James Scatliff
Jar In Ahn (Korea)	Derek Harwood-Nash	Joanna Seibert
Bernard Blumenthal	Guy Hicks	Frederick Silverman
Stephen Brown	Alan Hoffman	Joseph Smith
John Campbell	Marvin Kogutt	Thomas Sumner
Marie Capitanio	Alberto Larieu	Steven Taylor
Ernest Ferrell	Hajime Maeta (Japan)	Ina Tonkin
Barry Fletcher	Peter Moskowitz	Frances Toomey
Godfrey Gaese	Marcia Murakami	David Turner
Brit Gay, Jr.	Mary Ann Radkowski	Milton Wagner
Jeffrey Goldstein	Webster Riggs	Jon Williams
R. John Gould	Guillermo Sanchez	

Congenital Abnormalities of the Larynx, Trachea, Esophagus, Bronchi, and Lungs

Developmental anomalies of the larynx, trachea, esophagus, bronchi, and lungs usually produce severe neonatal distress in the first critical hours or days of life. If undiscovered and untreated, irreparable damage may result, most often from aspirated oral feedings or gastric contents. Approximately one-half of children born with these deformities have associated congenital anomalies, and half of these are fatal.

The three chapters in this section will focus on the radiographic expression of some of these anomalies. Effort is made to correlate the clinical and radiographic pictures with the embryologic etiologies. Whenever possible, pathologic specimens are included for emphasis, clarity, and interest.

Chapter 1 summarizes the major congenital anomalies caused by abnormal or incomplete septation of the primitive foregut. In general, these manifest as atresias, fistulas, and/or defects in the tracheoesophageal septum, or "party wall."

Chapter 2 considers congenital lesions that result from abnormal or aberrant lung bud development. Among these are ectopic bronchial connections, underdeveloped lungs, "sequestered" lobes, and cystic formations.

Chapter 3 contains a heterogeneous group of lesions in which the major aberrations involve parenchymal lung structures, such as alveoli, blood vessels, supporting stroma, and peripheral bronchial tree. It is difficult to trace the teratogenic roots of these lesions; some may actually be acquired rather than congenital.

Chapter 1

Abnormal Tracheoesophageal Development

1. Abnormal *differentiation* of the primitive foregut into the trachea, larynx, and/or esophagus
   a. Tracheal agenesis-atresia
   b. Esophageal atresia with or without tracheo-esophageal fistula
   c. Laryngotracheoesophageal cleft, esophago-trachea, H(N) fistula
2. Abnormal *maturation* and development of the trachea and larynx after normal differentiation has occurred
   a. Tracheomalacia
   b. Laryngomalacia
   c. Tracheal stenosis
   d. Tracheobronchomegaly

Abnormal Differentiation of the Primitive Foregut

Tracheal Agenesis-Atresia

Tracheal atresia is a rare anomaly that results when the trachea fails to develop; air reaches the lungs through esophageal communications. Floyd et al.[1] have classified tracheal agenesis-atresia into three types; type II is the most common (Figure 1-1). Pulmonary abnormalities in association with tracheal agenesis are unusual, but associated cardiac, gastrointestinal, and genitourinary anomalies are frequent.[2]

Tracheal Agenesis

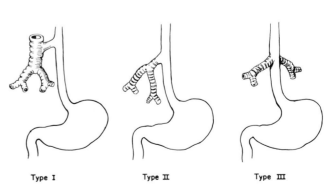

Type I   Type II   Type III

Figure 1-1 Tracheal agenesis. Type II is most common. (Adapted from Floyd et al.[1])

Because of the associated congenital defects, tracheal atresia may be considered within the group of anomalies referred to as the *VATER association* (vertebral, *a*nal, *t*racheal, *e*sophageal, and *r*enal defects).[3] *VACTERL association* is a term occasionally used to signify the additional presence of cardiac and limb abnormalities.

While almost universally fatal, sporadic cases of tracheal atresia have been reported in which surgical repair has prolonged survival from days to several months and beyond.[4,5]

Embryology

Tracheal agenesis results from abnormal embryogenesis between the twenty-first and twenty-fourth day of gestation. During this period, the primitive foregut differentiates into the trachea and esophagus (Figure 1-2). Simultaneously, the future airway arises as a midline, ventral diverticulum, or lung bud. In the ensuing 10 days, the lung bud divides, elongates, and branches while the lateral esophageal grooves and tracheoesophageal septum complete the separation of the primitive foregut into trachea and esophagus. Normally, these structures are completely developed by 34 days, and laryngeal differentiation follows shortly thereafter.

Bremer[6] has suggested that aberrant deviation of the tracheoesophageal septum causes esophageal and/or tracheal atresia, with or without fistulas. Dorsal deviation of the septum leads to esophageal atresia (Figure 1-2D), with or without tracheoesophageal

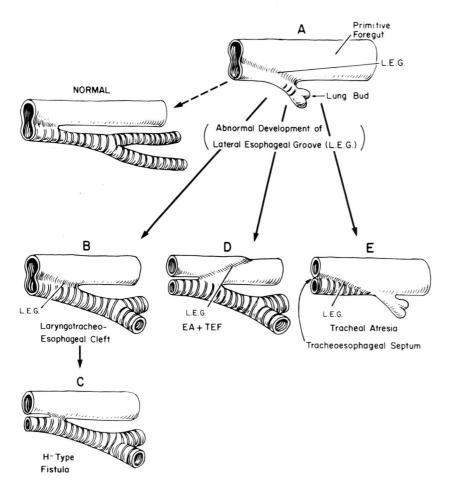

Figure 1-2 Diagram of normal and abnormal tracheoesophageal differentiation. A. At 21 to 24 days of gestation, the lateral esophageal grooves (LEG) appear and begin the separation of the foregut into trachea and esophagus. This process proceeds in a caudocranial direction until the entire tracheoesophageal septum is developed. As the foregut elongates, the ventral lung buds arise simultaneously, begin to branch, and ultimately give rise to the tracheobronchial tree. **B.** Failure of normal development and migration of the lateral esophageal grooves result in variable degrees of communication between the trachea and esophagus. (See Fig. 1-9.) **C.** The H(N) fistula probably results from a localized developmental defect in the tracheoesophageal septum (see Figure 1-3E). **D.** Localized overgrowth of the lateral esophageal grooves or dorsal deviation of the tracheoesophageal septum leads to the common form of esophageal atresia and tracheoesophageal fistula (see Figure 1-3A). **E.** Ventral deviation of the tracheoesophageal septum or abnormal development of the lateral esophageal groove may result in tracheal atresia (see Figure 1-3D). The simultaneous development of a caudal lung bud may give rise to esophagotracheal fistula or esophageal lung (see Figure 2-1). Oblique deviation of the tracheoesophageal septum is probably responsible for other combinations of abnormal bronchoesophageal attachments (see Figure 1-3B, C, F).

fistula, whereas ventral deviation produces tracheal atresia (Figure 1-2E). During this complicated developmental process, supernumerary or aberrant lung buds may give rise to esophageal bronchi or other anomalies (sequestration? bronchogenic cyst?). These anomalies of abnormal lung bud development are considered in more detail in Chapter 2. Disturbances in the sequence of septal deviation, esophageal elongation, and lung bud development probably account for the clinical variations of tracheal and esophageal atresias depicted in Figure 1-3. In addition to Bremer's theory of embryogenesis, other authorities have suggested that hypertrophic development of the lateral esophageal grooves plays a part in the genesis of these complex anomalies.[7]

Clinical Symptoms

Infants with tracheal agenesis present with cyanosis, severe respiratory distress, and lack of audible cry. Inability to intubate the trachea is a consistent feature. Hydramnios is frequently present, but oligohydramnios occurs with accompanying renal dysgenesis. Associated external congenital abnormalities may be evident, and, if the infant survives, additional developmental defects may become manifest. Tracheal intubation is impossible; the endotracheal tube usually enters the esophagus. Nevertheless, some oxygen delivered through a tube in the esophagus will reach the lungs via tracheoesophageal communication. Thus, life is sustained for a few hours or days. The larynx is usually well developed.

Radiologic Findings

In infants who have tracheal atresia and survive long enough to have film studies, the lungs may appear surprisingly well aerated.[2] Within a short time, generalized opacity, collapse, and pneumothoraxes appear (Figure 1-4A). The tracheal air column is not visible (Figure 1-5A), and endotracheal tubes usually are displaced into the esophagus and stomach. Contrast esophogram usually confirms the presence of bronchoesophageal communication (Figures 1-4B and 1-5C). The cardiac silhouette may or may not be abnormal, depending upon the presence and type of congenital heart defects, but the heart may appear normal at birth even in the presence of complex cardiac disease. Vertebral deformities occasionally occur in association with tracheal atresia.

Esophageal Atresia and Tracheoesophageal Fistula

The combination of esophageal atresia and tracheoesophageal fistula (EA/TEF) occurs once in every

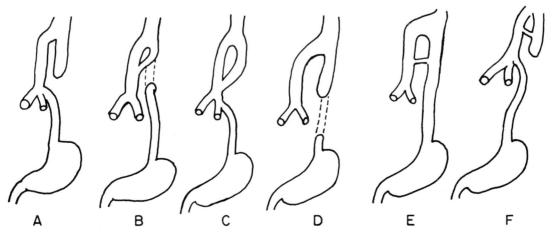

Figure 1-3   Diagram of tracheoesophageal abnormalities. Type A shows the most common abnormality, accounting for approximately 95 percent of cases.

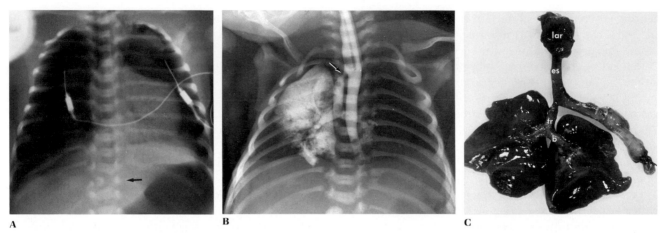

A   B   C

Figure 1-4   Tracheal agenesis (type I). This 2200-g infant could not be intubated. Tracheostomy was performed, but the patient died at approximately 6 h of age. Imperforate anus and polyhydramnios were additional complications. **A.** The only film study obtained shows bilateral pneumothoraxes and pneumomediastinum. There is gas in the stomach. *Note:* vertebral malformations (arrow). **B.** A postmortem contrast injection shows the tracheoesophageal connection (arrow). **C.** Autopsy specimen: The trachea (tr) originates directly from the midesophagus (es). The tracheal segment is narrow at its origin, but the tracheal rings in this region and distally are unremarkable. The larynx (lar) is well formed. (b) = bronchus.

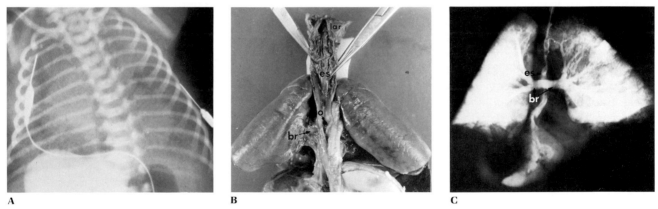

A   B   C

Figure 1-5   Tracheal agenesis (type III).   A. The lungs are generally opaque, but central air bronchograms are present. The tracheal air column is absent. **B.** The autopsy specimen, viewed from behind. The larynx (lar) is developed, but the trachea is absent. A single orifice (o) arises anteriorly from the opened esophagus (es) and gives rise to the stem bronchi (br). **C.** This radiograph of injected specimen shows both bronchi (br) arising from the esophagus (es).

3000 to 3500 live births. In contrast to tracheal atresia, this combination of anomalies is almost always amenable to surgical correction, but the prognosis for survival depends heavily upon associated congenital defects. Survival rates of 88 percent in infants with no additional congenital anomalies are reported.[8] Early recognition of this abnormality, accurate evaluation of the anatomic defect, and thorough

delineation of associated anomalies are critical for the survival of these infants.

Additional congenital anomalies occur in 50 percent of patients with EA/TEF; most commonly involved are the heart, anus, rectum, vertebrae, and gastrointestinal and genitourinary tracts (VATER-VACTERL associations). Thymic and parathyroid abnormalities also accompany EA/TEF, as in Di-

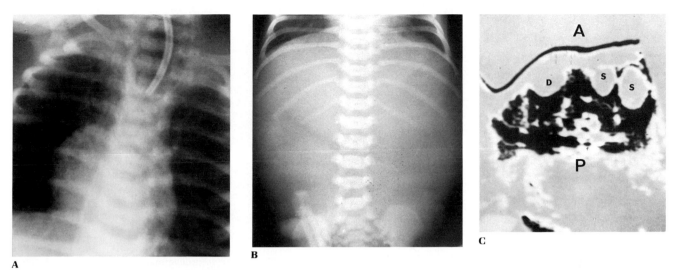

Figure 1-6   Esophageal atresia and duodenal atresia. A and **B.** Esophageal atresia is evident from the distended upper esophageal pouch, obstruction to passage of an esophageal tube, and absent gas in the abdomen. **C.** Ultrasound of the abdomen shows the fluid-filled stomach (S) with a peristaltic wave and the distended proximal duodenum (D). (From McCook TA, Felman AH: Esophageal atresia, duodenal atresia, and gastric distention: Report of two cases. *AJR* 131:167, 1978. © 1978, American Roentgen Ray Society. With permission.)

George's syndrome of thymic hypoplasia. Hypoplasia and atresia of the lung are uncommon, but when present provide a poor prognosis.[9]

Embryology

As with tracheal atresia, EA/TEF is probably caused by abnormal partition of the primitive foregut.[6] However, in contrast to tracheal atresia, which results when the folds of the lateral wall turn ventrad, esophageal atresia occurs when the folds of the lateral wall turn abruptly dorsad (Figure 1-2D). The proximal esophagus becomes atretic, but communication between the distal esophagus and trachea is preserved. The distal TEF may be located at any level below the larynx, but it is commonly found just above the tracheal bifurcation and less often at the carina or left stem bronchus.

Because of the critical timing of normal foregut septation and lung bud development during this vulnerable period of gestation, other forms of proximal EAs, with or without distal fistulous connections, are possible (Figure 1-3). The exact etiology of EA is not clear in all cases. In some, EA without fistula (Figure 1-6) may be acquired in utero from interruption of the blood supply, constricting vascular anomalies, or failure of recanalization. However, the frequent combination of EA with other congenital anomalies suggests that it is also a primary aberration of embryogenesis (Figure 1-6C).

Clinical Presentation

Difficulty with respiration and feedings after birth frequently signals the presence of congenital anomalies of tracheoesophageal structures. Excessive mucus, cough, stridor, and severe respiratory distress are prominent features. Polyhydramnios will occasionally provide an early clue, particularly in cases of isolated EA. Associated anomalies, previously described in the VACTERL association, may complicate the clinical picture.

Radiologic Findings

The diagnosis of isolated EA is confirmed when the abdomen is airless (Figure 1-6 A and B). Additional stenotic or atretic gastrointestinal tract lesions, com-

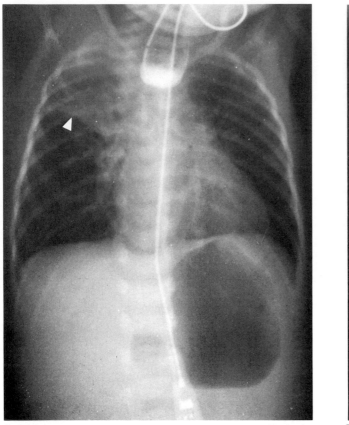

A

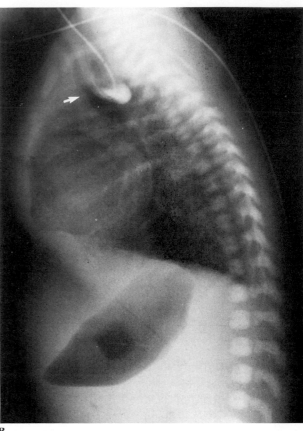

B

Figure 1-7   Esophageal atresia, tracheoesophageal fistula, and duodenal atresia. A. This is a frontal study with a small amount of barium-water mixture in the proximal esophageal pouch. Right upper lobe atelectasis is apparent; the horizontal fissure is bowed upward (arrowhead). **B.** The lateral film illustrates the bowed trachea (arrow) anterior to the distended esophageal pouch. *Note:* The "double bubble" sign of duodenal atresia is produced by the distended, air-filled stomach and proximal duodenum.

monly associated with EA/TEF, may be diagnosed with ultrasonography (Figure 1-6C).[10,11] Initial chest films often show generalized overaeration and scattered atelectasis (Figures 1-6A and 1-7A), a result of aspirated feeding or regurgitation of gastric contents. In the lateral projection, anterior displacement and bowing of the trachea by the distended, atretic upper esophageal pouch are helpful clues (Figure 1-7B).

Tracheoesophageal fistula accompanying EA is confirmed by the presence of air in the gastrointestinal tract. Duodenal stenosis and atresia are well-known companions of esophageal anomalies and are readily appreciated since the presence of a TEF

allows air to reach the gastrointestinal tract (Figure 1-7A). Ultrasonography is most handy in detecting the presence of renal anomalies, and plain films usually disclose associated vertebral deformities.

Attention must be paid to the thymic shadow in the first several days of life. A radiograph that shows an absence of thymic tissue should suggest the possibility of DiGeorge's syndrome, a condition in which the third and fourth pharyngeal pouch derivatives, including the parathyroid glands, are hypoplastic or absent. Early recognition of this condition is of great significance since immunohumoral mechanisms of treatment are now available (see Chapter 8).

Right-sided aortic arch occurs in 5 percent of patients with EA and TEF and may influence the surgical approach.[12,13] The use of high-kilovoltage technique is helpful in detecting this anomaly.[14] Computed tomography (CT) is also recommended for this procedure.[15] However, interpretation is often difficult in neonates because of the marked mediastinal mobility and the presence of pulmonary problems in the upper lobes.

In patients suspected of having EA and TEF, definitive diagnostic delineation of the defects depends partly on the desires of the surgeon and partly on the plain film findings. In some, the anatomy of the upper atretic pouch may be defined sufficiently on plain films with a radiopaque catheter passed to the point of atresia. In others, instillation of small amounts of nonirritating contrast material (barium-water, metrizamide) into the upper pouch through an end-hole rubber catheter under fluoroscopy may be necessary (Figure 1-7B). In addition to determining the level of EA, this procedure will identify a fistula between the upper pouch and trachea, when present (Figure 1-8). Identification of these fistulas is important as they are often not apparent at surgery. On rare occasions, a catheter may coil in a normal upper esophagus and mislead the initiated and uninitiated alike. Fluoroscopic examination and contrast study in these cases will avoid needless embarrassment and unnecessary expense.

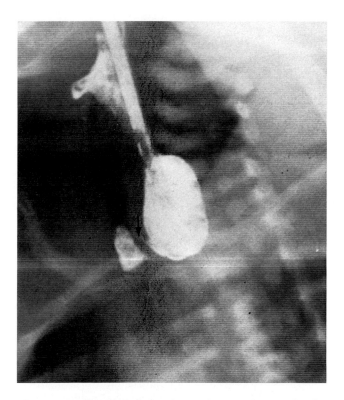

Figure 1-8 Esophageal atresia, tracheoesophageal fistula, and proximal H fistula. A barium-water mixture outlines the atretic esophagus and a fistula between the proximal pouch and the trachea (arrow).

Laryngotracheoesophageal Cleft, Esophagotrachea, H(N) Fistula

The H(N) fistula, in which a single communication remains between the esophagus and trachea, is the mildest form of incomplete tracheoesophageal septum, or "party wall" (Figure 1-9). Esophagotrachea is the most severe manifestation; there are intermediate varieties depending upon the degree of septal deficiency. Prognosis for the more severe forms is poor, but surgical correction is occasionally successful.[16]

Embryology

Incomplete differentiation of the foregut into the trachea and esophagus is the embryogenic fault responsible for the various forms of esophagotrachea. This condition occurs between 21 and 27 days of gestation (4- to 5-mm length), when bilateral indentations of the mesoderm begin to separate the anterior trachea from the posterior esophagus. Separation begins caudally and proceeds rostrally, reaching the level of the larynx by 33 days (9 to 10 mm). Failure of the tracheoesophageal septum to develop normally may prevent fusion of the cricoid cartilages, a necessity for normal function of the epiglottis and vocal cords. The severity of the defect, from the mildest (laryngeal cleft) to the most severe (complete esophagotrachea), depends on the stage at which the rostral advance of the tracheoesophageal septum is interrupted.

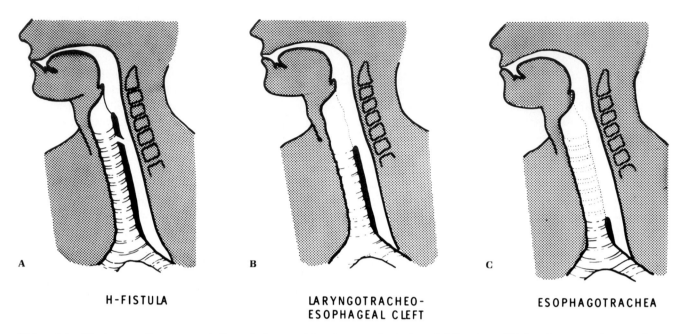

A H-FISTULA

B LARYNGOTRACHEO-
ESOPHAGEAL CLEFT

C ESOPHAGOTRACHEA

Figure 1-9   Diagrammatic representation of abnormal tracheoesophageal septal ("party wall") development. (From Felman and Talbert,[19] with permission.)

Clinical Presentation

The presenting symptoms depend primarily upon the anatomic configuration of the anomaly, and also upon the severity and number of accompanying malformations. Abnormal phonation, hoarse cry, excess mucous production, and cyanosis are typical, but not invariable, signs of a laryngeal cleft. Mild forms of laryngeal cleft, and even those with short segment defects of the tracheoesophageal septum, may escape detection in the first few days or weeks of life. H(N) fistulas often remain undiagnosed for the first weeks or months, only to be discovered later because of recurrent cough, pneumonia, and chronic lung disease. Infants with significant tracheoesophageal communications cough and choke at the first feedings, and these symptoms are exacerbated with additional food intake. If the defect remains undetected, the child may be aggravated by attacks of aspiration, atelectasis, and apnea. Progressive pulmonary infections invariably follow.

When laryngotracheal cleft is suspected, early laryngobronchoscopy should be performed. The ab-normality is usually well visualized by this technique, but short segments of nonfusion of the larynx and cricoid cartilages (Figure 1-9B) might escape detection as the edges remain approximated. Separation of the laryngeal cartilages by inserting the laryngoscope blade directly into the laryngeal cavity may be necessary to confirm the diagnosis.

Radiologic Findings

Plain chest films in neonates with tracheoesophageal septal defects are often characterized by pulmonary overaeration, diffuse infiltrates, and atelectasis (Figures 1-10A and 1-11A). Excessive air may accumulate in the esophagus and bowel as a result of the fistula. Vertebral anomalies are associated features in some infants.

In patients with a suspected H fistula, contrast esophogram using an opaque, end-hole rubber catheter is the diagnostic study of choice. The use of CT in the diagnosis of TEF has been reported.[17] Under

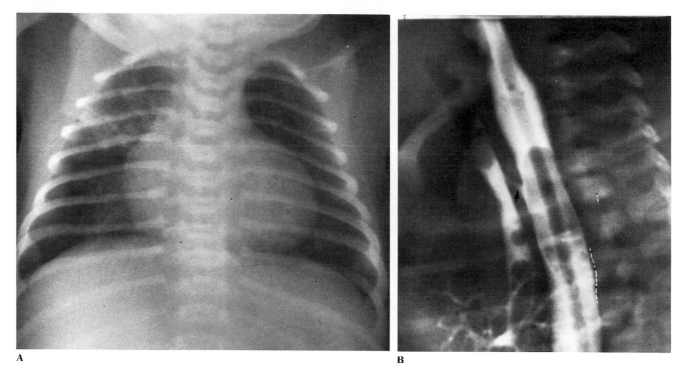

A   B

Figure 1-10   Tracheoesophageal fistula (H type). A. The right upper lobe infiltrate is a nonspecific finding but frequently accompanies tracheoesophageal abnormalities. **B.** A barium-water mixture, injected into the esophagus through a catheter, passes through a fistula (arrow) between the esophagus and the trachea.

fluoroscopic observation, with the child in the prone oblique position, the catheter should be inserted into the distal esophagus and small amounts of contrast material (barium-water, metrizamide) injected as it is withdrawn. An H fistula is outlined by the contrast flowing from the esophagus into the trachea (Figure 1-10B). Difficulty in filling the esophagus with barium may be encountered in some cases when air bubbles through at the site of the fistula. At other times, the fistula may not fill because of mucus plugging. When the index of suspicion is sufficiently high, repeat studies should be performed.

If the catheter study shows no fistula, a barium swallow should be carried out to exclude laryngotracheal aspiration and/or gastroesophageal reflux. Duodenal stenosis may accompany an H fistula, and the swallowed barium should be followed through this segment of bowel. Tracheal stenosis, an additional complication of an H fistula, should also be excluded.

The presence of laryngotracheoesophageal cleft should be suspected when esophageal and tracheal tubes assume unusual positions (Figure 1-11A). The endotracheal tube often fails to remain within the lumen of the trachea when viewed in the lateral projection. In this projection, the endotracheal and nasogastric tubes often assume a side-by-side position rather than the normal anteroposterior relationship.

If the clinical and/or radiologic features suggest the presence of this anomaly, direct laryngoscopic observation rather than contrast instillation is the best approach. Water-soluble, nonionic agents such as metrizamide have been demonstrated to be adequate substitutes for barium as a contrast material.[18] Studies to delineate these abnormalities should be performed with great care to prevent flooding the lungs (Figure 1-11B). The endotracheal tube should be placed within the trachea to maintain the child's respiratory integrity while the esophagus is carefully studied through an opaque tube.[19]

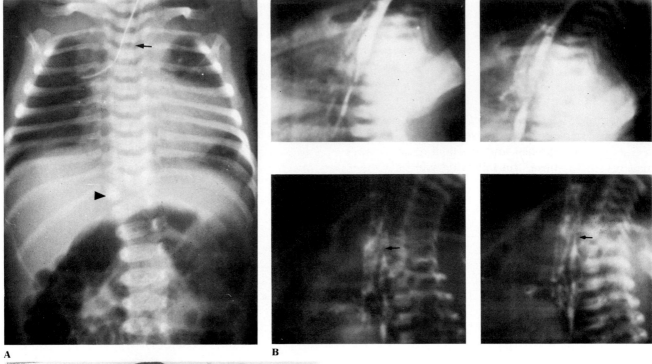

A

B

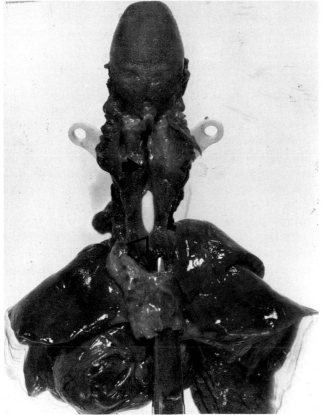

C

Figure 1-11 Laryngotracheoesophageal cleft. This full-term infant experienced immediate respiratory difficulty at birth, and therefore an endotracheal tube was used. Because of the unusual positions assumed by the endotracheal and naso-gastric tubes, as viewed on the initial chest radiographs, the presence of laryngotracheoesophageal cleft was suggested. Surgically uncorrectable cardiac disease was also present. **A.** In the frontal projection the endotracheal tube is positioned just proximal to the carina (arrow), and the nasogastric catheter extends into the right stem bronchus. Abnormal cardiac configurations and vertebral anomalies are noted (arrowhead). **B.** The contrast study of the esophagus demonstrates the passage of barium into the tracheobronchial tree at the thoracic inlet. A short tracheoesophageal septum can be identified distally; the superior edge of this septum lies against the inferior edge of the endotracheal tube (arrow). Note the excess air in the esophagus. **C.** Pathologic specimen. The laryngotracheoesophageal cleft viewed from behind (arrow). The white tracheostomy tube remains in place. A portion of the upper esophagus has been opened; the scissors tip lies in the distal esophageal lumen. The superior limit of the tracheoesophageal septum is indicated by the open arrow. No tracheal cartilages could be identified histologically. (From Felman and Talbert,[19] with permission.)

Abnormal Tracheal and Laryngeal Maturation

After normal differentiation of the trachea, larynx, and esophagus has occurred, several developmental and acquired laryngeal and tracheal abnormalities may result. Of these, the following will be considered:

1. Tracheomalacia
   a. Primary
   b. Secondary
2. Laryngomalacia
3. Tracheal stenosis
   a. Congenital
   b. Acquired
4. Tracheobronchomegaly

Tracheomalacia

Tracheomalacia is a clinical term used to describe generalized weakness or abnormal flaccidity of the tracheal wall, a condition that allows for excessive tracheal collapse during normal respiration. A precise definition of tracheomalacia is not well established, and accepted therapeutic measures are the subject of considerable debate.

Primary Tracheomalacia

Primary tracheomalacia refers to flaccidity of the tracheal wall in the absence of coexisting disease and is extremely rare as a significant clinical entity. In two cases reported with primary tracheomalacia, one patient was a 21-year-old in whom there were two additional areas of tracheal stenosis. A second patient, 6 years old, had been treated with radiation to the thymus in infancy.[20] Whittenborg et al.[21] found no documented reports of absent cartilage crescents or rings involving 17 infants with collapsing trachea at Boston Children's Hospital.

Secondary Tracheomalacia

This abnormality may exist secondary to, or in association with, other conditions that cause extrinsic compression on the trachea (i.e., vascular anomalies and mediastinal masses).[22] In addition, segmental tracheomalacia may follow tracheostomy and prolonged use of endotracheal tubes, particularly with cuffed attachments. Tracheomalacia may accompany other systemic diseases with cartilage–connective tissue abnormalities, such as relapsing polychondritis, cutis laxa, Ehlers-Danlos, and tracheobronchomegaly.[23] Tracheomalacia in association with TEF most often results from a deficiency of the tracheal cartilage.

The treatment of tracheomalacia is controversial. Benjamin et al.[24] advocate the use of "tracheopexy" for cases that are severe. These clinicians established the diagnosis primarily with bronchoscopy. In most of their patients, the abnormal area of collapse was limited to a 2- to 3-cm segment of the lower thoracic trachea.

The surgical treatment for tracheomalacia that is associated with vascular compression, following repair of TEF, is controversial. Schwartz and Filer[25] reported patients with tracheomalacia who developed episodes of apnea and "dying spells" following repair of TEF. The reasons for the apneic episodes could not be determined, but all infants were relieved by aortopexy. Benjamin et al.[24] reported similar cases and advocate the use of aortopexy for symptomatic tracheomalacia.

Innominate artery compression of the trachea is another condition thought to cause clinically symptomatic tracheomalacia in selected cases (see Chapter 12). Berdon and colleagues[26] do not advocate surgical intervention in patients with innominate artery compression unless accompanied by symptoms of stridor and apnea.

The diagnosis of fixed tracheal abnormalities is often aided by bronchoscopy,[27] but the presence of tracheomalacia is often a debatable issue between clinician and radiologist. Video fluoroscopic observation is the best radiographic tool in the diagnosis of tracheomalacia. This technique provides a clear picture of the tracheal dynamics and is not influenced by instrumentation or other extraneous factors. Bronchoscopic examination is subject to error because of the blockage of airflow by the bronchoscope. However, application of fiberoptic bronchoscopy has greatly improved the techniques of airway visualization.

The natural tendency for the trachea to stiffen with age is reason not to operate on most cases of tracheomalacia, but severe symptoms of localized tracheal collapse may be helped by surgery. Most of these conditions are associated with external compression, previous trauma, or repair of TEF.

Laryngomalacia

Laryngomalacia (infantile supraglottic hypermobility) is less of a clinical problem than tracheomalacia. Infants with this abnormality sound much worse than they really are. The voice is normal, but loud, stridorous breathing occurs when the infant is aggravated or upset.

Laryngomalacia is best confirmed fluoroscopically. In this procedure, the table should be raised to the upright position, the child placed supine on the step, and the laryngeal area monitored during quiet respiration. In the presence of laryngomalacia, the larynx "collapses" on inspiration because of inadequate cartilaginous support. Laryngoscopy should be reserved for atypical patients in whom laryngeal stenosis, vocal cord paralysis, or other obstructing lesions are suspected. As in tracheomalacia, laryn-

gomalacia is invariably a self-limited disease; rarely do patients need tracheostomy.

Tracheal Stenosis

Fixed narrowing of the tracheal air column results from developmental constriction, external compression, or intraluminal lesions. Developmental constrictions and congenital and acquired stenosis will be examined here. Disease processes which cause tracheal narrowing as a result of external pressure or intraluminal obstruction are discussed in Chapter 17.

Congenital Tracheal Stenosis

Congenital tracheal stenosis may take the form of a short, locally constricted segment; in other patients the entire trachea may be narrowed (Figure 1-12A). Less commonly, the tracheal lumen constricts as it descends toward the carina ("carrot shape") (Figure 1-12B).[28] Tracheal webs are uncommon lesions usually found just above the carina. Focal narrowing is often associated with tracheal rings that are frequently fragmented, increased in number, and often

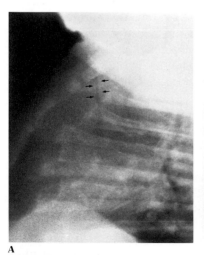
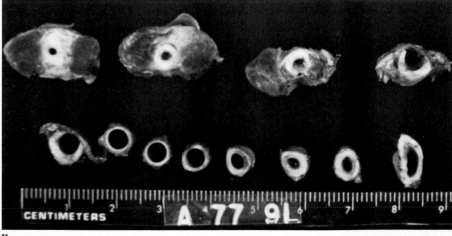

A

B

Figure 1-12   Tracheal stenosis. A. The lateral chest film shows a markedly narrowed tracheal air column (arrows) in a child with stridor. **B.** This child died suddenly, and the pathologic specimen shows complete cartilaginous rings instead of the normal C shape. The internal diameters vary from 0.3 to 0.5 cm.

complete (with no posterior membrane).[29] On occasion, absent cartilaginous rings in a segment of trachea contribute to intermittent collapse and obstruction.[30] Tracheal stenosis may also result from an embryologic aberration wherein esophageal tissue is sequestered in the trachea.[31,32]

Benjamin et al.[33] reported 21 patients with congenital tracheal stenosis; all but 2 were seen within the first year of life. Nineteen had associated anomalies that included tracheomalacia, congenital lobar emphysema, accessory diaphragm, diaphragmatic hernia, tracheal web, and laryngeal hypoplasia, as well as cardiac, skeletal, and limb anomalies. Other diseases associated with varieties of tracheal stenosis include the pulmonary vascular sling and certain chondrodystrophies, such as Ellis–van Creveld syndrome and congenital stippled epiphyses.[34,35]

Presenting symptoms of tracheal stenosis are quite variable. They include respiratory distress, persistent wheeze or stridor, recurrent croup, atypical bronchiolitis, and barking cough.

Recently developed surgical techniques hold some promise for correction of these serious and often lethal defects.[36,38] (See Chapter 17.)

Acquired Tracheal Stenosis

Most cases of acquired tracheal stenosis result from trauma. Tracheostomy and prolonged endotracheal intubation are among the most frequent causes. Although tracheostomies regularly heal without sequelae, posttracheostomy complications occur in 1.5 to 2.6 percent of patients.[39,40] Stenosis follows tracheal intubation in 0.9 to 5 percent.[40–42] Intubation of less than 24-h duration usually produces no change in the tracheal mucosa. However, microscopic mucosal alterations have been observed after 48 h, and epithelial metaplasia after a week.[43] The use of cuffed endotracheal tubes is in large measure responsible for these changes. Ulceration and necrosis at the site of the inflated cuff may occur within 4 days and produce granulation tissue, perichondrosis, fibrosis, and stenosis.[44–47] Symptoms of obstruction usually do not occur until the endotracheal tube has been removed. Laryngeal stenosis is a well-known but less common occurrence.

Acute airway obstruction is covered in Chapter 17.

Tracheobronchomegaly

Tracheobronchomegaly (Mounier-Kuhn syndrome, trachiectasis, tracheobronchiectasis), first described by Mounier-Kuhn in 1932, is characterized by marked dilatation of the trachea and major bronchi and by chronic respiratory tract infection.[48,49] While most individuals present at older ages, the abnormality has been reported in tots as young as 18 months of age.[50] A slight racial preference for blacks exists.

The disease is characterized by progressive tracheal enlargement that begins in children or young adults.[51,52] The trachea may reach a diameter as wide as the dorsal spine and assume a "corrugated" appearance as the lumen bulges between the cartilaginous rings (Figures 1-13 and 1-14). Marked dilatation on inspiration and collapse on expiration constitute important fluoroscopic findings.[53]

Tracheal diverticula occur in about one-third of cases; widespread cylindrical and saccular bronchiectasis are additional complications.[51] Pulmonary function tests usually show increased dead space, greater than normal tidal volume, and occasional evidence of obstructive airway disease.

Tracheobronchomegaly probably results from faulty development of connective tissues in the walls of the trachea and major bronchi. However, chronic infection may be a contributing cause in some cases. Patients have been reported in whom tracheobronchomegaly coexists with Ehlers-Danlos syndrome and cutis laxa, both of which have connective tissue abnormalities.[48,54,55] Associated anatomic aberrations of the airway have also been observed.[56,57] Two cases have been reported in siblings.[53]

The radiographic findings of tracheobronchomegaly may be extremely subtle in the early stages of disease. Chronic lung changes with focal or diffuse areas of atelectasis and bronchiectasis usually develop as the disease progresses. Serial film studies show gradual tracheal enlargement. The walls may assume a corrugated appearance (Figure 1-14A). Tra-

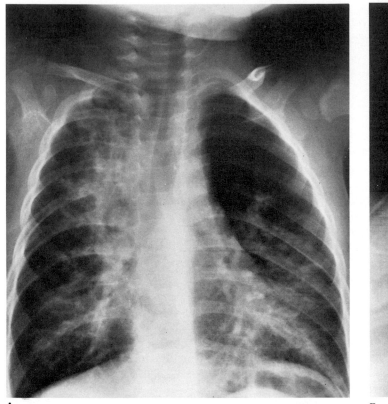
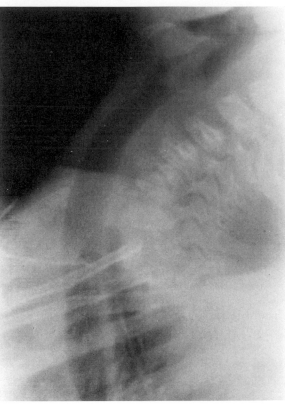

A

B

Figure 1-13   Tracheobronchomegaly (Mounier-Kuhn syndrome). This child developed symptoms of chronic pulmonary infection at 18 months of age. **A.** Films at 2 years of age show diffuse, bilateral, patchy, confluent opacities. Close inspection reveals evidence of peribronchial thickening and basal bronchiectasis. Gradual widening of the intrathoracic trachea is present from the thoracic inlet to the carina. **B.** The lateral projection shows generalized tracheomegaly.

cheal and laryngeal diverticula may also develop and are accentuated during respiration.

In rare cases, tracheobronchomegaly may result from chronic trauma of endotracheal intubation, especially in the newborn and infant (Figure 1-15).[58] This abnormality probably differs from that described by Mounier-Kuhn.

References

1. Floyd J, Campbell DC, Dominy DE: Agenesis of the trachea. *Am Rev Respir Dis* 86:557, 1962.

2. Effman EL, Spackman TJ, Berdon WE, et al: Tracheal agenesis. *AJR* 125:767, 1975.

3. Milstein JM, Lau M, Bickers RG: Tracheal agenesis in infants with VATER association. *Am J Dis Child* 139:77, 1985.

4. Buchino JJ, Meagher DP, Cox JJ: Tracheal agenesis: A clinical approach. *J Pediatr Surg* 17:132, 1982.

5. Sankaran K, Bhagirath CP, Bingham WT, et al: Tracheal atresia, proximal esophageal atresia, and distal tracheoesophageal fistula. Report of two cases and review of the literature. *Pediatrics* 71:821, 1983.

6. Bremer JL: *Congenital Anomalies of the Viscera: Their Embryological Basis.* Cambridge, Harvard University Press, 1957, p 27.

7. Smith EI: The early development of the trachea and esophagus in relation to atresia of the esophagus and

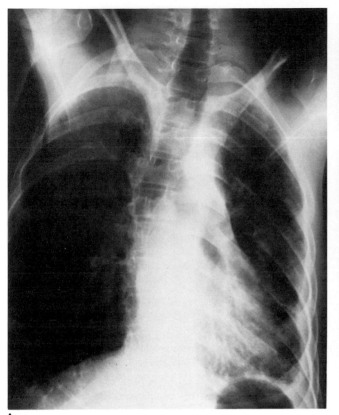

A

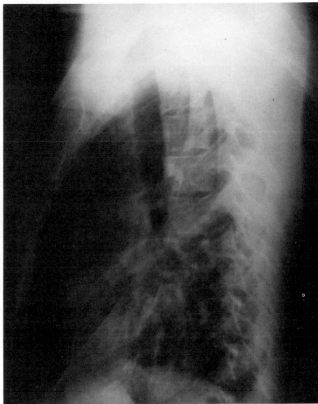

B

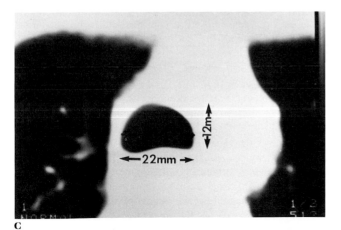

C

Figure 1-14 Tracheobronchomegaly (Mounier-Kuhn syndrome). A 21-year-old man had chronic lung disease and repeated hospital admissions for "pneumonia." **A.** The lungs have bibasal peribronchial disease characterized by bronchiectasis and atelectasis. The tracheal air column is dilated, and the walls appear corrugated. The stem bronchi are also ectatic. **B.** The lateral projection confirms the dilated, corrugated trachea as well as the posterobasal bronchiectasis. **C.** The computed tomogram confirms the enlarged tracheal caliber.

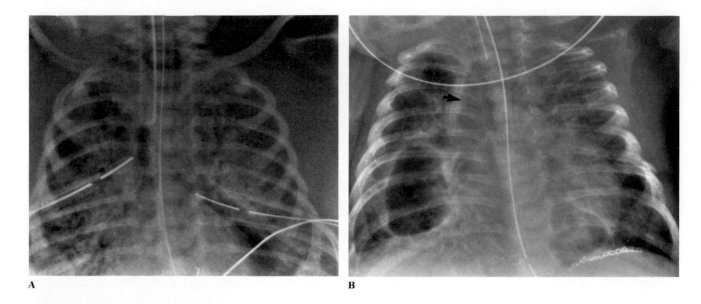

A   B

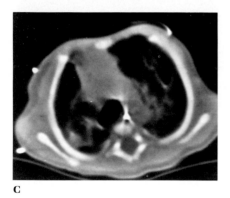

C

Figure 1-15   Tracheobronchomegaly—acquired. A. An infant at 3 weeks of age with chronic lung disease and normal-sized trachea. **B.** At age 3 months there is massive distension of the trachea below the tip of the endotracheal tube. **C.** Computed tomography taken at same time as part B confirms the tracheal dilatation. (Courtesy of Dr. Mervyn D. Cohen, Indianapolis, Indiana.)

tracheoesophageal fistula. Carnegie Institute of Washington Pub 611. *Contrib Embryol* 36:41, 1957.

8. Louhimo I, Lindahl H: Esophageal atresia: Primary results of 500 consecutively treated patients. *J Pediatr Surg* 18:217, 1983.

9. Brereton RJ, Rickwood AMK: Esophageal atresia with pulmonary agenesis. *J Pediatr Surg* 18:618, 1983.

10. McCook TA, Felman AH: Esophageal atresia, duodenal atresia and gastric distention: Report of two cases. *AJR* 131:167, 1978.

11. Spitz L, Ali N, Brereton RJ: Combined esophageal and duodenal atresia: Experience in 18 patients. *J Pediatr Surg* 16:4, 1981.

12. Berdon WE, Baker DH, Schullinger JN, et al: Plain film detection of right aortic arch in infants with esopha-

geal atresia and tracheoesophageal fistula. *J Pediatr Surg* 14:436, 1979.

13. Harrison MR, Hanson BA, Mahour GH, et al: The significance of right aortic arch in repair of esophageal atresia. *J Pediatr Surg* 12:861, 1977.

14. Joseph PM, Berdon WE, Baker DH, et al: Upper airway obstruction in infants and small children. Improved radiographic diagnosis by combining filtration, high kilovoltage and magnification. *Radiology* 121:143, 1976.

15. Day DL: Aortic arch in neonates with esophageal atresia: Preoperative assessment using CT. *Radiology* 155:99, 1985.

16. Donahoe PK, Gee PE: Complete laryngotracheoesophageal cleft: Management and repair. *J Pediatr Surg* 19:143, 1984.

17. Johnson JF, Sueoka BL, Mulligan ME, et al: Tracheo-esophageal fistula: Diagnosis with CT. *Pediatr Radiol* 15:134, 1985.

18. Belt T, Cohen MD: Metrizamide evaluation of the esophagus in infants. *AJR* 143:367, 1984.

19. Felman AH, Talbert JL: Laryngotracheoesophageal cleft. Description of a combined laryngoscopic and roentgenographic diagnostic technique and report of two cases. *Radiology* 103:641, 1972.

20. Cox WL, Shaw RR: Congenital chondromalacia of the trachea. *J Thorac Cardiovasc Surg* 49:1033, 1965.

21. Whittenborg MH, Gyepes MT, Crocker D: Tracheal dynamics in infants with respiratory distress, stridor, and collapsing trachea. *Radiology* 88:653, 1967.

22. Gross RE, Neuhauser EBD: Compression of the trachea or esophagus by vascular anomalies. *Pediatrics* 7:69, 1951.

23. Johner CH, Szauto PA: Polychondritis in a newborn presenting as tracheomalacia. *Ann Otol Rhinol Laryngol* 79:114, 1970.

24. Benjamin B, Cohen D, Glasson M: Tracheomalacia in association with congenital tracheoesophageal fistula. *Surgery* 79:504, 1976.

25. Schwartz MZ, Filer RM: Tracheal compression as a cause of apnea following repair of tracheoesophageal fistula: Treatment by aortopexy. *J Pediatr Surg* 15:842, 1980.

26. Berdon WE, Baker DH, Bordiuck J, et al: Innominate artery compression of the trachea in infants with stridor and apnea. *Radiology* 92:272, 1969.

27. Benjamin B: Endoscopy in congenital tracheal anomalies. *J Pediatr Surg* 15:164, 1980.

28. Kissane JM: *Pathology of Infancy and Childhood*, 2d ed. St Louis, CV Mosby, 1975, p. 457.

29. Wolman IJ: Congenital stenosis of the trachea. *Am J Dis Child* 61:1263, 1961.

30. Hirsch W, Loewenthal M, Swirsky S: Congenital stridor and malformations of the trachea. *Ann Paediatr* 182:1, 1954.

31. Lacosse JE, Reilly BJ, Mancer K: Segmental esophageal trachea: A potentially fatal type of tracheal stenosis. *AJR* 134:829, 1980.

32. Ishida M, Tsuchida Y, Saito S, et al: Congenital esophageal stenosis due to tracheobronchial remnants. *J Pediatr Surg* 4:339, 1969.

33. Benjamin B, Pitkin J, Cohen D: Congenital tracheal stenosis. *Ann Otol Rhinol Laryngol* 90:364, 1981.

34. Berdon WE, Baker DH, Wung JT: Complete cartilage-ring tracheal stenosis associated with anomalous left pulmonary artery: The ring-sling complex. *Radiology* 152:57, 1984.

35. Landing BH: Syndromes of congenital heart disease with tracheobronchial anomalies. *AJR* 123:679, 1975.

36. Idriss RS, Serafin YD, Ilbawi MN: Tracheoplasty with pericardial patch for extensive tracheal stenosis in infants and children. *J Thorac Cardiovasc Surg* 88:527, 1984.

37. Weber TR, Eigen H, Scott PH, et al: Resection of congenital tracheal stenosis involving the carina. *J Thorac Cardiovasc Surg* 84:200, 1982.

38. Aki BF, Yabek SM, Berman W Jr: Total tracheal reconstruction in a three-month old infant. *J Thorac Cardiovasc Surg* 87:543, 1984.

39. Scott JR, Kramer SS: Pediatric tracheostomy. I: Radiographic features of normal healing. *AJR* 130:887, 1978.

40. Scott JR, Kramer SS: Pediatric tracheostomy. II: Radiographic features of difficult decannulations. *AJR* 130:893, 1978.

41. Louhimo I, Grahne B, Pasila M, et al: Acquired laryngotracheal stenosis in children. *J Pediatr Surg* 6:730, 1971.

42. Lindholm CE: Prolonged endotracheal intubation. *Acta Anaesthesiol Scand* (Suppl) 33, 1969.

43. Van Duc T, Tsan Vink L, Huault G, et al: Laryngotracheal lesions induced by endotracheal intubation in children: Anatomic study of 53 cases. *Nouv Presse Med* 3:365, 1974.

44. Symchych PS, Cadotte M: Squamous metaplasia and necrosis of the trachea complicating prolonged naso-tracheal intubation of small newborn infants. *J Pediatr* 71:534, 1967.

45. Miller DR, Sethi G: Tracheal stenosis following prolonged cuffed intubation: Cause and prevention. *Ann Surg* 171:283, 1970.

46. Cooper JD, Grillo HC: The evolution of tracheal injury due to ventilatory assistance through cuffed tubes: A pathologic study. *Ann Surg* 169:334, 1969.

47. James AE Jr, MacMillan AS Jr, Eaton, SB, et al: Roentgenology of tracheal stenosis resulting from cuffed tracheostomy tubes. *AJR* 109:455, 1970.

48. Mounier-Kuhn D: Dilatation de la trachee. Constations radiographiques et bronchoscopiques. *Lyon Med* 150:106, 1932.

49. Katz I, Le Vine M, Herman P: Tracheobronchomegaly; the Mounier-Kuhn syndrome. *AJR* 88:1084, 1962.

50. Hunter TB, Kuhns LR, Roloff MA, et al: Tracheobronchomegaly in an 18 month old child. *AJR* 123:687, 1975.

51. Bateson EM, Woo-Ming M: Tracheobronchomegaly. *Clin Radiol* 24:354, 1973.

52. Hicks GM: Two cases of tracheal abnormality in teenagers presenting as obstructive lung disease. *Ann Radiol* 198:77, 1976.

53. Johnson RF, Green RA: Tracheobronchomegaly. *Am Rev Respir Dis* 91:35, 1965.

54. Aaby GV, Blake HA: Tracheobronchomegaly. *Ann Thorac Surg* 2:64, 1966.

55. Wanderer AA, Ellis EF, Goltz RW, et al: Tracheobronchomegaly and acquired cutis laxa in a child. *Pediatrics* 44:709, 1969.

56. Fiser F, Tomanek A, Rumanova V, et al: Tracheobronchomegaly. *Scand J Respir Dis* 50:147, 1969.

57. Lutz P: Tracheobronchiectasis and trachea incomplete duplex. *Klin Med* 6:422, 1951.

58. Bhutani VK, Ritchie WG, Schaffer TH: Acquired tracheomegaly in very preterm neonates. *Am J Dis Child* 140:449, 1986.

Chapter 2

Abnormal Lung Bud Development (Bronchopulmonary Foregut Malformation)

Congenital abnormalities that result from faulty lung bud development probably occur at 3 to 4 weeks of embryogenesis. At this time, while the foregut is dividing into the esophagus, trachea, and larynx, the lung bud appears as a ventral diverticulum. This lung bud, destined to become the tracheobronchial tree, grows into, and is surrounded by, mesenchymal tissue, blood vessels, and other future pulmonary structures. Repeated branching takes place until approximately 16 weeks of gestation, at which time the tracheobronchial and preacinar structures are established.[1]

Because of the complicated developmental process and the critical timing of events, a wide variety of defects are possible. Some of the better-known and well-defined complexes examined in this chapter are:

1. Bronchoesophageal fistula
2. Primary pulmonary hypoplasia syndromes
   a. Hypoplasia (uncomplicated)
   b. Scimitar syndrome
   c. Accessory diaphragm
   d. Horseshoe lung

3. Pulmonary sequestration
4. Abnormal systemic vessels
5. Bronchogenic cyst

Radiologists, embryologists, and similar types differ concerning the derivation and classification of these lesions. According to Cowart and Blumenthal,[2] more than 40 theories have been proposed to explain their origins.

One of the more popular theories, advanced initially by Gerle et al.,[3] suggests that most of these lesions can be explained on the basis of faulty lung bud and foregut development. Their term, *congenital bronchopulmonary foregut malformation*, has gathered a considerable following. Others have added more recent evidence to support this unified embryologic concept.[4]

Bronchopulmonary foregut malformations are not necessarily solitary. More often they are associated with other foregut anomalies such as ectopic pancreas, foregut duplication cysts, and gastroesophageal diverticula.[4,5] The clinical symptoms and radiographic findings will vary according to the particular anatomic features that exist. Among the most significant are cardiac anomalies and communications between lung, trachea, and/or esophagus. Superimposed infection may also complicate their behavior.

Bronchoesophageal Fistula (Esophageal Lung)

Bronchial communication from the esophagus to a lung, or portion of lung, is a rare congenital anomaly.

It apparently results when a supernumerary lung bud arises from the esophagus, remains patent, and communicates with a portion of lung. Most often, a lower lobe is aerated by this ectopic bronchus through its esophageal connection, but occasionally an entire lung may be involved (Figure 2-1).[6-9] In addition to this abnormal airway communication, the blood supply to the involved lung is often aberrant, and usually arises from the descending aorta or its branches. Venous drainage of the lung may enter

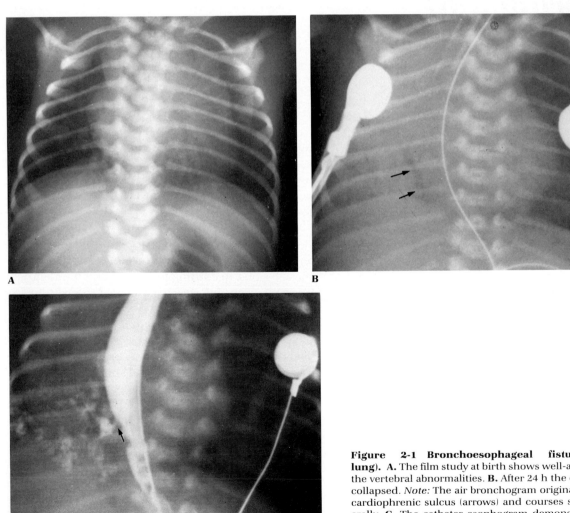

A

B

C

Figure 2-1 Bronchoesophageal fistula (esophageal lung). A. The film study at birth shows well-aerated lungs. Note the vertebral abnormalities. **B.** After 24 h the entire right lung is collapsed. *Note:* The air bronchogram originates from the right cardiophrenic sulcus (arrows) and courses superiorly and laterally. **C.** The catheter esophogram demonstrates the ectopic bronchus (arrow), which supplies the entire right lung. The right lung was removed, but the child died with associated pulmonary artery atresia.

the pulmonary or systemic system. Associated abnormalities include diaphragmatic hernia, cardiac anomalies, vertebral malformations, and genitourinary defects. The condition is found twice as often in females as in males.

When free communication exists between the lung and esophagus, symptoms of pulmonary infection usually present early in life. On occasion, however, the abnormality may not be discovered until adolescence or adulthood. When associated congenital defects are severe and crippling, they may overshadow the underlying pulmonary pathology.

Radiographic findings of bronchoesophageal fistula are inconsistent because of the spectrum of anatomic defects. If an entire lung is supplied by an aberrant bronchus, the normal radiographic pattern may be altered early in life (Figure 2-1B). However, isolated lobes or segments of lung may retain a normal or near-normal appearance for months or years. Various patterns of collapse, consolidation, cavitation, and cyst formation are the rule. Considerable improvement in the radiographic appearance may follow vigorous pulmonary toilet and antibiotic therapy, but return to normal is uncommon.

Bronchoesophageal fistula should be suspected when the atelectatic lung outlines a bronchus arising inferiorly to the hilum (Figure 2-1B). Contrast study of the esophagus with catheter technique will usually confirm this anomaly (Figure 2-1C), but failure to demonstrate the fistula does not always exclude its presence. Recurrent right upper lobe pneumonia is a complication that occurs with a particular type of tracheal bronchus, often seen in Down's syndrome and with rib anomalies.[10]

Primary Pulmonary Hypoplasia Syndromes

The embryogenic defect responsible for the primary pulmonary hypoplasia syndromes is not well established. In all probability, the lung bud arises from the normal location but, for an unknown reason(s), fails to reach normal development. Associated defects, though inconstant, may involve the heart, vertebrae, pulmonary vessels, and diaphragm.

Secondary hypoplasia of the lung usually results from conditions that deplete amniotic fluid or occupy the thoracic space into which the lung must grow. These conditions are covered in Chapter 3.

In a review of 33 children with congenital unilateral pulmonary hypoplasia, Currarino and William[11] observed the following association:

Simple hypoplasia:	9
Absence of pulmonary artery:	7
Anomalous venous return and scimitar syndrome:	8
Accessory diaphragm:	7
Pulmonary sequestration:	2

Only in simple hypoplasia and accessory diaphragm was a significant sex difference found, with females predominating in each. The association of unilateral pulmonary hypoplasia with laryngotracheoesophageal cleft and tracheal stenosis has also been seen in twins.[12]

Pulmonary Hypoplasia (Uncomplicated)

Uncomplicated pulmonary hypoplasia is frequently asymptomatic and is discovered as an incidental finding on chest radiograph (Figure 2-2A). The affected lung and hemithorax are smaller than normal; the heart is shifted to the ipsilateral side; and occasionally the cardiomediastinal border is ill-defined. Elevated hemidiaphragm, closer rib approximation, decreased vascular structures, and thickened apical pleural cap are additional radiographic findings. The pulmonary artery is absent in some patients (Figure 2-2B).[13] Inspiration-expiration films and/or fluoroscopic observations show normal diaphragmatic movement and mediastinal stability in contrast to conditions resulting from partially obstructed airflow. Fluoroscopy is also useful in evaluating tracheal dynamics. Increased mortality has been reported in patients with severe agenesis or hypoplasia of the right lung caused by tracheal compression from a normal aorta, which is deviated to the right.[13]

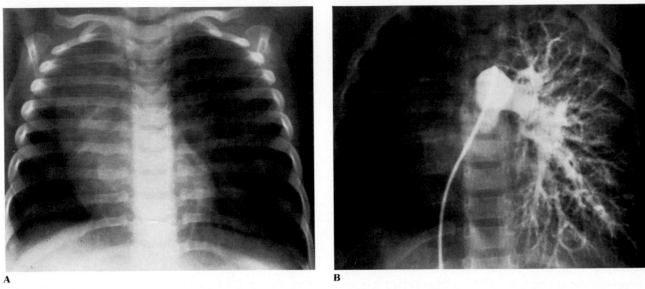

A   B

Figure 2-2   Hypoplastic lung—asymptomatic. A. The right hemithorax is smaller than the left, the ribs are closer together, the mediastinal structures are displaced to the right, and the right pulmonary blood flow is diminished. **B.** The pulmonary angiogram (early phase) shows decreased blood flow to the right lung.

Radionuclide perfusion scans have largely eliminated the need for pulmonary angiography in hypoplastic lungs.

Scimitar Syndrome (Pulmonary Hypoplasia with Abnormal Vascular Connections)

Pulmonary hypoplasia with the scimitar syndrome may cause few clinical symptoms. However, in some patients there may be serious accompanying congenital abnormalities, especially involving the heart. The severity of clinical symptoms results not so much from the pulmonary hypoplasia, as from the complex cardiac malformations.[14] Serious congenital heart disease occurs in approximately one-third of patients in the pediatric age group. Common lesions are ventricular septal defect, patent ductus arteriosus, coarctation of the aorta, and tetralogy of Fallot. The anomalous pulmonary venous return, after which the syndrome is named, is of little physiologic consequence. Recurrent pulmonary infection is a frequent complaint.

The scimitar syndrome often produces characteristic plain-film changes. The right lung is smaller than the left, and the mediastinal structures are shifted to the right (Figures 2-3A and 2-4A). The roentgenographic plain-film sign that separates this syndrome from uncomplicated pulmonary hypoplasia is a curvilinear shadow in the right lower lung field.[14] This shadow has been likened to a scimitar (saber) and represents an anomalous pulmonary vein draining the right lung or a portion thereof.

Venous drainage usually empties into the inferior vena cava or its junction with the right atrium, and less commonly into the right atrium, coronary sinus, and portal or hepatic vein.[11,15] The remaining pulmonary veins drain normally to the left atrium, but may connect to the superior vena cava or azygous system (Figures 2-3C and 2-4B).

In the scimitar syndrome, as in other hypoplastic lung complexes, the pulmonary artery to the involved lobe is often small or absent. A systemic arterial supply to the hypoplastic portion of lung, when present, originates from the descending aorta or one of its branches (Figure 2-4B). Dextroposition and dextrorotation of the heart are commonly associated features. Vertebral abnormalities regularly accompany the scimitar syndrome (Figure 2-3B).

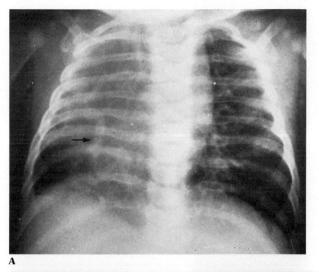

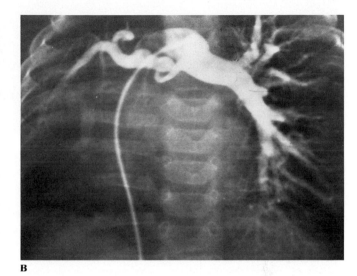

A

B

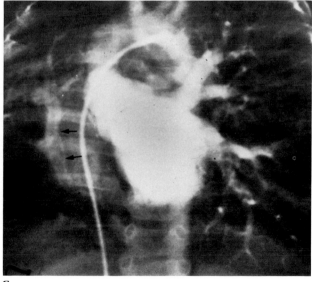

C

Figure 2-3 Scimitar syndrome. A. The right lung is hypoplastic; the curvilinear density (arrow) represents the anomalous pulmonary vein. The syndrome is named because of the similarity of this shadow to a scimitar. **B.** The pulmonary angiogram shows the hypoplastic right pulmonary artery to the upper lung. The remaining right lung is supplied by the aberrant systemic artery from the descending aorta. *Note:* There are lower thoracic vertebral anomalies. **C.** The levophase demonstrates return pulmonary flow through the aberrant pulmonary vein (arrows) into the right atrium.

Accessory Diaphragm

Accessory diaphragm is a distinct anomaly that may accompany hypoplastic lung.[16] Like the scimitar syndrome, it favors the right side, but left-sided cases are reported.[17,18]

This complex is caused by a fibromuscular diaphragm that originates from the anterior portion of the normal diaphragm and inserts somewhat higher and posteriorly, usually along the fifth to seventh rib.[18] The development of normal lung bud branching is altered by this abnormally developing septum.[19] The divided septum presumably gives rise to the accessory diaphragm, which is complete anteriorly and incomplete posteromedially. Pulmonary tissue is thus divided into two compartments by this additional diaphragm, which may have normal innervation.

Associated anomalies are present. They consist mainly of hypoplasia and maldevelopment of the ip-

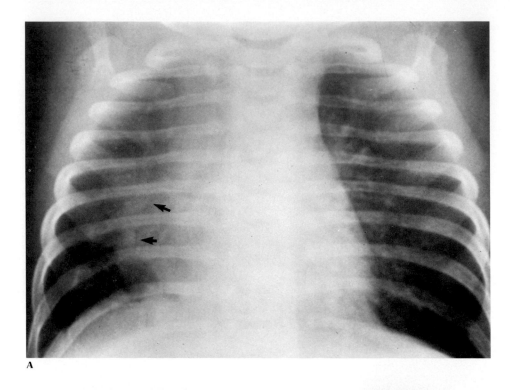

A

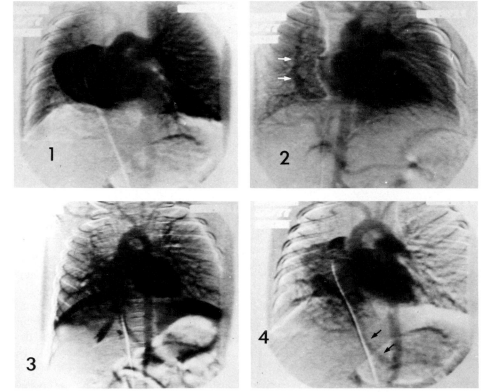

B

Figure 2-4 Scimitar syndrome—digital subtraction angiography. A. The right hemithorax is smaller than the left, and the right heart border is obscured. The scimitar shadow (arrows) is difficult to appreciate. **B.** Digital subtraction angiogram. (1) Right atrial injection with predominant flow to the left lung. (2) Pulmonary venous return via the aberrant right "scimitar" pulmonary vein (white arrows). (3,4) Levophase—an aberrant systemic vessel (arrows) from the descending aorta supplies the right lower lung. (Courtesy of Dr. Milton Wagner, Houston, Texas.)

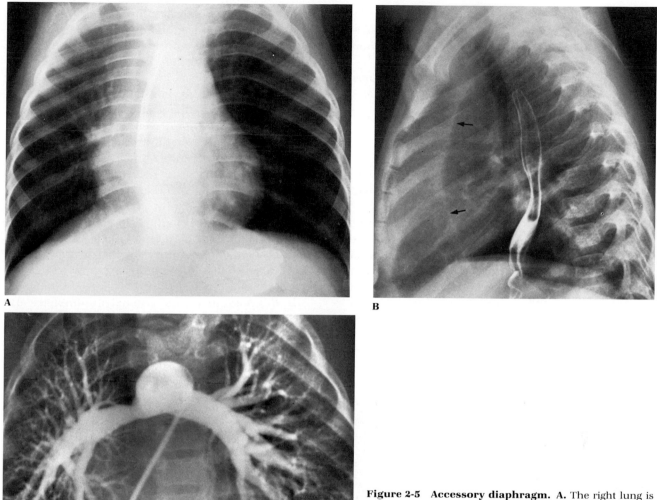

Figure 2-5   Accessory diaphragm. A. The right lung is smaller than the left, the right mediastinal border is obscured, and the mediastinum is shifted to the right. **B.** The lateral film shows a curvilinear interface (arrows) which demarcates the soft tissue interposed between the lung and anterior chest wall. This line is not the accessory diaphragm. **C.** The right pulmonary artery is mildly stenotic and hypoplastic. Note the upper thoracic vertebral anomalies.

silateral lung, vascular anomalies of pulmonary venous drainage and systemic arterial supply, congenital heart disease, diaphragmatic hernia, and occasional vertebral abnormalities.[17] A medial diaphragmatic hiatus is often present.

On the frontal radiograph, the affected hemithorax is small, the cardiac silhouette often ob-

scured, and the mediastinal structures shifted toward the involved side (Figure 2-5A). In the lateral projection, a characteristic radiopacity with a well-defined posterior convex margin is often visible along the anterior chest wall (Figure 2-5B). This opacity consists of loose areolar tissue that occupies the space between the hypoplastic lung and chest wall. It does not represent the accessory dia-phragm.[18] Rarely, the accessory diaphragm is visible as an additional thin, curved opacity above the nor-mal diaphragm in the lateral projection.[20]

As with the other hypoplastic lung syndromes, this roentgenographic pattern is quite characteristic, but not necessarily diagnostic.

Horseshoe Lung

Horseshoe lung is a term first used by Spencer to describe an unusual malformation wherein the right and left lungs are fused behind the pericardial sac.[21] Since his description, several additional patients have been reported.[22-24] Salient features include right lung hypoplasia, cardiac dextroversion, partial anomalous pulmonary venous return from the right lung to the inferior vena cava (scimitar shadow), and aberrant systemic arterial supply to all or a portion of the hypoplastic lung. In most, the aberrant sys-temic artery originates from the aorta or one of its branches, but the arterial supply to the lung may arise from the pulmonary artery.[22]

Patients with horseshoe lung suffer from recur-rent pulmonary infections more frequently than those with scimitar syndrome. Surgical removal of the hypoplastic lung has resulted in clinical im-provement in some cases.[23]

The radiographic findings of horseshoe lung sim-ulate those found in the scimitar syndrome, with a few subtle differences. A well-defined hyperlucent segment of lung is sometimes visible in the left car-diophrenic sulcus (Figure 2-6A). This represents the isthmus of lung extending behind the heart into the left hemithorax. The pleuroesophageal or posterior junction line is absent in some cases. A barium esophogram might well show lung tissue between the esophagus and cardiac shadow. Bilateral left-sided bronchial branching may be a feature of this complex, as well as the scimitar shadow of anoma-lous pulmonary venous return.[25]

In the horseshoe lung anomaly, pulmonary an-giography shows small branches of the pulmonary artery supplying the isthmus of lung coursing infe-romedially across the midline behind the heart (Fig-ure 2-6B). These branches are often small and easily

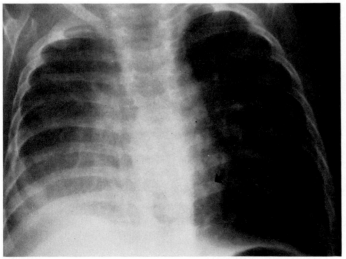 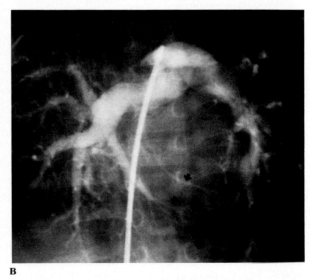

A   B

Figure 2-6   Horseshoe lung. A. This plain film of a child at 8 months of age shows a small right hemithorax, dextra position of the heart, obliteration of the right phrenic silhouette, and compensatory emphysema of the left lung. The triangular lucency (arrow) at the medial aspect of the left lung base probably results from underperfusion of this portion of lung. **B.** A pulmonary angiogram of the same child at 3½ years of age demonstrates right pulmonary artery branches crossing the midline to the left base (arrows). This exposure does not show the presence of aberrant aortic vessel to the right lung base and right pulmonary venous drainage into the inferior vena cava.

overlooked, but they identify the presence of lung fusion. Aberrant systemic vessels and anomalous pulmonary venous return are inconstant features.

Pulmonary Sequestration

Pulmonary sequestrations are traditionally considered as either extralobar or intralobar. Both varieties share at least three characteristics: (1) absent connection to the normal tracheobronchial tree, (2) aberrant vascular supply, usually from the aorta, less commonly from one or more of its branches, or rarely from one or both pulmonary arteries,[26] and (3) involvement with chronic recurrent infection.

Extralobar Sequestration

The embryologic concept of bronchopulmonary foregut malformation, described earlier, is useful when considering extralobar sequestration. In normal embryogenesis, the lung bud appears as an outgrowth of the ventral wall of the primitive foregut at approximately 5 weeks of gestation. As the foregut partitions and elongates, the lung bud divides, subdivides, and branches into the tracheobronchial tree. Extralobar sequestration results when a supernumerary lung bud arises caudally in relation to the normal lung bud. From its aberrant location, it clongates and is enveloped by mesenchymal lung tissue with a separate pleural covering.[11]

The following are distinguishing characteristics of extralobar sequestration:

1. A distinct pleural investment is present.
2. The arterial supply is usually systemic but may be pulmonary.
3. The venous drainage most often flows into azygous or hemiazygous veins, but may empty into pulmonary veins.
4. Ninety percent are left-sided.
5. There is a common association with diaphragmatic hernia or eventration and with other congenital abnormalities especially of the gastrointestinal tract.[27] These sequestrations may be found below the diaphragm.[3]
6. Presentation is most often in infancy or childhood.
7. Males are more commonly affected (80 percent).
8. Extralobar sequestrations usually present radiographically as triangular densities in the posterior and medial left base.

Intralobar Sequestration

Intralobar sequestrations demonstrate the following characteristics:

1. The mass is totally contained within the visceral pleura of the ipsilateral lung.
2. The arterial supply arises from the aorta or major branches.
3. The venous drainage usually flows into pulmonary veins and the left atrium.
4. Most are located in the posterior basal segments of the lower lobes, with approximately 60 percent on the left.
5. Patent communications with the gastrointestinal tract and other associated anomalies are rare.
6. Diagnosis is infrequent in infants and neonates; more than half are discovered in adolescent youngsters.
7. The sex incidence is equal.
8. The radiographic opacities produced are surrounded by aerated lung.

The exact origin of intralobar sequestration is still uncertain. Gerle and coworkers suggest that these lesions, like the extralobar type, also result from aberrant lung bud development.[3] Because of a critical difference in timing, the intralobar, in contrast to the extralobar, becomes enveloped within the visceral pleura and usually retains normal pulmonary venous drainage. Gerle's original concept has been supported by others, who agree that this abnormality represents one of a group of foregut malformations with a common embryology but with variable clinical and radiographic manifestations.[4,28–30] Less popular theories include (1) mechanical, (2) vascular traction, (3) vascular insufficiency, (4) coincidental occurrence, (5) idiopathic, and (6) acquired origins.

Gebaur and Mason[31] proposed that all cases of intralobar pulmonary sequestration are the result of acquired intrapulmonary pathology with secondary enlargement of bronchial and mediastinal arteries. They further suggest that pleural adhesions bridge the gap separating the intercostal and/or diaphragmatic vessels from the pulmonary vessels and lead to communication between these systems in some cases (Figure 2-7). Bronchial arteries may dilate and carry large amounts of blood in a variety of pulmonary conditions, notably chronic active pulmonary suppuration, bronchiectasis, cystic fibrosis, and foreign bodies. Pulmonary hemorrhage is an occasional complication.

Stocker and Malczak[32] published a compelling and comprehensive study that supports and advances the theory that intralobar sequestration is an acquired, chronic, inflammatory process that obtains its blood supply from systemic arteries located primarily within the pulmonary ligament (Figure 2-7B and C). They confirmed, moreover, that arteries are present normally in the pulmonary ligament of autopsied infants, and proposed that chronic infection caused these arteries to hypertrophy. This pathologic change simulates that which occurs with other chronic pulmonary infections such as bronchiectasis. Clearly, acquired intrapulmonary abnormalities that simulate intralobar sequestrations have been observed (Figure 2-7).[36]

In spite of these revelations, several questions that point to the congenital origin of intralobar sequestration remain unanswered. (1) Intralobar and extralobar sequestrations have been observed in the same patient.[29,33] (2) Bilateral intralobar sequestrations are reported.[34] (3) Intralobar sequestration may have fistulous connections with the gut. (4) A 14 percent incidence of associated congenital abnormalities has been reported.[35] Intralobar sequestration has also been observed in early infancy before the onset of infection. Dr. Felson's observation that pulmonary sequestrations have "many faces" seems secure, for at least the near future.

Radiologic Findings

Patients with intralobar pulmonary sequestration may have normal plain chest films in early life, but

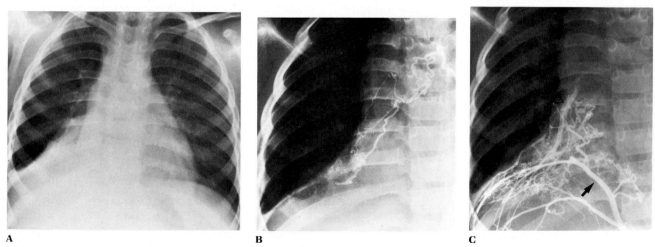

A   B   C

Figure 2-7   **"Acquired sequestration."** **A.** Chronic right lower lobe atelectasis is evident on this and multiple previous films. Bronchoscopy showed a markedly narrowed bronchus intermedius. **B.** A bronchial artery injection shows hypertrophied vessels. **C.** The diaphragmatic artery (solid arrow) gives rise to a plethora of branching vessels that supply the atelectatic lower lobe. This most likely represents satellite vascularization resulting from chronic pulmonary infection and should not be confused with congenital aberrant systemic supply to the lung. At surgery, considerable pleural adhesions were present between the chronically infected lower lobe and diaphragm. Note pulmonary venous drainage (open arrow).

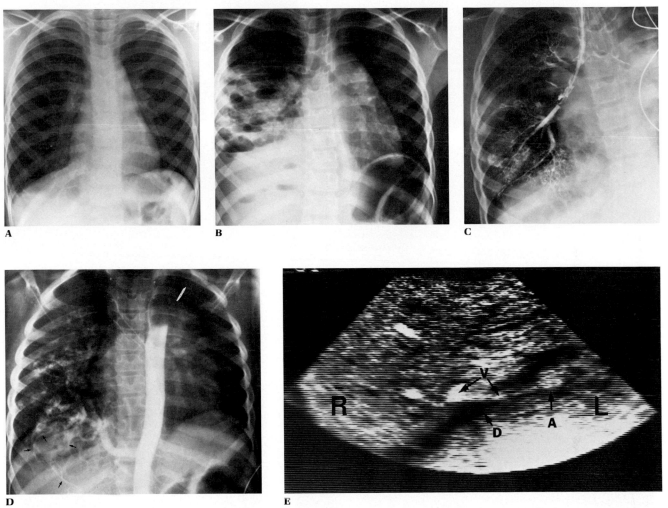

Figure 2-8 Pulmonary sequestration—recurrent pneumonia. A. The film study of this 7-year-old girl was exposed during a period of relative well-being; cystic changes are present in the overexpanded right lower lobe. These are best viewed through the hepatic shadow. **B.** On another occasion, these cystic structures are partially fluid-filled. **C.** Bronchography shows normal bronchi to portions of the lower lobe; the abnormal cystic lung is not in communication with the tracheobronchial tree. **D.** Aortic injection demonstrates a large systemic vessel arising from the descending aorta supplying the abnormal lung (arrows). **E.** Abdominal ultra-sonography shows the aberrant systemic vessel (V) arising from the aorta (A) and coursing through the diaphragm (D) into the liver.

recurrent, indolent infections eventually produce a persistent pulmonary process, often in the same location (Figures 2-8 to 2-10). Cystic changes, cavitations, and air-fluid levels usually superimpose upon the chronic underlying infiltrate (Figures 2-8 and 2-9). Less often, intralobar pulmonary sequestration begins as a cystic, multicystic, or solid lesion. Most

are posterior and basal in location, but with recurrent infections they may extend well beyond. Upper lobe presentation is rare, but reported.[2]

The shadow of an abnormal vessel entering the lung is occasionally visible. The large volume of blood shunting through the aberrant systemic vessel may induce cardiomegaly and congestive failure.[37,38]

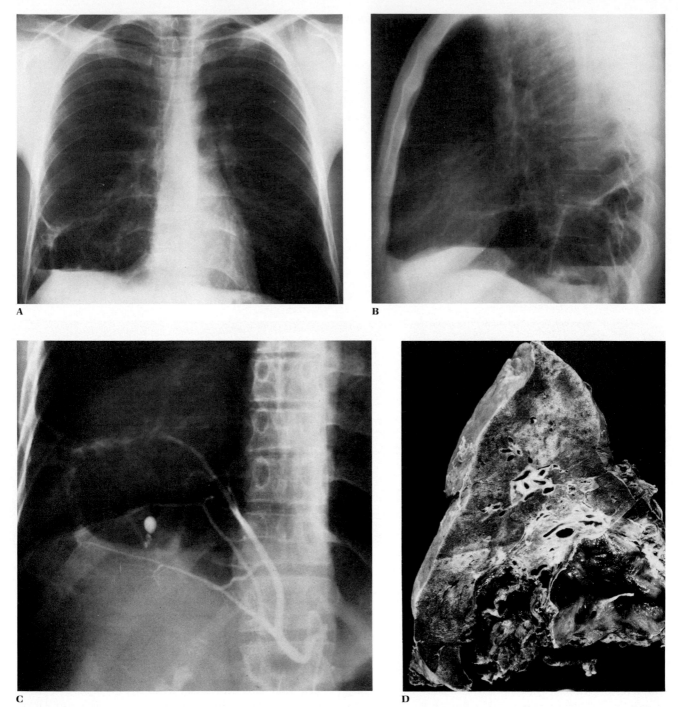

Figure 2-9 Pulmonary sequestration—acquired (?). A 21-year-old man in good health until the age of 19 when he developed right lower lobe "pneumonia" with abscess formation. This cleared with antibiotics, but symptoms recurred 2 years later. **A** and **B.** These chest films show numerous cavitary lesions containing air-fluid levels in right posterior lower lobe segments. **C.** This selective celiac arteriogram opacifies an aberrant vessel branching from the phrenic artery and entering the right lower lobe. *Note:* There is collection of contrast material in the "sequestered" lung from a previous bronchogram. **D.** The gross anatomic specimen of the right lower lobe confirms the presence of marked cavitary, necrotic basal segments. This area is supplied by the systemic branch of the celiac artery demonstrated in part C.

Diaphragmatic eventration and/or hernia are associated abnormalities that may accompany these lesions.

Recurrent, unresolved, pulmonary processes, especially basal and/or posterior in location, call for specialized radiographic procedures to confirm or exclude the presence of sequestration. Identification of systemic arterial supply to the involved lung, usually by arteriography, is presumptive evidence for the presence of sequestration (Figures 2-8D, 2-9C, and 2-10C). If a feeding vessel from the aorta is not identified, other branches of the aorta, including the celiac axis, must be opacified. The delineation of these feeding vessels is as important to the surgeon in mapping the operative approach as it is to the radiologist in making the initial diagnosis. Systemic vessels from the aorta or its branches may enter portions of normal lung, and these should not be confused with sequestration. (See the next section.) Attention to previous pulmonary patterns of infection and careful arteriography should eliminate the confusion between sequestration and pseudosequestration.

Bronchograms are rarely needed in the evaluation of patients with suspected sequestration (Figure 2-8C). While, by definition, intralobar sequestration is isolated from the normal tracheobronchial tree, if bronchography is performed, contrast material may enter the cystic cavities (Figure 2-9C). The broncho-

graphic contrast apparently passes through connections that develop from superimposed infection. Collateral communication between sequestration and normal lung has been shown by ventilation nuclear lung scan.[39]

The use of computed tomography (CT) has also been reported in the diagnosis of pulmonary sequestration.[33,40] Kaude and Laurin[41] have used ultrasound to identify the presence of sequestration, its relationship to lung and diaphragm, and the aberrant arterial supply. An aberrant artery has been identified with ultrasound in two additional patients (Figure 2-8E). Digital subtraction radiography is still another method for evaluation of these lesions (Figure 2-4B).

Pathologic Findings

Before significant infection has occurred, the sequestered lung may appear quite normal on histologic examination. As time passes, the changes of chronic infection appear, i.e., interstitial fibrosis, lymphoid follicles, and diffuse, chronic infiltrate. Cystic spaces representing destroyed parenchyma and dilated bronchioles are common findings (Figure 2-9D). These lesions usually have no true connection to the normal bronchial tree; however, bronchial isolation may not be complete.[42,43] On rare occasions, normal mucosal and submucosal conti-

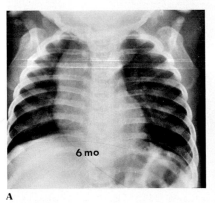
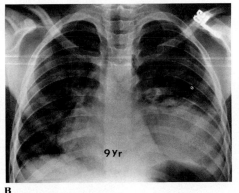
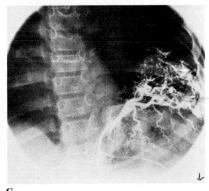

A   B   C

Figure 2-10 Intralobar pulmonary sequestration—congenital. A. This chest film discovered a multicystic lesion in the left lower lobe of this 6-month-old patient. **B.** The patient returned 9 years later with recurrent left lower lobe infection. **C.** The arteriogram shows two vessels from the descending aorta supplying the left lower lobe. (From Sanchez GR, et al: Radiologic case of the month. *Am J Dis Child* 139:207, 1985. Copyright 1985, American Medical Association. With permission.)

nuity between sequestered lung and bronchial tree has been observed without superimposed inflammatory change.[42,43]

Enteric duplications, diaphragmatic eventrations/hernias, ectopic pancreas, and other gastroenteric abnormalities are occasionally seen in association with sequestration. Surgical removal of intralobar sequestration is usually curative.

Pseudosequestration

Pseudosequestration is an abnormality in which a mass of liver tissue is herniated through the right hemidiaphragm. The right lower lobe, overlying the herniated liver, consists of normal or partially collapsed lung which is perfused by a systemic artery arising from the aorta. The underlying liver receives its arterial supply from normal sources. Abnormal pulmonary drainage into the azygous vein is present in some patients.[36]

Abnormal Systemic Vessels

Abnormal pulmonary and bronchial supply to the lungs develops with acquired infections as well as congenital malformations, i.e., pulmonary sequestration, scimitar syndrome, horseshoe lung, and hypoplastic lung with accessory diaphragm. Systemic arteries to the lung may also exist in the absence of any identifiable pulmonary abnormality.[44–47] This condition is usually asymptomatic, but the auscultation of a continuous murmur over the posterior chest may bring it to attention. Left heart enlargement, with or without florid congestive failure, may result if the systemic to pulmonary blood flow is of sufficient quantity (Figure 2-11).

The abnormal artery characteristically arises from the dorsal or abdominal aorta and enters the left chest, but it may be seen on the right (Figure 2-11B). On occasion, it may connect directly to a pulmonary artery.[48] In rare cases when the pulmonary

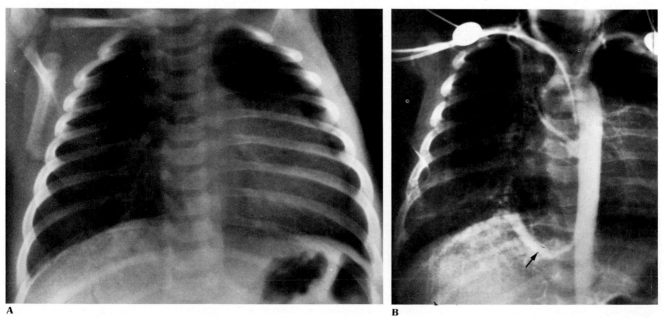

A   **B**

Figure 2-11   Systemic artery—pulmonary venous fistula. A. Cardiomegaly is present in this child with symptoms of heart failure. **B.** Aortic injection demonstrates an aberrant vessel into the right lower lung (arrow). Ligation of this vessel alleviated the symptoms. The surrounding lung was normal at surgery.

artery is absent or hypoplastic, the entire blood supply to a lung or portion of lung is furnished via systemic arteries.[49] Pulmonary venous drainage usually flows into the inferior pulmonary vein.

The presence of abnormal systemic vessels to the lung probably relates embryologically to the spectrum of bronchopulmonary foregut malformation. By 30 days of embryologic life, a vascular plexus surrounds the branching primary lung buds.[50] Vascular channels from the sixth primitive arches, as well as systemic connections from paired dorsal aortas, feed this plexus. The systemic channels from the aortas involute and remain as bronchial arteries, while those from the sixth arches persist to form the pulmonary arteries. An aberrant vessel to the lung results when a systemic artery retains its original embryonic size, character, and connection between the aorta and developing pulmonary parenchyma.[48] In these circumstances, the lungs are usually normal. However, these systemic arteries have the capability to enlarge in response to pulmonary infections or oligemia.

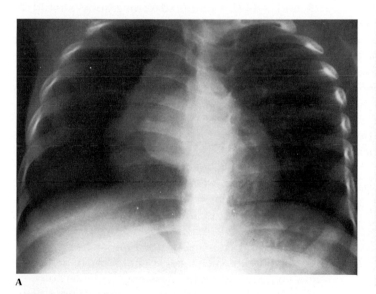

A

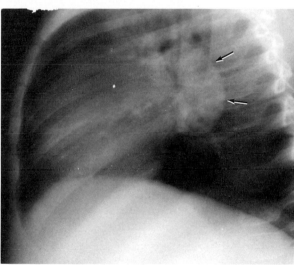

B

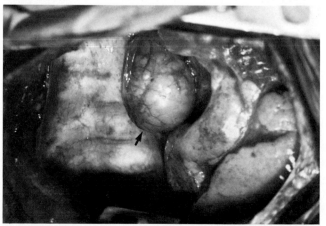

C

Figure 2-12 Bronchogenic cyst—asymptomatic. A. This frontal film (slightly rotated) reveals a rounded, subcarinal mass projecting to the right of the vertebrae. The heart, vertebrae, and remaining lung are normal. **B.** The posterior margin of the mass (arrows) is well outlined against the adjacent lung, the anterior margin is obscured. **C.** Thoracotomy shows the relation of the cyst (arrow) to the vertebral column and overlying lung.

Bronchogenic Cyst

Bronchogenic cysts are often discovered in older children and are commonly found in adults. However, because of their frequent proximity to the adjacent airway, bronchogenic cysts may cause respiratory distress, cough, and recurrent infections in very early life. Whereas most bronchogenic cysts reside near the trachea, stem bronchi, and carina (Figure 2-12), on occasion they stray into the neck or out into the lung parenchyma.

Although opinions vary regarding the origin of bronchogenic cysts, the most widely held view is that they represent ectopic lung buds that have closed their connection to the tracheobronchial tree and failed to incorporate into the primitive mesenchymal lung tissue. In some cases, the original connection to the esophagus is preserved as a fibrous stalk. Rarely, a patent communication with the esophagus persists in a manner similar to the bronchoesophageal anomalies. Associated congenital defects are rare, except when they occur in the cervical region where vertebral anomalies are sometimes present. Pericardial defects and gastric duplication associated with bronchial cysts have been reported.[34,51] Discovery of the cysts in the neonatal period and the presence of anomalous systemic blood supply support a congenital etiology.

When respiratory distress or swallowing difficulties are present, impingement on the tracheobronchial tree and/or esophagus should be suspected. Plain films will often disclose the presence of a rounded mass in proximity to the carina and stem bronchi. Barium esophogram is often helpful in outlining the margins of bronchogenic cysts (Figures 2-13 and 2-14B). Computed tomography should be performed to separate these lesions from solid masses (Figure 2-14C). However, confusion with a solid mass may occur when bronchogenic cysts exhibit high CT numbers as a result of previous infection, hemorrhage, or similar process.[52] Peripherally situated cysts cannot always be differentiated radiographically from other lesions such as tumors and lymph nodes (Figure 2-15).

Histologically, the walls of bronchogenic cysts contain bronchial elements such as cartilage, fibrovascular connective tissue, and pseudostratified columnar epithelium, as well as respiratory and seromucous glands (Figures 2-14D and 2-15D). These features help differentiate bronchogenic cysts from enteric and thymic cysts. However, microscopic differentiation between a congenital bronchogenic cyst and an acquired cystic mass may be hazardous, especially with a history of antecedent trauma or infection.

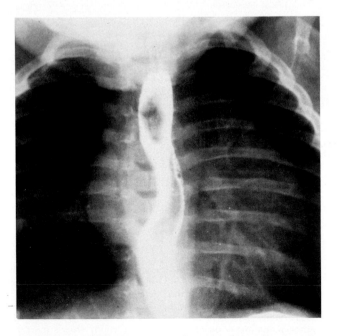

Figure 2-13 Bronchogenic cyst. Barium esophogram delimits the medial margin of the mass.

References

1. Reid L: The lung: Its growth and remodeling in health and disease. *AJR* 129:777, 1977.
2. Cowart MA, Blumenthal BI: Bronchopulmonary sequestration: An unusual presentation. *South Med J* 74:500, 1981.
3. Gerle RD, Jaretzki A, Ashley CA, et al: Congenital bronchopulmonary-foregut malformation. Pulmonary se-

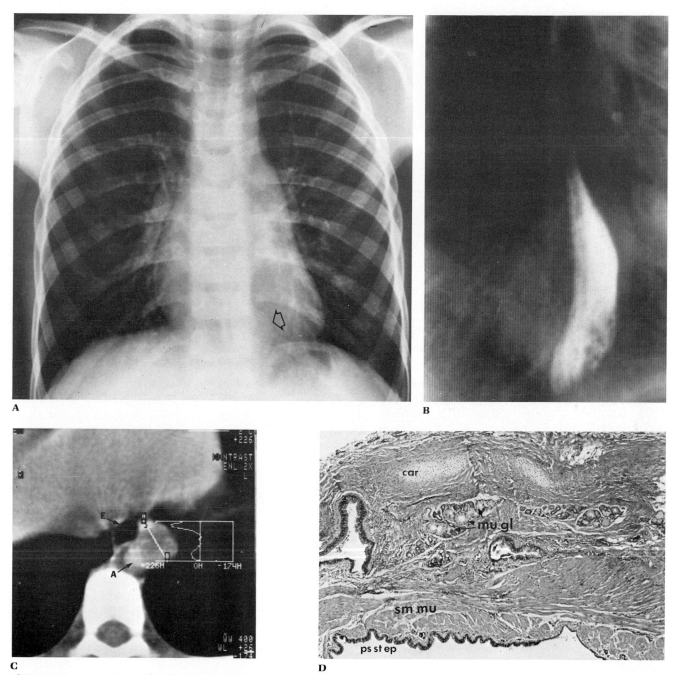

Figure 2-14   Bronchogenic cyst—asymptomatic. A. A round left paraspinous mass is present in this 4-year-old boy (arrow). **B.** The barium esophogram confirms the proximity of the mass to the esophagus. **C.** Computed tomography with contrast enhancement. The mass (A-B) measures 22 mm in diameter and lies astride the air-filled esophagus (E) and the aorta (A). The cystic nature of the mass is suggested by the low-density reading in the center. **D.** This histologic section of the wall demonstrates pseudostratified, ciliated, columnar epithelium (ps st ep). The submucosa contains smooth muscle (sm mu), mucous glands (mu gl), and foci of cartilage (car). These are characteristic histologic features of a bronchogenic cyst.

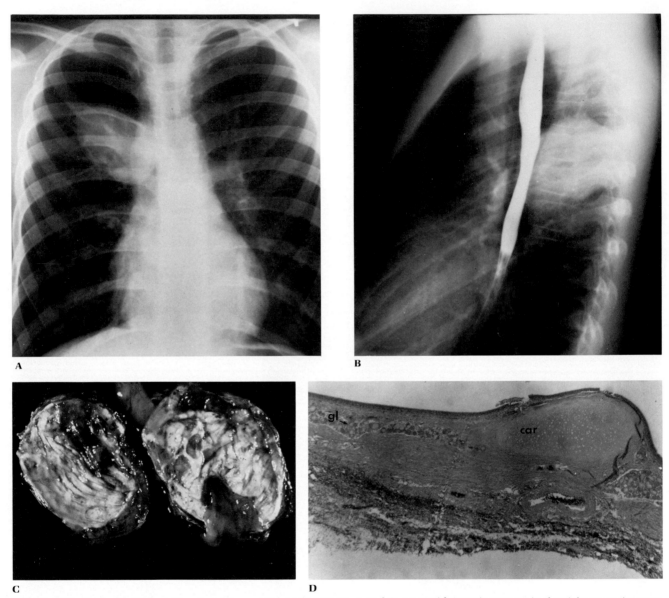

Figure 2-15   Bronchogenic cyst—simulates neurogenic tumor. A and **B.** An ovoid mass is present in the right posterior para-spinous region. **C.** This fluctuant unilocular cyst is 6 cm in diameter and contains yellow-brown viscous fluid. **D.** Nearly all the wall consists of fibrovascular connective tissue. The cyst lumen is lined by pseudostratified columnar respiratory epithelium beneath which are seromucous glands (gl) and cartilage (car), typical histologic features of bronchi.

questration communicating with the gastrointestinal tract. *N Engl J Med* 278:1413, 1968.

4. Heithoff KB, Sane SM, Williams HJ, et al: Bronchopulmonary foregut malformations. A unifying etiological concept. *AJR* 126:46, 1976.

5. Beskin CA: Intralobar enteric sequestration of the lung containing aberrant pancreas. *J Thorac Cardiovasc Surg* 41:314, 1961.

6. Nikaidoh H, Swenson O: The ectopic origin of the right main bronchus from the esophagus. A case of pneumonectomy in a neonate. *J Thorac Cardiovasc Surg* 62:151, 1971.

7. Bates M: Total unilateral pulmonary sequestration. *Thorax* 23:311, 1968.

8. Hanna EA: Broncho-esophageal fistula with total sequestration of the right lung. *Ann Surg* 159:599, 1964.

9. Thompson NB, Aquino T: Anomalous origin of the right main-stem bronchus. *Surgery* 51:668, 1962.

10. McLaughlin FJ, Streider DJ, Harris GBC, et al: Tracheal bronchus: Association with respiratory morbidity in childhood. *J Pediatr* 106:751, 1985.

11. Currarino G, William B: Causes of congenital unilateral pulmonary hypoplasia: A study of 33 cases. *Pediatr Radiol* 15:15, 1985.

12. Novak RW: Laryngotracheoesophageal cleft and unilateral pulmonary hypoplasia in twins. *Pediatrics* 67:732, 1981.

13. Werber J, Ramilo JL, London, R, et al: Unilateral absence of a pulmonary artery. *Chest* 84:729, 1983

14. Jue KL, Amplatz K, Adams, P Jr, et al: Anomalies of great vessels associated with lung hypoplasia. The scimitar syndrome. *Am J Dis Child* 111:35, 1966.

15. Felson B: Pulmonary agenesis and related anomalies. *Semin Roentgenol* 7:17, 1972.

16. Haeberlin P: Eine seltene Zwerchfellmissbildung (partielle einseitige doppelbildung). *Schweiz Med Wochenschr* 75:509, 1945.

17. Kenanoglu A, Tuncbilek E: Accessory diaphragm in the left side. *Pediatr Radiol* 7:172, 1978.

18. Davis WA, Allen RP: Accessory diaphragm: Duplication of the diaphragm. *Radiol Clin North Am* VI:253, 1968.

19. Drake EH, Lynch JB: Bronchiectasis associated with anomaly of the right pulmonary vein and right diaphragm. *J Thorac Surg* 19:453, 1950.

20. Gwinn JL, Lee FA: Radiological case of the month. *Am J Dis Child* 128:367, 1974.

21. Spencer H: *Pathology of the Lung*, 2d ed. Oxford, Pergamon Press, Inc, 1968, p 72.

22. Dische MR, Tiexeira ML, Winchester PN, et al: Horseshoe lung associated with a variant of the "scimitar" syndrome. *Br Heart J* 36:617, 1974.

23. Orzan F, Angelini P, Oglietti J, et al: Horseshoe lung: Report of two cases. *Am Heart J* 93:501, 1977.

24. Frank JL, Poole CA: Clinical and radiographic features of horseshoe lung. *Proc Soc Pediatr Radiol* 1981.

25. Halasz NA, Halloran KH, Liebow AA: Bronchial and arterial anomalies with drainage of the right lung into the inferior vena cava. *Circulation* 14:826, 1956.

26. Pryce DM, Sellors TH, Blair LG: Intralobar sequestration of lung associated with an abnormal pulmonary artery. *Br J Surg* 35:18, 1947.

27. Flye NW, Izant RJ: Extralobar pulmonary sequestration with esophageal communication and complete duplication of the colon. *Surgery* 71:744, 1972.

28. Sade RM, Clouse M, Ellis FH Jr: The spectrum of pulmonary sequestration. *Ann Thorac Surg* 18:644, 1974.

29. Pendse P, Alexander J, Khademi M, et al: Pulmonary sequestration. Coexisting classic intralobar and extralobar types in a child. *J Thorac Cardiovasc Surg* 64:127, 1972.

30. Carter R: Pulmonary sequestration. *Ann Thorac Surg* 7:68, 1969.

31. Gebaur PW, Mason CB: Intralobar pulmonary sequestration associated with anomalous pulmonary vessels: A nonentity. *Dis Chest* 30:282, 1959.

32. Stocker JT, Malczak HT: A study of pulmonary ligament arteries. Relationship to intralobar pulmonary sequestration. *Chest* 86:611, 1984.

33. Kafka V, Beco V: Simultaneous intra- and extrapulmonary sequestration. *Arch Dis Child* 35:51, 1960.

34. Wimbish KJ, Agha FB, Brady TM: Bilateral pulmonary sequestration: Computed tomographic appearance. *AJR* 140:689, 1983.

35. Thornhill BA, Kyunghee CC, Morehouse HT: Gastric duplication associated with pulmonary sequestration: CT manifestations. *AJR* 138:1168, 1982.

36. MacPherson RI, Whytehead L: Pseudosequestration. *J Can Assoc Radiol* 28:17, 1977.

37. Ranson JM, Norton JB, Williams GD: Pulmonary sequestration presenting as congestive failure. *J Thorac Cardiovasc Surg* 76:378, 1978.

38. Goldblatt E, Vimpani G, Brown JH: Extralobar sequestration: Presentation as an arteriovenous aneurysm with cardiac failure in infancy. *Am J Cardiol* 29:100, 1972.

39. Hopkins RL, Levine SD, Waring WW: Intralobar sequestration—Demonstration of collateral ventilation by nuclear lung scan. *Chest* 82:192, 1983.

40. Baker EL, Gore RM, Moss AA: Retroperitoneal pulmonary sequestration: Computed tomographic findings. *AJR* 138:956, 1982.

41. Kaude, JV, Laurin, S: Ultrasonographic demonstration of systemic artery feeding extrapulmonary sequestration. *Pediatr Radiol* 14:226, 1984.

42. Takahashi M, Ohno M, Mihara K, et al: Pulmonary sequestration. *Radiology* 114:543, 1975.

43. Groot H: Lung sequestration. *Radiol Clin (Basel)* 45:49, 1975.

44. Campbell DC Jr, Murney JA, Dominy DE: Systemic arterial blood supply to a normal lung. *JAMA* 182:497, 1962.

45. Ernst MPG, Bruschke, AVG: An aberrant systemic artery to the right lung with normal pulmonary tissue. *Chest* 60:606, 1971.

46. Kirks DR, Kane PE, Free EA, et al: Systemic arterial supply to normal basilar segments of the left lower lobe. *AJR* 126:817, 1976.

47. Currarino G, Willis K, Miller W: Congenital fistula between an aberrant systemic artery and a pulmonary vein without sequestration. A report of three cases. *J Pediatr* 87:554, 1975.

48. Hessell EA, Boyden EA, Stamm SJ, et al: High systemic origin of the sole artery to the basal segments of the left lung: Findings, surgical treatment and embryologic interpretation. *Surgery* 67:624, 1970.

49. Maier HC: Absence or hypoplasia of a pulmonary artery with anomalous systemic arteries to the lung. *J Thorac Cardiovasc Surg* 28:145, 1954.

50. Boyden EA: Developmental anomalies of lungs. *Am J Surg* 89:79, 1955.

51. Jones P: Developmental defects in the lungs. *Thorax* 10:205, 1955.

52. Mendelson DS, Rose JS, Efremidis, SC, et al: Bronchogenic cysts with high C.T. numbers. *AJR* 140:463, 1983.

Chapter 3

Abnormal Bronchial, Parenchymal, and Vascular Development

The congenital pulmonary abnormalities to be examined in this chapter are difficult to categorize. In all probability, they are caused by defective embryogenesis of lung parenchymal structures (bronchi, blood vessels, lymphatics, and supporting stroma) after normal foregut and tracheoesophageal differentiation and maturation are completed. In general, they exist as isolated defects and are rarely associated with deformity of the trachea and esophagus. Although invariably present at birth, some may be thought of as acquired in utero rather than true embryologic deformities.

In this chapter the following abnormalities will be described:

1. Congenital (infantile) lobar emphysema
2. Cystic adenomatoid malformation of the lung
3. Bronchial atresia
4. Pulmonary arteriovenous malformation
5. Pulmonary lymphangiectasia
6. Secondary pulmonary hypoplasia
   a. Oligohydramnios
   b. Inadequate thoracic space (diaphragmatic hernia, eventration and phrenic paralysis)
7. Esophageal duplication
8. Neurenteric (gastroenteric) cyst

Congenital (Infantile) Lobar Emphysema

Congenital, or infantile, lobar emphysema (CLE) is a recognizable pathologic abnormality with unusual patterns of clinical and radiographic expression. The origin of this lesion is not completely understood, and it is possible that several different varieties exist. In approximately half the cases, no anatomic abnormality is found other than an emphysematous lobe. Reduced size and number of bronchial cartilage plates are thought to be responsible in some cases.[1] Bronchial constriction by anomalous vessels or adjacent masses or cysts is implicated in others. Redundant mucosal folds and bronchomalacia are additional possible causes.

Studies have emphasized the importance of lung fluid in the development of the normal fetal lung.[2] It is known that retention of fetal lung fluid in a portion of lung leads to hyperplasia of the involved segment A similar mechanism may be instrumental in the development of CLE. On the contrary, rapid loss of fluid from the lung in utero causes hypoplasia.

Clinical Presentation

Early onset of respiratory distress is the rule in cases of CLE, where 81 percent of patients have symptoms within the first 6 months of life; however, discovery as late as 8 years of age has been reported.[3] The association of cardiac abnormalities, particularly ventricular septal defect (VSD) and patent ductus arteriosus (PDA), has been reported in 10 to 30 percent of patients with CLE (Figure 3-1). The clinical manifestations of the cardiac defects may overshadow the pulmonary symptoms, and in most of these cases the overexpanded lung may be secondary to abnormal pulmonary vascularity rather than to bronchial obstruction. Other abnormalities affecting the ribs, chest, kidneys, and limbs have been reported in association with CLE. Males are affected almost 2 to 1 over females; the disease has been reported in a mother and daughter.[4]

On occasion, the abnormality is recognized as an incidental finding on chest films taken for other reasons (Figures 3-2 and 3-3). While prompt surgical removal is the usual treatment, long-term nonoperative management is occasionally acceptable.[5]

Radiologic Findings

The radiographic appearance of CLE depends upon the patient's age, location within the lung, degree of overdistension, and fluid content of the diseased lobe or lobes. Overaeration of a lobe or multiple lobes usually causes compression of the adjacent lung, localized spreading of the ribs, and mediastinal shift. In more severe cases the lung herniates across the midline (Figure 3-4A). The emphysematous lung often assumes a hyperlucent appearance because of the displacement of pulmonary vascular markings over a larger area. This hyperlucency is further accentuated by vascular constriction brought on by regional pulmonary hypoxia.

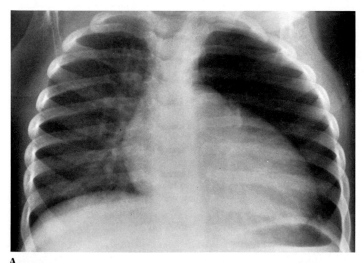

A

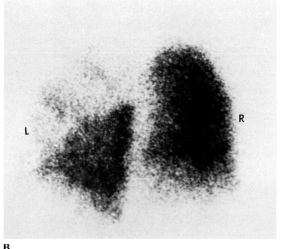

B

Figure 3-1 Lobar emphysema with ventricular septal defect. A. The left upper lobe is overexpanded and hyperlucent, and increased blood flows to the remaining lung. Minimal contralateral mediastinal shift, compression of lower lobe vessels, and cardiomegaly are also evident. **B.** Technetium-99m MAA lung scan shows decreased perfusion to the left upper lobe. *Note:* Lobar emphysema in the presence of left to right intracardiac shunt is not uncommon, generally is well tolerated, and probably differs in its pathophysiology from the congenital variety.

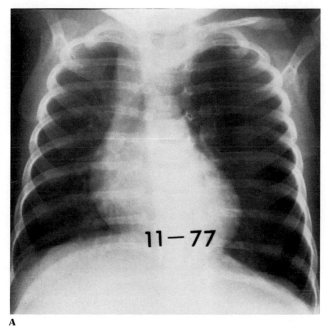

A

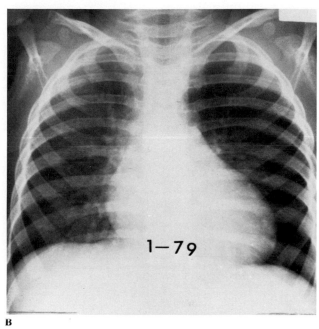

B

Figure 3-2 Lobar emphysema (long-term follow-up). A. An overaerated left upper lung was discovered incidentally in this asymptomatic child. Mediastinal displacement, herniation of the lung across the midline, and compression of the lower lobe vessels are apparent. **B.** Fourteen months later, mild hyperaeration persists in the left upper lobe, but the mediastinal shift and herniated lung are no longer evident.

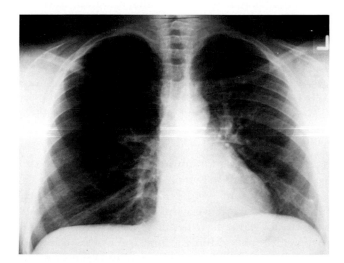

Figure 3-3 Adult lobar emphysema. Congenital, mild, asymptomatic right upper lobe emphysema is identified by subtle signs, e.g., depressed right hilum; slightly bowed, midline trachea; and hyperlucent right upper lung field.

In rare cases, the overdistended lobe is fluid-filled and appears radiopaque on initial films taken shortly after birth (Figure 3-4A).[6-9] However, lobar enlargement and compression of adjacent structures should suggest the diagnosis. Sequential film studies usually disclose an overdistended, hyperlucent lobe as the fluid clears (Figure 3-4B).

Pathologic Findings

Single lobe involvement is most common; approximately 50 percent occur in the left upper lobe (Figure 3-1), 24 percent in the right middle lobe (Figure 3-5), and 18 percent in the right upper lobe (Figure 3-3). Lower lobe and multiple lobe involvement is less frequent.[3] The affected lobe is overinflated and fails to deflate after excision (Figure 3-5B). Histologically, the alveoli are overdistended with minimal, if any, interstitial involvement (Figure 3-5C and D).

Hislop and Reid[10] reported on three patients with clinical and radiographic features of lobar emphy-

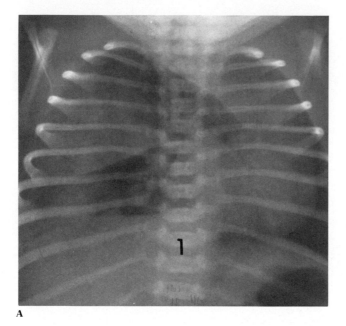

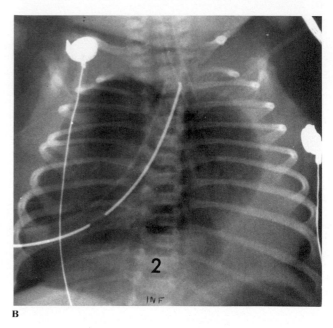

A   B

Figure 3-4   Congenital lobar emphysema (fluid-filled). A. Films taken on the first day of life show a partially fluid-filled overdistended lobe herniating across the midline. A right thoracotomy disclosed a boggy, edematous lobe, which was not resected. **B.** On the second day, the right upper lobe is air-filled and has the classical appearance of congenital lobar emphysema. Surgical removal of an emphysematous right upper lobe was performed. (Courtesy of Dr. Frederick N. Silverman, Stanford, California.)

sema, but with a different histological appearance. In contrast to the overdistended, emphysematous alveoli of CLE, their patients had normal-sized alveoli that were present in increased numbers. They referred to this as gigantism of the alveolar region and suggested the term *polyalveolar lobe with emphysema.* The bronchial tree in the involved segments was normal.

Congenital Cystic Adenomatoid Malformation of the Lung

Congenital cystic adenomatoid malformation (CCAM) of the lung was first recognized as a distinct abnormality by Chin and Tang.[11] It is an uncommon lesion, but prompt recognition is important since most cases have an excellent prognosis following surgical removal.[12]

Congenital cystic adenomatoid malformation is caused by abnormal overgrowth of distal bronchial

and pulmonary tissue. Communication with the tracheobronchial tree is usually retained, and the vascular supply and venous drainage are normal with few exceptions. These lesions occur with equal frequency in either right or left lung, but they have a slight predilection for the upper lobes. Lobar involvement is most often seen, but multiple lobes may be affected.

Clinical Presentation

The clinical presentation in CCAM of the lung depends largely upon which of the three pathologic types are present (Figure 3-6).[13] Type I lesions are most common and carry the best prognosis. The vast majority of patients with this type develop respiratory symptoms within the first 6 months of life; 90 percent develop symptoms by 1 year. Other congenital abnormalities often occur, especially in association with Stocker et al. type II abnormalities.[13] Of their 33 patients with CCAM, 10 had additional mal-

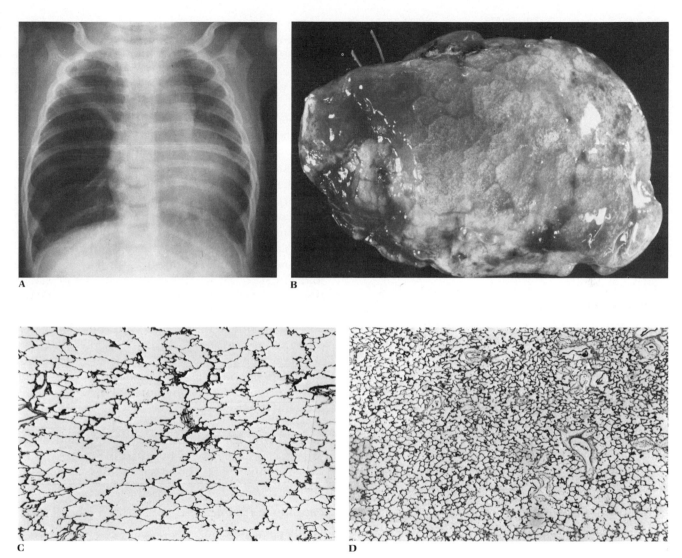

Figure 3-5 Congenital lobar emphysema (right middle lobe). A. The right middle lobe is overexpanded and hyperlucent. Adjacent parenchyma and pulmonary vessels are compressed and splayed about the emphysematous lung. Minimal contralateral mediastinal shift and mild cardiomegaly are present. The right middle lobe was removed. **B.** The specimen was perfused at 30-cm water pressure through the resected bronchus to avoid overdistension. Individual segments of distended superficial emphysematous foci are evident. **C.** Histologic section shows enormous alveolar spaces. **D.** Comparison normal at the same magnification.

formations, and 9 of these occurred in type II lesions. The most commonly associated anomalies are renal (cystic disease, agenesis, dysgenesis), intestinal (atresias), cardiac, and osseous. Type III abnormalities are extremely rare and carry a poor prognosis.

Occasionally, patients with CCAM are discovered in later life, usually as a result of chronic or recurrent pulmonary infection.[14] The sex incidence is equal. Maternal hydramnios occurs in some patients, and infants may be stillborn or hydropic at birth.

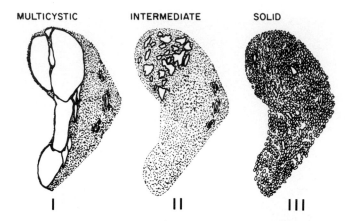

MULTICYSTIC   INTERMEDIATE   SOLID

I   II   III

Figure 3-6   Diagrammatic representation of three major types of cystic adenomatoid malformations. Type I is most common. (From Stocker et al.,[13] with permission.)

Radiologic Findings

The major radiologic feature in CCAM is an expanded lobe or lung. The criteria for pulmonary expansion are similar to those seen with congenital lobar emphysema, i.e., shift of the mediastinum, herniation of the lung across the midline, compression of the adjacent lung, and spreading of the ribs (Figures 3-7A and B and 3-8).[15]

In the most common type I lesion, cystic spaces are visible within the involved lobe. These appear as round lucencies, bordered by the circular configuration of vessels, bronchi, and atelectatic adjacent lung (Figure 3-7B and C). Occasionally, one large dominant cyst is surrounded by smaller cysts and inhomogeneous lung. Solid densities and air-fluid levels within the cysts are less common observations. The radiographic pattern of CCAM does not always conform to the anatomic specimen (Figure 3-7D).

Patients with type II lesions rarely survive long enough to be radiographed. The few that have been studied have shown a nonhomogeneous mass that is consistent with the gross anatomic specimen which consists of numerous, evenly spaced cysts, usually less than 1 cm in diameter. CCAM presenting with a spontaneous pneumothorax is a rare, but recognized, complication.[16] Type III lesions usually appear completely solid (Figure 3-9).

The precise configuration and anatomic extent of lobar involvement may be difficult to ascertain from plain films. Bronchography and arteriography have been reliable tools in the past, but are of less value with the development of ultrasound, computed tomography, nuclear magnetic resonance, and perfusion-ventilation lung scans. Foreign bodies, intraluminal tumors, or extrinsic bronchial constriction may produce radiographic findings similar to CCAM. In these situations, bronchoscopic evaluation before definitive surgery is of value.

Ultrasonography has been shown to be of value in the prenatal diagnosis of CCAM.[17–19] The features that suggest the presence of CCAM include hydramnios, placental edema, fetal hydrops, and a cystic intrathoracic mass. Postnatal ultrasound may be of use in delineating the internal cystic structure of lesions that present radiographically as solid masses (Figure 3-10).[20]

Diaphragmatic hernia and congenital lobar emphysema are the most common lesions that may simulate type I CCAM radiographically. Absence or decreased subphrenic bowel should provide a clue to the presence of diaphragmatic hernia. However, congenital lobar emphysema may be more difficult to distinguish. Since the differentiation between these two is often impossible and the surgical approach essentially the same, pursuing costly and invasive identifying procedures is of little value.

Pathologic Findings

Type I CCAM, the most common form, is composed of variable-sized cysts lined by cuboidal to low columnar epithelium (Figure 3-8C). One or more dominant cysts may prevail, surrounded by alveoli, bronchi, and occasional bronchioles. The intermediate, or type II, lesions have many thin-walled small cysts with ciliated, cuboidal, epithelial lining that are separated by clusters of tubular structures resembling respiratory bronchioles. The solid form, or type III lesion, may not appear cystic to the naked eye; microscopically it is similar to early fetal lung. Multiple small, cuboidal lined cysts are present and range in size from that of a normal alveolus to slightly larger than normal terminal bronchioles.

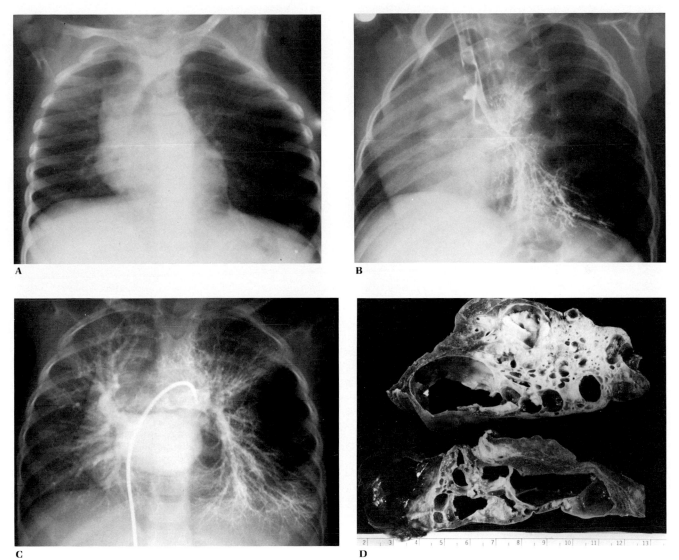

Figure 3-7   Adenomatoid malformation (late onset—type 1). This previously well 2-year-old girl presented with a 2-month history of cough. **A.** The left lung is hyperaerated, herniated across the midline, and devoid of vasculature in its midportion. **B.** The bronchogram shows compressed and displaced lower and upper lobe bronchi which are draped about the hyperlucent midlung. **C.** The pulmonary angiogram in the frontal projection shows similar findings. *Note:* The central lower lobe vessels are curved around cystic lung structures. **D.** The left lower lobe contains one dominant cyst and several smaller cysts, within a honeycomb-textured specimen. (Compare with Figure 3-6, type I.)

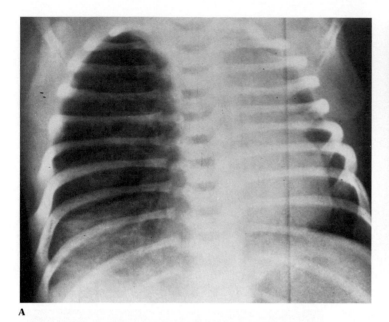

A

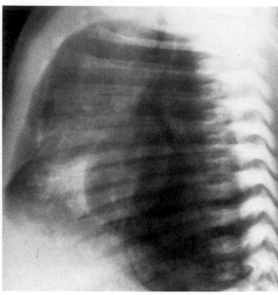

B

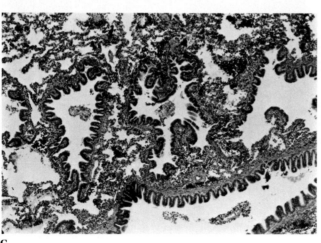

C

Figure 3-8   Cystic adenomatoid malformation (early onset and recurrent—type I). This 3020-g boy presented with increasing dyspnea at 5 days of age. **A.** The right upper lung is markedly overexpanded but contains areas of patchy radiopacity. **B.** The lateral view confirms the overaeration but does not help localize the abnormality. At surgery, the emphysematous right lower lobe was removed. Symptoms recurred after 6 weeks and a repeat radiograph showed recurrent emphysema. The right middle and upper lobes were resected and the child has done well since. **C.** The histologic section shows cystic dilated spaces lined by bronchiolar epithelium underlaid by thin fibrous or smooth muscular layers. Patches of alveoli may connect directly to such segments or be interspaced within large fields of proliferated bronchiolar structures.

Kwittken and Reines[21] have summarized the pathologic features of CCAM of the lung as follows:

1. An adenomatoid increase of terminal respiratory structures as manifested by cysts of various sizes communicating with each other and variably lined with either a pseudostratified or ciliated columnar (bronchial-type) epithelium
2. Polypoid configuration of the mucosa and in-

creased amounts of elastic tissue in the walls of the cystic portions lined with bronchial-type epithelium
3. An absence of cartilage plates in the cystic parenchyma, except as constituents of nondeformed bronchial structures trapped within the diseased lung
4. Occasional groups of alveoli lined with mucogenic cells
5. Absence of inflammation

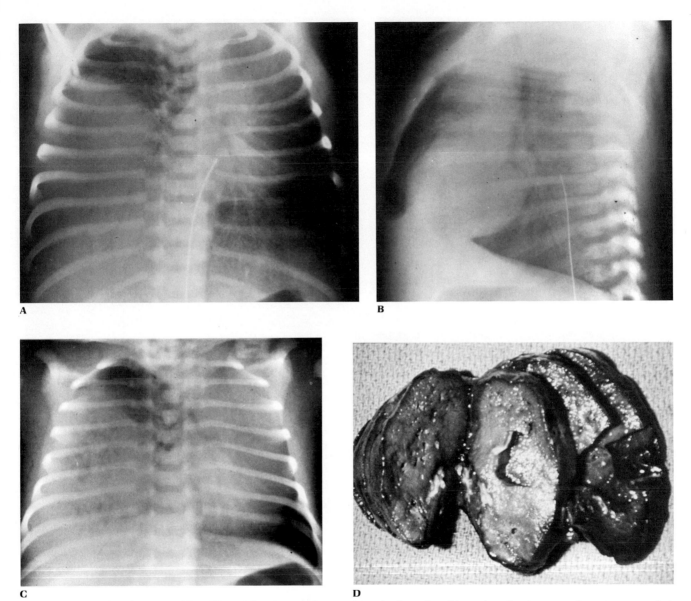

Figure 3-9 Cystic adenomatoid malformation (type III). A and **B.** The frontal and lateral projections reveal an overexpanded, opaque right lower lobe. **C.** Later film shows enlargement and minimal aeration of the affected lobe. **D.** The pathologic specimen is a solid (type III) adenomatoid malformation. (Courtesy of Dr. Bernard Blumenthal, Jackson, Mississippi.)

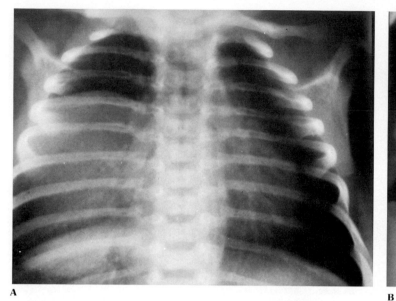

A

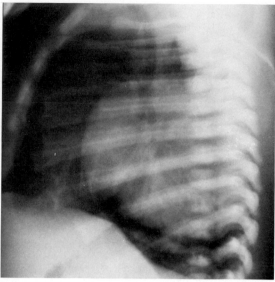

B

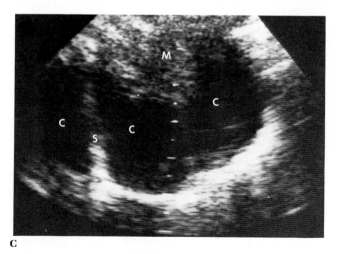

C

Figure 3-10 Cystic adenomatoid malformation—ultraso-nography. A and **B.** Frontal and lateral chest films show a large water-density mass lesion in the right, posterior hemithorax adjacent to the chest wall. **C.** Transverse thoracic sonograms obtained through the right posterior chest wall (chest wall is at top). The malformation consists of fluid-filled cystic spaces (C), internal septation (S), and solid tissue components (M). (From Hartenberg MA, Brewer WH: Cystic adenomatoid malformation of the lung: Identification by sonography. *AJR* 140:693, 1983. © by American Roentgen Ray Society, 1983. With permission.)

Bronchial Atresia

Bronchial atresia is an uncommon congenital abnormality, usually limited to a single bronchus. Normal bronchial development beyond the point of atresia suggests that the lesion is acquired in utero, after the fifteenth week of gestation when the tracheobronchial tree is fully developed. A traumatic intrauterine event, resulting in compromised vascular supply to the bronchus, is one etiologic theory advanced.[22] The

lesion may occur anywhere in the lung, but prefers the upper lobes.[23]

Clinical symptoms are nonspecific. Signs of recurrent infection and wheezing may bring the condition to attention.

Radiographic examination will often reveal (1) an overaerated lung distal to the atresia, (2) a round or linear-ovoid opacity just beyond the atretic bronchus, and (3) an amputated bronchus to this portion of lung on bronchography (Figure 3-11A).

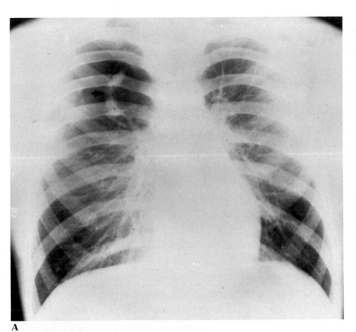

A

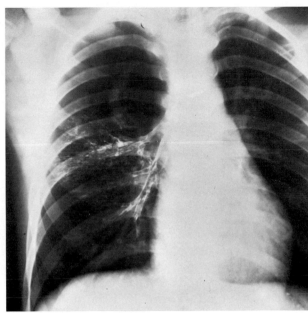

B

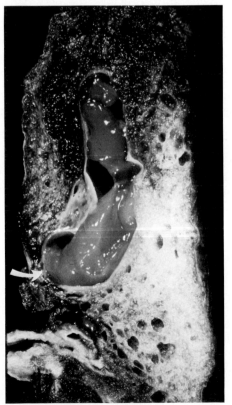

C

Figure 3-11   Bronchial atresia. This asymptomatic 14-year-old boy was followed from age 4 because of an opacity in the right upper lobe. **A.** A curvilinear radiopacity (arrow) is present within a relatively lucent right upper lobe. **B.** Bronchography fails to fill any upper lobe segments. The radiopacity is oriented in a manner similar to a normal right-upper lobe bronchus. **C.** The pathologic specimen shows the mucoid impaction distal to the atretic bronchus (arrow). (Courtesy of Dr. James Scatliff, Chapel Hill, North Carolina.)

On gross examination, the bronchial lumen is obliterated and plugged with mucus (Figure 3-11C).[23] The lung beyond is usually air-filled as a result of communication via the pores of Kohn. In some circumstances, the peripheral lung may be overaerated. An etiologic relationship between this lesion and congenital lobar emphysema may exist.

Surgical resection of these lesions is usually curative.

Pulmonary Arteriovenous Malformation

Pulmonary arteriovenous malformation (AVM) is a congenital vascular communication between the pulmonary artery (or arteries) and vein (or veins) without an intervening capillary bed. Unoxygenated blood is delivered directly from the pulmonary to the systemic circulation without passing through the alveolar capillaries. Between 25 and 50 percent of patients with this condition are symptomatic, depending upon the amount of shunted blood. Although many cases are discovered in adult life, symptoms can be traced to childhood in more than half.[24] Rare cases of pulmonary AVM are reported in neonates.[25,26] A higher probability of cyanosis and congestive heart failure is expected in neonates because of the relatively high pulmonary vascular resistance at this age.

Pulmonary AVM may exist in several different forms: (1) as a solitary lesion, (2) as multiple, discrete lesions with one dominant lesion, (3) as multiple and discrete fistulas of approximately equal size, and (4) as diffuse "telangiectatic" lesions.[27] More than half are solitary, most occur in the lower lobes, and there is no side preference. Approximately one-half of patients have an associated familial syndrome of telangiectasias and hemangiomas of the skin and mucous membranes (Osler-Weber-Rendu disease), an autosomal-dominant disease with high penetrance. Osler-Weber-Rendu disease, as well as the AVM with multiple, discrete fistulas and a dominant lesion, is most likely to be discovered in childhood.[27]

Clinical symptoms, more severe with multiple lesions,[28] are caused when 25 percent or more pulmonary blood shunts to the systemic circulation. The symptoms include cyanosis, dyspnea, hemoptysis or epistaxis, and exercise intolerance. Patients exhibit physical signs of digital clubbing, rubor, hemorrhagic conjunctiva, and systolic or continuous murmurs over the area of involved lung. Polycythemia is an additional regular feature. Cerebrovascular accidents may result from periods of ischemia, from bouts of anoxia, or from emboli that gain entrance to the systemic circulation through the fistula. Infected emboli, suppuration, and spontaneous rupture are additional disadvantages.[29]

The diagnosis, when suspected clinically, may be confirmed with the roentgen ray. Plain chest studies often show single or multiple discrete, unchanging opacities with linear, vascular shadows in proximity (Figure 3-12A). Tomograms may better define the linear vascular shadows entering or leaving the lesion. Cardiomegaly and pulmonary artery dilation reflect the increased blood volume traversing the heart.

Pulmonary angiography provides the best definition of the anatomy (Figure 3-12B). Computed tomography with contrast enhancement is a less invasive, but reliable, way to differentiate between vascular malformations and other pulmonary masses.[30]

Most pulmonary AVMs are subpleural in location and are accessible to local resection. Staged, bilateral thoracotomies have been employed to remove as many as 23 fistulas.[31] Small, asymptomatic fistulas, in the absence of hereditary telangiectasia, should not be removed.[32] Embolotherapy with detachable balloons is an alternative method of treatment.[33]

Acquired pulmonary arteriovenous fistulas, sufficiently extensive to produce clinical clubbing, may occur with acute and chronic liver disease.[34–36] They may remain and cause persistent symptoms after resolution of the liver dysfunction. Multiple pulmonary artery aneurysms and peripheral venous thrombosis (Hughes-Stovin syndrome) constitute an additional rare abnormality of the pulmonary vasculature that may be confused with multiple AVMs (Figure 3-13).[37] Pulmonary varix is yet another vascular abnormality akin to AVMs and aneurysms. It may simulate a mass lesion on chest film (Figure 3-14).

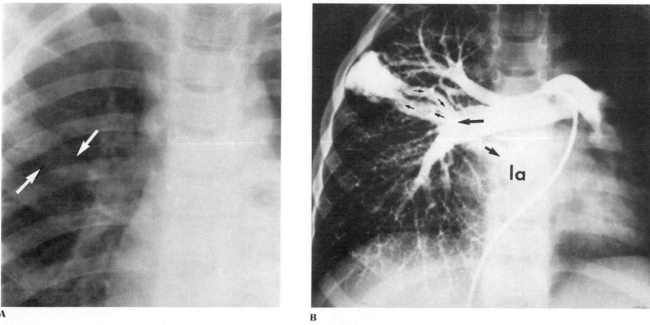

A   B

Figure 3-12   Pulmonary arteriovenous malformation. A. Poorly defined radiopacity in the right upper lobe is connected to the hilum by structures that appear vascular (arrows). **B.** The arterial phase of the pulmonary arteriogram shows the malformation being supplied by a branch of the main pulmonary artery, with early venous drainage into the left atrium (la).

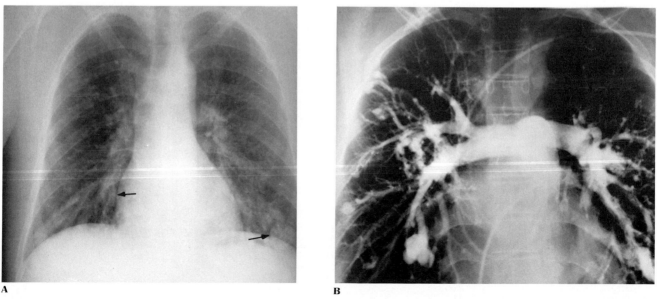

A   B

Figure 3-13   Multiple pulmonary artery aneurysms and peripheral venous thromboses (Hughes-Stovin syndrome). A. Several irregularly shaped, rounded shadows (arrows) are scattered throughout the lungs. They appear in relation to pulmonary vessels. **B.** The pulmonary angiogram confirms the presence of multiple, focal, aneurysmic dilatations of pulmonary artery branches. (From Roberts et al.,[37] with permission.)

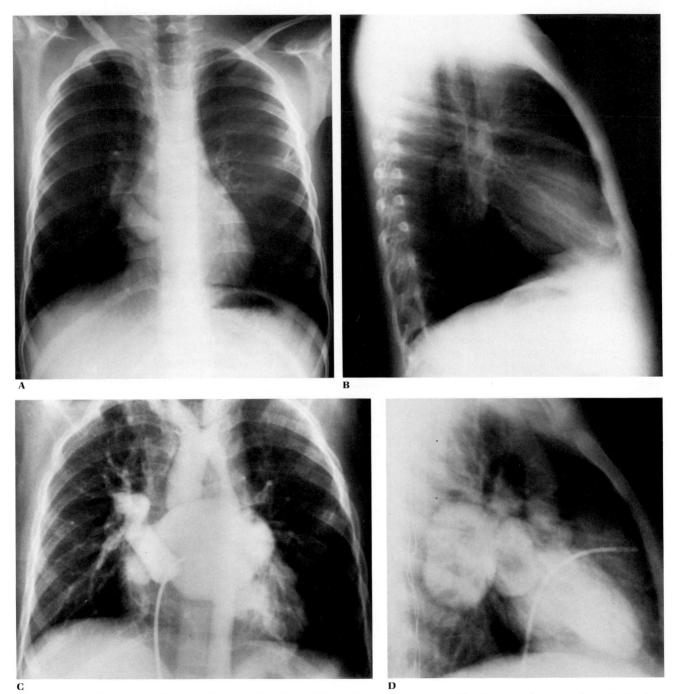

A

B

C

D

Figure 3-14   Pulmonary varix. A and **B.** Frontal and lateral films disclose the presence of a circuitous, "sausage-shaped" structure in the right hilar region that has the appearance of a blood vessel. **C** and **D.** The levophase of the right ventricular injection confirms the vascular nature of this structure, which represents a varicose right pulmonary vein. (From Chilton,[37a] with permission.)

Pulmonary Lymphangiectasia

Congenital pulmonary lymphangiectasia is thought to result from abnormal lung development that probably occurs between the fourteenth and twentieth week of gestation. During this phase of intrauterine life, the pulmonary lymphatics are quite large and situated in the subpleural and interlobular connective tissue. In the normal course of events, the fetal lung lobulations become less prominent, the connective tissue diminishes in amount, and the lymphatics become much narrower. Congenital pulmonary lymphangiectasia results when the interlobular connective tissue fails to involute as lung growth continues. Therefore, the lymphatics retain their enlarged 12- to 16-week gestational proportions within otherwise normal lung parenchyma.[38]

Approximately one-third of the reported cases of pulmonary lymphangiectasia occur in association with, or secondary to, congenital cardiac defects that cause pulmonary venous obstruction (Figure 3-15).[33,38] In others, the pulmonary lymphatic abnormality is apparently present at birth. Most infants with this form of lymphangiectasia will die within the first 24 h of life.[38–40] Markedly dilated intralobular and subpleural lymphatics have been reported in another group of children, who expired with severe lung disease in later infancy.[40] In these children, an underlying abnormality of lymphatic drainage may be a predisposing factor in the development of pulmonary disease. The possibility that the pulmonary lymphangiectasia was acquired postnatally as a result of infection, obstruction, or other unknown factors has been suggested.[40]

Confusion has developed over the proper identification of dilated lymphatics in patients with lung disease and extraalveolar air found at autopsy. Beverly Wood and her associates have shown dilated, air-filled lymphatics in newborns treated with assisted ventilation and elevated end expiratory pressure.[41] Pulmonary interstitial emphysema was present on the radiographs of their patients. Figure 6-1 in Chapter 6 illustrates a patient with findings quite similar to those described by Wood. Older children and adults may develop interstitial air, localized mainly within dilated lymphatics, which might be confused at autopsy with congenital lymphangiectasia. With the life-support systems presently in use, the correct histopathologic definition of congenital lung abnormalities may be impossible in patients who survive days or weeks with ventilatory assistance and drug therapy.

Secondary Pulmonary Hypoplasia

Pulmonary hypoplasia may be considered as (1) primary—a result of abnormal embryogenesis—or (2) secondary—from either (a) an inadequate supply of amniotic or fetal lung fluid (oligohydramnios) or (b) an insufficient thoracic space for lung growth. The primary hypoplastic lung syndromes are covered in Chapter 2; the secondary causes are discussed below.

Oligohydramnios

Whereas all preacinar airways are formed by the sixteenth week of intrauterine life, pulmonary alveoli continue to develop until birth and multiply further until the eighth year of life. Decreased amount of fetal lung or amniotic fluid, as occurs with amniotic leak or dysplastic kidneys, contributes to pulmonary hypoplasia. Thoracic compression, from oligohydramnios, will also constrict the thoracic space and further compromise lung growth.[41,42] After birth, infants with hypoplastic lungs aerate poorly, and attempts to ventilate them mechanically often cause extravasation of air, pneumomediastinum, pneumothorax, and interstitial emphysema (Figure 3-16).

The presence of renal disease should always be suspected when difficult pulmonary ventilation is encountered in the absence of underlying lung abnormality. Renal dysplasia or urinary tract obstruction and secondary oligohydramnios are often evident by prenatal ultrasound (Figure 3-16B and C).

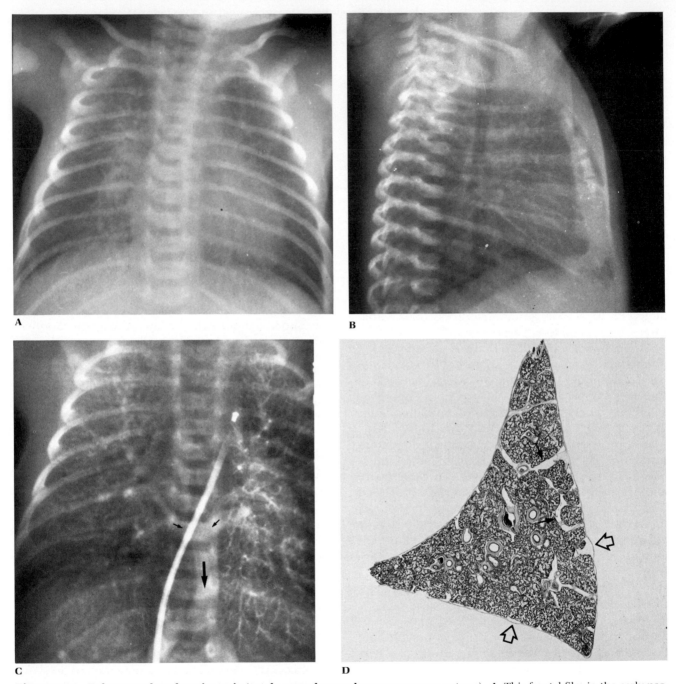

A

B

C

D

Figure 3-15 Pulmonary lymphangiectasia (total anomalous pulmonary venous return). A. This frontal film in the early neonatal period shows mild cardiomegaly and diffuse interstitial densities that obscure the normal intrapulmonary vasculature. **B.** The lateral view illustrates the generalized, random, fine, linear markings produced by swollen intralobular lymphatics. The major fissure also is thickened. **C.** The delayed phase of the pulmonary artery injection shows the venous return to the common pulmonary vein and portal vein (see Figure 4-11C). **D.** The whole lung mount shows moderate dilatation of the septal (solid arrows) and subpleural (open arrows) lymphatics. These dilated lymphatics closely resemble the pattern of pulmonary interstitial emphysema (Figures 6-1A and 6-2) but with lymphangiectasia, there is less disruption of the interstitial tissue. (From Felman AH, Rhatigan R, Pierson KK: Pulmonary lymphangiectasia. Observations in 17 patients and proposed classification. *AJR* 116:548, 1972. © 1972 American Roentgen Ray Society. With permission.)

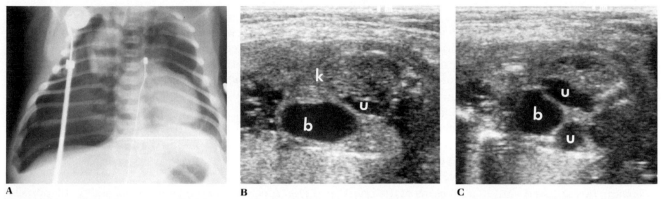

Figure 3-16 Hypoplastic lungs (oligohydramnios-posterior urethral valves). A. Pneumomediastinum and bilateral pneumo-thoraxes complicate the life of this newborn. Resuscitative efforts failed, and the child expired within 24 h of birth. **B.** Prenatal sonography at 21 weeks of gestation indicates the presence of a dilated bladder (b), dilated ureter (u), and well-formed kidney (k). No amniotic fluid is seen. **C.** Sonogram from a different view shows bladder (b) and dilated ureters (u). Posterior urethral valves were present. (Sonography is courtesy of Dr. Ernest Ferrell, Jacksonville, Florida.)

Inadequate Thoracic Space

Congenital diaphragmatic hernia is often accompanied by significant pulmonary hypoplasia of the ipsilateral, and sometimes contralateral, lung (Figure 3-17). The severity of pulmonary hypoplasia depends, in large measure, upon the size and timing of the herniation. Herniations that occur before completion of development of the tracheobronchial tree will compromise the lungs much more severely than those that occur later, after this development is complete. Later-developing hernias may compromise the pulmonary alveolar maturation. However, the potential for continued alveolar growth after birth and well

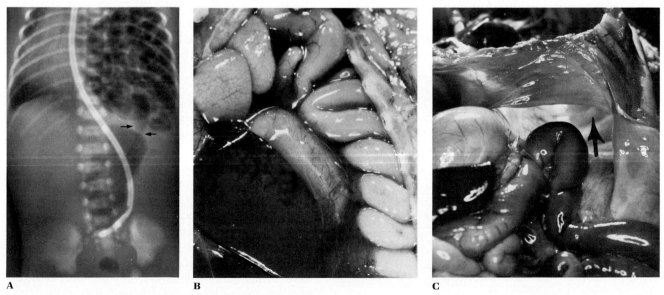

Figure 3-17 Hypoplastic lungs (congenital diaphragmatic hernia). A. The mediastinum is displaced to the right by bowel which is herniated through the left hemidiaphragm (arrows). *Note:* There is an absence of a gas-filled bowel in the abdomen. **B.** Autopsy photograph of another patient showing bowel herniated into the chest. **C.** Diaphragmatic defect after bowel has been withdrawn (arrow).

into childhood is responsible for a better prognosis in these cases.

Diaphragmatic eventration is usually quite evident on plain films. Almost always anterior, the eventration contour usually blends into the diaphragmatic silhouette. When a significant portion of liver is contained within the eventration, the lower hepatic edge is higher than normal. Ultrasound and hepatic scintigraphy are reliable confirming studies.[43] (See Chapter 12, Figures 12-18C and 12-19C.)

Diaphragmatic hernia and eventration may, on occasion, be confused with mass lesions of the chest or mediastinum. When the diagnosis of diaphragmatic hernia is in doubt, a carefully controlled contrast esophogram will confirm the condition.

In spite of early and adequate surgical repair of diaphragmatic hernia, approximately one-half of all children with respiratory distress in the first 12 hours of life will die. Postoperative pulmonary hypertension, after a brief "honeymoon" period, contributes to sudden deterioration of arterial blood gases, which, despite intense pharmacologic treatment, is usually fatal.[44,45]

In an attempt to predict the prognosis for patients with diaphragmatic hernia, Touloukian and Markowitz[46] developed certain risk factors for radiographic variables. They published a grading system

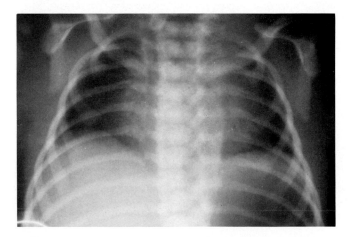

Figure 3-18 Hypoplastic lungs (diaphragmatic denervation). This chest film demonstrates small thoracic volume and diaphragmatic elevation. (From Goldstein and Reid,[48] with permission.)

to help identify high-risk patients likely to need intensive pharmacologic therapy and possible extracorporeal membrane oxygenation.[47]

Abnormal phrenic innervation will also contribute to pulmonary hypoplasia (Figure 3-18).[48]

Esophageal Duplication

The precise embryogenic abnormality responsible for esophageal duplication remains controversial. Some experts consider esophageal duplication and neurenteric cyst to be variations of the same embryogenic aberration (split notochord syndrome).[49] Others hold that bronchogenic cysts, esophageal duplications, and esophageal cysts are close embryologic relatives of pulmonary sequestration.[50,51] Still others trace the origin of esophageal duplications to remnants of the dorsal neurenteric canal.[52] Communication between these lesions and the gastrointestinal tract is rare. However, in some cases the presence of a connection supports the theory of gastroenteric duplication.[53,54]

Approximately 10 to 15 percent of all gastroenteric duplications are located in the thorax adjacent to the esophagus.[55] More than one-half of these malformations are discovered by 1 year of age. Presenting symptoms usually are related to respiratory distress and less often to difficult swallowing. Chronic cough may be caused by esophageal duplication as well as by other lesions located in proximity to the respiratory tract. Stimulation of neural pathways involved in the cough reflex probably explains this symptom rather than direct irritation or mechanical impingement of the cyst on the airway.[56] Patients with duplications occasionally show evidence of infection, abscess, draining sinus, and recurrent pneumonia, but many are asymptomatic at the time of discovery. Older children with these anomalies often have symptoms of anemia, melena, hematemesis, and substernal and epigastric pain.[53]

The radiographic manifestations of esophageal duplications may be obscured when the lesions are buried within the normal soft tissue of the mediastinum. When visible, they usually have a perfectly smooth outline in contrast to neurogenic tumors, which tend to be irregular. Deviation of or impingement upon adjacent structures such as the trachea and esophagus occurs in some cases. Barium esophogram is usually helpful in the delineation of these lesions. Vertebral abnormalities are present in some patients.

Differentiation from other mass lesions, particularly lymphadenopathy and bronchogenic cysts, is not always possible with conventional film studies. Enteric cysts tend to be larger and posterior in relation to bronchogenic cysts.[51] Computed tomography will identify the lesion but cannot always distinguish between bronchogenic cyst and enteric duplication unless oral contrast enters the enteric cyst.

Duplications, or enteric cysts, often attain large sizes, up to 10 cm or more. The contents may be clear, watery, mucoid, or hemorrhagic; the walls are composed of smooth muscle with or without chronic inflammation. The cysts are lined by primitive esophageal, gastric, or intestinal mucosa. Mucous-secreting columnar epithelium with gastric glands and parietal cells are identifying features of these lesions. Cysts that contain cartilage are thought of as bronchogenic in origin, and those with no distinguishing features are most likely respira-

tory.[51] Connections to structures below the diaphragm should be suspected, especially when the mass presents in the right chest.

Neurenteric (Gastroenteric) Cyst

Neurenteric cysts are also known as gastroenteric cysts, dorsal enteric remnants, enteric duplications with vertebral anomaly, and possibly other names. Much of the confusion in terminology derives from controversy over the exact origin of these lesions. Bentley and Smith[49] used the term *split notochord syndrome* to describe the relation of these anomalies to abnormal notochord development. Another explanation is that endodermal structures fail to separate normally from the notochord and cause diverticula or cysts and vertebral malformations to occur simultaneously.[57]

The most widely accepted embryologic explanation of neurenteric cyst anomaly relates to a failure of normal development and involution of the neurenteric canal of Kovalevsky (Figure 3-19A).[58] In early fetal development this canal appears transiently as a structure in association with the notochord. The

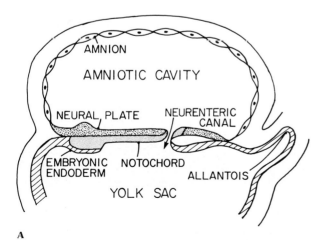

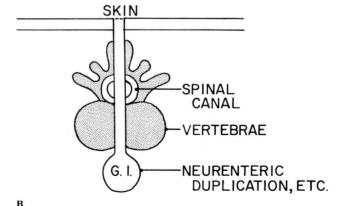

A   B

Figure 3-19   Neurenteric malformations. A. Diagrammatic representation of the neurenteric canal (Kovalevsky) embryogenesis at 14 to 15 days of gestation. **B.** Relationship of the neurenteric canal to the developing spine and gastrointestinal tract. Abnormal involution of this canal is the most likely explanation for neurenteric cyst.

canal passes between the primitive intestinal tract (yolk sac) and the amniotic cavity. The normal, primary, neurenteric canal usually resides at the tip of the coccyx. Accessory canals may develop cranially along the spine, and neurenteric cysts, with associated anomalies of the vertebrae, may result from incomplete involution of these accessory canals. Abnormal connections between the dorsal skin, spinal canal, cystic enteric structures, and vertebral deformities are the end result of this embryologic aberration. In almost all cases, a fibrous stalk joins the mass to the spine (Figure 3-19B).

The complex of vertebral malformations in association with a soft tissue mass in the posterior mediastinum is virtually pathognomonic of this abnormality (Figure 3-20). The vertebral deformities are usually found in a more cranial location to the mass and consist of widened spinal canal, anterior and/or posterior defects, and assorted malsegmentation deformities.

The soft tissue masses usually occupy the posterior mediastinum in close proximity to the spine.

They may be large enough to extend into the middle and anterior chest. Diaphragmatic hernias may accompany this condition. Superina and coworkers[59] have emphasized the association of spinal cysts with vertebral abnormalities. They found a spinal component accompanying mediastinal cysts in as many as 20 percent of the patients in their study. Neurologic symptoms deriving from vertebral abnormalities usually do not appear until several years after the discovery of the mediastinal mass. The authors suggest that myelography and computed tomography be used to determine the presence of spinal anomalies. Others have also advocated the use of computed tomography in these cases.[60]

Neurenteric cysts may grow to immense proportions before they are recognized or produce clinical symptoms. They are lined with enteric mucosa and often contain gastric glands, parietal cells, squamous epithelium, and layers of smooth muscle. Ulceration and chronic inflammation may develop in cysts that contain rennin, pepsin, chlorides, and free hydrochloric acid.

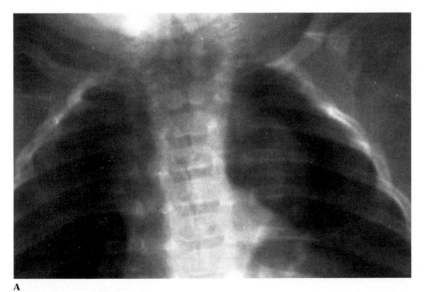

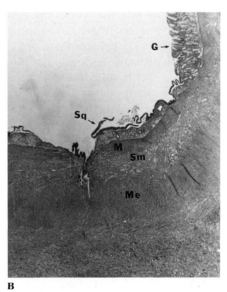

A

B

Figure 3-20   Neurenteric cyst. A. A posterior mass occupies the left paraspinous area. *Note:* There are multiple vertebral abnormalities at the lower cervical, upper thoracic levels. **B.** The mass, 2 cm in diameter, has a thick wall lined by gastric mucosa (G) and metaplastic squamous epithelium (Sq). Beneath lies an abnormally formed muscularis mucosa (M), fibrous submucosa (Sm), and apparently normal muscularis externa (Me). The central cleft connects with the vertebrae.

References

1. Campbell PE: Congenital lobar emphysema. *Aust Paediatr J* 5:226, 1969.
2. Reid L: The lung: Its growth and remodeling in health and disease. *AJR* 129:777, 1977.
3. Stocker JT, Drake RM, Madewell JE: Cystic and congenital lung disease in the newborn. *Perspect Pediatr Pathol* 4:93, 1978.
4. Wall MA, Eisenberg JD, Campbell JR: Congenital lobar emphysema in a mother and daughter. *Pediatrics* 70:131, 1982.
5. Roghair GD: Nonoperative management of lobar emphysema. Long-term follow-up. *Radiology* 102:125, 1972.
6. Eagen CJ, Swischuk LE: The opaque lung in lobar emphysema. *AJR* 114:300, 1972.
7. Allen RP, Taylor, Reiquam CW: Congenital lobar emphysema with dilated septal lymphatics. *Radiology* 86:929, 1966.
8. Franken E Jr, Buehl I: Infantile lobar emphysema: A report of two cases with unusual roentgenographic manifestations. *AJR* 98:354, 1966.
9. Griscom NT, Harris GBC, Wohl MEB, et al: Fluid filled lung due to airway obstruction in newborn. *Pediatrics* 43:383, 1969.
10. Hislop A, Reid L: New pathological findings in emphysema of childhood. I. Polyalveolar lobe with emphysema. *Thorax* 25:682, 1970.
11. Chin KY, Tang MY: Congenital adenomatoid malformation of one lobe of lung with general anasarca. *Arch Pathol* 4P:221, 1949.
12. Nishibayashi SW, Andrassy RJ, Woolley MM: Congenital cystic malformation of the lung: A 30 year experience. *J Pediatr Surg* 16:704, 1981.
13. Stocker JT, Madewell JE, Drake RM: Congenital cystic adenomatoid malformation of the lung. Classification and morphologic spectrum. *Hum Pathol* 8:155, 1977.
14. Wexler HA, Valdes Dapena M: Congenital cystic adenomatoid malformation: A report of three unusual cases. *Radiology* 126:737, 1978.
15. Craig JM, Kirkpatrick J, Neuhauser EBD: Congenital cystic adenomatoid malformation of the lung in infants. *AJR* 76:516, 1956.
16. Gaise G, Sang Oh K: Spontaneous pneumothorax in congenital cystic adenomatoid malformation. *Pediatr Radiol* 13:281, 1983.
17. Stauffer UG, Savoldelli G, Meith D: Antenatal ultrasound diagnosis in congenital cystic adenomatoid malformation—Case report. *J Pediatr Surg* 19:141, 1984.
18. Johnson JA, Rumack CM, Johnson ML, et al: Cystic adenomatoid malformation: Antenatal demonstration. *AJR* 142:483, 1984.
19. Graham D, Winn K, Dex W, et al: Prenatal diagnosis of congenital cystic adenomatoid malformation. *J Ultrasound Med* 1:9, 1982.
20. Hartenberg MA, Brewer WH: Congenital cystic adenomatoid malformation: Identification by sonography. *AJR* 140:693, 1983.
21. Kwittken J, Reines L: Congenital cystic adenomatoid malformation of the lung. *Pediatrics* 30:759, 1962.
22. Waddel JA, Simon G, Reid L: Bronchial atresia of the left upper lobe. *Thorax* 20:214, 1965.
23. Schuster SR, Harris GBC, Williams A, et al: Bronchial atresia: A recognizable entity in the pediatric age group. *J Pediatr Surg* 13:682, 1978.
24. Utzon F, Brandrup F: Pulmonary arteriovenous fistulas in children. A review with special reference to the diffuse telangiectatic type, illustrated by report of a case. *Acta Paediatr Scand* 62:422, 1973.
25. Taylor GA: Pulmonary arteriovenous malformation: An uncommon cause for cyanosis in the newborn. *Pediatr Radiol* 13:339, 1983.
26. Hall RJ, Nelson WP, Blake HA, et al: Massive pulmonary arteriovenous fistula in the newborn. A correctable form of "Cyanotic Heart Disease": An additional cause of cyanosis with left axis deviation. *Circulation* 31:762, 1965.
27. Higgins CB, Wexler L: Clinical and angiographic features of pulmonary arteriovenous fistulas in children. *Radiology* 119:171, 1976.
28. Moyer JH, Glantz G, Brest AN: Pulmonary arteriovenous fistulas: Physiologic and clinical considerations. *Am J Med* 32:417, 1962.
29. Schumacker HB Jr, Waldhausen JA: Pulmonary arteriovenous fistulas in children. *Ann Surg* 158:713, 1963.
30. Godwin JD, Webb WR: Dynamic computed tomography in the evaluation of vascular lung lesions. *Radiology* 138:629, 1981.
31. Brown SE, Wright DW, Renner JW et al: Staged bilateral thoracotomies for multiple pulmonary arteriovenous malformations complicating hereditary hemorrhagic telangiectasia. *J Thorac Cardiovasc Surg* 83:285, 1982.

32. Gomes MR, Bernatz PE, Dines DE: Pulmonary arteriovenous fistulas. *Ann Thorac Surg* 7:582, 1969.

33. Barth KH, White RI, Kaufman SL: Embolotherapy of pulmonary arteriovenous malformations with detachable balloons. *Radiology* 142:599, 1982.

34. Kravath RE, Scarpelli EM, Bernstein J: Hepathogenic cyanosis: Arteriovenous shunts in chronic active hepatitis. *J Pediatr* 78:238, 1971.

35. Silverman A, Cooper MD, Moller JH, et al: Syndrome of cyanosis, digital clubbing, and hepatic disease in siblings. *J Pediatr* 72:70, 1968.

36. Mac Hee W, Buist T, Finlayson NDC: Multiple microscopic pulmonary arteriovenous connections in the lungs presenting as cyanosis. *Thorax* 40:316, 1985.

37. Roberts DH, Jimenez JF, Golladay ES: Multiple pulmonary artery aneurysms and peripheral venous thromboses—The Hughes-Stovin syndrome. *Pediatr Radiol* 12:214, 1982.

37a. Chilton SJ, Campbell JB: Pulmonary varix. *Radiology* 129:400, 1978.

38. Laurence KM: Congenital pulmonary cystic lymphangiectasis. *J Pathol Bacteriol* 70:325, 1970.

39. Rywlin AM, Fojaco, RM: Congenital pulmonary lymphangiectasis associated with blind common pulmonary vein. *Pediatrics* 41:931, 1968.

40. Felman AH, Rhatigan R, Pierson KK: Pulmonary lymphangiectasia. Observations in 17 patients and proposed classification. *AJR* 116:548, 1972.

41. Wood BP, Anderson VM, Maulk JE, et al: Pulmonary lymphatic air: Locating "Pulmonary Interstitial Emphysema" in the premature infant. *AJR* 138:809, 1982.

42. Thibeault DW, Beatty EC Jr, Hall RT, et al: Neonatal pulmonary hypoplasia with premature rupture of fetal membranes and oligohydramnios. *J Pediatr* 107:278, 1985.

43. Moccia WA, Kaude JV, Felman AH: Congenital eventration of the diaphragm. Diagnosis by ultrasound. *Pediatr Radiol* 10:198, 1981.

44. Adzick NS, Harrison MR, Glick PL, et al: Diaphragmatic hernia in the fetus: Prenatal diagnosis and outcome in 94 cases. *J Pediatr Surg* 20:357, 1985.

45. Geggel RL, Murphy JD, Langleben D, et al: Congenital diaphragmatic hernia: Arterial structural changes and persistent pulmonary hypertension after surgical repair. *J Pediatr* 107:457, 1985.

46. Touloukian RJ, Markowitz RI: A preoperative x-ray scoring system for risk assessment of newborns with congenital diaphragmatic hernia. *J Pediatr Surg* 19:252, 1984.

47. German JC, Gazzaniga AB, Amlie R, et al: Management of pulmonary insufficiency in diaphragmatic hernia using extracorporeal circulation with a membrane oxygenator (ECMO). *J Pediatr Surg* 12:705, 1977.

48. Goldstein JD, Reid LM: Pulmonary hypoplasia resulting from phrenic nerve agenesis and diaphragmatic amyoplasia. *J Pediatr* 97:282, 1980.

49. Bentley JFR, Smith JR: Development of posterior enteric remnant and spinal malformations. The split notochord syndrome. *Arch Dis Child* 35:75, 1960.

50. Heithoff KB, Sane SM, Williams HJ, et al: Bronchopulmonary foregut malformations—A unifying etiologic concept. *AJR* 126:46, 1976.

51. Reed JC, Sobonya RE: Morphologic analysis of foregut cysts in the thorax. *AJR* 120:851, 1974.

52. Smith JR: Accessory enteric formations—A classification and nomenclature. *Arch Dis Child* 35:87, 1960.

53. Pokorny WJ, Goldstein IR: Enteric thoracic duplications in children. *J Thorac Cardiovasc Surg*, 87:821, 1984.

54. Shepherd MR: Thoracic, thoracoabdominal and abdominal duplication *Thorax* 20:82, 1965.

55. Grosfeld JL, O'Neill JA, Clatworthy HW: Enteric duplication in infancy and childhood: An 18 year review. *Ann Surg* 172:83, 1970.

56. Bowden DL, Katz PO: Esophageal cyst as a cause of chronic cough. *Chest* 86:150, 1984.

57. Fallon M, Gordon ARG, Lindrum, AC: Mediastinal cysts of foregut origin associated with vertebral anomalies. *Br J Surg* 41:520, 1954.

58. Neuhauser EBD, Harris GBC, Barrett A: Roentgenographic features of neurenteric cysts. *AJR* 79:235, 1958.

59. Superina RA, Ein SH, Humphreys RP: Cystic duplications of the esophagus and neurenteric cysts. *J Pediatr Surg* 19:527, 1984.

60. James HE, Oliff M: Computed tomography in spinal dysraphism. *J Comput Assist Tomogr* 1:391, 1977.

Section II

Neonatal Pulmonary Disorders

The cause for respiratory distress in a newborn is often suggested from initial clinical appearance and examination. Laboratory and blood gas analyses are of inestimable value, but radiographic studies play an important role in the initial diagnostic delineation and future follow-up of these infants. Radiographic studies of the newborn are obtained for the following reasons:

1. To aid in initial clinical diagnosis
2. To define the positions of life-support tubes and catheters
3. To document complications of the disease or treatment methods
4. To evaluate the progress of therapy and evaluate residual changes

Methods and techniques for obtaining and displaying neonatal intensive care radiographs depend largely upon local conditions. By its nature, neonatal critical care demands a multidisciplinary approach involving many different medical and paramedical personnel. The following criteria for radiologic support of neonatal intensive care nurseries are essential:

1. Twenty-four-hour radiologic service should include traditional radiographic studies, as well as all imaging techniques.
2. Film studies should be interpreted by radiologists who are familiar

with the diseases of the newborn and who are able to provide and interpret special imaging procedures.

3. Radiographs should be displayed in an area convenient to radiologists, as well as neonatologists and other consultants.
4. A mechanism for regular communication and consultation between clinicians and radiologists is mandatory for proper diagnosis and management.

The risk of radiation exposure to nursery and ancillary personnel is always of concern. Improved film screen combinations, proper collimation, and other technical factors should be employed to minimize radiation exposure. With proper attention to standard protection devices, there should be no danger.[1] However, improved knowledge of neonatal disease and better understanding of the role of radiography should reduce the number of films needed and thus the amount of radiation received.

Radiographic Technique

Initial chest films should be obtained with the infant supine, the arms away from the chest, and the head in the neutral position. Proper positioning is especially important when trying to identify the location of an orotracheal or nasotracheal tube; these may change when the head is moved.[2] Magnification films may be of some value in selected cases.

Frontal film studies are exposed at the longest tube-film distance possible and should be coned to the area of interest. It is acceptable to include the upper abdomen on a chest film to identify catheter positions and detect the presence of pneumoperitoneum.[3] Total body films should be avoided.

Lateral chest films are recommended as part of the initial radiographic evaluation. These should be taken with a horizontal beam and the infant supine. The following information may be gained from the lateral projection:

1. The state of lung aeration
2. Anteroposterior dimensions of the chest and heart
3. The presence (or absence) of thymic tissue
4. Vertebral anomalies
5. Tracheal anatomy and caliber
6. Hilar vascular detail

7. Small collections of extrapulmonary air in the mediastinum, anterior thorax, or upper abdomen
8. Verification of the position of intravascular catheters and endotracheal tubes

The following is offered to help recall the various causes for neonatal respiratory distress. The mnemonic is NACHAS: N—*p*neumonia, all organisms; A—*a*spiration, meconium; C—*c*ardiac, congenital anomalies; H—*h*yaline membranes, hypertension-pulmonary; A—*a*irway, paralyzed vocal cords, webs, cysts; S—*s*urgical lesions.

References

1. Sabau MN, Radkowski MA, Vyborny CJ: Radiation exposure due to scatter in neonatal radiographic procedures. *AJR* 144:811, 1985.
2. Brasch RC, Hildt GA, Heckt S: A new position-dependent cause of endotracheal tube obstruction. 66th Scientific Meeting, Radiological Society of North America, Dallas, 1980.
3. Gfeller-Varga D, Felman AH: Pneumoperitoneum. Diagnosis from chest radiographs. *Clin Pediatr* 19:761, 1980.

Chapter 4

Noninfectious Disorders

A wide variety of noninfectious disorders are capable of causing respiratory distress in the full-term and premature infant. The following abnormalities are covered in this chapter.

1. Respiratory distress syndrome (RDS; hyaline membrane disease, HMD)
2. Transient tachypnea of the newborn (TTN)
3. Persistent fetal circulation (PFC)
4. Pulmonary hemorrhage

Respiratory Distress Syndrome (Hyaline Membrane Disease)

Respiratory distress syndrome, or clinical hyaline membrane disease, is the most common cause of severe respiratory distress of the newborn. It is confined almost exclusively to premature babies. However, HMD also afflicts infants of diabetic or toxemic mothers, those born by cesarean section, and less often, term infants weighing more than 2500 g.

Clinical signs of HMD may begin at or shortly after birth. Tachypnea, grunting respirations, cyanosis, and sternal retractions are typical signs. The diagnosis is often suspected from physical examination and blood gas analysis.

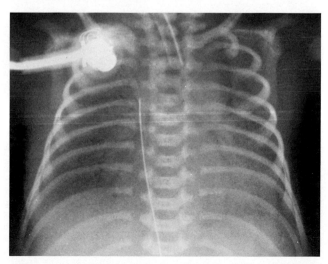

Figure 4-1   Hyaline membrane disease. Diffuse granularity, air bronchograms, and underaeration are well illustrated. *Note:* The catheter is in the superior vena cava.

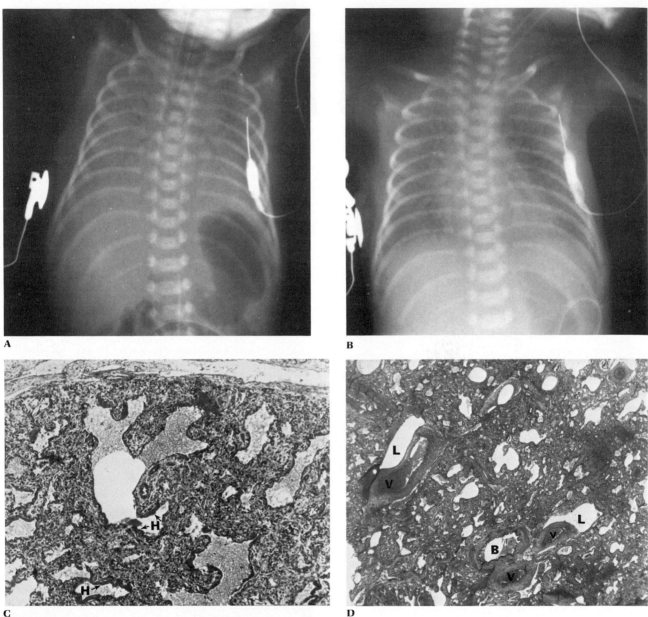

Figure 4-2   Hyaline membrane disease. A. The initial film demonstrates diffusely opaque lung fields, air bronchograms, and underaeration. **B.** Four hours later a small hyperlucent area is present in the left midlung field. **C.** The infant died shortly thereafter, and the histologic section illustrates immature lungs with thickened alveolar septa. The alveoli are lined with hyaline membranes (H) and filled with protein-rich edema fluid. **D.** This histologic section is taken from the area of hyperlucency in the left lung (A). It shows markedly distended, air-filled perivascular lymphatics (L) representing pulmonary interstitial (lymphatic) emphysema. *Note:* There is a close approximation of lymphatics (L), blood vessels (V), and bronchus (B).

Radiographic features are usually quite distinctive within the first hour (Figures 4-1 and 4-2).[1] Early radiographic examination is imperative to identify surgically correctable conditions such as diaphragmatic hernia and other congenital malformations. Radiographic examination is also necessary to exclude pulmonary disease in patients with other causes for respiratory distress, such as sepsis, intracranial hemorrhage, intrauterine infections, and maternal drug ingestion.

While the pathogenesis and prevention of HMD remain elusive, several therapeutic modalities have shown some promise. At least temporary radiographic improvement has been observed in infants treated with human and bovine surfactant.[2,3] Partial venoarterial bypass with extracorporeal membrane oxygenation is an additional technique used to support neonates with respiratory failure.[4,5] High-frequency jet ventilation may be of use in selected patients.[5a]

Radiologic Findings

Certain buzzwords such as *granular, ground glass, white out,* and *reticular-granular* are commonly used to describe the radiographic appearance of HMD.[6–11] While of some use, these terms often mean different things to different people and are frequently confusing to the novice. In order to avoid these semantic pitfalls, the following radiographic criteria are proposed for the evaluation of HMD:

Blood vessel definition
Degree of expansion

Generalized granularity
Persistent abnormality

Air bronchograms present
Certain findings absent

Blood Vessel Definition

Pulmonary vessels are important landmarks of the lung. Loss of normal vascular shadows is one of the earliest radiographic features of HMD.

Degree of Expansion

Hyaline membranes cause generalized pulmonary atelectasis and underaeration of the lungs. However, underaerated lungs may occur in disease processes other than HMD (pulmonary hemorrhage, pulmonary edema, and non-group A beta-hemolytic streptococcal pneumonia). The presence of hyperaeration in nonventilated infants virtually excludes HMD.

Underaeration in neonates will, on occasion, produce a chest film which resembles a bell (Figure 4-3). The etiology of a "bell-shaped" chest has traditionally been associated only with neonatal "depression" from neurologic damage and/or decreased muscle tone. However, immature lungs and prematurity also diminish muscle tone, resulting in a bell-shaped chest.

Generalized Granularity

The granular pattern associated with HMD is a relatively late radiographic finding. Its appearance is caused by admixtures of collapsed alveoli and air-bearing bronchioles.

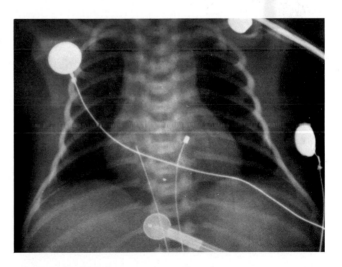

Figure 4-3 Hypotonia. The chest demonstrates a bell-shaped configuration. Lungs are normal.

Persistent Abnormality

During the course of illness, the chest radiograph should remain relatively unchanged until resolution begins. If the film suddenly takes on a generalized opacity, the possibility of superimposed hemorrhage should be suspected. However, an expiration exposure will also appear generally opaque, making differentiation from hemorrhage, edema, or severe HMD extremely difficult. Air bronchograms located in the center chest favor an expiration film, whereas preserved bronchograms in the periphery suggest HMD.

Air Bronchograms Present

Air bronchograms are well-known radiographic criteria of air space disease and/or atelectasis. They usually appear in well-established HMD, but may also occur normally in the central lung and left lower lobes.

Certain Findings Absent

1. Localized involvement. The disease should not be localized to one area of lung, although asymmetrical involvement may occur early.[13,14] Careful inspection of good-quality films over a period of several hours should reveal changes throughout the lungs.
2. Pleural edema and fluid. The appearance of pleural edema and fluid indicates possible superimposed complications, such as congestive heart failure, mostly with patent ductus arteriosus (PDA),[15] and non-group A beta-hemolytic streptococcal infection.
3. Spontaneous pneumothorax. This complication can occur in untreated HMD, but its presence should raise concern for congenital renal dysplasia, intrauterine pneumonia, or aspiration.

Additional Observations

Attaching prognostic significance to the early radiographic findings in HMD may be hazardous. Unpredictable clinical variables render such an opinion of little value. Once treatment is begun, especially with ventilatory assistance, endotracheal intubation, and positive end expiratory pressure (PEEP, C-PAP, etc.), the radiographic pattern of HMD is altered (Figure 4-4). Positive end expiratory pressure artificially expands the collapsed alveoli, creating a pseudoclearing pattern.[16] This pseudoclearing may be deceiving and suggest spurious radiologic improvement. Superimposed pulmonary interstitial emphysema (PIE) will contribute, on occasion, to a false picture of radiographic clearing.

The radiographic patterns that develop during the course of treatment for HMD will vary considerably, depending upon the therapeutic measures employed and the complications that occur. The lungs usually attain their maximum radiopacity between 3 and 5 days, after which gradual clearing ensues. Redefinition of pulmonary vessels is often the first sign of recovery.

Delay in the appearance of normal blood vessels and lung markings, and/or the development of other residual opacities, portends possible problems. One of the more feared is the onset of interstitial fibrosis and bronchopulmonary dysplasia (BPD) (Figure 4-5). Once begun, BPD may progress, arrest, or regress. (See Chapter 7, Figures 7-2 to 7-4.)

In smaller infants and those with more severe disease, the ductus arteriosus may remain patent. Jones and Pickering[17] reported a 31 percent mortality in infants with HMD and complicating PDA, compared with 17 percent mortality in those without PDA. These and other clinicians suggest that prolonged ductal patency may contribute to difficult weaning from oxygen and ventilatory assistance.[15] In addition, PDA may play a roll in the development of BPD (see Chapter 7, Figure 7-2) and intracranial hemorrhage.[17-20]

Clinical signs of patent ductus—murmur, bounding pulses, and signs of congestive failure—are sometimes difficult to assess. The need for increased ventilatory assistance and oxygen is suggestive of a PDA. Delayed clearing of HMD is an additional early clue.[13]

Radiographic changes of PDA may precede the murmur and clinical signs by 24 to 48 h. These al-

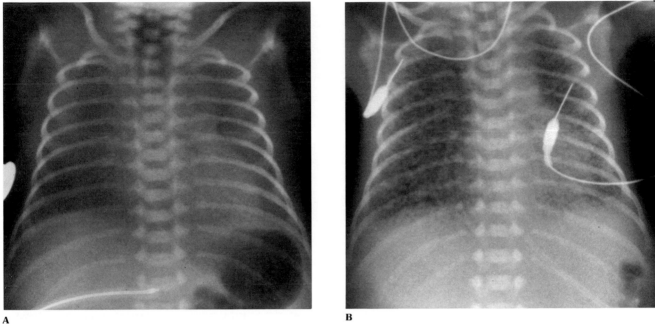

A   **B**

Figure 4-4   Hyaline membrane disease—pseudoclearing. A. Typical HMD. **B.** After 24 h, the film shows hyperaeration and right-sided PIE, giving the appearance of radiographic clearing.

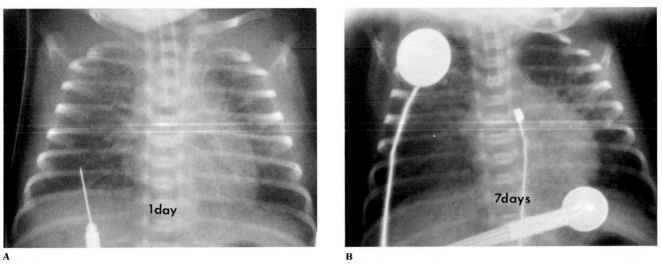

A   **B**

Figure 4-5   Hyaline membrane disease—bronchopulmonary dysplasia. A. Hyaline membrane disease treated with mechanical ventilation on the first day of life. **B.** By 7 days, the lungs retain diffuse opacities that represent unresolved HMD and early BPD. Mild cardiomegaly and ill-defined pulmonary vascularity suggest the presence of arterial PDA.

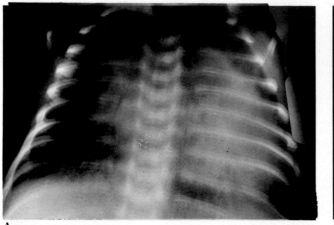
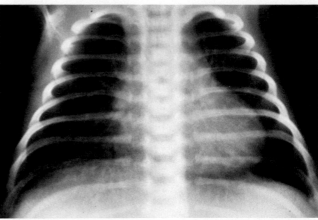

A   B

Figure 4-6   Patent ductus arteriosus. A. The initial film shows marked cardiomegaly and pulmonary edema. **B.** After 1 week of conservative management, the PDA closed spontaneously, and the lungs returned to normal with possible borderline cardiomegaly.

terations are often quite subtle, and interpretation is frequently complicated by the underlying lung changes (Figures 4-5B and 4-6). Evaluation of all interval films, not just the most recent, is frequently needed to discern subtle changes in cardiac size. Ratio of the heart size to chest width is notoriously misleading in neonates and infants. Measurements are for tailors, not for radiologists.

Fluid retention and subcutaneous edema, caused by decreased renal function and diminished cardiac output, may complicate the course of HMD.[21] This is best appreciated over the shoulders and along the chest wall. Fluid accumulation in the lungs may gravitate to the most dependent portion and, if the patient has been supine, will appear as increased posterior opacity on lateral film (Figure 4-7).

Long-term sequela in patients with HMD has changed in recent years. Outerbridge et al.[22] found that 21 percent of patients who recovered from HMD clinically and biochemically developed an increased incidence of lower respiratory tract illness requiring hospital admission. In their series, the infants had not necessarily been treated with mechanical ventilatory assistance, and their chest films showed no changes of BPD. Others have reported episodes of bronchiolitis and respiratory infection that required hospitalization in 17 to 33 percent of HMD survi-

vors.[23,24] Stahlman et al.,[25] reviewing patients treated for HMD between 1961 and 1970, found that long-term pulmonary complications were infrequent. However, their patients were not treated for long periods of time with positive pressure ventilators.

Careful clinical and radiologic follow-up of patients who survive HMD is necessary if residual pulmonary disease is to be identified and treated.

Transient Tachypnea of the Newborn

Transient tachypnea of the newborn is a complex of symptoms described by Avery and coworkers in 1966.[26] Disease states that resemble and might be identical to TTN have been reported under a variety of names: transient respiratory distress of the newborn (TRDN),[27] wet-lung disease,[28] type II respiratory distress syndrome,[29,30] and transient neonatal tachypnea.[31] Unfortunately, TTN, by any other name, still looks pretty much the same. The conditions named above may represent separate diseases, variants of the same disease, or diseases with closely allied pathophysiologic aberrations. They all share the same clinicoradiographic pattern which, if recog-

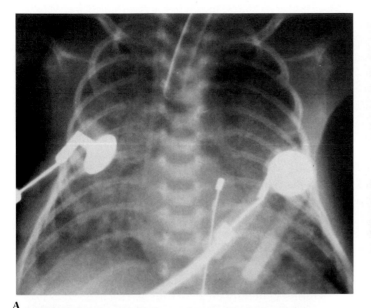

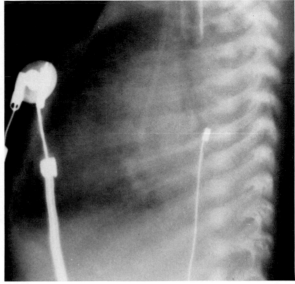

A

B

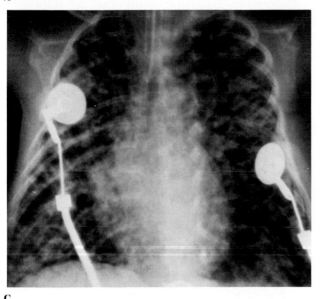

C

Figure 4-7 Pulmonary edema—gravitational shift and PIE. A.
Diffuse radiopacity with central confluence is suggestive of edema.
B. Posterior lung fields are selectively opaque, a reflection of fluid
gravitation in the supine attitude. **C.** Sudden onset of pulmonary interstitial emphysema occurred in the same patient several days later
causing a generalized admixture of ramifying black and white shadows that are well defined. Contrast this pattern with BPD (see Chapter 7).

nized, should lead to proper therapy. In the interest
of consistency and simplicity, the term *transient
tachypnea of the newborn* (TTN) will be used in de-
ference to the clinicians who first described the
complete clinical picture.

The clinical parameters of TTN are not well
standardized, possibly because of the lack of understanding of the basic underlying pathophysiology.
Patients with TTN have typically been reported
weighing less than 3000 g. However, Rawlings and
Smith[32] found an average birth weight of 3723 g in
100 patients. Most clinicians agree that prolonged labor and cesarean section increase the risk of developing TTN, but difference of opinion exists over the

etiologic role of maternal sedation.[32,33] Most infants with TTN are less than 38 weeks of gestation and have physical signs of immaturity but not prematurity. Size is usually appropriate for gestational age. Intrauterine pneumonia and meconium aspiration may present similar clinical features and should be excluded.

Patients with TTN characteristically develop extreme tachypnea in the first minutes or hours after birth. The tachypnea may be accompanied by expiratory grunting and mild to moderate intercostal and substernal retractions. This condition slowly improves in the ensuing 2 to 5 days. Minimal cyanosis may be present in room air but is usually relieved by mask oxygen. Normal pH and P_{CO_2} are the rule.[9] The cardiovascular system shows no abnormalities.[30]

Delayed resorption of fetal lung fluid probably causes this symptom complex and accounts for most of the following radiographic alterations (Figure 4-8): (1) indistinct pulmonary vessels, (2) thickened fissures (sometimes a normal finding), (3) free-flowing pleural effusions, (4) swollen subpleural lymphatics, and (5) alveolar opacities. Mild overaeration and patchy, confluent infiltrates may be present (Figure 4-9). These changes, however, are more compatible with meconium aspiration or pneumonia, but their presence does not exclude TTN. Indeed, TTN and meconium aspiration share many clinical and radiographic features.[34,35]

The differential diagnosis of TTN includes mild HMD, pneumonia-aspiration syndrome, congenital heart disease with failure, polycythemia, non-group A beta-hemolytic streptococcal infection, persistent fetal cardiopulmonary circulation, paroxysmal auricular tachycardia (Figure 4-10), and/or venous obstruction (Figure 4-11).[36] Mild HMD may be difficult to distinguish from TTN, and indeed the two may coexist. However, patients with TTN require less ventilatory support, and their symptoms and radiographs generally clear within 48 to 72 h.

Pneumonia-aspiration syndrome, as indicated previously, may also be confused with TTN, but this condition generally causes more severe clinical symptoms. The radiographs show extensive infiltration, shifting atelectasis, and frequent pneumo-

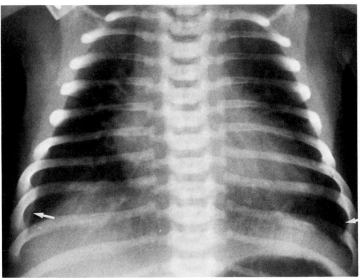

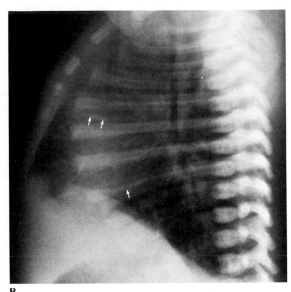

A

B

Figure 4-8   Transient tachypnea of the newborn. A. The intrapulmonary vessels are indistinct, subpleural edema is evident bilaterally (arrows), and the heart is slightly enlarged. The lungs are normal to slightly overaerated. **B.** Mild thickening of fissures (arrows) and fine, linear opaque lines are seen behind the sternum. These are produced by swollen interlobular septa.

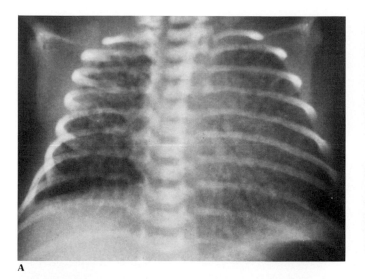

A

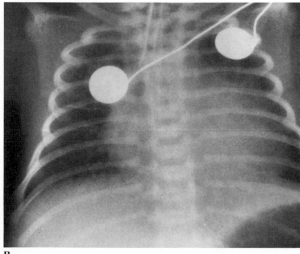

B

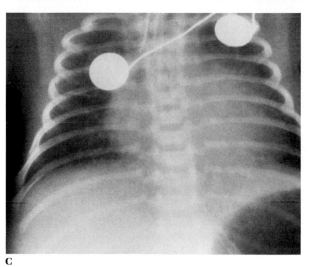

C

Figure 4-9 Transient tachypnea of the newborn. A. The initial film shows a diffuse pattern of linear densities, obscure thickened vessels, moderate overaeration, and cardiomegaly. Air bronchograms behind the heart indicate alveolar fluid. Differential diagnosis should include meconium-amniotic fluid aspiration, intrauterine pneumonia, obstructed venous return, and pulmonary lymphangiectasia. **B.** Twenty-four hours later the lungs remain mildly abnormal, but considerable improvement has occurred. This case represents a combination of transient tachypnea and amniotic fluid aspiration. **C.** Film at 48 h continues to show clearing of the lung fields, but mild cardiomegaly remains. The presence of an orotracheal tube indicates greater severity of disease than expected, but total recovery ensued.

thorax. On occasion, the diagnosis of TTN must be made in retrospect or by exclusion.

Persistent Fetal Circulation

Persistent fetal circulation (PFC) in the newborn should be suspected when there is distress and cyanosis out of proportion to relatively mild, nonspe-

cific, radiographic changes. In the eleven patients reported by Merten et al.,[37] four had an HMD pattern, four had a pattern of aspiration syndrome (Figure 4-12), and two had a wet-lung appearance. In nine, cardiomegaly was evident. Marked cardiomegaly and signs of congestive failure were observed by Nielson et al.,[38] but this presentation seems to be the exception rather than the rule.

Pathologic examination of the lungs in some infants who die with PFC shows increased muscular

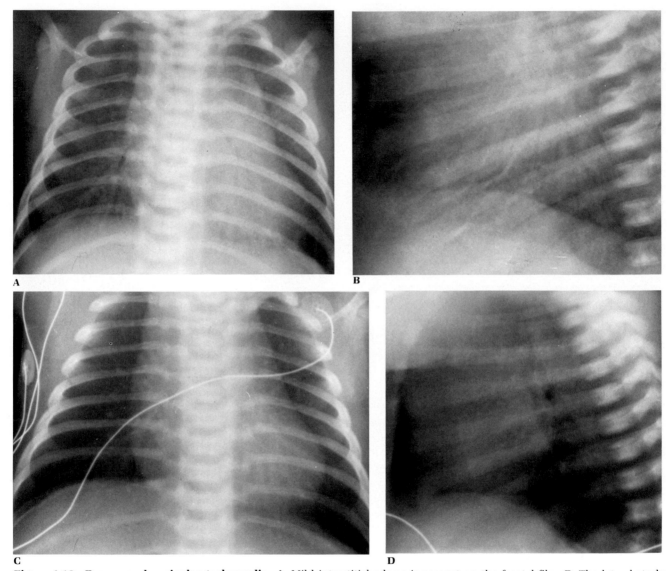

Figure 4-10   Paroxysmal auricular tachycardia. A. Mild interstitial edema is present on the frontal film. **B.** The lateral study confirms the interstitial edema with swollen fissures and intralobular septa. **C** and **D.** Films after conversion to normal rhythm are free of edema.

thickness of intraacinar pulmonary arteries and extension of muscle into more peripheral arteries, not normally muscularized at birth.[39–41]

As yet, the exact cause for PFC is not well delineated. Murphy and coworkers[41] suggest the possibility of prenatal influences including (1) increased sensitivity to intrauterine hypoxia, (2) altered flow in the fetal pulmonary vascular bed, and (3) failure of the usual mechanisms regulating arterial muscularization of the vascular bed.

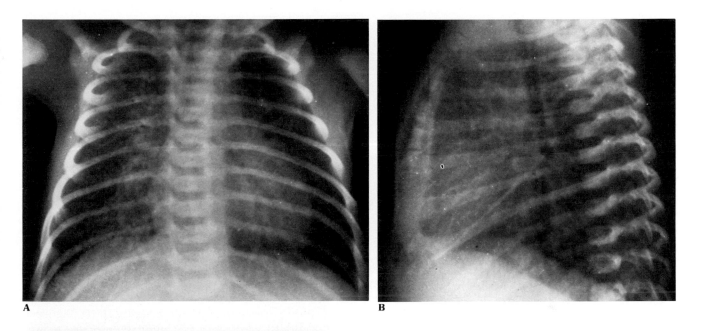

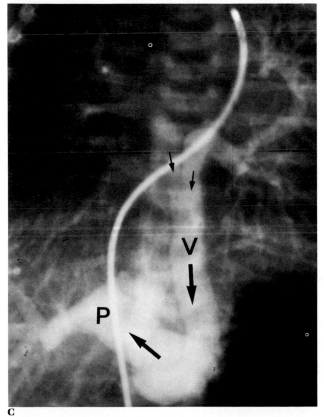

Figure 4-11 Total anomalous pulmonary venous return (TAPVR). A. The pulmonary vessels are prominent and ill-defined in this newborn. There is minimal subpleural edema on the right. The heart does not appear enlarged. **B.** Moderate hyperaeration is present, and the swollen major fissures and interlobular septa are evident. **C.** The pulmonary angiogram outlines the pulmonary venous drainage to the portal vein (P) via the common pulmonary vein (V). Arrows depict the direction of blood flow. TAPVR below the diaphragm is a rare occurrence, but may present a radiographic pattern similar to transient tachypnea of the newborn in the first few days of life. Coarctation of the aorta and other left heart obstructive lesions may do the same.

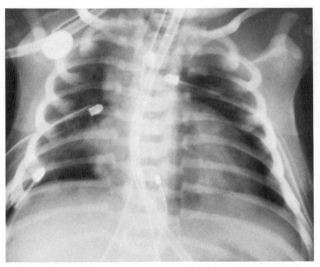

Figure 4-12 Persistent fetal circulation with meconium aspiration. This child was born with clinical and radiologic features of meconium aspiration and treated for bilateral thoraxes. Persistent fetal circulation complicated the clinical course and could not be controlled. The infant expired after the first week of life.

Quite possibly, PFC is only a transitory physiologic aberration with several different underlying causes.

Pulmonary Hemorrhage

The significance of pulmonary hemorrhage in the overall spectrum of neonatal respiratory distress is difficult to assess because the methods and criteria for diagnosis are not uniform. In addition, HMD and other underlying neonatal pulmonary processes are often present in association with pulmonary hemorrhage. The clinical symptoms—retractions, tachypnea, and cyanosis—are features common to both hemorrhage and HMD.

Respiratory distress begins within 3 h of birth in the large majority of infants who develop pulmonary hemorrhage. Bleeding from the airway occurs in somewhat less than half of patients.[42-44] In some infants, no premonitory signs occur. Sudden occurrences of extreme respiratory distress, shock, and respiratory failure are the first signs of disease in a previously asymptomatic infant.[45] Most deaths from pulmonary hemorrhage occur within the first 48 h of life.

Prematurity predisposes infants to pulmonary hemorrhage, but the duration of survival is not related to birth weight.[46] When present in full-term infants, pulmonary hemorrhage often complicates other abnormalities, such as congenital heart disease, intrauterine hypoxia, pneumothorax, and aspiration pneumonia.[42]

The radiographic findings in acute pulmonary hemorrhage are often colored by underlying lung disease. Rowe and Avery[42] reported several radiographic features including a reticular-granular pattern, coarse irregular densities, nodular patchy shadows, and homogeneous opacification. In most cases, pulmonary hemorrhage cannot be diagnosed solely by the roentgen ray. However, a sudden opacification superimposed on a clearing HMD (Figure 4-13) should serve as a red light. Pulmonary edema from other causes may produce a similar radiographic appearance.

References

1. Peterson HG Jr, Pendleton MD: Contrasting roentgenographic pulmonary patterns of the hyaline membrane and fetal aspiration syndrome. *AJR* 74:800, 1955.
2. Smyth JA, Metcalfe IL, Duffty P, et al: Hyaline membrane disease treated with bovine surfactant. *Pediatrics* 71:913, 1983.
3. Hallman M, Merritt TA, Schneider H: Isolation of human surfactant from amniotic fluid and a pilot study of its efficacy in respiratory distress syndrome. *Pediatrics* 71:473, 1983.
4. Hall JA Jr, Hartenberg MA, Kodroff MB: Chest radiographic findings in neonates on extracorporeal membrane oxygenation. *Radiology* 157:75, 1985.
5. Bartlett RH, Gazzaniga AB, Fong SW: Extracorporeal membrane oxygenator support for cardiopulmonary failure. *J Thorac Cardiovasc Surg* 73:375, 1977.
5a. Boros SJ, Mammel MO, Coleman JM, et al: Neonatal high-frequency jet ventilation: Four years experience. *Pediatrics* 75:657, 1985.
6. Singleton EB: Respiratory distress syndrome. *Progress in Pediatric Radiology.* New York, S Karger, 1967, vol 1, 135.

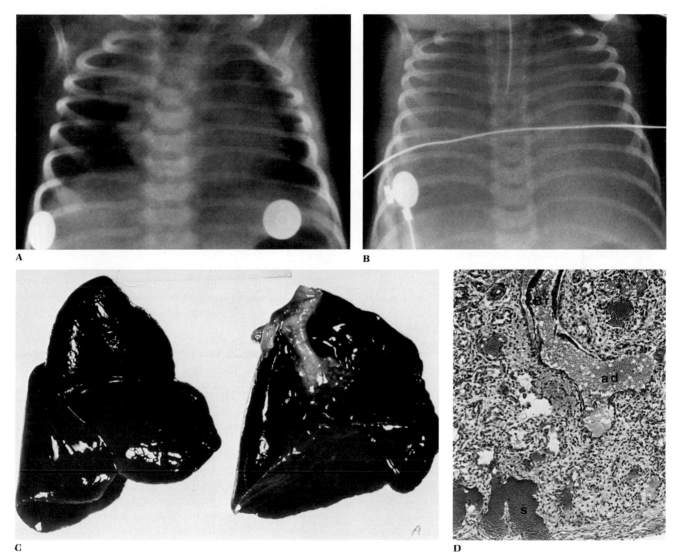

Figure 4-13   Pulmonary hemorrhage. A. The initial film study is unremarkable except for the right pneumothorax. **B.** Four days later total opacification of the lungs appears just before death. **C.** Pulmonary hemorrhage was discovered at autopsy, but a specific cause could not be identified. These dense, airless lungs are dark purple and fleshy. When sectioned, they resemble a soft blood clot. **D.** Erythrocyte ghosts fill the bronchioles (Br), alveolar duct (ad), and alveolar saccule (s). Nearby saccules are collapsed in this immature lung.

7. Feinberg SB, Goldberg ME: Hyaline membrane disease: Preclinical roentgen diagnosis. *Radiology* 68:185, 1957.

8. Schultze G: Chest film findings in neonatal respiratory distress. *Radiology* 70:230, 1958.

9. Avery ME, Fletcher BD Jr: *The Lung and Its Disorders in the Newborn Infant.* Philadelphia, WB Saunders Co, 1974, pp 40, 268.

10. Currarino G, Silverman FN: Roentgen diagnosis of pulmonary disease of the newborn infants. *Pediatr Clin North Am* 4:27, 1959.

11. Wolfson SI, Frech R, Hewitt C, et al: Radiologic diagnosis of hyaline membrane disease. *Radiology* 93:339, 1969.

12. Johnson JF, Dean BL: The expiratory film in hya-

line membrane disease: Preliminary observations. *AJR* 139:31, 1982.

13. Rudhe U, Margolin FR, Robertson B: Atypical roentgen appearance of the lung in hyaline membrane disease of the newborn. *Acta Radiol* 10:57, 1970.

14. Tchow CS, Fletcher BD, Franke P, et al: Asymmetric distribution of the roentgen pattern in hyaline membrane disease. *J Can Assoc Radiol* 23:85, 1972.

15. Slovis TL, Shankarer S: Patent ductus arteriosus in hyaline membrane disease: Chest radiography. *AJR* 135:307, 1980.

16. Giedion A, Haefliger H, Dangel P: Acute pulmonary x-ray changes in hyaline membrane disease treated with artificial ventilation and positive end-expiratory pressure (PEEP). *Pediatr Radiol* 1:145, 1973.

17. Jones RWA, Pickering D: Persistent ductus arteriosus complicating respiratory distress syndrome. *Arch Dis Child* 52:274, 1977.

18. Gupta JM, Fisk GC, Wright JS: Ductus ligation in respiratory distress syndrome. *J Thorac Cardiovasc Surg* 63:642, 1972.

19. Gay JH, Daily WJR, Meyer BHP, et al: Ligation of the patent ductus arteriosus in premature infants. Report of 45 cases. *J Pediatr Surg* 8:667, 1973.

20. Jacob J, Gluck L, Di Sessa T, et al: The contribution of PDA in the neonate with severe RDS. *J Pediatr* 96:79, 1980.

21. Guignard JP, Torrado SM, Mazouni SM: Renal function in respiratory distress syndrome. *J Pediatr* 88:845, 1976.

22. Outerbridge EW, Nogrady B, Beaudry PH, et al: Idiopathic respiratory distress syndrome. Recurrent respiratory illness in survivors. *Am J Dis Child* 123:99, 1972.

23. Lewis S: A follow-up study of the respiratory distress syndrome. *Proc R Soc Med* 61:771, 1968.

24. Shepard FM, Johnston RB Jr, Klatte EC, et al: Residual pulmonary findings in clinical hyaline membrane disease. *N Engl J Med* 279:1063, 1968.

25. Stahlman M, Hedvall G, Lindstrom D, et al: Role of hyaline membrane disease in production of later childhood lung abnormalities. *Pediatrics* 69:572, 1982.

26. Avery ME, Gatewood OB, Brumley G: Transient tachypnea of the newborn: Possible delayed resorption of fluid at birth. *Am J Dis Child* 111:380, 1966.

27. Swischuck L: Transient respiratory distress of the newborn. A temporary disturbance of a normal phenomenon. *AJR* 108:557, 1970.

28. Wesenberg RI, Graven SN, McCabe FB: Radiological findings in wet-lung disease. *Radiology* 98:69, 1971.

29. Prod'hom LS, Levinson H, Cherry RB, et al: Adjustment of ventilation, intrapulmonary gas exchange, and acid-base balance during the first day of life. Infants with early respiratory distress. *Pediatrics* 35:662, 1965.

30. Sundell H, Garrott J, Blankenship WJ, et al: Studies on infants with type II respiratory distress syndrome. *J Pediatr* 78:754, 1971.

31. Malan AF: Neonatal tachypnea. *Aus Paediatr J* 3:159, 1966.

32. Rawlings JS, Smith FR: Transient tachypnea of the newborn. An analysis of neonatal and obstetric risk factors. *Am J Dis Child* 138:869, 1984.

33. Stahlman MT, Kendig EL, Chernick V: *Disorders of the Respiratory Tract in Children*. Philadelphia, WB Saunders Co, 1977, p 196.

34. Steele RW, Copeland GA: Delayed resorption of pulmonary alveolar fluid in the neonate. *Radiology* 103:637, 1972.

35. Northway WH Jr, Daily WJR, Parker BR, et al: Perinatal pulmonary study. *Invest Radiol* 6:354, 1971.

36. Bucciarelli RL, Egan EA, Gessner IH, et al: Persistence of fetal cardiopulmonary circulation: One manifestation of transient tachypnea of the newborn. *Pediatrics* 58:192, 1976.

37. Merten DF, Goetzman BW, Wennberg RP: Persistent fetal circulation; an evolving clinical and radiographic concept of pulmonary hypertension of the newborn. *Pediatr Radiol* 6:74, 1977.

38. Nielson HC, Riemenschneider TA, Jaffe RB: Persistent transitional circulation. Roentgenographic findings in thirteen infants. *Radiology* 120:649, 1976.

39. Haworth SG, Reid L: Persistent fetal circulation: Newly recognized structural features. *J Pediatr* 88:614, 1976.

40. Siassi S, Goldberg SJ, Emmanouilides GC, et al: Persistent pulmonary vascular obstruction in newborn infants. *J Pediatr* 78:610, 1971.

41. Murphy JD, Rabinovitch M, Goldstein JD: The structural basis of persistent pulmonary hypertension of the newborn infant. *J Pediatr* 98:962, 1981.

42. Rowe S, Avery ME: Massive pulmonary hemorrhage in the newborn, II. Clinical consideration. *J Pediatr* 69:12, 1966.

43. Ahvenainen EK: Massive pulmonary hemorrhage in the newborn. *Ann Paediatr Fenniae* 2:44, 1956.

44. Thorburn MJ: Neonatal death and massive pulmonary hemorrhage in Jamaica. *Arch Dis Child* 38:589, 1963.

45. Stahlman MT: Respiratory disorders in the newborn, in Kendig EL Jr, Chernick V (eds): *Disorders of the Respiratory Tract in Children*. Philadelphia, WB Saunders Co, 1977, p 290.

46. Esterly JR, Oppenheimer EH: Massive pulmonary hemorrhage in the newborn. I. Pathological considerations. *J Pediatr* 69:3, 1966.

Chapter 5

Infectious Disorders

Pneumonia is the most common serious infection of newborn infants, accounting for 9 to 23 percent of deaths.[12] Infection may be acquired in utero, usually from premature rupture of maternal membranes with secondary amnionitis. Difficult passage through the birth canal, especially in abnormal or prolonged labor, increases the susceptibility to pneumonia. The immediate postnatal period is an especially dangerous time for the development of pulmonary infection.

Hematogenous placentofetal infection is an additional method for the acquisition of intrauterine pneumonia. These infections are most often caused by a group of unusual organisms including *toxoplasma*, *rubella*, *cytomegalovirus*, and *herpes* simplex. The mnemonic ToRCH is frequently used to designate this group of organisms. Bacteria responsible for transplacental infection include *Escherichia coli*, staphylococci, streptococci, pneumococci, and *Listeria monocytogenes*.[3] Tuberculosis and syphilis are rare causes, but may be increasing in incidence.

Infants may be contaminated during passage through the birth canal. Group B streptococci, herpes simplex, herpes zoster varicellosus, and *Chlamydia trachomatis* are common causes of pneumonia acquired in this manner. Staphylococcus, streptococcus, and *E. coli* are additional causes for perinatal pneumonia. Less common, but reported, causes include *Haemophilus influenzae* and *Pneumocystis carinii*.[4-6]

Aspirated material, which frequently contaminates the tracheobronchial tree, often contributes to respiratory distress and complicates the therapy of pulmonary infection in these vulnerable new citizens.

Few clinical clues help separate these entities from one another, and radiographic differentiation may also be impossible.[7] However, when taken together, the clinical-radiologic picture is usually sufficiently specific to institute proper therapy.

Intrauterine Pneumonia (Amniotic Infection Syndrome)

Intrauterine bacterial pneumonia (Figure 5-1) and neonatal sepsis are likely sequelae of premature rupture of fetal membranes with secondary amniotic fluid infection.[8] Prolonged and sometimes inert labor, abnormal delivery, old mothers, maternal pyrexia, fetal distress, and prematurity all increase risk for intrauterine infection. The contribution of aspirated infected amniotic fluid or infected meconium to the production of pulmonary damage is unknown.[9] Davis and Aherne[9] found little histologic evidence for pulmonary inflammation in congenital pneumonia and concluded that it is a passive condition, caused only by aspiration of maternal inflammatory cells. Naeye et al.,[2] in autopsied infants with congenital pneumonia, found no etiologic agent in 3 percent of cases. A more traditional concept argues that neonatal pneumonia is caused by bacterial invasion of the lung from aspiration of infected amniotic fluid.[10–12] Sherman and coworkers,[11] by using Gram's stains of tracheal secretions, demonstrated a coexistence between congenital pneumonia and bacteremia.

Foul, purulent amniotic fluid and vaginal discharge in a feverish mother with prepartum ruptured membranes should suggest the possibility of congenital pneumonia. In addition to the usual nonspecific clinical signs of lower respiratory tract disease (retractions, grunting, and air hunger), infants with congenital pneumonia often show neurologic signs of increased limb tone, irritability, and convulsions.[9] Fever, hypothermia, and delayed onset of respirations are additional features.

Tracheal aspiration and blood culture are the most reliable methods of identifying a causative organism.[11] In most cases, the infections occur with gram-negative rods of the colon group; proteus and *Pseudomonas aeruginosa* are occasional invaders in addition to the more common *E. coli* and streptococci. Group B beta-hemolytic streptococcus infections, thought to be acquired from passage through the birth canal, are assuming greater importance and will be discussed separately.

Meconium Aspiration Pneumonia

Whereas hyaline membrane disease (HMD) occurs most often in prematures, meconium aspiration is a disease of term and postterm infants. Spillage of me-

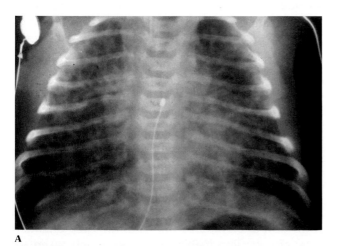 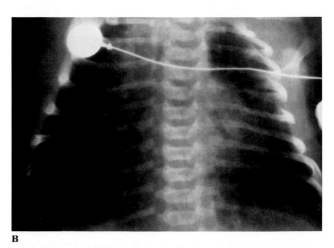

A   B

Figure 5-1   Intrauterine pneumonia. Premature rupture of fetal membranes and infected amniotic fluid. **A.** The lungs are hyperaerated and contain generalized irregular nondescript radiopacities with some areas of coalescence. **B.** After 48 h the lungs are improved but still abnormal. (See Chapter 4, Figure 4-9.)

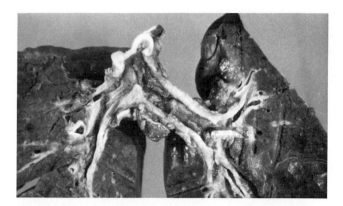

Figure 5-2 Meconium aspiration. Note the presence of copious amounts of meconium in the bronchial lumina.

conium into the amniotic fluid usually results from fetal distress, hypoxia, or difficult prolonged labor. Fetal respiration and initial inspiratory efforts after birth draw meconium into the trachea (Figure 5-2). Prompt removal of this tenacious material before the infant initiates respiration may diminish the severity of the pulmonary insult.[13] Although vigorous suction will partially clear the tracheal lumen, some meconium is already present in the peripheral respiratory tract before birth.[14]

The respiratory symptoms caused by aspirated meconium depend largely upon the amount of material that reaches the peripheral bronchial tree. Meconium is confined to the trachea in just over half of meconium-stained patients; one-third of these will develop respiratory distress. Clinical symptoms are caused mostly from mechanical obstruction of the airway by particles of meconium or squamous epithelial cells.[15] However, meconium also acts as a chemical irritant and contributes to inflammation, infection, and possibly irreversible pulmonary damage.

Persistent pulmonary arterial hypertension, or persistent fetal circulation (PFC), has been reported in patients with fatal meconium aspiration syndrome.[16] Excessive muscularization of the pulmonary artery microcirculation is present histologically and presumed to be developmental in origin. Persistent fetal circulation is discussed further in Chapter 4.

Thorough tracheal suction should be carried out to establish patency of the airway and to remove as much material as possible before instituting ventilatory assistance. Emptying the stomach will help avoid further regurgitation and aspiration. Gram's staining of tracheal secretions has been shown to help in predicting the onset of neonatal bacteremia.[17] Otherwise, the treatment is largely supportive. Avery[18] suggests antibiotic coverage because of the difficulty in separating uncomplicated meconium aspiration from infectious pneumonia.

Radiologic Findings

The radiographic changes of meconium aspiration differ little, if any, from those produced by congenital or intrauterine pneumonia. It is reasonable to use the term *pneumonia-aspiration syndrome* when referring to this clinicoradiographic complex. Both are often accompanied by tracheobronchial accumulations of tenacious material which cause random blockage of central and peripheral airways.

Meconium aspiration is characterized by generalized and/or unequal pulmonary overaeration and coarse, patchy, radiating infiltrates (Figure 5-3). This contrasts with HMD, which produces a homogeneous, finely granular pattern with underaerated lungs.[19] On occasion, there may be considerable overlapping of the radiographic features. Haney and coworkers,[7] in an analysis of 30 infants with autopsy-proven neonatal pneumonia, reported radiographic alterations that suggested transient tachypnea of the newborn in 17 percent of cases and HMD in 13 percent. Generalized alveolar opacities occurred in 77 percent of cases and dense bilateral alveolar changes with air bronchograms in 33 percent. Transient cardiomegaly is an additional feature in selected cases.

In patients with pneumonia-aspiration syndrome, pneumomediastinum or pneumothorax, or both, occur spontaneously in 10 to 44 percent of affected newborns (Figure 5-4).[7,20,21] These complications, if present, are usually manifest in the first hours of life. When pneumomediastinum or pneumothorax (or both) occurs in the absence of pulmonary abnormality, the possibility of abnormal renal

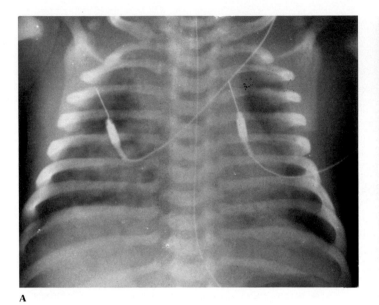

A

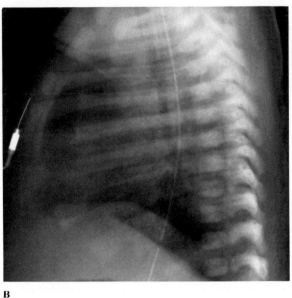

B

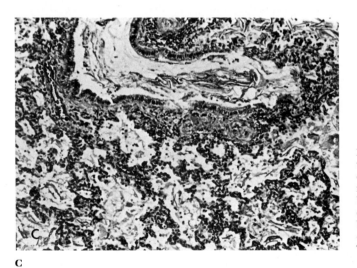

C

Figure 5-3 Neonatal pneumonia (meconium aspiration). This full-term infant, born by cesarean section, was covered with thick meconium. He died within 24 h of birth. **A.** The frontal film shows several areas of patchy confluent opacity in both lower lung fields. **B.** The lateral film confirms the presence of mild to moderate overaeration. **C.** The alveoli and nearby bronchioles contain amniotic fluid squamae and granular meconium-stained debris. The interstitial capillaries are engorged. The process involves the entire lung.

development should be considered.[22] (See Chapter 3, Figure 3-16.)

In uncomplicated meconium aspiration, rapid clearing is to be expected, with return to normal or near normal lungs within 3 to 5 days. Slower resolution, as well as the development of persistent atelectasis and other chronic alterations, implies superimposed pulmonary infection.

Group B Beta-Hemolytic Streptococcus Pneumonia

Between the years 1969 and 1978, rates of infections in newborns with group B beta-hemolytic streptococcus pneumonia ranged from 27.7 to 39.2 percent.[23] In 1979 they accounted for 25 percent of neonatal sepsis in a series from the Boston City Hos-

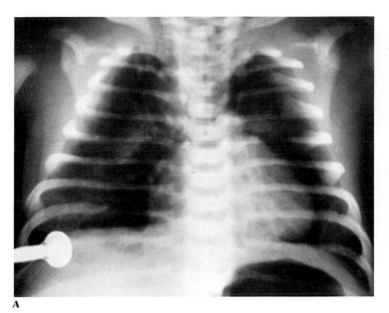
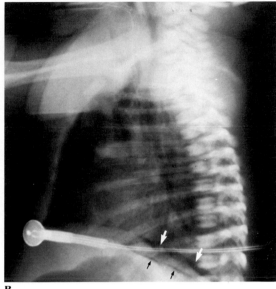

A   B

Figure 5-4 Pneumonia-aspiration syndrome. A. Pneumomediastinum and pneumothoraxes are apparent on the initial film study. **B.** Free air occupies the anterior mediastinum. *Note:* There is air between the diaphragm and lung (arrows).

pital.[24] There is no evidence to indicate that group B streptococcal disease is declining.

Two distinct clinical patterns of group B streptococcal infection have been reported.[25–30] Early-onset infection (before 7 to 10 days) is associated with maternal colonization and may result from obstetrical complications, i.e., amnionitis, premature delivery, and contamination during passage through the birth canal.[31] Late-onset disease is probably acquired by nosocomial infection.

With early-onset infections, infants may appear deceptively asymptomatic at birth and then develop sudden signs of profound pulmonary involvement within the first few hours of life. Tachypnea, tachycardia, metabolic acidosis, poor peripheral perfusion, and cytotoxic shock are the principal clinical features that herald the onset of pneumonia and/or bacteremia. Mortality rates of 60 to 75 percent may result despite adequate therapy.[32] Periventricular leukomalacia is an associated complication in surviving infants.[33]

Group B streptococcal pneumonia may produce few if any radiographic alterations. A fine, granular

pattern similar to HMD, with bronchial tree demarcation, diffuse air bronchograms, and interstitial air, has been reported in small premature infants (Figure 5-5).[34] Typical consolidations and lobar infiltrates occur in less than half of patients.[35] Cardiomegaly, venous congestion, pleural effusion, and signs of delayed fluid resorption are additional findings.[35,36] In spite of the above, there are no radiologic features that distinguish this disease from other causes of respiratory distress in the newborn.[37] Infants with clinical and radiologic appearances of HMD should always be suspect for group B streptococcal infections.

Persistent fetal circulation is a reported companion of group B streptococcus pneumonia.[38] One theory advanced to explain this relationship suggests that pulmonary hypoxemia and acidosis stimulate pulmonary vasoconstriction, thus causing blood to shunt from right to left through a patent ductus arteriosus.[38] Not limited to group B streptococcal pneumonia, PFC has been reported in the company of meconium aspiration, though possibly for different reasons.[16]

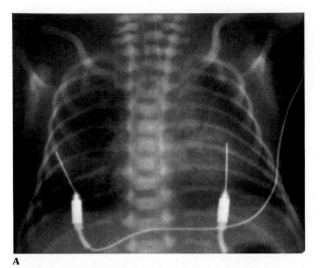
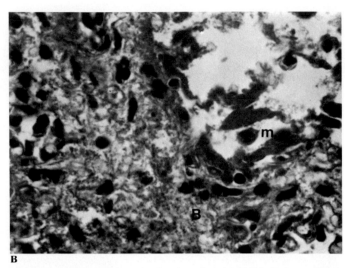

Figure 5-5   Group B beta-hemolytic streptococcal pneumonia. This 1400-g white male developed respiratory distress shortly after birth. Cyanosis and hypotension ensued rapidly, and the child expired within the first 24 h of life. Postmortem blood cultures were positive for group B beta-hemolytic streptococci. **A.** This chest film exposed shortly before death is characterized by ill-defined vessels, minimal granularity, a few basal air bronchograms, and mild cardiomegaly. **B.** Fragments of hyaline membranes (m) partly fill the alveolar duct. Bacteria (B) lie amid collagen fragments of the intersaccular septum.

Right-sided Bochdalek hernia with group B streptococcal sepsis and pneumonia is a rare but well-known association.[39] Ashcraft and colleagues[39] have suggested that diminished motility of the diaphragm in the region of the hernia and underaeration of the adjacent lobe create a potential for pulmonary infection with group B streptococcus. Unlike infants with congenital diaphragmatic hernia, patients with this complication tend to do well once the diagnosis is established and the infection brought under control. A large pleural effusion, on the right side of the chest in an infant with group B streptococcal septicemia, should suggest the presence of a diaphragmatic hernia.

Late-onset group B streptococcal disease, which usually begins after 7 days (mean 24 days of age) is characterized by meningitis and focal infections, such as otitis, conjunctivitis, cellulitis, abscess, endocarditis, and pericarditis. Septic arthritis and osteomyelitis are additional complications. On occasion, these may be extremely indolent, and result in extensive bone destruction before clinical symptoms are manifest (see Chapter 13, Figure 13-2).[40] The humerus is the most common bone involved; adjacent

septic arthritis is not unusual. Pneumonia, a characteristic of early-onset group B streptococcal infection, is also a feature of the late-onset disease.

Cytomegalic Inclusion Pneumonia

Cytomegalic inclusion disease is a systemic infection caused by one group of cytomegaloviruses (CMVs), formerly labeled human salivary gland viruses. Several serologic types exist, and the organism may infect animals, including monkeys and rodents. More than 9 percent of pregnant women excrete the virus from their cervices in progressively increasing amounts during pregnancy.[41]

Mothers with infections acquired before becoming pregnant usually do not transmit the disease to their offspring. Primary infection of the mother during gestation is probably necessary for fetal involvement, but in some cases the fetus may escape the disease.[42] While the bulk of evidence favors intrauterine placentofetal transmission, infection may begin

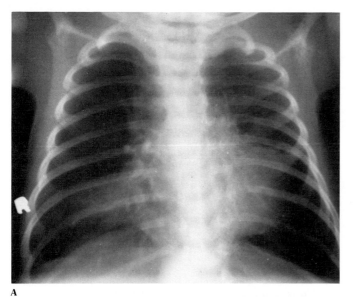

A

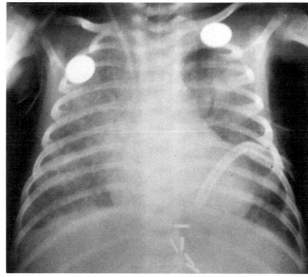

B

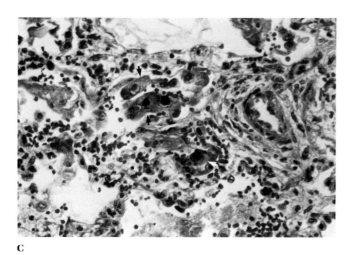

C

Figure 5-6 Cytomegalic inclusion pneumonia. A. This infant developed nasal congestion at 2 weeks of age, followed by increasing respiratory difficulty and radiographic findings of pneumonia. After another month of complicated illness, the patient expired without a definitive diagnosis. **B.** This film study obtained before death shows diffuse chronic lung disease which had developed over the previous month. The radiographic pattern, while not specific, is more homogeneous than the patchy irregularity of bronchopulmonary dysplasia. **C.** Intranuclear CMV inclusion is the hallmark of this infection. One can appreciate the considerably greater size of these infected cells in comparison with uninfected cells (arrows).

with passage through an infected birth canal.[43] Infection may also be acquired from other infants or nursery personnel and from transfusion of infected blood.[44,45] Yaeger[46] estimates that blood transfusions may account for CMV infection in one out of every seven transfused infants. Three to four percent of premature infants excrete CMV at birth, a fact that suggests congenital infection.

Characteristic features of intrauterine infection with CMV include hepatosplenomegaly, hepatitis, jaundice, petechiae, purpura, thrombocytopenia, microcephaly, cerebral calcification, chorioretinitis, and brain damage.[47] Some infected infants manifest quite subtle symptoms, such as mild, transient hepatomegaly.[48]

The radiographic expression of CMV infection is nonspecific; intracerebral calcification, microcephaly, and hepatosplenomegaly are typical. Bone changes akin to those of rubella have been described.[49–51] These consist of linear, longitudinally oriented, alternating radiolucencies and radiopacities in the metaphyses of the femurs and humeri. The metaphyseal ends are serrated, and periosteal reaction is absent. By 8 weeks the bones have usually resumed their normal appearance. Osseous changes, similar to those described above, occur in other neonatal infections, such as syphilis, smallpox, vaccinia, and erythroblastosis. Patients with rubella have delayed osseous maturation of the knee, whereas CMV patients do not.[52]

The chest film findings in CMV pneumonia are characterized by gentle overaeration and slowly evolving, diffuse, indolent, nonspecific opacities (Figure 5-6). These changes are not sufficiently characteristic to establish a firm diagnosis of CMV, but when accompanied by the typical proximal humeral osseous abnormalities, the disease may be suggested from the chest study.

Listeria monocytogenes Pneumonia

Listeria monocytogenes is a pleomorphic gram-positive rod that is a well-known cause of animal illness. The disease has become a recognized threat in humans, because of greater awareness in bacteriologic laboratories. Critical isolation techniques are necessary to distinguish this organism from diphtheroids, atypical pneumococcus, streptococcus, or other contaminants.

The organism inhabits the cervix and vagina and has an affinity for the fetoplacental unit.[53-55] Thus, infection may develop in utero from placental and fetal membrane invasion or by contamination during birth. Hematogenous spread in the infant also results from infection of mucous membranes.

Listeria monocytogenes infection closely resembles other forms of neonatal sepsis and pneumonia, particularly those of group B streptococcus infections.

Fever and infected amniotic fluid are consistent features of prenatal infections. Symptoms, which may occur within the first 4 days of life or later, are characterized by profound signs of nervous system

infection, cyanosis, jaundice, petechial rash, myocarditis, hepatomegaly, and apnea. Later-onset disease is probably acquired from human contacts and is characterized by fever, irritability, and meningitis.

Radiographic evidence of pneumonia is present in more than half of patients with congenital listeriosis.[56] Overaeration, confluent infiltrates, atelectasis, and medium to large miliary lesions are salient features. Pleural effusions occur infrequently. Confusion with other forms of neonatal pneumonia is possible, but the presence of miliary granulomas should suggest the diagnosis of listeriosis in the absence of a clear history of aspiration, tuberculosis, or syphilis.[56]

Pneumocystis carinii Pneumonia

Pneumocystis carinii pneumonia, a disease usually seen in compromised hosts, occasionally attacks immunologically competent newborns. Pulmonary infestation is characterized by tachypnea, cough, and intercostal retractions; clinical symptoms that are indistinguishable from infections with chlamydia, cytomegalovirus, and other similar organisms. Affected infants are often severely ill, but usually afebrile.

Most infections are acquired after birth. However, transmission of the organism to the fetus is supported by reports of children of the same infected mother, each of whom manifested disease in the immediate postnatal period.[57] Others have reported occurrence of the disease within family units.[58]

Radiographic differentiation of neonatal pneumocystis pneumonia from other infections is not possible.

Viral Pneumonia

A variety of viral organisms may cause neonatal pneumonia. Among these are parainfluenza[59-61] and respiratory syncytial viruses.

Rubella virus may produce pneumonia as well as generalized infection in the fetus.[62] When the lungs are involved, the chest radiographs show diffuse interstitial infiltrates with some areas of patchy consolidations.[18] Because of the frequent association of congenital heart disease with rubella infection, differentiation between pneumonia and congestive heart failure in an infant with rubella cardiopathy may be difficult. Histologically, rubella lungs demonstrate acute and chronic changes which suggest long-standing intrauterine involvement.

Venereal herpes virus is an additional etiologic agent of neonatal pneumonia and sepsis. Generalized symptomatic herpes simplex infection of the newborn is often fatal; 50 percent of survivors have significant neurologic sequelae.

Herpes simplex virus is also capable of causing pneumonia in the newborn. Herpes simplex pneumonia may present with a chest film that appears normal and progress rapidly to one with prominent perihilar interstitial markings and coalescent areas of pulmonary infiltrates (white-out lungs). Hyperinflation, in contrast to aspiration pneumonia, is not characteristic. Pleural effusions may be present.

References

1. Driscoll SG, Smith CA: Neonatal pulmonary disorders. Meconium aspiration. *Pediatr Clin North Am* 9:325, 1962.

2. Naeye RL, Dellinger WS, Blank WA: Fetal and maternal features of antenatal bacterial infections. *J Pediatr* 69:733, 1971.

3. Blank WA: Pathways of fetal and early neonatal infection. *J Pediatr* 59:473, 1961.

4. Kuhn JP, Lee SB: Pneumatoceles associated with *E. coli* pneumonia in the newborn. *Pediatrics* 51:1008, 1973.

5. Lilien LD, Yeh TF, Novak GM, et al: Early onset *Haemophilus sepsis* in newborn: Clinical, roentgenographic, and pathologic features. *Pediatrics* 62:299, 1978.

6. Stagno S, Pifer LL, Hughes WT, et al: Pneumocystis carinii pneumonitis in young immunocompetent infants. *Pediatrics* 66:56, 1980.

7. Haney PJ, Bohlman M, Sun CCJ: Radiographic findings in neonatal pneumonia. *AJR* 143:23, 1984.

8. Bada HS, Alojipan LC, Andrews BF: Premature rupture of membranes and its effect on the newborn. *Pediatr Clin North Am* 24:441, 1977.

9. Davis PA, Aherne W: Congenital pneumonia. *Arch Dis Child* 37:598, 1962.

10. Bernstein J, Wang J: Pathology of neonatal pneumonia. *Am J Dis Child* 101:330, 1961.

11. Sherman MP, Goetzman BW, Ahlfors CE, et al: Tracheal aspiration and its clinical correlates in the diagnosis of congenital pneumonia. *J Pediatr* 65:258, 1980.

12. Stahlman MT, in Kendig EL Jr, Chernick V (eds): *Disorders of the Respiratory Tract in Children*. Philadelphia, WB Saunders Co, 1977, p. 292.

13. Gregory GA, Gooding CA, Phibbs RH, et al: Meconium aspiration in infants: A prospective study. *J Pediatr* 85:848, 1974.

14. Gooding CA, Gregory GA: Roentgenographic analysis of meconium aspiration of the newborn. *Radiology* 100:131, 1971.

15. Bacsik, RD: Meconium aspiration syndrome. *Radiol Clin North Am* 24:463, 1977.

16. Murphy JD, Vawter GF, Reid LM: Pulmonary vascular disease in fatal meconium aspiration. *J Pediatr* 104:758, 1984.

17. Sherman MD, Chance KH, Goetzman BW: Gram's stains of tracheal secretions predict neonatal bacteremia. *Am J Dis Child* 138:848, 1984.

18. Avery ME, Fletcher BD: *The Lung and Its Disorders in the Newborn Infant*. Philadelphia, WB Saunders Co, 1974, pp 188, 268.

19. Peterson HG Jr, Pendleton ME: Contrasting roentgenographic pulmonary patterns of the hyaline membrane and fetal aspiration syndromes. *AJR* 74:800, 1955.

20. Hoffman RR Jr, Campbell RE, Decker JP: Fetal aspiration syndrome. Clinical, roentgenographic, and pathologic features. *AJR* 122:90, 1974.

21. Gooding CA, Gregory GA, Taber P, et al: An experimental model for the study of meconium aspiration of the newborn. *Radiology* 100:137, 1971.

22. Renert WA, Berdon WE, Baker DN, et al: Obstructive urologic malformations of fetus and infant; relation to neonatal pneumomediastinum and pneumothorax: Air-block. *Radiology* 105:97, 1972.

23. Baker CJ: Group B streptococcal infections in neonates. *Pediatrics in Review* 1:5, 1979.

24. Eickhoff TC, Klein JO, Daly AK, et al: Neonatal sepsis and other infections due to group B beta-hemolytic streptococci. *N Engl J Med* 2(71):1221, 1964.

25. Franciosi RA, Knostman JD, Zimmerman RA: Group B streptococcal neonatal and infant infections. *J Pediatr* 82:707, 1973.

26. McCracken GH: Group B streptococci: The new challenge in neonatal infections. *J Pediatr* 82:703, 1973.

27. Barton LL, Faigin RD, Lins R: Group B beta-hemolytic streptococcal meningitis in infants. *J Pediatr* 82:719, 1973.

28. Baker CJ, Barrett FF, Gordon RC, et al: Suppurative meningitis due to streptococci of Lancefield group B: A study of 33 infants. *J Pediatr* 82:724, 1973.

29. Quirante J, Ceballos R, Cassady G: Group B beta-hemolytic streptococcal infection in the newborn. 1. Early onset infection. *Am J Dis Child* 128:659, 1974.

30. Horn KA, Zimmerman RA, Knostman JD, et al: Neurological sequelae of group B streptococcal neonatal infection. *Pediatrics* 53:501, 1974.

31. Baker CJ, Barrett FL: Transmission of group B streptococci among parturient women and their neonates. *J Pediatr* 83:919, 1973.

32. Gotoff SP: Emergence of group B streptococci as major perinatal pathogens. *Hosp Pract* Sept 85, 1977.

33. Faix RG, Donn SM: Association of septic shock caused by early-onset group B streptococcal sepsis and periventricular leukomalacia in the preterm infant. *Pediatrics* 76:415, 1985.

34. Ablow RC, Effman EL, Vany R, et al: The radiographic features of early onset group B streptococcal neonatal sepsis. *Radiology* 124:771, 1977.

35. Leonidas JC, Hall RT, Beatty EC, et al: Radiologic findings in early onset neonatal group B streptococcal septicemia. *Pediatrics* 59:1006, 1977.

36. Weller MH, Katzenstein AA: Radiological findings in group B streptococcal sepsis. *Radiology* 118:385, 1976.

37. Lilien LD, Harris VJ, Pildes RS: Significance of radiographic findings in early onset group B streptococcal infection. *Pediatrics* 60:360, 1977.

38. Shankaran S, Farooki ZQ, Desai R: B hemolytic streptococcal infection appearing as persistent fetal circulation. *Am J Dis Child* 136:725, 1982.

39. Ashkraft KW, Holder TM, Amoury RA, et al: Diagnosis and treatment of right Bochdalek hernia associated with group B streptococcal pneumonia and sepsis in the neonate. *J Pediatr Surg* 18:480, 1983.

40. McCook TA, Felman AH, Ayoub E: Group B beta-hemolytic streptococcal infections of bone and joints. *AJR* 130:456, 1978.

41. Howard WA: Cytomegalic inclusion disease, in Kendig EL Jr, Chernick V (eds): *Disorders of the Respiratory Tract in Children.* Philadelphia, WB Saunders Co, 1977, p 436.

42. Hayes K, Gibas H: Placental cytomegalovirus infection without fetal involvement following primary infection in pregnancy. *J Pediatr* 79:401, 1971.

43. Whitley RJ, Brassfield D, Reynolds DW, et al: Protracted pneumonitis in young infants associated with perinatally acquired cytomegaloviral infection. *J Pediatr* 89:16, 1976.

44. Spector SA, Schmidt K, Ticknor W, et al: Cytomegaloviruria in older infants in intensive care nurseries. *J Pediatr* 95:444, 1979.

45. Ballard RA, Drew WL, Hufnagh KG, et al: Acquired cytomegalovirus infection in preterm infants. *Am J Dis Child* 133:482, 1971.

46. Yaeger A: Editorial comment. *Yearbook Pediatr* 37, 1981.

47. Hanshaw JB: Congenital and acquired cytomegalovirus infection. *Pediatr Clin North Am* 13:279, 1966.

48. Birnbaum G, Lynch JI, Margileth AM et al: Cytomegalovirus infections in newborn infants. *J Pediatr* 75:789, 1969.

49. Merten DF, Gooding CA: Skeletal manifestations of cytomegalic inclusion disease. *Radiology* 95:333, 1970.

50. Graham CB, Thal A, Wassum CS: Rubella-like bone changes in congenital cytomegalic inclusion disease. *Radiology* 94:39, 1970.

51. Rudolph AJ, Singleton EB, Rosenberg HS, et al: Osseous manifestations of the congenital rubella syndrome. *Am J Dis Child* 110:428, 1965.

52. Kuhns LR, Slovis T, Hernandez R, et al: Knee maturation as a differentiating sign between rubella and cytomegalovirus infection. *Pediatr Radiol* 6:36, 1977.

53. Ahlfors CE, Goetzman BW, Halsted CC, et al: Neonatal listeriosis. *Am J Dis Child* 131:405, 1977.

54. Ray CG, Wedgewood RJ: Neonatal listeriosis. Six case reports and a review of the literature. *Pediatrics* 34:378, 1964.

55. Driscoll SG, Gorbach A, Feldman D: Congenital listeriosis: Diagnosis from placental studies. *Obstet Gynecol* 20:216, 1962.

56. Willich E: The radiological appearance of pulmonary listeriosis. *Prog Pediatr Radiol* 1:160, 1967.

57. Bazaz GR, Manfredi OL, Howard RG, et al: *Pneumocystis carinii* pneumonia in three full term siblings. *J Pediatr* 76:767, 1970.

58. Gentry LO, Remington JS: *Pneumocystis carinii* pneumonia in siblings. *J Pediatr* 76:769, 1970.

59. Moscovici C, La Placa M, Amer J: Respiratory illness in

prematures and children. Illness caused by parainfluenza type 3 virus. *Am J Dis Child* 102:91, 1961.

60. Sano T, Niitsu I, Nakagawa I: Newborn virus pneumonitis (type Sendai). I. Report: Clinical observation of a new virus pneumonitis of the newborn. *Yokohama Med Bull* 4:199, 1953.

61. Kuroya M, Ishida N: Newborn virus pneumonitis (type Sendai). II. Report: The isolation of a new virus possessing hemagglutinin activity. *Yokohama Med Bull* 4:217, 1953.

62. Phelan P, Campbell P: Pulmonary complications of rubella embryopathy. *J Pediatr* 75:202, 1969.

Chapter 6

Complications of Air Leak

The treatment of neonatal respiratory distress has been advanced by the use of positive pressure ventilation delivered through an endotracheal tube or face mask. This therapy helps combat atelectasis and facilitates gaseous exchange. However, the placement of endotracheal tubes may lead to complications, such as tracheal stenosis, perforation, and mechanical blockage of stem bronchi. Extravasation of air from the normal confines of the lung and tracheobronchial tree is an occasional finding in asymptomatic newborns. However, in infants being treated with mechanical ventilation, leakage of air into the mediastinum, pericardium, pleural space, soft tissues, peritoneum, and vascular system may be life-threatening.

Several mechanisms are thought to be responsible for the production of pneumomediastinum, pneumopericardium, and pneumothorax. In 1939, Macklin[1] proposed a theory whereby overdistended alveoli rupture, allowing extravasated air to enter the perivascular sheaths, dissect centrifugally, and break into the mediastinum and/or thoracic cavity. Other clinicians have suggested that the extravasated air

is confined to the interstitial pulmonary lymphatics.[2-4] While the Macklin theory has remained popular and may well be correct in some patients, it does not adequately account for the occurrence of pneumothorax without a preexisting pneumomediastinum. The development of pneumothorax without pneumomediastinum suggests rupture of air from the subpleural lymphatics directly into the pleural space (Figure 6-1).[2-4]

In spite of the possibility that extravasated air is confined within lymphatics, the conventional radiographic terminology, *pulmonary interstitial emphysema* (PIE), will be retained (at least for this edition).

Pulmonary Interstitial Emphysema

Mechanical ventilation used to treat neonatal respiratory diseases has markedly increased the incidence of air leak; 40 percent of infants with hyaline membrane disease (HMD) may be expected to develop PIE.[5]

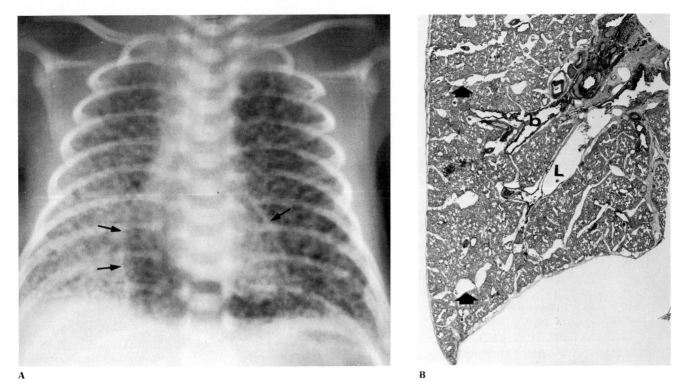

Figure 6-1 Pulmonary interstitial (intralymphatic) emphysema. A. This frontal chest film was the only one taken before death. The random, irregularly shaped radiolucencies scattered diffusely throughout both lung fields are pathognomonic for pulmonary interstitial emphysema. They should not be confused with air bronchograms, which are much more linear, branching, discrete, tapering structures. The central collection of air, outlining the heart and pericardium, represents a pneumopericardium (arrows). **B.** This histologic section through an entire lobe discloses the presence of extravasated air in septal, subpleural, peribronchial, and perivascular lymphatics (L = lymphatic; b = bronchus). (Compare with Figure 3-14D.)

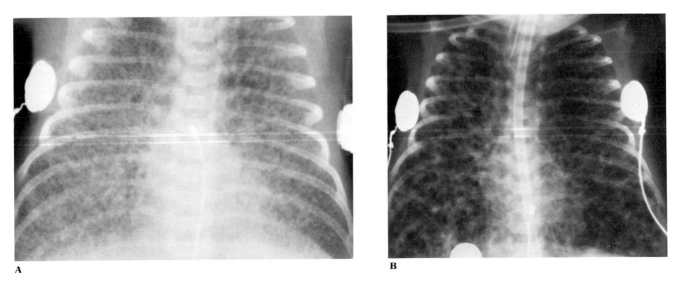

Figure 6-2 Pulmonary interstitial emphysema. A. The lung fields are characterized by disseminated, homogeneous background containing myriad small, irregular, disorganized lucencies representing extravasated interstitial air. **B.** Within 48 h, these have enlarged to produce a coarse, bubbly pattern not unlike bronchopulmonary dysplasia. (See Chapter 7.)

When air remains within the interstitium or lymphatics of the lung, a characteristic roentgenographic appearance of PIE is often produced (Figure 6-1). This extravasated interstitial air is characterized by random, small "bubbles," admixed with an irregular network of branching radiolucencies (Figures 6-1 and 6-2).[6-8] Some of these lines resemble air-filled bronchi, but on closer examination, they do not maintain the predictable bronchial pattern of branching and tapering. Frequently, interstitial air may be identified by blood vessels that appear as small white dots surrounded by a lucent halo.

Interstitial air may occupy both lungs, one lung, or any combination thereof (Figure 6-3). Small areas of PIE may be evanescent or remain localized (Figure 6-4). Pulmonary interstitial emphysema may disappear within hours and never return, or suddenly reappear in a different location. This unpredictable shifting pattern, peculiar to PIE, must be appreciated as potentially problematic, often the prologue to pneumothorax or pneumomediastinum (Figure 6-4).

On occasion, the radiologic appearance of persistent generalized PIE may simulate chronic fibrosis and/or bronchopulmonary dysplasia (BPD). Pulmonary interstitial emphysema usually produces a stark pattern of contrasting black (air) and white (lung tissue) markings, whereas in BPD softer shades of gray prevail (Figure 6-5). Sequential film studies are usually helpful in difficult cases.

Localized Pulmonary Interstitial Emphysema (Acquired Lobar Emphysema)

Extraalveolar air may expand into the interstitium and develop air-filled cysts of variable shapes and sizes. An entire lung, a lobe, or portion thereof may be transformed into an emphysematous, multicystic structure (Figure 6-6). The radiographic pattern thus produced often simulates that of congenital lobar emphysema or adenomatoid malformation. However, judicious review of previous film studies usually clarifies any confusion (Figure 6-7A and B). While localized PIE usually resolves spontaneously, persistent, expanded collections may remain and inhibit adequate ventilation and development of the adjacent lung.[9]

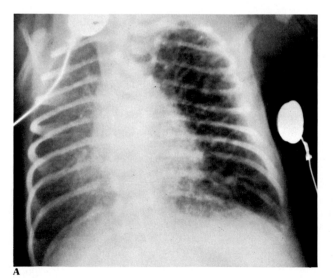
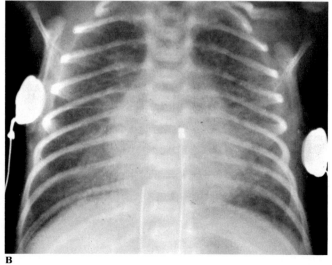

A   B

Figure 6-3   Pulmonary interstitial emphysema—localized. A. The left lung, expanded by PIE, shifts the mediastinum. **B.** Film taken 5 days later shows residual lung disease but no interstitial emphysema.

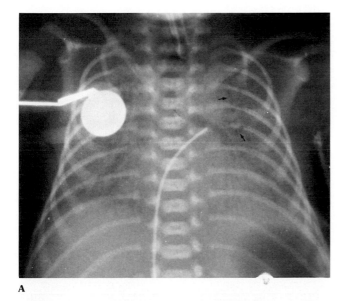

A

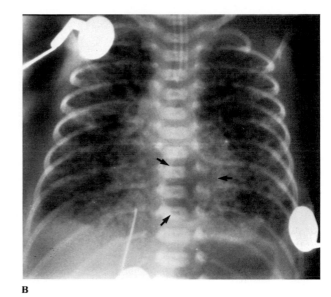

B

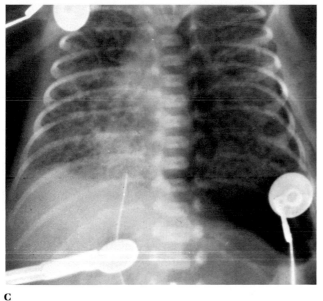

C

Figure 6-4   Pulmonary interstitial emphysema. A. The initial film shows the typical homogeneous pattern of HMD with several small pockets of extravasated air in the left upper lung (arrows). **B.** Twenty-four hours later diffuse interstitial emphysema has developed. Note the postcardiac air collection (arrows), probably a localized pneumothorax behind the pulmonary ligament. **C.** Three hours later, obvious left-sided tension pneumothorax has accumulated. The right lung has lost most of its interstitial emphysema in the interval.

Several therapeutic approaches to PIE have been advanced. Administration of 100% oxygen for short periods of time when an associated pneumothorax exists is one method of treatment.[10] Others have reported success by selective intubation of the contralateral bronchus, thus bypassing the abnormal area of localized emphysema (Figure 6-8).[11,12] Serial radiographs are necessary for evaluation of the effective-

ness of this procedure and for the detection of complications in the ventilated lung and hemithorax. In rare cases, mucoid impaction of major bronchi may prevent selective intubation (Figure 6-9).

Surgical removal of fixed lobar emphysema is now an established procedure.[3–5,13–15] According to Schneider and coworkers,[16] PIE is the most common indication for pulmonary resection in the newborn.

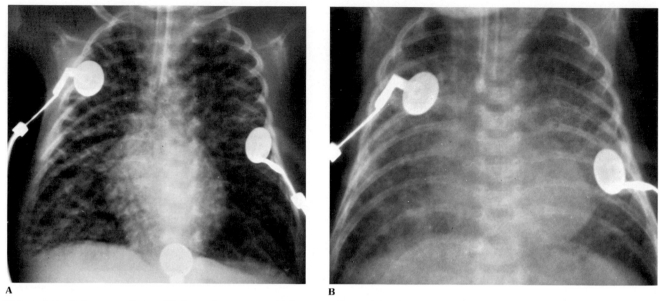

A   B

Figure 6-5   Pulmonary interstitial emphysema and BPD. A. A disseminated, coarse, "lacy" pattern compatible with PIE or BPD. **B.** This film study, several days later, is typical of BPD. *Note:* This study emphasizes the importance of sequential film analysis in circumstances of considerable radiographic overlap.

Lobectomy is necessary in some patients, while in others, a wedge resection is sufficient.

More conservative procedures, such as saline instillation and suctioning, are sometimes successful.[17] Positioning of the child in the lateral decubitus with the affected lung dependent may be of use in selected patients.[18] Spontaneous resolution of PIE results from conservative management and general support in the majority of cases (Figure 6-10).[19]

Pneumomediastinum

Spontaneous pneumomediastinum may occur in otherwise healthy infants but is more often seen in association with HMD, meconium aspiration syndrome, or difficult delivery requiring resuscitation or ventilatory support (Figure 6-11). This complication has been reported in 25 out of 10,000 births and usually causes no problems for the majority of patients.[20] Extravasation of air from alveoli into the interstitium,

followed by retrograde dissection and rupture into the mediastinum, is the accepted pathogenesis of pneumomediastinum. Direct trauma to the trachea, bronchus, or esophagus during difficult intubation or resuscitation may produce similar changes (Figure 6-12).[21-23]

Clinical symptoms of pneumomediastinum are often inapparent except when air dissects into the soft tissues of the neck and chest causing subcutaneous emphysema. Pneumomediastinum of small or moderate degree is usually well tolerated and demands no specific treatment in most infants. However, the development of pneumothorax is a constant danger.

The radiographic features of pneumomediastinum are usually obvious. However, when pneumothorax and pneumomediastinum coexist, differentiation between the two is sometimes difficult or impossible. Horizontal beam decubitus films may help, but critical differentiation is not always necessary so long as the pneumothorax is recognized and treated adequately.

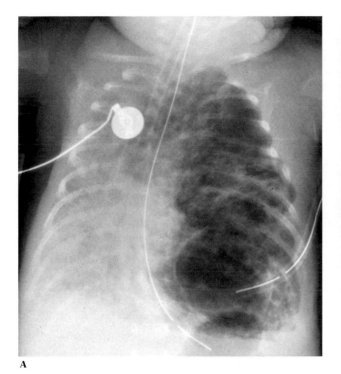

A

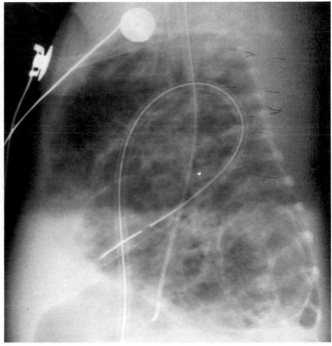

B

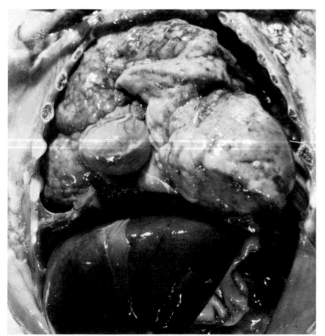

C

Figure 6-6 Pulmonary interstitial emphysema. A and **B.**
These film studies, obtained shortly before death, represent the
final of a long series of examinations. There is severe shift of
mediastinal structures to the right. The left lung is overdistended and contains extensive interstitial emphysema. The curvilinear densities in the inferior portions surround acquired
bullae. This radiographic pattern remained unchanged for approximately 2 weeks before death. **C.** The lungs are white-tan
and cobbled and have the texture of a dry sponge. The bulging
left lower lobe has several tense, large emphysematous bullae.
The apex of the hypertrophied heart points anteriorly.

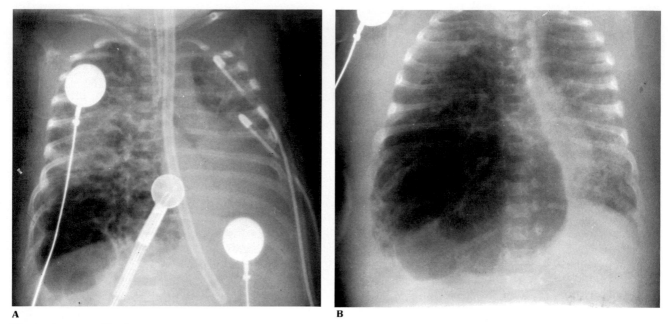

A   B

Figure 6-7   Localized PIE. A. Localized, expansile PIE is present in the right lower lung field. Note the soft tissue edema of the chest wall. **B.** One week later, just before demise, massive right lower lobe emphysema has developed along with marked soft tissue edema.

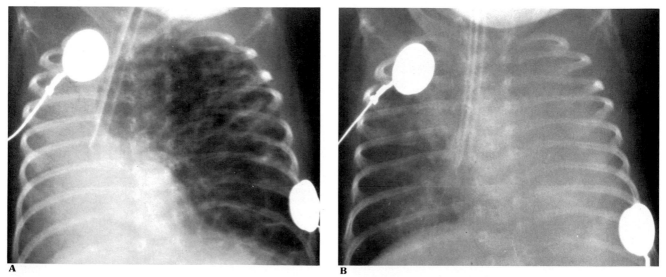

A   B

Figure 6-8   Pulmonary interstitial emphysema—endotracheal tube bypass. A. Massive left-sided PIE is encroaching upon the collapsed right lung. The endotracheal tube, positioned in the right stem bronchus, bypasses the stem orifice. **B.** Twenty-four hours later, the left lung is collapsed, and the right is hyperaerated.

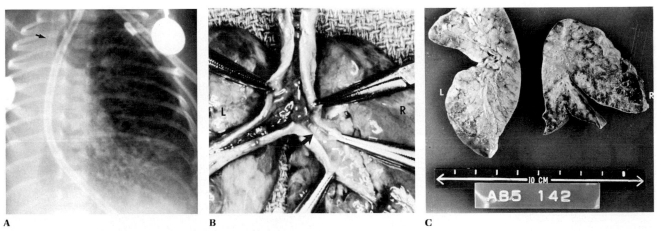

A   **B**   **C**

Figure 6-9 Tracheobronchial impactions. A. Long-standing left-sided pulmonary interstitial emphysema. Repeated attempts to pass an endotracheal tube (arrow) into the right stem bronchus were unsuccessful, and the child expired. **B.** The gross anatomic specimen seen from behind, shows complete mucoid impaction of the right stem bronchus (arrow). The trachea and left stem bronchus are filled with necrotic, mucoid debris. Extensive epithelial hyperplasia of the trachea and stem bronchus is present on histologic examination. **C.** Photographs of gross specimens demonstrate marked asymmetry between the small right and large left lungs. Changes of bronchopulmonary dysplasia and pulmonary interstitial emphysema are present throughout the left lung.

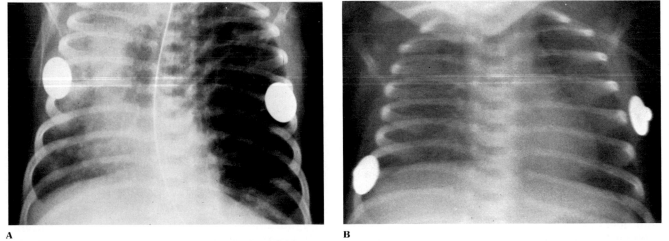

A   **B**

Figure 6-10 Pulmonary interstitial emphysema—spontaneous resolution. A. Extensive PIE of the left chest is evident. **B.** Spontaneous resolution occurred within 1 week.

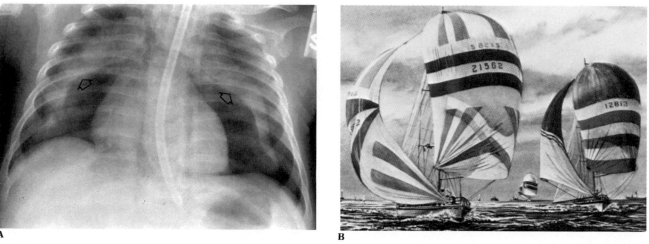

A   **B**

Figure 6-11   Pneumomediastinum—spontaneous.   A. The pneumomediastinum is identified by the presence of air separating the thymus (arrows) from the heart (spinnaker sail sign). Bilateral pneumothoraxes are also evident. **B.** Large striped sails are spinnakers.

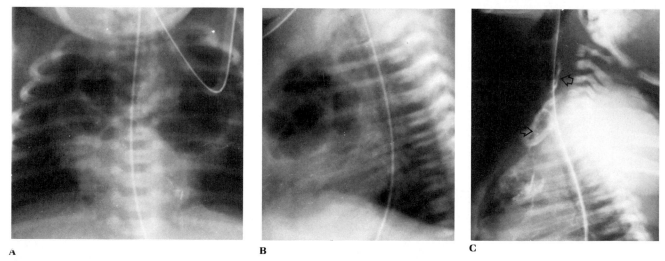

A   **B**   **C**

Figure 6-12   Pneumomediastinum—traumatic.   A. The anterior mediastinum contains multiple air pockets following difficult re-suscitation efforts. **B.** The anterior position of the air is noted. **C.** The barium esophogram with catheter instillation outlines a sinus tract (arrows) leading into the anterior mediastinum. Surgical drainage resulted in a complete cure. (From Talbert et al., with permission.[21])

Pneumopericardium

Pneumopericardium (PPC) is not common and sel-dom occurs spontaneously. It usually accompanies air leaks in other compartments of the thorax.[24] Burt and Lester[25] reported PPC in 1.3 percent of patients

admitted to the nursery intensive care unit at some-time during their hospitalization. The most likely pathophysiologic explanation for PPC, as for pneu-momediastinum, suggests that extravasated air, dis-secting along perivascular sheaths, ruptures into the pericardium through the pleural reflections sur-rounding the great vessels. Abnormal endotracheal tube placement, especially in the right stem bronchus, may contribute to this complication.

As air accumulates in the pericardium, tamponade may ensue and compromise cardiac output.[26] Bradycardia, cyanosis, muffled heart tones, hypotension, and reduction of the electrocardiographic voltage pattern are recognized clinical signs. However, PPC is asymptomatic in approximately 75 percent of patients.[25]

Pneumopericardium has several characteristic radiographic findings. In most cases, the heart is encircled by a halo of air and the continuity of the cardiohepatic shadow is interrupted (Figure 6-13). When pneumomediastinum is also present, a "pericardial line" is produced by the pericardium, outlined by air on either side. This line should not extend cranially beyond the attachments of the great vessels. Decubitus films may record a shift of intra-

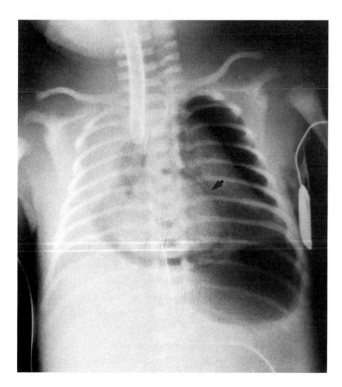

Figure 6-13 Pneumopericardium. Air can be seen completely surrounding the heart (halo sign). A tension pneumothorax is also present. *Note:* The pericardial line is indicated by the arrow.

pericardial air from one side of the heart to the other. Infracardiac air is another helpful roentgenographic feature.

Patients with PPC must be observed religiously for the development of cardiac tamponade necessitating lifesaving pericardiocentesis. The placement of suction catheters in the pericardium is often helpful in preventing recurrence of this complication.

Pneumothorax

Pneumothorax occurs spontaneously in 1.3 percent of vaginally delivered term infants and rises to 6 percent following intubation.[27] A 35 percent incidence may be expected in patients on mechanical ventilatory assistance. Pneumothorax is usually seen in association with, or as a complication of, pneumomediastinum.

The roentgenographic diagnosis of pneumothorax is usually straightforward. However, free air often collects anteriorly and centrally in supine infants, creating an atypical appearance. This "anterior-central" pneumothorax may be suspected from a sharply marginated, well-defined heart border in the frontal projection (Figure 6-14). Cross-table lateral films will help define an anterior pneumothorax when the lung is collapsed against the posterior chest wall (Figure 6-15).[28] Careful technique is necessary since the anterior lung edge, a sign of anterior pneumothorax, may be simulated by sternal retraction, anterior rib ends, axillary soft tissue, and atelectasis.

Skin folds, underlying drapes, and other artifacts may be mistaken for pneumothorax in the frontal projection. When the diagnosis of pneumothorax is in doubt, repeat films in the decubitus position are usually helpful.

The tension in pneumothoraxes that accompany HMD may be most dangerous in every respect. The lung, because of its inherent "stiffness," frequently remains expanded in the face of increased intrathoracic pressure (Figures 6-15 and 6-16). However,

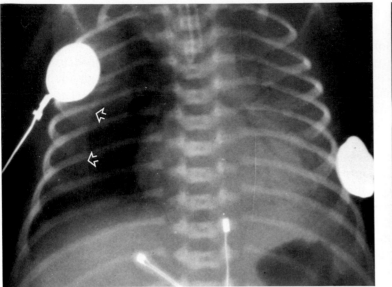 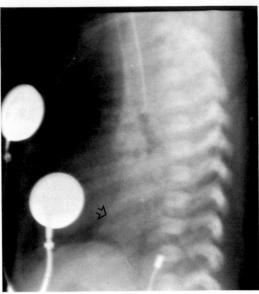

A   **B**

Figure 6-14   Pneumothorax—anterocentral. A. A well-defined radiolucency is present in the right hemithorax. Mild intrathoracic tension is suggested by minimal mediastinal shift, depressed right hemidiaphragm, and separated right ribs. The anteromedial lung edge is outlined (arrows), and the right heart border is sharply defined by adjacent air. **B.** The lateral projection confirms the anterior position of the pneumothorax; the lung is collapsed posteriorly (arrow). (Compare with Figure 6-15.)

when there are findings of depressed hemidiaphragm, spread ribs, and contralateral mediastinal shift, tension pneumothorax should not be ignored just because the underlying lung fails to collapse. In the frontal projection, the lung may appear remarkably well aerated, and markings often extend to the chest wall.

Chest tubes often fail to evacuate an anterior pneumothorax because of the posterior position of the end hole. Allen et al.[29] recommend that chest tubes be placed in an anterosuperior position through the first to third intercostal space, rather than through the conventional lateral fourth to sixth intercostal space. Noninvasive methods for the treatment of pneumothorax include repositioning the patient in the prone position, or with the affected side up (Figure 6-16). Selective bronchial intubation of the normal side, thus bypassing the abnormal, has also had success in a limited number of patients (Figure 6-8A and B).[30] Administration of 100% oxygen for short periods of time also has several distinguished advocates.[10]

A cause-effect relationship between intracranial bleeding and tension pneumothorax in the premature infant is thought to exist.

Venous Air Embolism

Venous air embolism is usually a terminal affair and only diagnosed on radiographs taken immediately before death or shortly thereafter (Figure 6-17). One survivor of venous air embolism has been reported.[31] Rupture of alveoli into the pulmonary veins is thought to account for the embolism.[32] This explanation is supported by the work of Chin et al.,[33] who studied pulmonary venous pressures and concluded that a bronchopulmonary pressure gradient appears to favor air embolism.

Similar pathophysiologic air-block mechanisms are probably responsible for air emboli in patients with cystic fibrosis, bronchial asthma, or other pul-

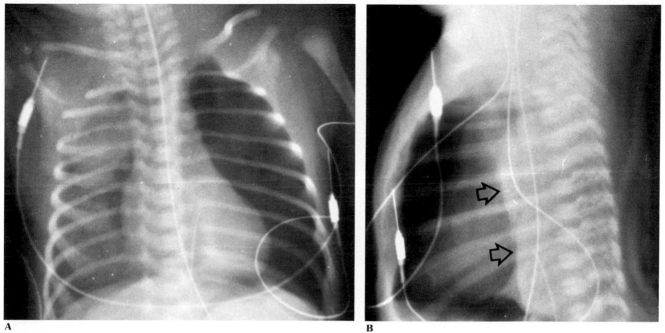

A   B

Figure 6-15   Anterior pneumothorax. A. A tension pneumothorax is present on the left and can be recognized by the enlarged and hyperlucent hemithorax, depressed left hemidiaphragm, spread left ribs, and sharply defined left heart border. *Note:* The left lung edge is not visible. A small medial pneumothorax is present on the right. **B.** The cross-table lateral projection shows the anterior position of the extrapulmonary air and a sharp anterior margin of compressed lung tissue (arrows).

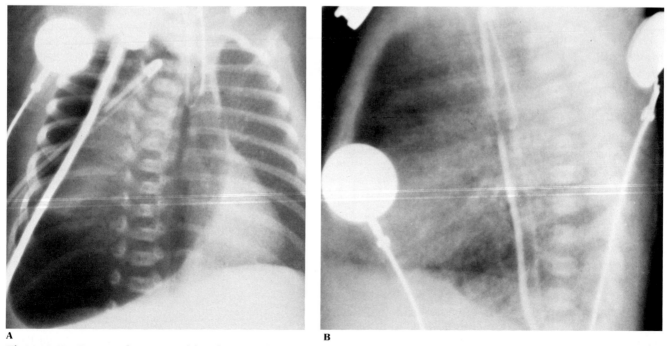

A   B

Figure 6-16   Pneumothorax—positional evacuation. A. An extremely significant right-sided pneumothorax has accumulated in spite of chest tube drainage. **B.** This left-side-down lateral film taken at the same time shows marked resolution of the pneumothorax. *Note:* Pneumothoraxes will frequently drain after repositioning of the infant.

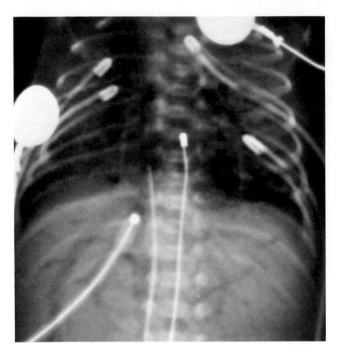

Figure 6-17   Venous air embolism. Air is visible in the cardiac chamber and hepatic veins.

monary diseases which obstruct airway lumina. Individuals with these chest conditions who ascend to high elevations or participate in deep-sea diving are at risk.

When air embolism occurs in older patients, it is accompanied by sudden onset of air hunger, dyspnea, cough, and chest pain. In addition to physical signs of tachypnea, tachycardia, and hypotension, a "mill-wheel" murmur is produced by air in the old bloodstream.

Pneumoperitoneum

In ventilated infants who develop thoracic air leak and pneumoperitoneum, pneumoperitoneum usually occurs as a result of air dissection from the chest.[34] However, perforation of a viscus also occurs in debilitated infants, and the differentiation be-

tween a pneumoperitoneum from bowel perforation and one from air dissection is frequently difficult. Unfortunately, pneumoperitoneum may occur from perforation in infants who manifest thoracic air leak; and in contrast, neonates may develop pneumoperitoneum without perforation or thoracic air leak.[35]

Cohen and coworkers[35] advocate the use of a water-soluble agent (metrizamide) to exclude perforation of a viscus in infants with pneumoperitoneum. They reported on four patients with pneumoperitoneum from dissected thoracic air in whom no radiographically evident pneumothorax or pneumomediastinum was present. Knight and Abdenour,[36] in a review of 13 neonates with pneumoperitoneum, found that pneumothorax and/or pneumomediastinum were present in all patients with pneumoperitoneum from dissected air and in none with perforated viscus. These authors also concluded that the presence or absence of peritoneal fluid levels was of little help in establishing the diagnosis of perforated viscus. Knight and Abdenour did find, however, that there was a considerable difference in the mechanical pressure settings between the children with intestinal perforations and those with dissected air. Mean peak inspiratory pressure was 34- to 38-cmH$_2$O in all children with dissected air and 5.2- to 19.3-cmH$_2$O in those with perforation.

In cases where a decision between dissected air and perforated viscus cannot be made, needle aspiration of the peritoneum may be of help.

The radiographic signs of pneumoperitoneum should be quite obvious, but they may be missed on supine films. When pneumoperitoneum is present, it should be recognized on chest studies that include a portion of the upper abdomen (Figure 6-18).[37]

References

1. Macklin CC: Transport of air along sheaths of pulmonic blood vessels from alveoli to mediastinum: Clinical implications. *Arch Int Med* 64:913, 1939.
2. Wood BP, Anderson VM, Mauk JE, et al: Pulmonary lymphatic air: Locating "pulmonary interstitial emphysema of the premature infant." *AJR* 138:809, 1982.

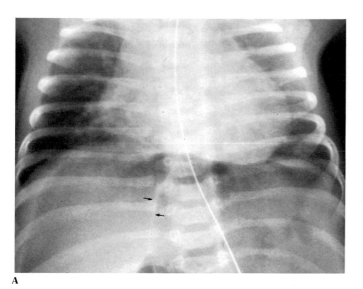
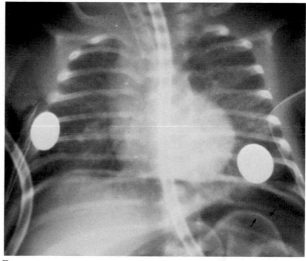

A   B

Figure 6-18   Pneumoperitoneum. Two cases are presented to illustrate pneumoperitoneum visible on supine chest film. **A.** Central air collection outlines a vertical white line, the falciform ligament (arrows). **B.** Air is present under both diaphragmatic leaves, along the inferior heart border, and on either side of the bowel loops (arrows).

3. Leonidas JC, Bhan I, McCauley RGK: Persistent localized pulmonary interstitial emphysema and lymphangiectasia: A causal relationship? *Pediatrics* 64:105, 1979.

4. Fletcher BC, Outerbridge EW, Youssef S, et al: Pulmonary interstitial emphysema in a newborn treated by lobectomy. *Pediatrics* 54:808, 1974.

5. Stocker JT, Madewell JE: Persistent interstitial pulmonary emphysema: Another complication of respiratory disease syndrome. *Pediatrics* 59:847, 1977.

6. MacPherson RI, Chernick V, Reed M: The complication of respiratory therapy in the newborn. *J Can Assoc Radiol* 23:91, 1972.

7. Swischuk LE: Bubbles in hyaline membrane disease. Differentiation of three types. *Radiology* 122:417, 1977.

8. Kirkpatrick BV, Felman AH, Eitzman DV: Complications of ventilator therapy in respiratory distress syndrome. Recognition and management of acute air leaks. *AM J Dis Child* 128:496, 1974.

9. Smith TH, Currarino G, Rutledge JC: Spontaneous occurrence of localized pulmonary interstitial emphysema and endolymphatic emphysema in infancy. *Pediatr Radiol* 14:142, 1984.

10. Chernick V, Avery ME: Spontaneous alveolar rupture at birth. *Pediatrics* 32:816, 1963.

11. Brooks JG, Bustamante SA, Koops BL, et al: Selective bronchial intubation for the treatment of severe local-ized pulmonary interstitial emphysema in newborn infants. *J Pediatr* 91:648, 1977.

12. Vahey TN, Pratt, GB, Baum RS: Treatment of localized pulmonary emphysema with selective bronchial intubation. *AJR* 140:1107, 1983.

13. Magilner AD, Capitanio MA, Wertheimer I, et al: Persistent localized intrapulmonary emphysema: An observation in three infants. *Radiology* 111:379, 1974.

14. Drew JH, Landau LI, Actor CM, et al: Pulmonary interstitial emphysema requiring lobectomy. Complication of assisted ventilation. *Arch Dis Child* 53:424, 1978.

15. Martinez-Frontanilla LA, Hernandez J, Haase G, et al: Surgery of acquired lobar emphysema in the neonate. *J Pediatr Surg* 19:375, 1984.

16. Schneider JR, St Cyr JA, Thompson TR: The changing spectrum of cystic pulmonary lesions requiring surgical resection in infants. *J Thorac Cardiovasc Surg* 89:332, 1985.

17. Leonidas JC, Hall RT, Rhodes PG: Conservative management of unilateral pulmonary interstitial emphysema under tension. *J Pediatr* 87:776, 1975.

18. Cohen RS, Smith DW, Stevenson DK: Lateral decubitus position as therapy for persistent focal pulmonary interstitial emphysema in neonates: A preliminary report. *J Pediatr* 104:441, 1984.

19. Lopez JB, Campbell RE, Bishop HC, et al: Non-opera-

tive resolution of prolonged localized intrapulmonary interstitial emphysema associated with hyaline membrane disease. *J Pediatr* 94:653, 1977.

20. Morrow G III, Hope JW, Boggs TR Jr: Pneumomediastinum, a silent lesion in the newborn. *J Pediatr* 70:554, 1967.

21. Talbert JL, Rodgers BM, Felman AH, et al: Traumatic perforation of the hypopharynx in infants. *J Thorac Cardiovasc Surg* 74:152, 1977.

22. Purohit DM, Lorenzo RL, Bradford BF: Bronchial laceration in the newborn with persistent posterior pneumomediastinum. *J Pediatr Surg* 20:82, 1985.

23. Harrell GS, Friedland GW, Daily WJ, et al: Neonatal Boerhaave's syndrome. *Radiology* 95:665, 1976.

24. Matthieu JM, Nussle D, Torrado A, et al: Pneumopericardium in the newborn. *Pediatrics* 46:117, 1970.

25. Burt TB, Lester PD: Neonatal pneumopericardium. *Radiology* 142:82, 1982.

26. Maurer ER, Mendez FL Jr, Finkelstein M, et al: Cardiovascular dynamics in pneumopericardium and hydropericardium. *Angiology* 9:176, 1958.

27. Steele RW, Metz JR, Bass JW, et al: Pneumothorax and pneumomediastinum in the newborn. *Radiology* 98:629, 1971.

28. Hoffer FA, Ablow RC: The cross-table lateral view in neonatal pneumothorax. *AJR* 142:1283, 1984.

29. Allen RW, Jung AL, Lester PD: Effectiveness of tube evacuation of pneumothorax in neonates. *J Pediatr* 99:629, 1981.

30. Mathew OP, Bhatia J: Management of persistent pneumothorax: An innovative approach. *J Pediatr* 103:117, 1983.

31. Kogut MS: Systemic air embolism secondary to respiratory therapy in the neonate: Six cases including one survivor. *AJR* 131:425, 1978.

32. Van Allen CM, Hardina LS, Clark J: Air embolism from the pulmonary vein. A clinical and experimental study. *Arch Surg* 19:567, 1929.

33. Chin, CJ, Golding MR, Linder JB, et al: Pulmonary venous air embolism: A hemodynamic reappraisal. *Surgery* 61:816, 1967.

34. Joannides M, Tsoulos GD: The etiology of interstitial and mediastinal emphysema: Experimental production of air embolism, acute pneumothorax, acute pneumoperitoneum, interstitial, mediastinal, and retroperitoneal emphysema. *Arch Surg* 21:333, 1930.

35. Cohen MD, Schreiner RS, Lemons J: Neonatal pneumoperitoneum without significant adventitious pulmonary air: Use of metrizamide to rule out perforation of bowel. *Pediatrics* 69:587, 1982.

36. Knight PJ, Abdenour G: Pneumoperitoneum in the ventilated neonate: Respiratory or gastrointestinal origin? *J Pediatr* 98:972, 1981.

37. Gfeller-Varga DA, Felman AH: Pneumoperitoneum. Diagnosis from chest radiographs. *Clin Pediatr* 19:761, 1980.

Chapter 7

Chronic Lung Disease

Life-support systems which have been developed to treat neonatal respiratory distress employ a variety of methods to oxygenate the lungs. Most of these use different combinations of equipment that are designed to deliver oxygen through an endotracheal tube to the alveoli at increased pressure. While these methods are responsible in large measure for improved infant survival, they are also guilty, at least as accessories, in the development of chronic pulmonary disease that has in the past been unknown or overlooked.

The most significant and well-studied forms of chronic lung disease in premature infants are (1) pulmonary dysmaturity (Wilson-Mikity or Mikity-Wilson syndrome) and (2) bronchopulmonary dysplasia (BPD). There is considerable overlap in the clinical, radiographic, and pathologic features of these two conditions, and with the advances in newborn therapy, it probably is incorrect to try to separate the two. The above notwithstanding, this chapter will consider the two as separate, but not equal, diseases.

In addition to these well-described syndromes, many other factors color the picture of intensive neonatal therapy, not the least of which is a host of infecting organisms that always seem to germinate in intensive care nurseries.

Pulmonary Dysmaturity (Wilson-Mikity Syndrome)

In 1960, Wilson and Mikity[1] described a unique type of chronic lung disease in premature infants. Their patients developed generalized, cystlike changes on chest radiograph several weeks after birth. The children had not been treated with mechanical ventilation or significant oxygen, and though mildly distressed at birth, they did not suffer from hyaline membrane disease (HMD). The lung changes were usually self-limited, but in patients who died, characteristic pathologic findings were observed. Since Wilson and Mikity's original study, additional similar cases have been reported.[2,3]

With the development of improved methods for treating HMD, most infants with significant neonatal respiratory distress are treated with oxygen and mechanical ventilation. Therefore, the true incidence of Wilson-Mikity syndrome is quite low, and radiographic distinction between this syndrome and BPD is virtually impossible.

Bronchopulmonary Dysplasia

In 1967, Northway, Rosan, and Porter[4] described a group of infants in whom lung changes appeared after treatment for HMD with oxygen, endotracheal intubation, and mechanical ventilation. They labeled this condition *bronchopulmonary dysplasia*. Originally reported only after severe HMD, it is now recognized that BPD may complicate other types of neonatal lung disease. Among these are meconium aspiration syndrome, neonatal pneumonia, congenital heart disease, and immature lung.

Since Northway and his colleagues' original report, extensive literature on the subject has been generated; one of the more complete reviews is in the *Journal of Pediatrics*.[5] In spite of a prodigious effort directed at an understanding of this enigmatic disease, whether or not to report BPD is a question that often faces radiologists involved with neonates.

It should be emphasized that BPD is, above all else, an iatrogenic disease. As preventive and therapeutic measures used to treat neonatal respiratory distress continue to evolve, changes may be expected in the clinical, radiologic, and pathologic patterns of BPD. Indeed, the present manifestations of BPD are significantly different from those originally reported.[6,7]

The cause, or causes, of BPD is incompletely understood at present, but the administration of oxygen probably plays a key role. The mechanism of oxygen damage remains unclear.[8] However, for the changes of BPD to occur, oxygen must be administered through an endotracheal tube at increased atmospheric pressures to an already damaged lung (as in HMD).

Other factors undoubtedly contribute to the development of BPD, but their significance cannot always be determined. Patent ductus arteriosus,[9] excess fluid,[10,11] severity of underlying disease, and interstitial emphysema may play a role.[12]

Pulmonary maturation is basic to the pathogenesis of chronic lung disease of the newborn. Clinically significant BPD usually does not develop in smaller infants (less than 1000 g) who display little or no respiratory distress at birth. The lungs of these patients may assume a diffuse opacity, with streaky infiltrates. The radiographic lung changes are related, in some way, to markedly immature pulmonary development. However, this process does not usually progress through the stages of HMD and BPD.[6] The majority of these infants recover, and their chest studies return to normal. The "full-blown" picture of BPD is more often seen in infants who weigh more than 1000 g at birth (Figure 7-1).[4,6]

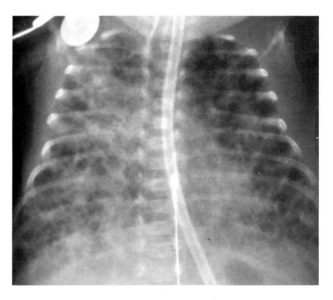

Figure 7-1 Bronchopulmonary dysplasia. Film studies such as this are familiar sights around pediatric neonatal units where oxygen is available. Once infection and a few rare congenital abnormalities have been excluded, the diagnosis of BPD can be made from this film study with reasonable certainty. The lungs are generally hyperaerated, the left lung slightly more than the right. The parenchyma is completely replaced by a disorganized pattern of random opacities and lucencies with some areas of coalescence, especially on the right. There is little thymic tissue. Heart borders are completely obliterated by adjacent atelectatic or infiltrated lung.

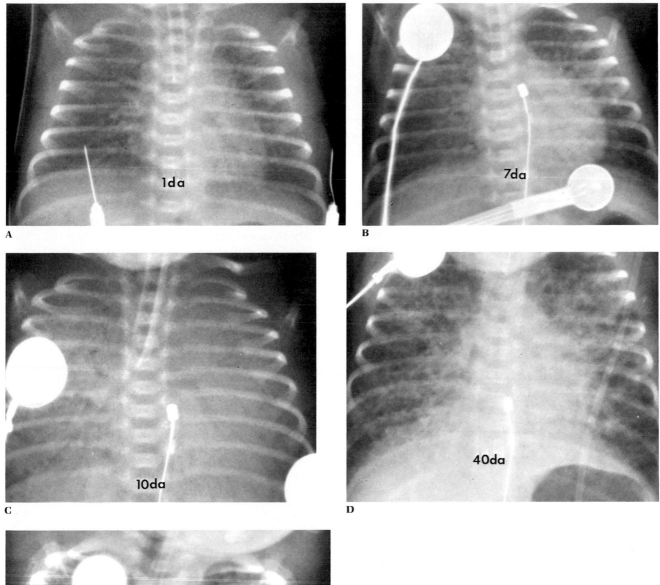

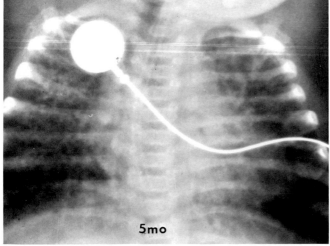

Figure 7-2 Bronchopulmonary dysplasia—typical progression. A. A patient with typical radiographic features of HMD on mechanical ventilation. **B.** After 7 days the lungs have failed to clear normally, and the central vasculature is ill-defined and suggests the presence of a shunt to the lungs. Patent ductus arteriosus was suspected at this time. **C.** Three days later, the lungs are completely opaque with pulmonary edema. Patent ductus arteriosus was ligated. **D.** One month later, a typical pattern of BPD is established. **E.** Three months later, the pattern is unchanged, with no radiographic progression. *Note:* In all likelihood, the presence of a PDA contributed to the development of BPD in this patient.

The typical radiographic alterations of HMD show early pulmonary involvement which progresses over 2 to 3 days (Figure 7-2). If no complications ensue, the lungs begin to clear within 4 to 7 days. Reappearance of vascular detail is the first revelation of roentgenographic resolution. Within 6 to 8 days the lungs should return to normal. If the radiopacity of the lungs fail to resolve and vascular shadows do not reappear, several possibilities should be entertained. One is that the HMD process is slow to recover, for whatever reason. Another cause for delayed radiographic clearing is the development of early BPD (stage I or II). Up to this time the condition is reversible, and the chest studies may return to normal or near normal. During this transition, it is often impossible to separate early-stage BPD from persistent HMD solely on the basis of film studies.

If a generalized pulmonary opacity is accompanied by signs of cardiomegaly and pulmonary edema (indistinct vessels, thickened fissures), the possibility of a complicating patent ductus arteriosus (PDA) should be considered (Figure 7-2B and C). Other causes for generalized opacification, in addition to PDA and congestive failure, include fluid overload and/or diminished renal output, pulmonary hemorrhage, massive aspiration, and infection, especially with non-group A beta streptococci. Clinical correlation with the radiographic appearance

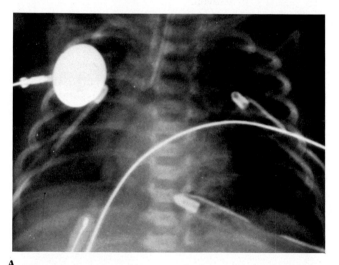

A

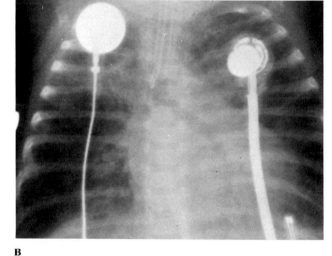

B

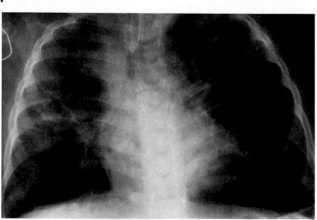

C

Figure 7-3 Bronchopulmonary dysplasia—end-stage lung. A. This film demonstrates multiple tube thoracotomies and developing chronic lung disease. **B.** Six weeks later, the patient is stable but remains on respiratory therapy. The lungs retain their appearance of chronic disease. **C.** Seven months later, end-stage lungs have developed, the patient remains on ventilatory therapy, and is fed through a gastrostomy.

will often help separate these various underlying processes. Patients with PDA are usually slow to wean from the respirator.

In those unfortunate patients destined to develop progressive BPD, the lungs assume the unhappy appearance of coarse, irregular, linear densities, admixed with lucent, cystlike foci (Figures 7-1 and 7-2D and E). Within a fortnight or two, generalized hyperaeration ensues, often accompanied by focal, shifting atelectasis. Episodes of aspiration, fluid overload, and/or congestive failure often complicate this radiographic portrait (Figure 7-2C). In most patients, the disease stabilizes and may even improve (Figure 7-2D and E). In others, the process marches inexorably to its ultimate outcome of end-stage lung (Figure 7-3). Superimposed pneumonia is a constant threat, and when present, is often masked by the underlying lung disease. Cor pulmonale is an unfortunate complication, but right heart enlargement is difficult to assess radiographically (Figure 7-4).

Not uncommonly, in the course of treatment of HMD, pulmonary interstitial emphysema (PIE) supervenes. The radiographic pattern of PIE may prove difficult to distinguish from BPD (see Chapter 6, Figure 6-5) and depends upon its severity and duration. A survey of sequential studies often helps solve this difficult differential dilemma (see Chapter 6).

Attempts have been made to standardize the radiographic findings of BPD.[13] Wide variations in both the radiographic and clinical presentations of BPD limit the usefulness of scoring systems. Also, in the early stages of disease (stages I and II), the radiographic appearance of BPD correlates poorly with the pathologic findings in any given patient.[14] As later stages occur (III and IV), radiologic-pathologic correlation improves.

Pathologic Findings

The microscopic appearance of BPD is usually characteristic. Although changes in the treatment and

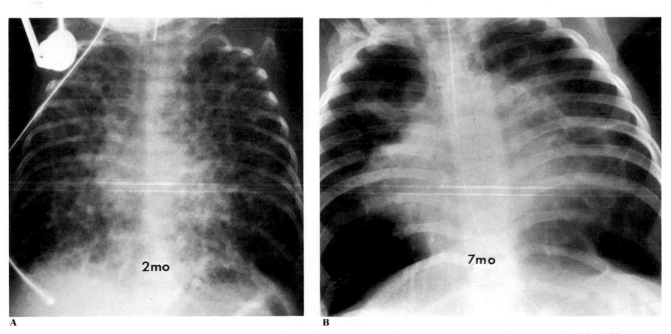

Figure 7-4 Bronchopulmonary dysplasia—cor pulmonale. A. Advanced BPD is present in this 2-month-old child. **B.** Five months later, the cardiac silhouette is markedly enlarged, the peripheral lung fields are emphysematous, and the cardiopericardial silhouette is obliterated by the adjacent collapsed lung. This child died shortly thereafter, and autopsy revealed right heart dilatation from cor pulmonale.

longevity of patients have markedly influenced the histologic material available from those who die of BPD, the following characterization of pathologic

stages, originally suggested by Rosan in 1975,[15] is still valid. The divisions between stages are not well de-

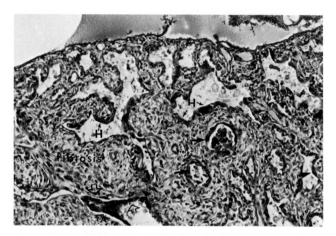

Figure 7-5   Bronchopulmonary dysplasia—stage II. Most areas of the underdeveloped lung have persistent hyaline membrane fragments (H). Regeneration of alveolar epithelial cells is taking place (arrows). Bronchiolar epithelial metaplasia is also evident (open arrows). Pronounced immature interstitial fibrosis separates the alveolar sacs. This histologic section illustrates the three major components of BPD: (1) alveolar cell hyperplasia, (2) bronchiolar hyperplasia, and (3) interstitial fibrosis.

	Pathology
Stage I (0–4 days)	Hyaline membranes, hyperemia, atelectasis, lymphatic dilatation, patchy loss of ciliated cells, and necrosis of bronchiolar mucosa
Stage II (4–10 days)	Persisting hyaline membranes, bronchiolar necrosis, eosinophilic exudate into lumen, squamous metaplasia, and interstitial edema (Figures 7-5 and 7-6)
Stage III (10–20 days)	Fewer hyaline membranes, persisting alveolar epithelial injury, bronchial and bronchiolar mucosal metaplasia, irregular aeration with emphysematous and atelectatic alveoli (Figures 7-7 and 7-8)
Stage IV (> 1 month)	Focally circumscribed groups of emphysematous alveoli; marked separation of capillaries from alveolar epithelia; increased collagen fibers; tortuous, dilated lymphatics; early vascular lesions of pulmonary hypertension; and right ventricular hypertrophy

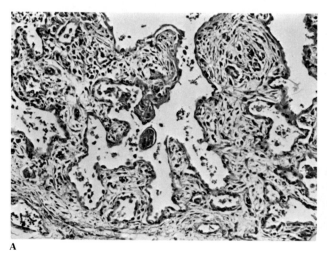

A

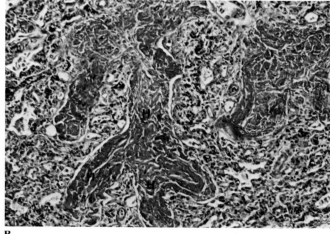

B

Figure 7-6   Bronchopulmonary dysplasia—stage II. A. Cell fragments and debris are scattered throughout the saccular lumina. The alveolar lining epithelium is regenerative and locally hyperplastic. The interstitium is thickened with immature fibroblastic activity. **B.** Different section of the same patient. Alveolar ducts and saccules (H) are filled with desquamated hyaline membrane fragments and necrotic epithelium.

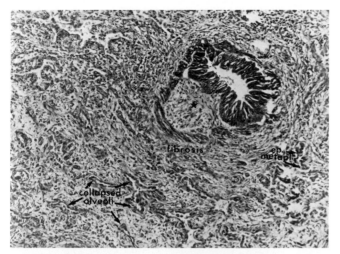

Figure 7-7 Bronchopulmonary dysplasia—stage III. This bronchiole has severe hyperplasia(∗). The alveolar saccular spaces are reduced to narrow slits because of collapse and severe interstitial fibrosis. Some regeneration and alveolar epithelial metaplasia are taking place. This histologic pattern is comparable with that shown in Figures 7-2D and 7-4A.

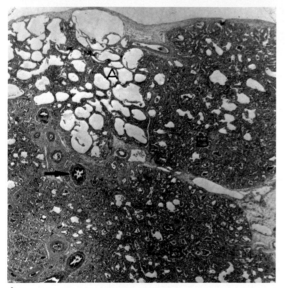

A

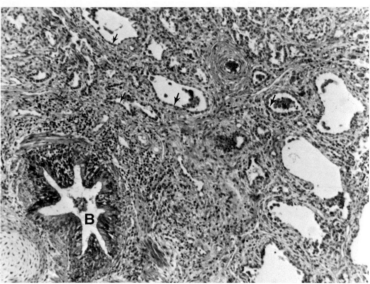

B

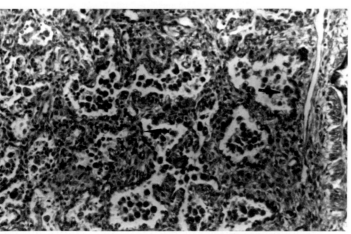

C

Figure 7-8 Bronchopulmonary dysplasia—stage III. A. This low-power view contains a markedly emphysematous section (A) adjacent to collapsed regions (B) in which alveolar saccules have thick walls and airways that are focally dilated. A bronchiole (arrow) has marked squamous metaplasia. **B.** This section contains a small bronchiole with adjacent cartilage and nearby alveolar saccules. The bronchus (B) has moderate epithelial metaplastic change. The type II pneumocytes of the alveoli are hyperplastic (arrow). Note the thick fibrous walls between these regions. The combination of epithelial hyperplasia, alveolar wall thickening, and metaplastic change in the bronchioles is typical of the long-term stage for bronchopulmonary dysplasia. **C.** The alveolar-saccular walls are thick and cellular. Type II alveolar pneumocytes (arrows) are hyperplastic, and many have desquamated into the saccular space.

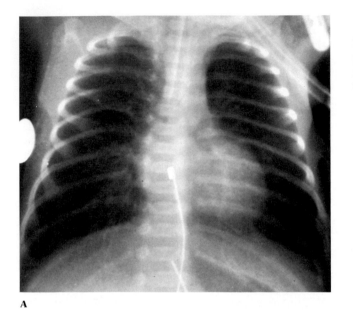

A

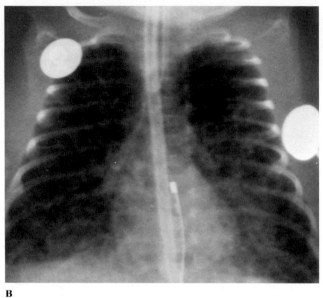

B

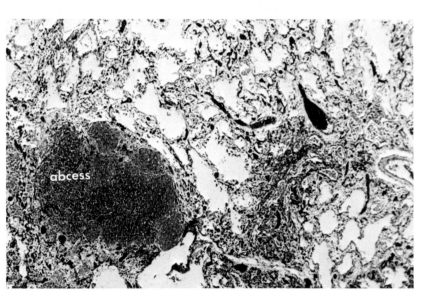

C

Figure 7-9   Focal interstitial fibrosis—superimposed infection. A. The lungs show little abnormality, but the patient demanded ventilatory assistance. **B.** Three weeks later, the lungs have a generalized pattern of coarse, irregular opacities resembling BPD. Note the extreme soft tissue edema. The patient expired after this film study. **C.** The histologic section of the lung shows focal interstitial fibrosis with areas of atelectasis and emphysema. Well-defined microabscesses are scattered throughout the lungs. *Pseudomonas* organisms were cultured from the blood and from these lesions.

fined, however, and radiologic-pathologic correlation is unreliable in the early stages.

Before concluding this chapter, it should again be emphasized that the lung, especially in small children, reacts in a limited way to a variety of acute or chronic insults. While certain radiographic patterns suggest the presence of specific diseases, such as BPD, close clinical correlation is mandatory for adequate diagnosis and therapy.

Acute and chronic infections (bacterial, protozoal, and/or viral) may superimpose upon the underlying disease process and not be readily appreciated on chest films alone (Figure 7-9). Chronic aspiration and recurrent congestive failure are additional conditions that may be masked by BPD. Pulmonary lymphangiectasia (congenital or acquired), cystic fibrosis, deficient host defense syndromes, tracheoesophageal fistula, and possibly other complicating abnormalities are occasionally discovered at the autopsy suite instead of in the radiology department.

References

1. Wilson MG, Mikity VG: A new form of respiratory disease in premature infants. *Am J Dis Child* 99:489, 1960.
2. Baghdassarian OM, Avery ME, Neuhauser EBD: A form of pulmonary insufficiency in premature infants. *AJR* 89:1020, 1963.
3. Grossman H, Berdon WE, Mizrahi A, et al: Neonatal focal hyperaeration of the lungs (Wilson-Mikity syndrome). *Radiology* 85:409, 1965.
4. Northway WH Jr, Rosan RC, Porter DY: Pulmonary disease following respiratory therapy of hyaline membrane disease. *N Engl J Med* 276:357, 1967.
5. Chernick V (moderator): Workshop on bronchopulmonary dysplasia. *J Pediatr* 85:1979.
6. Wung JT, Koons AH, Driscoll JM Jr, et al: Changing incidence of bronchopulmonary dysplasia. *J Pediatr* 95:845, 1979.
7. Edwards DK: Radiographic aspects of bronchopulmonary dysplasia. *J Pediatr* 95:823, 1979.
8. Stern L: The role of respirators in the etiology and pathogenesis of bronchopulmonary dysplasia. *J Pediatr* 95:867, 1979.
9. Brown E: Increased risk of bronchopulmonary dysplasia in infants with patent ductus arteriosus. *J Pediatr* 95:865, 1979.
10. Brown ER, Stark A, Sosenko I, Lawson EE, Avery ME: Bronchopulmonary dysplasia: Possible relationship to pulmonary edema. *J Pediatr* 92:982, 1978.
11. McCann EM, Lewis K, Deming DD, et al: Controlled trial of furosemide therapy in infants with chronic lung disease. *J Pediatr* 106:957, 1985.
12. Stahlman MT, Cheatham W, Gray ME: The role of air dissection in bronchopulmonary dysplasia. *J Pediatr* 95:878, 1979.
13. Toce SS, Farrell PM, Leavitt LA, et al: Clinical and roentgenographic scoring systems for assessing bronchopulmonary dysplasia. *Am J Dis Child* 138:581, 1984.
14. Edwards DK, Colby TV, Northway WH Jr: Radiographic-pathologic correlation in bronchopulmonary dysplasia. *J Pediatr* 95:834, 1979.
15. Rosan RC: Hyaline membrane disease and a related spectrum of neonatal pneumopathies. *Perspect Pediatr Pathol* 2:15, 1975.

Section III

Mediastinum

In the mediastinum, vital structures are gathered in close proximity so that pathologic alterations of any one are likely to affect others. The mediastinum is considered anatomically as that portion of the body within the thoracic cage located between the pleural spaces. For the purposes of radiologic localization, it is convenient to subdivide the mediastinum into anterior, middle, and posterior compartments, although authorities differ over the exact boundaries. In addition, a superior mediastinal compartment is sometimes identified. The development of computed tomography and magnetic resonance imaging has improved the accuracy of anatomic placement of lesions within the mediastinum (see Section VII).

The precise location of mediastinal lesions often helps to predict the existing pathosis.

Anterior	Middle
Germ cell tumor	Aneurysm
Teratoma	Pericardial cyst
Thymus	Duplication
Thymic neoplasm	Lymph nodes
Lymphoma	Bronchogenic cyst
Pericardial cyst	Thymus
Bronchogenic cyst	
Intrathoracic goiter	
Diaphragmatic hernia	

Posterior	Superior
Neural tumor	Vascular lesion
Neurenteric cyst	Cystic hygroma
Duplication	Neural tumor
Diaphragmatic hernia	Thymus
Thymus	Bronchogenic cyst
Bronchogenic cyst	
Lipomatosis	
Vertebral infection	

The clinical features of mediastinal disease depend upon (1) the type of the pathology present, (2) the rate of development, (3) the location of the disease, and (4) the age of the patient. In spite of the closely packed anatomy, it is not unusual for advanced mediastinal disease to be discovered before any significant clinical signs are manifest. Also, signs and symptoms of generalized disease (e.g., leukemia, lymphoma) may overshadow their mediastinal components and thus delay the diagnosis.

A feeling of pain, ache, or discomfort within the chest may result from mediastinal lesions that impinge upon nerves or pleural structures. Horner's syndrome will occur when cervical sympathetic nerves are involved. Posterior mediastinal tumors have a tendency to involve the intervertebral foramina and nerves, as well as the spinal canal, sometimes leading to paresis or paralysis.

Gastrointestinal symptoms are unusual, and when present, often relate to swallowing. Dysphagia and painful or unusual swallowing sensations may result from processes that interfere with peristaltic activity, whereas marked deviation of the esophagus may go unnoticed. While traction diverticula from adjacent inflammatory lesions may lead to retained food substances, vomiting is distinctly uncommon.

Stridorous breathing, chronic cough, and like symptoms of respiratory distress often accompany mediastinal mass lesions. Respiratory symptomatology often relates to the location, size, and physical character of the mass or infection, as well as the age of the patient.

Rib attenuation and osseous erosion are signs of long-standing posterior mediastinal processes. Enlarged intervertebral foramina and thinned vertebral pedicles suggest the presence of a neurogenic tumor. Calcification within such lesions strongly implies an origin from the sympathetic nervous tissue, i.e., neuroblastoma and ganglioneuroma. Malformations of vertebral bodies and adjacent ribs are often found in association with developmental defects in the primitive neurenteric canal and may accompany neurenteric cyst or esophageal duplication.

The following are mediastinal abnormalities and disease conditions to be covered in this section:

1. Tumors and tumor-like conditions
   a. Thymus (normal—hyperplasia)
   b. Thymoma
   c. Germ cell (teratoma, seminoma, yolk sac)
   d. Cardiac
   e. Pericardium
   f. Neurogenic
   g. Lymphoma—leukemia
   h. Endobronchial
   i. Vascular
   j. Lymphangioma
2. Congenital abnormalities
   a. Thymus
   b. Diaphragmatic hernia
   c. Diaphragmatic eventration
3. Inflammatory processes
   a. Tuberculosis
   b. Atypical tuberculosis
   c. Histoplasmosis
   d. Traumatic
   e. Osteomyelitis

Chapter 8

Thymus

The thymus is a complex organ which, because of its function, biologic behavior, and frequently unusual radiologic appearance, often presents challenging situations to pediatricians, surgeons, radiologists, and similar types. Embryologically, the thymus develops from the third pharyngeal pouch during the sixth week of fetal life. Its lymphocytes arise from hematopoietic stem cells that colonize the epithelial thymic anlage during the third month of fetal development. At birth, it is an anterior, midline, thoracic organ, totally enclosed within a fibrous capsule.

This chapter will cover the following thymic-related conditions:

1. Normal thymus
2. Thymic hypoplasia-aplasia
3. Thymic hyperplasia
4. Intrathymic hemorrhage
5. Thymic neoplasms
    a. Thymoma
    b. Thymic cyst

Normal Thymus

The thymus is partially responsible for developing and maintaining cell-mediated immune responses, such as graft-host rejection and delayed hypersensitivity. T lymphocytes, produced in the thymus, also play a role in the production of humoral antibodies. Through these pathways, the thymus plays a protective role in the development of resistance to infections, malignancy, and immune disorders.

The roentgenographic appearance of the thymus is often quite variable and can be best understood when the anatomic and physical characteristics of the gland are appreciated. As a bilobed, pyramidal structure, the thymus occupies the anterosuperior mediastinum and frequently extends beyond the edges of the cardiac shadow. On lateral projection, it is seen filling the anterior or retrosternal clear space, frequently displaying a well-defined inferior border. Because of its soft physical characteristics, the normal thymus will often change shape during respiration.

The "sail" sign and "wave" sign are markers which help chart the thymus (Figure 8-1A and B). These are often seen to better advantage on films exposed at a slight heel or obliquity (Figure 8-2). In difficult cases, inspiration-expiration films may be of help (Figure 8-3), and, as in so many similar situations, old film studies frequently bail out the radiologist. Fluoroscopic evaluation offers yet another convenient method of anchoring the diagnosis.

Differentiation between thymus and heart may cause problems when the two appear as a confluent shadow. A "notch," seen along the left cardiothymic

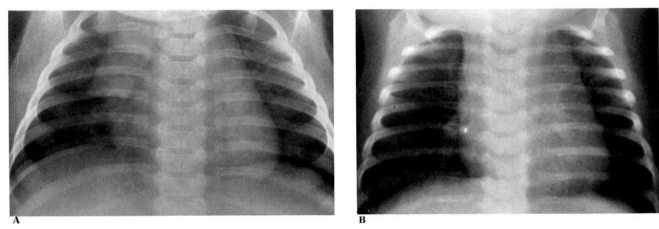

A   **B**

Figure 8-1   Normal thymus. A. "Sail" sign. The normal thymus is seen as a triangular density extending into the right upper hemithorax. It resembles a jib or main sail; not to be confused with the spinnaker sail sign of the pneumomediastinum (see Figure 6-11). **B.** "Wave" sign. The scalloped margin of the left upper mediastinal opacity identifies this as thymus; the indentations are produced by rib impressions on the soft thymic tissue.

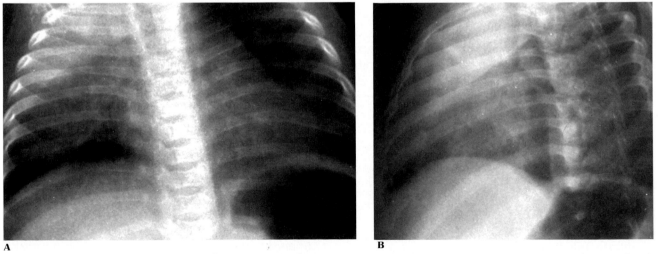

A   **B**

Figure 8-2   Normal thymus—oblique view. A. The frontal film demonstrates a shadow of double density in the right upper hemithorax. Part of this shadow is well demarcated by the adjacent lung; the remainder fades into the mediastinum. This was initially considered to be pneumonia, but the nonanatomic distribution, absence of air bronchograms, and general gestalt favor thymus. **B.** The left anterior oblique film confirms the findings on the frontal film and supports the diagnosis of normal thymus. The patient received no treatment.

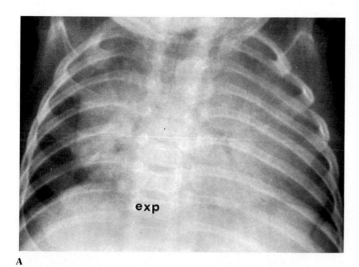 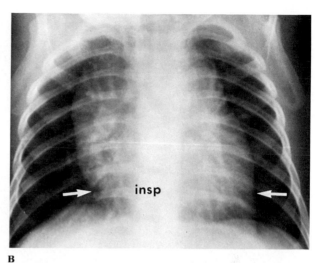

A   B

Figure 8-3   Normal thymus—inspiration-expiration (supine). A. The expiration film (buckled trachea) shows most of the thorax occupied by the cardiothymic silhouette. **B.** The inspiration film stretches out the malleable thymus (straight trachea). Bilateral cardiothymic notches (arrows) are described in Figure 8-4. *Note:* Supine films tend to be less well aerated and therefore often show larger cardiothymic shadow. This is the preferred position for children unable to sit alone, and in any event, a child with a large thymus who is able to empty the lungs cannot be too sick.

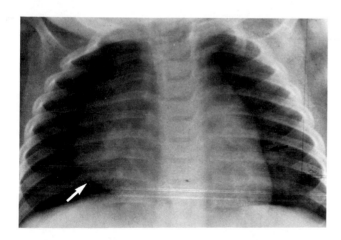

Figure 8-4   Normal cardiothymic notches. The indentation (black arrow) along the left cardiac border designates the junction of the thymus and heart. *Note:* There is a wavy contour of the right thymic edge (positive wave sign). The white arrow identifies the right cardiothymic interface.

border, delineates the junction of heart and thymus in selected patients (Figure 8-4). In the lateral projection, the thymus usually occupies the upper anterior mediastinum, filling in the retrosternal clear space, in contrast to an enlarged heart that more often pro-

jects posteriorly. Normal pulmonary vascularity is additional evidence of a normal heart. Congestion or engorgement of pulmonary vessels is best observed in the lateral projection in the presence of a large thymus. (See Chapter 4, Figures 4-7 and 4-8.)

In young children (up to 2 + years) the thymus is often a barometer of well-being. Well-nourished children in this age group often have generous thymic tissue, whereas a large, normal thymus in a thin, poorly nourished, chronically ill child would be unlikely. The general state of nutrition may also be gauged by the amount of subcutaneous fat and the thickness of soft tissue of the chest wall, especially anterior to the sternum.

Occasionally the thymus, or portion of thymus, fails to migrate from its cervical origin to the mediastinum. This ectopic, cervical, thymic tissue often becomes cystic and may impinge upon the cervical trachea and esophagus.[1] On rare occasions, the thymus may change course and dock in the posterior or middle mediastinum (Figure 8-5). Recognition of this may be aided by the use of computed tomography (CT).[2] (See Chapter 26, Figure 26-3.)

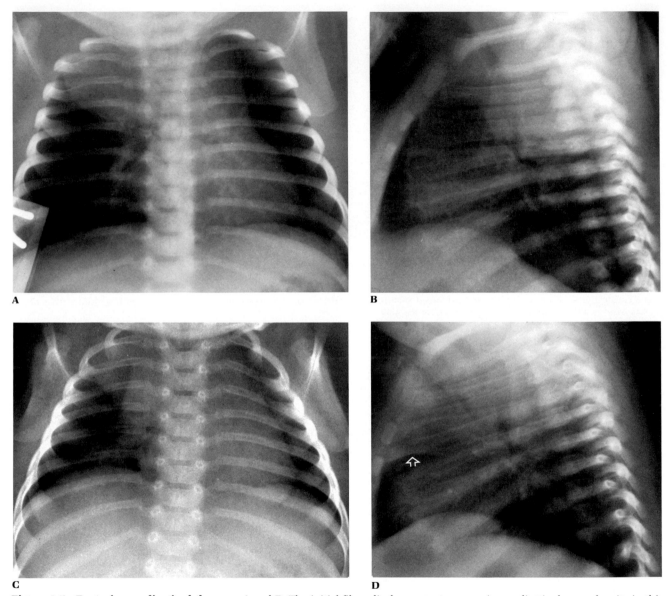

A

B

C

D

Figure 8-5   Posterior mediastinal thymus. **A** and **B.** The initial films disclose a posterosuperior mediastinal mass density in this asymptomatic child. **C.** One month later, the opacity has the characteristic anterior mediastinal thymic sail sign. **D.** The lateral film reveals substernal thymic tissue and typical pulmonary interface (arrow). (Courtesy of Dr. Mary Ann Radkowski, Chicago, Illinois.)

Thymic tissue, while most visible radiographically in early childhood, reaches its peak volume at puberty. Evidence of thymic tissue is expected on chest films of children up to 2 or 3 years of age. Thereafter, it is seen with decreasing frequency, but the presence of significant thymic tissue beyond this age is sometimes normal (Figure 8-6). Some functioning thymus tissue is present throughout life in the absence of marked stress involution. Small amounts of thymic tissue are regularly identified on CT well into adulthood. Various disease states including hyperthyroidism, Addison's disease, and neoplasm will cause the thymus to enlarge abnormally.

The use of CT for the identification and evaluation of the thymus has been advocated (see Chapter 26). Francis and coworkers,[3] in a study of 309 normal patients studied with CT, found that the anatomic shape of the normal gland as compared with abnormal processes was the most reliable differentiating feature (Figure 8-7). Ultrasonography is also of use in the definition of the thymus and other anterior mediastinal masses.

Rapid involution of the thymus often accompanies periods of illness or systemic stress, and may be induced by the administration of corticosteriods. Differentiation between thymus and other mass lesions of the anterior mediastinum with the administration of steroids has been advocated but is not always reliable. Tumors, especially lymphomas, will also regress with steroid therapy. Recovery from stress allows the thymus to return to normal over a period of several weeks to months; on occasion, the thymus will overgrow in these recovery periods. (See Chapter 26, Figure 26-37).

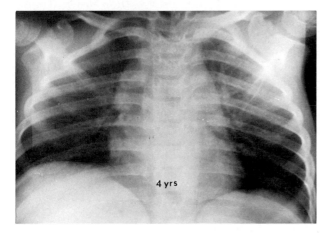

Figure 8-6 Normal thymus—older child. Prominent thymic tissue projects to the right of the mediastinal shadow in this asymptomatic 4-year-old child.

Thymic Hypoplasia-Aplasia

Hypoplasia of the Thymus

The thymus may be hypoplastic at birth, especially in premature infants. However, depleted thymic tissue in the larger neonate should raise the question of an immunodeficiency syndrome. Diseases in which the thymus is hypoplastic include Nezelof's disease, reticular dysgenesis, Swiss-type agammaglobulinemia, thymic alymphoplasia, ataxia telan-

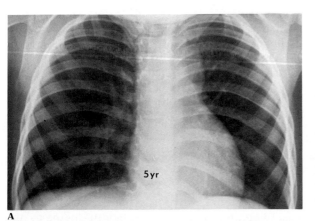

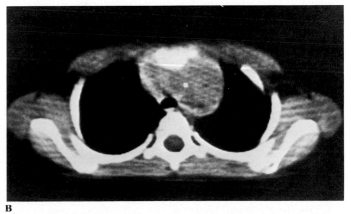

A   B

Figure 8-7 Normal thymus—older child. A. This mediastinal mass was discovered on chest film taken for mild pulmonary symptoms in a 5-year-old child. **B.** Computed tomography shows a mass of homogeneous density conforming to normal thymus configuration. The child has remained asymptomatic.

giectasia, and Wiskott-Aldrich syndrome. Many of these conditions have nonspecific clinical presentations and inconstant radiologic features.

Aplasia of the Thymus (DiGeorge's Syndrome, Third-Fourth Pharyngeal Pouch Syndrome)

Angelo DiGeorge (pediatrician, endocrinologist, and senior raconteur of St. Christopher's Hospital for Children in Philadelphia) and his coworkers originally called attention to abnormalities associated with aplasia of the thymus.[4-6] In classic DiGeorge's syndrome, infants are born with little or no thymic tissue and absent hypoparathyroid glands. Additional features of this syndrome include cardiac and great vessel abnormalities (tetralogy of Fallot, persistent truncus arteriosus, transposition of the great vessels, ventricular septal defect, and absent pulmonary valve).[7-9] Defects involving the esophagus and trachea, the pinna of the ear, and part of the mandible and aortic arch occur with less frequency.

The structures that are absent or hypoplastic in DiGeorge's syndrome all trace their origin, totally or in part, from the third and fourth pharyngeal pouches which develop between 6 and 12 weeks of gestational life.

While DiGeorge's syndrome usually occurs sporadically, it has been reported in association with chromosomal abnormalities and, rarely, has been reported in siblings.[10] Ammann and coworkers[11] have suggested that maternal alcoholism may play a role in the genesis of DiGeorge's syndrome; it shares many features with the fetal alcohol syndrome.

In the neonatal period, the symptoms of thymic deficiency are often overshadowed by the accompanying congenital anomalies. Neonatal tetany results from decreased parathyroid activity and hypocalcemia, a hallmark of the syndrome. However, the onset of neonatal tetany is often delayed until several days or weeks after birth.

Since cardiorespiratory distress from associated anomalies frequently accompanies DiGeorge's syndrome, chest radiographs are often obtained (Figure 8-8).[6] Inadequate soft tissue in the retrosternal space, as seen on the lateral projection (Figure 8-8A), should raise suspicion of congenital thymic defi-

ciency or DiGeorge's syndrome. When accompanied by cardiovascular abnormalities, great vessel deformities, and/or tracheoesophageal defects, the diagnosis is more compelling.

Several pitfalls in the radiographic evaluation of thymic tissue in the neonate must be avoided. Premature infants normally have little, if any, thymic tissue visible on early chest films. Involution of the thymus in response to intrauterine stress may occur in some newborns, and neonatal illness may deplete the thymus within the first few days of life. Therefore, films with absent thymic tissue after several days of illness are of little value in supporting the diagnosis of DiGeorge's syndrome.

Because of the potential for future thymic tissue transplantation, early recognition of DiGeorge's syndrome and radiographic evaluation of the presence or absence of thymic tissue are critical before administering blood or blood products.[6]

Thymic Hyperplasia

At birth, the thymus is largest in proportion to overall body size than at any other time in life. Its mass increases throughout childhood and reaches its maximum size at puberty. Thereafter, the thymus decreases in weight but maintains a presence throughout life.[3,12] True thymic hyperplasia, a process that involves both the cortex and the medulla, does not alter its histologic appearance.[13] The thymus may enlarge for no apparent reason (thymomegaly) or as a "rebound" phenomenon following previous involution (see Chapter 26, Figure 26-37). Enlargement also occurs in hyperthyroid patients and in children under therapy for hypothyroidism who have become euthyroid.[14,15] Rarely, thymic enlargement accompanies Addison's disease, collagen vascular illness, and liver diseases including hepatic cirrhosis.

Massive thymic hyperplasia probably never causes respiratory distress of sufficient degree to necessitate treatment, although occasional case reports of this complication have been published.[16]

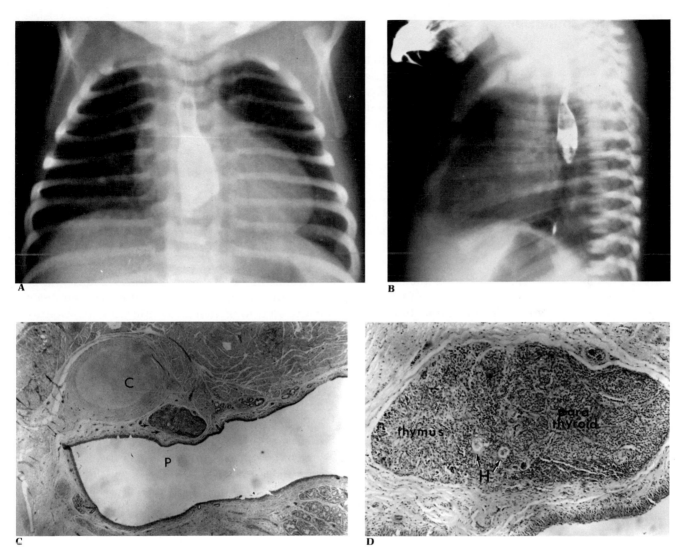

Figure 8-8   Thymic aplasia-hypoplasia (DiGeorge's syndrome). This infant was hypotonic at birth and soon after developed hypocalcemia. He died within the first week with sepsis. At autopsy, multiple cardiac abnormalities including truncus arteriosus, right aortic arch, and anomalous left subclavian artery were found. **A** and **B.** At 1 day of age, frontal and lateral films show cardiomegaly, right-sided arch, and posterior indentation on the esophagus from the aberrant subclavian artery. *Note:* The clear retrosternal space on the lateral film indicates depleted thymic tissue. **C.** This view shows the histologic section from the neck tissue block. The nodule in the center (arrows) is composed of thymus and parathyroid tissue. It is one of a symmetrical pair found in only one of 23 blocks examined. The nodule lies immediately below the epithelium of the pharyngeal lumen (P). The cartilaginous nodule (C) is the superior cornu of the thyroid cartilage. **D.** In this high-power view, the nodule consists of both parathyroid tissue and thymus. The parathyroid is distinguished by well-defined, rounded, organized collections of small cells separated by strands of fibrous stroma. This thymic tissue composed of epithelioid cells and several Hassall's corpuscles (H) was all that was found. *Note:* This patient may be considered to have "partial" DiGeorge's syndrome because of the presence of minimal thyroid and parathyroid tissue. These organs were of insufficient size to sustain their normal functions.

Intrathymic Hemorrhage

The suspicion of intrathymic hemorrhage should be raised with the onset of acute chest pain, respiratory distress, and evidence of a rapidly enlarging mediastinal mass on chest films. In the newly born child, thymic hemorrhage may accompany birth trauma or bleeding disorders. In older children, hemorrhage occurs in normal glands, thymic cysts, cystic thymomas, and cystic teratomas.

Thymic Neoplasms

Thymoma

Thymomas and tumor-like lesions of the thymus, other than malignant lymphomas, account for between 5 and 8 percent of all mediastinal tumors in childhood.[17,18] While most children with thymoma are over 10 years of age at the time of diagnosis, a case has been described in a 9-month-old child.[19] Males and females are equally affected.

Approximately one-half of all thymomas are discovered incidentally on chest film or at autopsy. The remainder present with local symptoms, often related to respiratory distress. The onset of systemic manifestations, usually myasthenia gravis, may be the first indication of thymoma in adults. Approximately 30 percent of patients with thymoma have associated myasthenia gravis, and 8 to 15 percent of those with myasthenia gravis have thymoma. In children, however, the association of thymoma with myasthenia gravis is rare or nonexistent.

The radiographic differentiation between thymoma and other causes of thymic enlargement (cyst, thymolipoma, teratoma, benign hyperplasia) may be difficult or impossible on conventional radiographs. Anterior mediastinal adenopathy may also simulate thymomegaly.[20]

Most thymomas are located in the anterior mediastinum and often appear lobulated. Calcification occurs in approximately 10 percent of cases (Figure 8-9).[20,21] Linear calcification is found in the walls of noninvasive cystic thymomas or in the fibrous capsules of well-demarcated lesions. Scattered calcifications are also present.[20] Mediastinal teratomas also show calcific densities, but in contrast to thymomas, these calcifications are typically homogeneous or solid, and they occasionally resemble teeth or bony structures. The presence of calcification excludes lymphoma, unless there has been previous radiation therapy.

Plain chest radiographs are of little or no help in determining the presence of thymoma.[22] Ultrasonography may be of use in isolated cases.[21] Computed tomography is of proven value in the recognition of myasthenia gravis–associated thymoma,[23–25] in the determination of tumor encapsulation, and in the evaluation of adjacent tissue invasion.

Malignant thymomas of similar microscopic appearance manifest different clinical behavior. In general, tumors with epithelial and mixed cell components tend to be more invasive, while thymomas in patients with myasthenia gravis are not as locally aggressive. Since invasion of adjacent tissues is the most consistent anatomic feature of malignant behavior, evaluation of the presence and extent of local spread is of extreme importance.

When metastasis occurs, it usually follows mesothelial surfaces, with tumor implanting upon pleura, pericardium, and diaphragm. While spread beyond the mediastinum is extremely rare, cases have been known to involve the neck, retroperitoneum, and liver.[20] Malignant thymomas are extremely rare in children, but they have been reported.[26,27]

Thymomas are classified histologically into four categories based upon their predominant cell types.

1. *Lymphocytic.* Lymphocytic tumors are generally smaller in size, with 33 percent under 5 cm. Approximately 25 percent are solid, 25 percent cystic, and 25 percent invasive.
2. *Epithelial.* Tumors with epithelial cells as the predominant cell type tend to be more invasive and are about equally divided in size and cystic structure.
3. *Mixed.* Mixed cell lesions are also more invasive and larger in size. Approximately 16 percent are cystic.

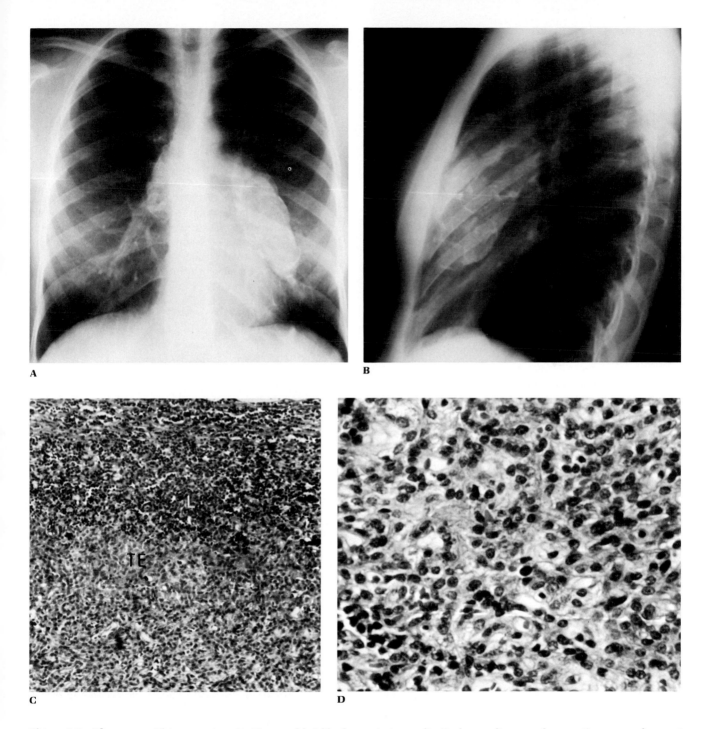

Figure 8-9 Thymoma. This asymptomatic 18-year-old girl had an anterior mediastinal mass discovered on routine preemployment radiography. **A** and **B.** A lobulated anterior mediastinal mass is present with its major component adjacent to the left heart border. Curvilinear calcifications are present about the margins and throughout the substance of the mass. **C.** In this medium-power view, most of the tumor shows fields of thymic epithelial cells (TE) and scattered mature lymphocytes (L). **D.** In this high-power view, the section illustrates the hallmark of thymoma: round to oval neoplastic epithelial cells lying in gently curved ribbons. The field contains few lymphocytes. The patient has remained well following surgical removal.

4. *Spindle.* Tumors consisting of spindle cells generally achieve the largest sizes but tend to be less invasive.[18]

No histologic difference exists between thymomas with or without myasthenia gravis.[18] Hyperplasia and germinal activity have been noted, however, in thymus glands removed for myasthenia gravis.[26]

Patients under 20 years of age with myasthenia gravis may expect good results from thymectomy.[27-29] However, prognosis is best in females with rapidly progressive, short-duration illness and increasing dependence on medication.[30,31] Transcervical resection is usually successful, eliminating the necessity of the more invasive and debilitating transsternal approach.[31]

Thymic Cyst

Thymic cysts are rare developmental abnormalities representing persistent tubular elements of the third pharyngeal pouch. They may occur anywhere along the course of embryologic thymic descent from the mandible to the diaphragm. As indicated previously, ectopic cervical thymus is more likely to become cystic and cause symptoms of tracheal or esophageal compression.[1] When located within the mediastinum, the cysts are usually asymptomatic.

References

1. Shackelford GD, McAlister WH: The aberrantly positioned thymus. A cause of mediastinal or neck masses in children. *AJR* 120:291, 1974.
2. Cohen MD, Weber TR, Sequeira FW: The diagnostic dilemma of the posterior mediastinal thymus: CT manifestations. *Radiology* 146:691, 1983.
3. Francis IR, Glazer GM, Bookstein FL, et al: The thymus: Reexamination of age-related changes in size and shape. *AJR* 145:249, 1985.
4. DiGeorge AM: Discussions on new concepts of cellular basis of immunity. *J Pediatr* 67:907, 1965.
5. DiGeorge AM, Dacou E, Lischner HW, et al: Program and Abstracts. 76th Meeting of American Pediatric Society, Atlantic City, April 27–29, 1966.
6. Kirkpatrick JA Jr, DiGeorge AM: Congenital absence of the thymus. *AJR* 103:32, 1968.
7. Rose JS, Levin DC, Goldstein S, et al: Congenital absence of the pulmonary valve associated with congenital aplasia of the thymus (DiGeorge's syndrome). *AJR* 122:97, 1974.
8. Freedom RM, Rosen JS, Nadas AS: Congenital cardiovascular disease and anomalies of third and fourth pharyngeal pouch. *Circulation* 46:165, 1972.
9. Cameron AH: Malformations of thymus and cardiovascular system. *Arch Dis Child* 40:334, 1965.
10. Raatikha M, Rapola J, Leena T, et al: Familial third and fourth pharyngeal pouch syndrome with truncus arteriosus: DiGeorge syndrome. *Pediatrics* 67:166, 1981.
11. Ammann AJ, Wara DW, Cowan MJ, et al: The DiGeorge syndrome and the fetal alcohol syndrome. *Am J Dis Child* 136:906, 1982.
12. Lack EE: Thymic hyperplasia with massive enlargement: Report of two cases with review of diagnostic criteria. *J Thorac Cardiovasc Surg* 81:741, 1981.
13. Day DL, Gedgaudas E: The thymus. *Radiol Clin North Am* 22:519, 1984.
14. Yulish BS, Owens RD: Thymic enlargement in a child during therapy for primary hypothyroidism. *AJR* 135:157, 1980.
15. Rose JS, Lam C: Thymic enlargement in association with hyperthyroidism. *Pediatr Radiol* 12:37, 1982.
16. Parker LA, Gaisie G, Scatliff JH: Computerized tomography and ultrasonographic finding in massive thymic hyperplasia. Case discussion and review of current concepts. *Clin Pediatr* 24:90, 1985.
17. Dehner LP: *Pediatric Surgical Pathology.* St. Louis, CV Mosby, 1975, pp 183–193.
18. Grosfeld JL, et al: Primary mediastinal neoplasms in infants and children. *Am J Thorac Surg* 12:179, 1971.
19. Matoni A, Dretsus C: Familial occurrence of thymoma. *Arch Pathol* 95:90, 1973.
20. Bernatz PE, Harrison EG, Clagett OT: Thymoma: A clinical pathologic study. *J Thorac Cardiovasc Surg* 42:424, 1961.
21. Rose JS, McCarthy J, Muthler RW, et al: Thymoma in childhood. *NY State J Med* 78:82, 1978.
22. Thurmond AS, Brash RC: Radiologic evaluation of the thymus in juvenile myasthenia gravis. *Pediatr Radiol* 7:136, 1978.
23. Mink JH, Bein ME, Sukov R, et al: Computed tomography of the anterior mediastinum in patients with myasthenia gravis and suspected thymoma. *AJR* 130:239, 1978.
24. Moore AV, Korobkin M, Powers B, et al: Thymoma de-

tection by mediastinal CT: Patients with myasthenia gravis. *AJR* 138:217, 1982.

25. Brown LR, Muhm JR, Sheedy PF, et al: The value of computed tomography in myasthenia gravis. *AJR* 140:31, 1983.

26. De Muth WF Jr, Smith J: Malignant thymoma in a child. *Am Surgeon* 37:742, 1971.

27. Gross RE: *The Surgery of Infancy and Childhood.* Philadelphia, WB Saunders Co, 1971.

28. Clarke RR, Van de Velde RL: Congenital myasthenia gravis. A case report with thymectomy and electron microscopic study of resected thymus. *Am J Dis Child* 122:356, 1971.

29. Fonkalsrud EW, Herrmann C Jr, Mulder DG: Thymectomy for myasthenia gravis in children. *J Pediatr Surg* 5:157, 1970.

30. Youssef S: Thymectomy for myasthenia gravis in children. *J Pediatr Surg* 18:537, 1983.

31. Campbell JR, Bisio JM, Harrison MW: Surgical treatment of myasthenia gravis in childhood. *J Pediatr Surg* 18:857, 1983.

Chapter 9

Neoplasms

Primary mediastinal masses, though uncommon in childhood, represent a heterogeneous group of cysts, congenital anomalies, and neoplasms. Dehner[1] and Bower[2] found that neurogenic tumors account for one-third of all mediastinal neoplasms. In other studies, lymphoma was determined to be the most common.[3,4] In a study by King et al., of 188 patients, approximately 75 percent of mediastinal tumors were malignant and 25 percent were benign.[3]

Clinical Presentations

Initial clinical symptoms depend on the size, location, age of patient, rapidity of growth, and pathologic characteristics of the tumors. The following is a simplified summation of the clinical presentations:

Age, yr	Benign	Malignant
< 2	Symptomatic	Asymptomatic
> 2	Asymptomatic	Symptomatic

In a study of a group of children with primary mediastinal tumors, reported by Heimberger and Battersby,[5] one-third were asymptomatic when discovered, and one-half presented with respiratory symptoms. Children less than 2 years old with benign lesions tend to present with symptoms of tracheal compression. Those more than 2 years old are usually asymptomatic. Children with malignant lesions show the opposite. Those under 2 years are more likely to be asymptomatic when discovered, while those more than 2 years often present with symptoms of fever, cough, and shortness of breath.

Mediastinal tumors may develop extremely large dimensions before the patient becomes aware of their presence. Symptoms of cough, stridor, dyspnea, and/or wheezing are caused by the mass impinging on the airway (Figure 9-1). Hoarseness and brassy cough may result from damage to the recurrent laryngeal nerve. Hemoptysis is more common in adults than in children.[6] Superior vena caval obstruction[3] and recurrent infections of the lower respiratory tract also occur.

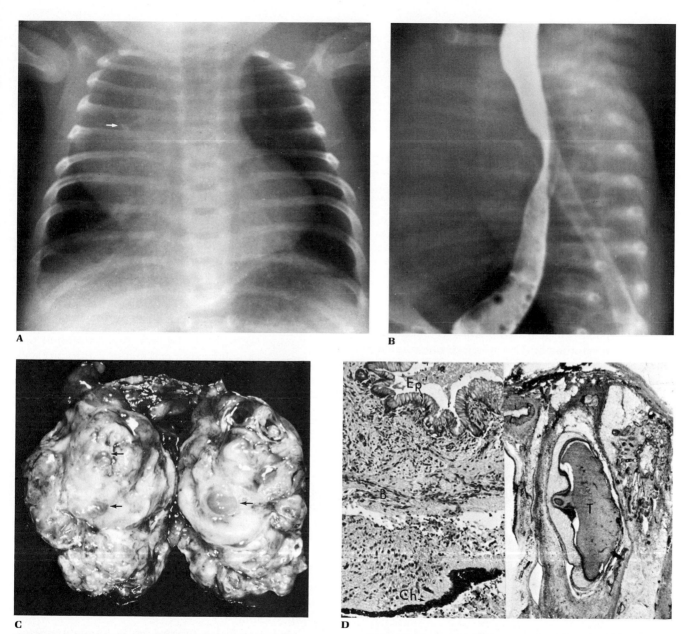

Figure 9-1   Mediastinal teratoma with respiratory distress.   A 6-week-old child presented with crouplike respiratory distress. **A.** The frontal chest film reveals a large mediastinal mass projecting into the right hemithorax containing a small calcific density (arrow). **B.** The mass is anterior and pressing upon the barium-filled esophagus and trachea. **C.** The tumor weighs 45 g and measures 6 × 4 × 4 cm. Its center has multiple thin-walled cysts (arrows) in soft surrounding tissue. **D.** Ectodermal derivatives include brain (B) and choroid of the retina (Ch). The tooth bud (T) is mesodermal in origin, and the mucous-secreting columnar epithelium (Ep) is of endodermal heritage.

The tumors discussed in this chapter are:

1. Germ cell tumors (GCTs)
   a. Teratomas
   b. Seminomas
   c. Endodermal sinus (yolk sac) tumors
2. Neurogenic tumors

Tumors arising in the thymus are covered in Chapter 8, lesions arising in or from cardiovascular structures are reviewed in Chapter 10, and lymphoid tissue neoplasms are discussed in Chapter 11.

Germ Cell Tumors

Primary GCTs arise most commonly from gonadal tissue. Those of clinical significance in childhood include (1) teratomas and teratocarcinomas, (2) seminomas, (3) embryonal carcinomas, (4) choriocarcinomas, and (5) endodermal sinus (yolk sac) tumors.[7] In addition to the usual site of origin in the gonads and less commonly in the mediastinum, GCTs have been found in the head (pineal), nasopharynx, oropharynx, neck, pericardium, lung, liver, stomach, kidney, retroperitoneum, and sacrococcygeal area.[8] Tumors in these ectopic locations probably originate from primordial germ cells that failed to complete their migration from the urogenital ridge to the gonads during embryogenesis. Of the malignant GCTs, pure seminomas have a better prognosis compared with those with nonseminomatous elements (teratocarcinoma, choriocarcinoma, endodermal sinus).[9]

Teratomas

Aside from normal or hyperplastic thymus, teratomas are the most common mass lesions found in the anterior mediastinum; they constitute 80 to 90 percent of all germ cell tumors in that location. In children, 12 percent of teratomas are mediastinal, while most others (68 percent) are sacrococcygeal.[10]

The terminology of these lesions is perplexing. Hope et al.[11] suggested the term *teratoma* (*benign or malignant*) to define lesions composed of all three germ layers. The older designation of *dermoid cyst*, used to describe a benign tumor of ectodermal derivatives only, has been abandoned.[6,10,12]

Teratomas fall into two major histologic types: (1) malignant and (2) benign.

1. Malignant teratoma or teratocarcinoma: These tumors are extremely rare and virtually restricted to males. Extension and local invasion are usually present at the time of discovery. The prognosis for patients with teratocarcinoma of the mediastinum is uniformly poor. However, reports of successful treatments combining chemotherapy and critically timed surgery are modestly encouraging.[9,13] Malignant teratomas elaborate alpha fetoprotein and human chorionic gonadotropin, substances not produced by seminoma and benign teratoma.
2. Benign teratoma: In infancy, this type often presents as a solid mass, capable of producing substernal chest pain, dyspnea, wheezing, and, rarely, superior vena caval obstruction (Figure 9-1).[6,14] In contrast, older children may develop extremely large lesions before they are discovered (Figures 9-2 and 9-3).[12,15]

On occasion, cystic teratomas rupture into the pleural space or pericardium. Trichoptysis may result from spillage into the tracheobronchial tree.[6,16] A red-haired teratoma has allegedly never been observed. Pancreatic tissue, included within some teratomas, may exude enzymes into the pleural space and cause a reaction or effusion (Figure 9-3). Insulin-producing mediastinal teratomas, containing islet cell tissue, may cause asymptomatic hypoglycemia.[17]

While mediastinal teratomas are usually present at birth,[6] Edge and Glennie[18] have reported two patients with mediastinal teratomas that were removed 2 and 4 years after the exposure of previously normal chest roentgenograms (Figure 9-4). Both male and female preponderance has been reported,[6,10] but most reports mention an approximately equal sex ratio.[15,19]

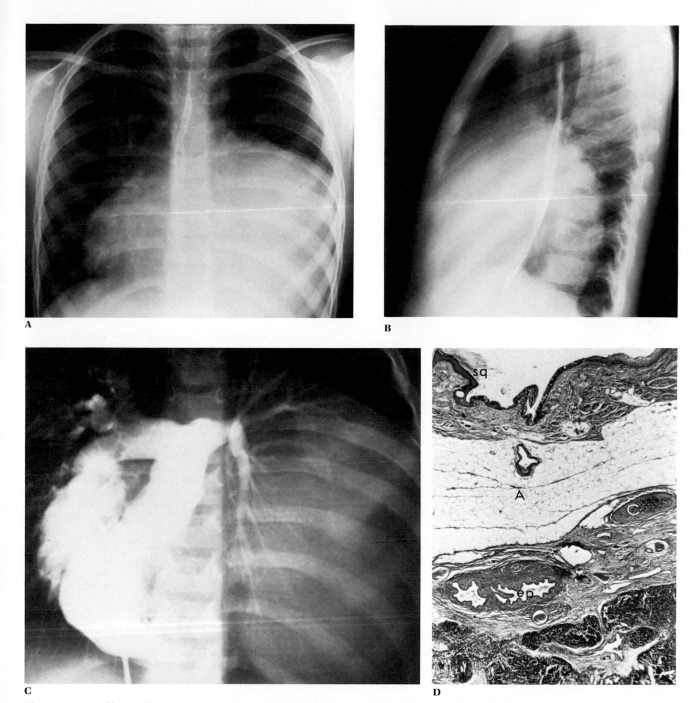

Figure 9-2 Mediastinal teratoma—asymptomatic. Except for a slight cough during the previous 3 to 4 months, this 6-year-old boy was in good health. **A** and **B.** The central silhouette is markedly enlarged in the frontal and lateral projections. **C.** The right ventriculogram shows marked displacement of the right ventricle and main pulmonary artery. The left pulmonary artery is compressed, and its branches are splayed about the mass. **D.** The three typical tissue elements in teratoma, derived from ectoderm, mesoderm, and endoderm, are illustrated in this histologic section taken from the mass. The ectodermal elements of this tumor include the keratinizing squamous epithelium (sq) lining the inner wall of the sac. Mesodermal elements are represented by adipose tissue (A) and cartilage (C). The endodermal elements consist of mucin-secreting epithelium (ep).

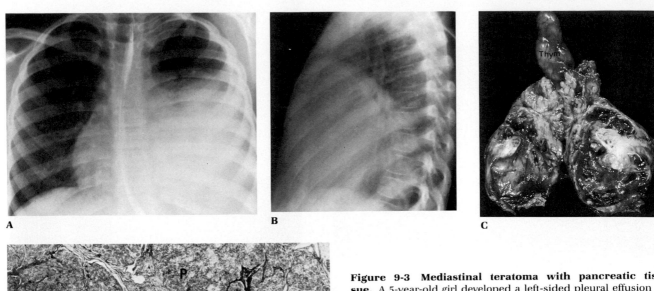

A

B

C

D

Figure 9-3 Mediastinal teratoma with pancreatic tissue. A 5-year-old girl developed a left-sided pleural effusion 2 weeks after minor chest trauma. In spite of repeated pleural taps, the fluid continued to accumulate. **A.** The left thoracic radiopacity is composed of pleural effusion and a mass lesion projecting superiorly. Slight mediastinal shift to the right is evident. **B.** The anterior mass lesion is better appreciated in the lateral projection. **C.** The gross specimen shows thymic tissue (Thym) connected to a teratoma containing solid and cystic components. **D.** The histologic section at low magnification shows that nearly three-fourths of this teratoma consists of pancreatic tissue (P); the ductular structures in the center resemble the mucosa and lamina propria of the colon. The broad fields to each side are mature pancreas. (Masson's trichrome.) *Note:* An amylase study on the pleural fluid would probably have been elevated.

In children less than 2 years old, the roentgen ray may be incapable of separating a teratoma from a normal or hypertrophied thymus. The close embryologic origin of thymus and teratomas compounds the difficulty.[19] Teratomas usually have lobulated and sharply defined silhouettes. Unlike the normal thymus, their configuration and size are not usually influenced by normal respiratory movement (see Chapter 8, Figure 8-3). Normal thymus often varies in size and configuration during periods of illness or stress; a teratoma should remain unchanged or enlarge gradually. Tracheal compression, a common symptom of teratoma in infancy, is distinctly uncommon but not unheard of with thymic hyperplasia.

Many teratomas reside at the base of the heart. However, they may occupy almost any location in the chest, including the cardiophrenic sulcus and the lung parenchyma. Teratomas rarely develop in the posterior mediastinum, but occasionally occur in the pericardial sac (see Chapter 10). Mediastinal teratomas may recur in the chest years after previous removal.[20]

Calcific densities within a teratoma often assume the configuration of rudimentary teeth or bone, in contrast to thymomas where the calcifications are more often linear or curvilinear (see Chapter 8, Figure 8-9). Lymphoreticular disease does not usually calcify except after radiation therapy.

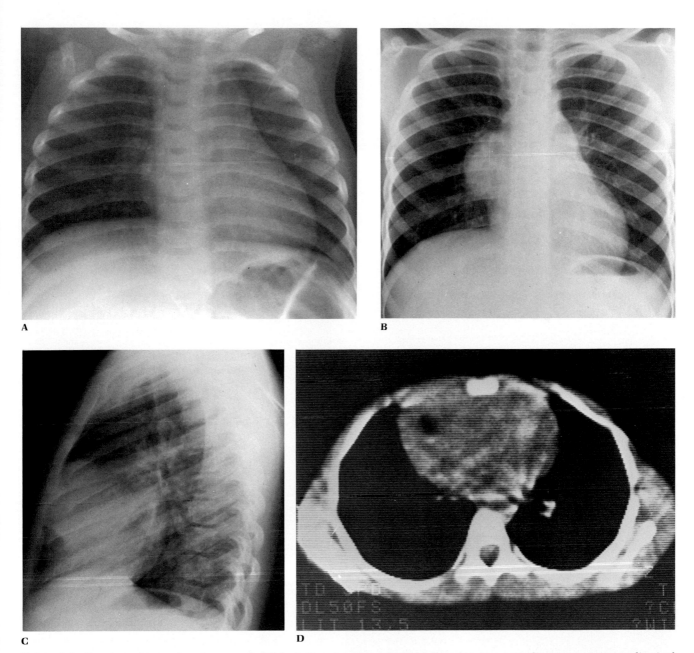

Figure 9-4   Teratoma in previously normal child. A. The chest film is normal. **B** and **C.** Five years later an anterior mediastinal mass has appeared. **D.** Computed tomography demonstrates the mass containing mixed densities characteristic of teratoma. A teratoma was resected.

The differentiation between mediastinal masses is often expedited by computed tomography (CT). In addition to defining the nature of the mass, CT may be helpful in separating tumor from normal thymus (Figures 9-4D and 9-5; also see Chapter 26, Figure 26-34).[21]

The pathologic features of teratoma are well defined. Benign solid teratomas are usually well differentiated histologically and easily separated from their malignant counterparts. Remarkably well-formed skin, teeth, and nerve tissue are common features. Hair follicles, well-developed sebaceous

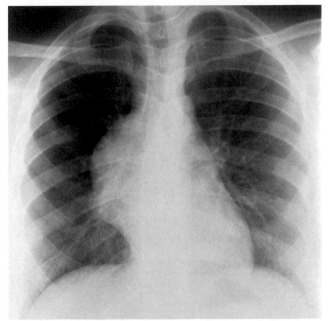

A

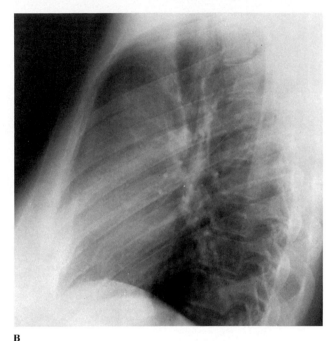

B

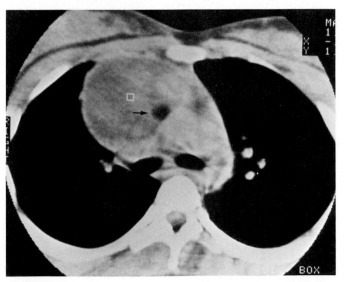

C

Figure 9-5 Teratoma—CT. A and **B.** A lobulated anterior mediastinal mass is apparent from this frontal and lateral film study. **C.** A representative section from a contrast-enhanced CT demonstrates a mass with tissues of mixed densities in the anterior mediastinum to the right of midline. The cursor reads water density; an area of fat is also visible (arrow).

glands, and apocrine sweat glands are often present in their normal relationship. Organoid patterns of mesodermal derivatives such as bone, cartilage, and connective tissues are common (Figures 9-1D and 9-2D). Smooth muscle and bronchial walls may be apparent, and entodermal structures, when present, may include intestinal and pancreatic tissues (Figure 9-3D).

Cystic teratomas are more common than their solid counterparts, but undergo malignant degeneration less often. The cysts contain a preponderance of ectodermal tissues such as hair, sweat glands, sebaceous cysts, and teeth; mesodermal and entodermal derivatives are also found on careful examination. Dehner[1] considers the mature, cystic teratoma as an extragonadal germ cell tumor. Differentiation between primary malignant teratoma of the mediastinum and metastatic disease from another primary lesion is of great importance. When malignant degeneration develops in a previously benign tumor, it usually involves one cell type. The possibility of malignant degeneration makes removal of any mediastinal teratoma mandatory at the time of discovery. When solid teratoid tumors are malignant, the presenting symptoms frequently relate to invasion of adjacent organs.

Seminomas

Primary seminoma of the mediastinum is a rare tumor; as of 1979, only 103 cases had been reported in the English literature.[22] Nevertheless, the understanding of therapy in these cases has improved.[9,23] The intimate association of seminoma with the thymus can probably be explained by germ cell dislocation during embryonic life.[24,25]

When a seminoma of the mediastinum is discovered, the possibility of metastasis from a primary tumor in the testis must be considered and excluded.[26] However, metastatic testicular seminoma traditionally bypasses the mediastinum and spreads via the retroperitoneal lymph nodes to the supraclavicular region. When the mediastinum is involved with testicular seminoma metastasis, the anterior mediastinal lymph nodes are rarely occupied.

The majority of seminomas occur in men, although occasional cases have been reported in women.[21,27] Most patients contract their illnesses in the third or fourth decades, but children are not exempt. Like other mediastinal tumors, approximately one-third are asymptomatic at the time of initial discovery. Seminoma, in contrast to yolk sac tumor, does not produce elevated alpha fetoproteins.

While all malignant germ cell tumors are bad actors, patients with seminoma are usually better off than those with malignant teratoma, choriocarcinoma, or yolk sac tumor.[1] As many as three-fourths may survive 5 years or more. Most seminomas are not resectable, but with adjunct radiation therapy, even the presence of metastatic spread does not exclude a cure.[28,29] The role of chemotherapy in the treatment of this tumor has not been defined.[9,30,31]

Primary mediastinal seminoma cannot be differentiated radiographically from other tumors in the same location. Invariably found in the anterior mediastinum, the tumor is usually large with lobulated borders. Calcification has not been demonstrated with plain films or tomograms.[21] Deviation of the tracheobronchial tree may occur with lesions of sufficient size.[32,33] Superior vena caval obstruction is reported in 10 percent of patients with seminoma. As with lymphomas and small cell undifferentiated carcinomas of the lung, rapid resolution is the rule following radiation therapy.

Mediastinal and testicular seminomas, histologically identical tumors, are characterized by nests of large, atypical cells with abundant cytoplasm, large nuclei, and prominent nucleoli.[22,26] Electron microscopy is sometimes helpful in distinguishing seminoma from thymoma and lymphoma.

Metastatic spread is most often confined within the thorax and may involve the lungs and regional lymph nodes. Systemic dissemination of seminoma to the skin, spleen, spinal cord, tonsils, thyroid, adrenal glands, skeleton, and central nervous system is less frequent.[22]

Endodermal Sinus (Yolk Sac) Tumors

Endodermal sinus tumors are extremely malignant lesions. Most have already metastasized when discovered, and local recurrences are common follow-ing treatment. In a series of yolk sac tumors studied by O'Sullivan et al.,[34] the sacrococcygeal region was the single most common site.

Yolk sac tumors are the least common primary mediastinal germ cell neoplasms.[35,36] Whereas semi-nomas are thought to arise directly from germ cells, endodermal sinus tumors probably spring from poorly differentiated embryonal carcinoma.[37] Teilum[38,39] first suggested a germ cell origin for these tumors, which were later found to be similar to the intraplacental perivascular structures known as en-dodermal sinuses of Duval. Because of this associa-tion, they are called *endodermal sinus tumors;* their origin in yolk sac endoderm has spawned the addi-tional term *yolk sac tumors.*

The presence of alpha fetoprotein in the serum of patients with these tumors strengthens the con-cept of their origin from yolk sac endoderm.[40] Ele-vated serum levels of alpha fetoprotein aid in the in-itial diagnosis and follow-up of this tumor.[41]

All anterior mediastinal yolk sac tumors to date have been reported in males between the ages of 13 and 49 years.[35] Unlike other mediastinal germ cell tu-mors, they characteristically produce significant sys-temic symptoms such as fever, fatigue, chest pain, and dyspnea. These symptoms, in a patient with an anterior mediastinal mass and elevated serum alpha fetoprotein, render the diagnosis of yolk sac tumor most tenable.

Patients with mediastinal yolk sac tumors have a poor prognosis, but remarkable results using a regi-men of radical resection, radiation, and chemother-apy were recently reported by Rusch et al.[42] A small number of patients have benefited from treatment with a combination of cytoreductive surgery and CEBA (cisplatin, etoposide, bleomycin, and adria-mycin).[43]

Neurogenic Tumors

Neurogenic tumors represent the largest group of posterior mediastinal lesions in childhood. In Deh-ner's review of 283 mediastinal tumors and tumor-like disorders of childhood, 35 percent were of neu-rogenic origin.[1]

Neurogenic tumors of the posterior mediastinum originate from two anlagen: (1) nerve sheath and (2) sympathetic nervous system:

1. Nerve sheath tumors
   a. Neurofibroma
   b. Neurilemmoma
   c. Malignant schwannoma
2. Sympathetic nervous system tumors
   a. Neuroblastoma
   b. Ganglioneuroma
   c. Ganglioneuroblastoma
   d. Pigmented neuroectodermal tumor (mela-notic progonoma, paraganglioma)
   e. Mediastinal pheochromocytoma

Of the above tabulated tumors, neuroblastoma, ganglioneuroma, and ganglioneuroblastoma occur most commonly in childhood. Neuroblastoma, the most aggravating of the three, is frequently discov-ered as a mass in an otherwise asymptomatic infant, while in others, the tumor gains attention because of metastatic disease. Ganglioneuroma, the benign counterpart, is usually uncovered as an asympto-matic lesion in older individuals, between 6 and 20 years of age (Figure 9-6).[44] This tumor is often discov-ered as a calcified mass on a radiograph taken for some unrelated reason. Ganglioneuroblastoma is dif-ficult to categorize, as this tumor contains elements of both neuroblastoma and ganglioneuroma. Like neuroblastoma, its behavior is erratic.

Neuroblastoma

It is safe to say that no one would ever get rich bet-ting on the outcome of neuroblastoma; odds on their finish are very hard to figure. Nevertheless, several clinical features that influence survival are recog-nized as follows: site of origin, histology, age, stage, clinical findings, radiologic findings, and pathologic findings.

Site of Origin

Thoracic and pelvic neuroblastomas have a better prognosis than those in the abdomen and adrenal gland.

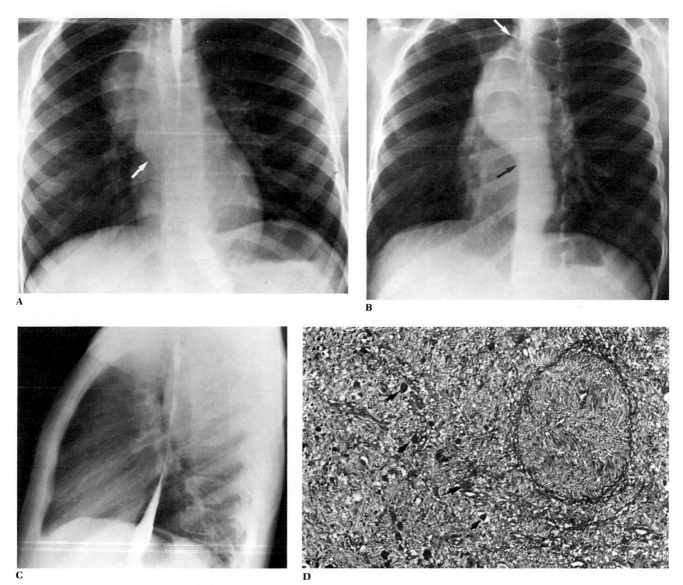

Figure 9-6   Ganglioneuroma—asymptomatic. A. Frontal **B.** left anterior oblique and **C.** lateral exposures confirm the posterior, paraspinal location of a mass density. A typical extrapleural configuration (arrows) is apparent in the frontal and oblique projections. **D.** In this histologic section taken at low magnification, numerous ganglion cells are visible (arrows), along with a segment of a small nerve trunk. (Masson's trichrome.)

Histology

Neuroblastomas may display variable histology throughout, depending upon the area that is sectioned. Therefore, careful histologic examination of the entire specimen is necessary. Those tumors with primitive, undifferentiated histology have a poorer prognosis than the more differentiated types. Tumors with high lymphocyte counts may be less ugly than others; infants less than 1 year old with tumors of this type and elevated blood lymphocytes may also have a better outlook.[45 – 48]

Age

Survival rates are related to age in the following manner:[49]

Age of Discovery	Survival
< 1 year	82% for 2 years
	50% for 3 years
1–2 years	30–50%
< 2 years	10–15%

Patients less than 6 weeks of age with Stage IV-S disease have a poor prognosis.[46]

Stage

The staging of neuroblastoma is based primarily upon the extent of tumor spread, as determined by surgical exploration and histologic confirmation. Therefore, the stage-dependent survival rates should not change as a result of newer imaging modalities such as ultrasonography, CT, and magnetic resonance imaging.[50–52]

The staging categories, developed originally by D'Angio and Evans, have formed the basis for treatment and are used in estimating prognosis and survival.[46,49,53]

Stage	Survival
I. Tumor is confined to the organ or structure of origin.	80%
II. Tumor extends in continuity beyond the organ or structure of origin but does not cross the midline. Homolateral regional lymph nodes may be involved.	60%
III. Tumor extends in continuity beyond the midline. Bilateral regional lymph nodes may be involved.	10%
IV. There is remote disease involving skeleton, parenchymatous organs, soft tissues, or distant lymph node groups.	5%
IV-S. (Special category) Patients are placed in this category if they satisfy the following criteria: a. One year of age or less b. Tumor stage I or II c. Remote disease in one or more of the following sites: liver, skin, or bone marrow d. Negative bone scan and/or radiographic survey	75%

While it is obvious from the above data that children with stage III and stage IV tumors are decidedly overmatched, one of the important and surprising findings of the original study by D'Angio et al.,[49] which has been confirmed by subsequent experience, is the relatively good prognosis in patients with stage IV-S disease. The presence of clumps of neuroblastoma cells in the bone marrow, originally thought to be inconsequential, is now considered more significant, and chemotherapy is recommended for these patients.[46,49,54] In infants (under a year of age) with stage IV-S neuroblastoma and negative bone marrow, removal of the primary tumor is usually curative.

Clinical Findings

Abdominal swelling is the most common presenting symptom in young patients. Clinical signs include pyrexia, malaise, kinesalgia, opsoclonus, ataxia, and myoclonic encephalopathy.[55–57] Paresis or paralysis indicates the probability of spinal cord compression. Many cases of neuroblastoma are discovered on chest or abdominal film examinations obtained for unrelated reasons.

Two percent of neuroblastomas may be multicentric in origin.[58] However, one-fourth of patients with familial neuroblastoma may have multicentric tumors.[59]

Soft tissue lesions, often involving the extremities, represent an unusual variant of neuroblastoma that occurs in older children and adults. In general, the prognosis for these tumors is good. Differentiating neuroblastomas from other round cell tumors in these locations may be difficult or impossible without the use of electron microscopy.[60]

Radiologic Findings

Many neuroblastomas and ganglioneuromas are detected on chest films obtained for unrelated reasons. Typically, they appear as a smooth, well-defined, posterior, paraspinous mass with single or multiple lobulations. Most are unilateral, but many cross the midline to involve the contralateral paraspinal region and, in so doing, displace adjacent structures, especially the esophagus. Mediastinal lesions may extend along the spine inferiorly to the retroperitoneal space and superiorly into the cervical region. Occasional tumors arise in the retropharyngeal space and dislocate the trachea and esophagus anteriorly.

Osseous changes are valuable clues to the identification of neuroblastoma and other neurogenic tumors. In the thorax, thinning and erosion of ribs are common findings (Figure 9-7). These changes are often quite subtle and best appreciated when compared with the opposite side. Enlarged intervertebral foramina, thinning of pedicles, scalloping of vertebral bodies, and widening of the spinal canal are additional alterations to be expected.[61]

The presence of calcific densities within a paraspinal mass is virtually pathognomonic of a neurogenic tumor, although teratomas may occasionally sneak into this location. On the contrary, the absence of calcium does not exclude a neurogenic tumor, or teratoma for that matter. Magnification films and CT are sometimes of value in the delineation of calcium content.

Once a tumor mass is discovered, the extent of local and metastatic spread must be delineated for the planning of proper treatment. Tumor size, involvement of adjacent structures, spread to regional lymph nodes, and extension across the midline are factors best defined by a combination of plain films, CT (see Chapter 26, Figures 26-32 and 26-35), ultrasound, and, occasionally, contrast esophogram.

Intraspinal extension should be evaluated before surgery.[61-63] Metrizamide-assisted CT of the subarachnoid space is necessary to determine the presence and/or extent of intraspinal tumor (Figures 9-8 and 9-9).[64-66] Magnetic resonance imaging is also a well-suited modality for determining the intraspinal extent of neuroblastoma.

Patients with neuroblastoma must also be evaluated for tumor dissemination. The most likely organs to be involved with metastatic disease, aside from local or regional lymph nodes, are the liver and skeleton. Radionuclide liver scan is a reliable and easily obtained imaging technique for evaluating metastatic involvement. In some cases, CT with contrast enhancement is as good, and possibly more sensitive.

Identification of skeletal metastasis is probably best determined with radioscintigraphy, a technique that is more sensitive than skeletal survey. Areas of positive radionuclide uptake should be radiographed to exclude lesions other than metastatic tumor.[67,68] False-negative bone scans in metastatic neu-

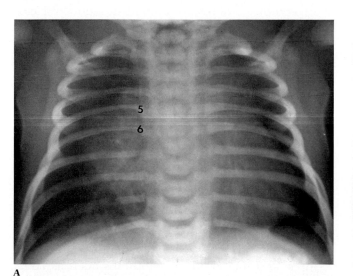

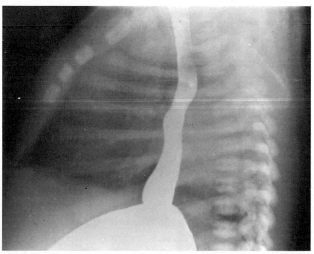

A   **B**

Figure 9-7   Neuroblastoma—rib erosion. A. The right paramediastinal opacity is difficult to localize on the frontal film. However, the erosion and thinning of the right fifth, sixth, and possibly seventh ribs place the lesion posteriorly, most probably extrapleural. **B.** The lateral projection confirms the posterior location.

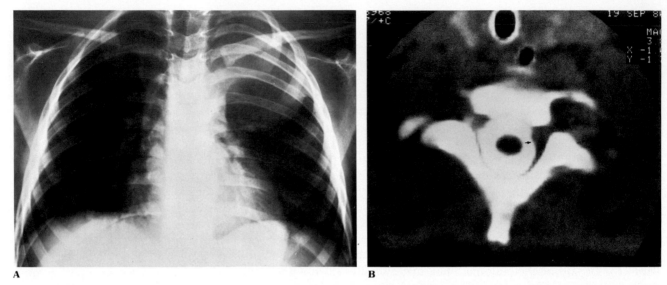

A   B

Figure 9-8   Neuroblastoma—intraspinal extension. A. The frontal film of a 6-year-old girl shows a clinically latent left apical mass extending into the neck. **B.** Computed tomography with metrizamide shows distortion of the seventh cervical vertebrae at the neural foramen with expansion of the transverse process. The metrizamide-filled subarachnoid space is flattened (arrow) by tumor extension. The patient had no neurologic problems. (Courtesy of Dr. Derek Harwood-Nash, Toronto, Canada.)

roblastoma have been reported.[69] Radionuclides, including ^{67}Ga citrates and Tc diphosphonate, may be taken up by neuroblastoma tissue.[70,71] In small infants, and occasionally small children, skeletal survey may still be the most efficacious way to begin the search for skeletal metastases.

Arteriography for the evaluation of patients with suspected neuroblastoma has lost popularity; this technique cannot distinguish between neuroblastoma and ganglioneuroma.[72] However, arteriography, or digital subtraction angiography, may provide valuable information to the surgeon, who must know the vascular supply before attempting a resection.

Pathologic Findings

Malignant neuroblastoma is formed from primitive neuroblasts derived from the neural crest. They originate from either the adrenal medulla or some part of the cervical, thoracic, abdominal, or pelvic autonomic ganglia. Extraadrenal sites also include the organ of Zuckerkandl and, rarely, the extremities. Some clinicians consider this tumor in the category of a neurocristopathy, along with von Recklinghausen's

disease, pheochromocytoma, nonchromaffin paragangliomas, and Hirschsprung's disease.[73]

Mediastinal neuroblastomas are softer and often have more hemorrhagic and necrotic character than their abdominal counterparts. Histologically, they are composed of relatively small, mononuclear cells with hyperchromatic nuclei and scant cytoplasm. Cellular differentiation is sometimes poor. Eosinophilic fibrillar structures make up the intracellular stroma. Pseudorosettes, characteristic of neuroblastoma, may or may not be present.

Ganglioneuromas

Ganglioneuromas are benign tumors of the sympathetic nervous system and are the best differentiated of neural crest origin. Rare in infancy, most are discovered between the ages of 6 and 20 years as asymptomatic masses in the posterior mediastinum and paravertebral regions. Many extend along the nerve roots into the intervertebral foramina and spinal canal. They grow slowly, compress local structures, and may produce symptoms such as cough (Figure 9-10).

Ovoid to round or dumbbell-shaped, they are

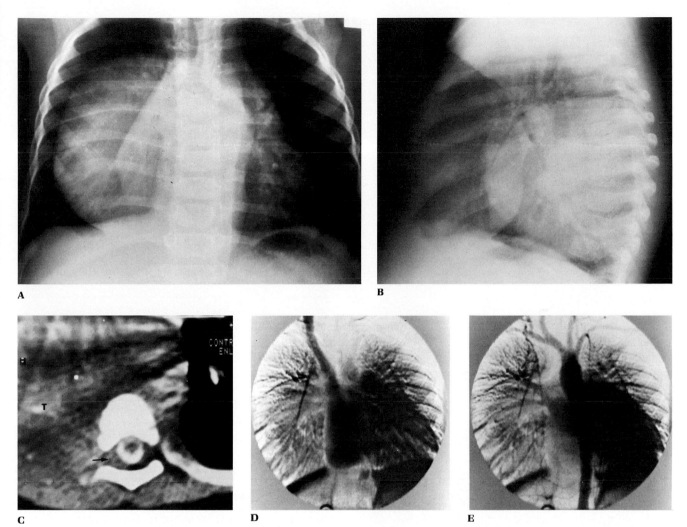

Figure 9-9   Neuroblastoma—intraspinal extension. A. A large paraspinous mass is present in this asymptomatic 13-month-old. The mass crosses the midline and produces a left paraspinous shadow. The right seventh and eighth ribs are thinned (see Figure 9-7). **B.** The lateral film shows anterior displacement of the right stem bronchus by the mass. No vertebral changes are apparent. **C.** Computed tomography with metrizamide shows the large tumor mass (T) extending into the spinal canal (arrow). The subarachnoid space, seen as a white circle around the dark spinal cord, is not compressed or distorted by the adjacent tumor mass that has penetrated the neural foramen. **D.** Subtraction intravenous angiogram shows the superior vena cava and right atrium deviated slightly to the left. **E.** The arterial phase demonstrates mild deviation of the descending aorta.

usually rubbery, are yellow to tan in color, and have a whorled character with occasional small cysts and flecks of calcium. Histologically, they are characterized by fine fibrillary stroma, occasional nerves, swathes of collagen fibers, and clusters of ganglion cells. The latter may appear normal; but large, binu-

cleate and multinucleated forms, as well as smaller, angulated obviously differentiating ganglion cells, may be found. The tumor should be generously sampled in search of small, angulated, immature ganglion cells that signal the presence of ganglioneuroblastoma, the malignant counterpart.

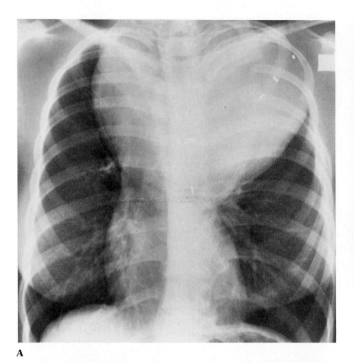

A

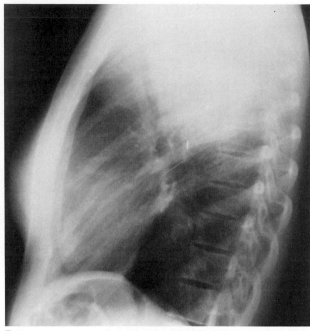

B

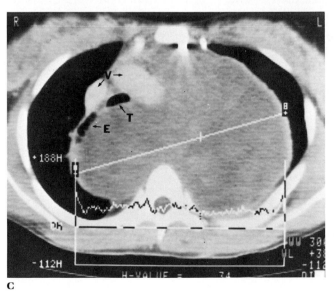

C

Figure 9-10   Neurofibroma—benign. A 16-year-old girl had a large tumor partially removed from the left chest. The tumor that was not removed continued to enlarge. The patient had mild symptoms. **A.** A large mass occupies the entire superior mediastinum. **B.** In the lateral projection the trachea is bowed forward. **C.** Computed tomography shows the mass to be 16 cm in diameter. It has a homogeneous character and displaces the trachea (T), esophagus (E), and great vessels (V). The entire mass was resected and proved to be a neurofibroma on light as well as electron microscopy. The size and rapid growth of this lesion belie its benign histologic appearance. This mediastinal mass created few symptoms in spite of its size and pressure on adjacent structures.

Ganglioneuroblastoma

Ganglioneuroblastoma shares histologic features of both neuroblastoma and ganglioneuroma. Different portions of the tumor may contain elements which are compatible with the histology of either. "Maturation" from malignant neuroblastoma to benign ganglioneuroma is well known.

Spontaneous regression of neuroblastoma is also well documented.[74,75] This maturation and regression is particularly evident in infants with metastatic disease to the liver and skin (stage IV-S)[53] and in cases of congenital neuroblastoma.[76]

Other tumors of infancy showing benign or regressive tendencies include:

1. Sacrococcygeal teratoma before 4 months of age
2. Yolk sac carcinoma of infantile testis before 2 years of age
3. Hepatoblastoma before 1 year of age
4. Congenital leukemia
5. Burkitt's lymphoma before 1 year of age
6. Retinoblastoma

References

1. Dehner LP: *Pediatric Surgical Pathology* St. Louis, CV Mosby, 1975, pp 183, 190, and 601.
2. Bower RJ, Kiesewetter WB: Mediastinal masses in infants and children. *Arch Surg* 112:1003, 1977.
3. King RM, Telander RL, Smithson WA, et al: Primary mediastinal tumors in children. *J Pediatr Surg* 17:512, 1982.
4. Elder JS, Touloukian RJ: Surgical diagnosis of mediastinal lymphoma of childhood. *Arch Surg* 114:54, 1979.
5. Heimberger IL, Battersby SJ: Primary mediastinal tumors in childhood. *J Thorac Cardiovasc Surg* 90:92, 1965.
6. Brooks JW: Tumors of the chest, in Kendig EL Jr, Chernick V (eds): *Disorders of the Respiratory Tract in Children.* Philadelphia, WB Saunders Co, 1977, p 711.
7. Mattin N, Golbey RB, Hajdu SI, et al: Primary mediastinal germ cell tumors. *Cancer* 33:763, 1974.
8. Dehner LP: Intrarenal teratoma occurring in infancy: Report of a case with discussion of extragonadal germ cell tumors in infancy. *J Pediatr Surg* 8:369, 1969.
9. Economou JE, Trump DL, Holmes EC: Management of primary germ cell tumors of the mediastinum. *J Thorac Cardiovasc Surg* 83:643, 1982.
10. Grosfeld JL, Ballantine TVN, Lowe D, et al: Benign and malignant teratomas in children: Analysis of 85 patients. *Surgery* 80:297, 1976.
11. Hope JW, Borns PF, Koop CE: Radiologic diagnosis of mediastinal masses in infants and children. *Radiol Clin North Am* 1:17, 1963.
12. Haller JA Jr, Mazur DO, Morgan WW Jr: Diagnosis and management of mediastinal masses in children. *J Thorac Cardiovasc Surg* 58:385, 1969.
13. Parker D, Holford CP, Begent RHJ, et al: Effective treatment for malignant mediastinal teratoma. *Thorax* 38:897, 1983.
14. Seibert JJ, Marvin WJ Jr, Rose EF, et al: Mediastinal teratoma: A rare cause of severe respiratory distress in the newborn. *J Pediatr Surg* 11:253, 1976.
15. Lewis BD, Hurt RD, Payne WS, et al: Benign teratomas of the mediastinum. *J Thorac Cardiovasc Surg* 86:727, 1983.
16. Thompson DP, Moore TC: Acute thoracic distress in childhood due to spontaneous rupture of a large mediastinal teratoma. *J Pediatr Surg* 4:416, 1969.
17. Honicky RE, dePapp EW: Mediastinal teratoma with endocrine function. *Am J Dis Child* 126:650, 1973.
18. Edge JR, Glennie JS: Teratoid tumors of the mediastinum found despite previous normal chest radiography. *J Thorac Cardiovasc Surg* 40:172, 1960.
19. Carney JA, Thompson DP, Johnson CL: Teratomas in children: Clinical and pathological aspects. *J Pediatr Surg* 7:271, 1972.
20. Prauer HW, Mack D, Babic R: Intrapulmonary teratoma 10 years after removal of a mediastinal teratoma in a young man. *Thorax* 38:632, 1983.
21. Francis IR, Glazer GM, Bookstein FL, et al: The thymus: Reexamination of age-related changes in size and shape. *AJR* 145:249, 1985.
22. Polanski SM, Barwick KW, Ravin CE: Primary mediastinal seminoma. *AJR* 132:21, 1979.
23. Slawson R, Aygun C, Carbone D: Primary mediastinal seminoma. *Radiographics* 3:100, 1983.
24. Friedman NB: Thymoma: A review and reclassification. *Am J Pathol* 32:695, 1956.
25. Schlumberger HG: Teratoma of the anterior mediastinum in a group of military age: Study of 16 cases and review of theory of genesis. *Arch Pathol* 41:398, 1946.
26. Meares EM Jr, Briggs EM: Occult seminoma of the testis masquerading as primary extragonadal germinal neoplasms. *Cancer* 30:300, 1972.

27. El-Domeiri AA, Hulter RVP, Pool JL, et al: Seminoma of the anterior mediastinum. *Ann Thorac Surg* 6:513, 1968.

28. Bagshaw MA, McLaughlin WT, Earle JD: Definitive radiotherapy of primary mediastinal seminoma. *AJR* 105:86, 1969.

29. Besznyak I, Sebesteny M, Kucher F: Primary mediastinal seminoma. A case report and review of the literature. *J Thorac Cardiovasc Surg* 65:930, 1973.

30. Feun LG, Samson MK, Stephens RL: Vinblastine (VLB), bleomycin (BLEO), cis-diamminedichloroplatinum (DDP) in disseminated extragonadal germ cell tumors: A Southwest Oncology Group study. *Cancer* 45:2543, 1980.

31. Reynolds TF, Yagoda A, Vugrin D, et al: Chemotherapy of mediastinal germ cell tumors. *Semin Oncol* 6:113, 1979.

32. Oberman HA, Libke JH: Malignant germinal neoplasms of the mediastinum. *Cancer* 17:498, 1964.

33. Kleitsch WP, Taricco A, Halsam, GJ: Primary seminoma (germinoma) of the mediastinum. *Ann Thorac Surg* 4:249, 1967.

34. O'Sullivan PO, Daneman A, Chan HSL, et al: Extragonadal endodermal sinus tumors in children: A review of 24 cases. *Pediatr Radiol* 13:249, 1983.

35. Fox MA, Vix VA: Endodermal sinus (yolk sac) tumors of the anterior mediastinum. *AJR* 135:291, 1980.

36. Mukai K, Adams WR: Yolk sac tumors of the anterior mediastinum: Case report with light and electron-microscopy examination and immunohistochemical study of alphafetoprotein. *Am J Surg Pathol* 3:77, 1974.

37. Teilum G: The concept of endodermal sinus (yolk sac) tumor. *Scand J Immunol* (suppl 8) 8:75, 1978.

38. Teilum G: Mesonephroma ovarii (Schiller): Extra-embryonic mesoblastoma of germ cell origin in the ovary and testis. *Acta Pathol Microbiol Scand* 27:249, 1950.

39. Teilum G: Endodermal sinus tumors of the ovary and testis, comparative morphogenesis of the so-called mesonephroma ovarii (Schiller) and extra embryonic (yolk sac-allantoic) structure in the rat's placenta. *Cancer* 12:1092, 1959.

40. Rimbaut C, Cailland JM, Cullon B, et al: Alpha-1-fetoprotein (AFP) in germ cell tumors: Biological and histological correlation. *Scand J Immunol* (suppl 8), 201, 1978.

41. Gitlin D, Perricelli A: Synthesis of serum albumin, prealbumin, alphafetoprotein, alpha l-antitrypsin and transferrin by the human yolk sac. *Nature* 228:995, 1970.

42. Rusch VW, Logothetis C, Samuels M: Endodermal sinus tumor of the mediastinum: Report of apparent cure in two patients with extensive disease. *Chest* 86:745, 1984.

43. Vogelzang J, Anderson RW, Kennedy BJ: Successful treatment of mediastinal germ cell/endodermal sinus tumors. *Chest* 88:64, 1985.

44. Abell MR, Hast WR, Olson JR: Tumors of the peripheral nervous system. *Hum Pathol* 1:503, 1970.

45. Evans AE, Hummeler K: The significance of primitive cells in marrow aspiration in children with neuroblastoma. *Cancer* 32:906, 1973.

46. Grosfeld JL, Schatzlein M, Ballantine TVN, et al: Metastatic neuroblastoma: Factors influencing survival. *J Pediatr Surg* 13:59, 1978.

47. Lander I, Aherne W: The significance of lymphocyte infiltration in neuroblastoma. *Br J Cancer* 26:321, 1972.

48. Bill AH, Morgan A: Evidence for immune reactions to neuroblastoma and future possibilities for investigation. *J Pediatr Surg* 5:111, 1970.

49. D'Angio GJ, Evans AE, Koop CE: Special pattern of widespread neuroblastoma with a favorable prognosis. *Lancet* 1:1046, 1971.

50. Berger PE, Kuhn JP, Manschauer RW: Computed tomography in abdominal mass lesions in children. *Radiology* 128:633, 1978.

51. Bolat DW, Reilly BJ: Computed tomography in abdominal mass lesions in children. *Radiology* 124:371, 1977.

52. Shkolnich A: Gray scale ultrasound of the pediatric abdomen and pelvis. *Curr Prob Diagn Radiol* 8:1, 1977.

53. Evans AE, D'Angio, GJ, Randolph, JG: A proposed staging for children in neuroblastoma. *Cancer* 27:374, 1971.

54. Koop CE, Schnaufer L: Management of abdominal neuroblastoma. *Cancer* 35:905, 1975.

55. Solomon GE, Chutorian AM: Opsoclonus and occult neuroblastoma. *N Engl J Med* 279:475, 1968.

56. Korobkin M, Clark RE, Palubiskas AJ: Occult neuroblastoma in acute cerebellar ataxia in childhood. *Radiology* 102:151, 1972.

57. Leonidas JC, Brill CB, Aron, AM: Neuroblastoma presenting with myoclonic encephalopathy. *Radiology* 102:87, 1972.

58. Gross RE, Farber S, Martin L: Neuroblastoma sympathicum: A study and report of 217 cases. *Pediatrics* 22:1179, 1959.

59. Roberts FF, Lee KR: Familial neuroblastoma presenting as multiple tumors. *Radiology* 116:133, 1975.

60. Mackay B, Luna MA, Butler JJ: Adult neuroblastoma—electron microscopic observations in nine cases. *Cancer* 37:1334, 1976.

61. Holgersen LO, Santulli TV, Schullinger JN: Neuroblastoma with intraspinal (dumbbell) extension. *J Pediatr Surg* 18:4, 1983.

62. Kirks DR, Korobkin M: Computed tomography for chest examinations in children. *Pediatr Ann* 9:192, 1980.

63. Berger PE, Kuhn JP, Munschaver, RW: Computed tomography and ultrasound in the diagnosis and management of neuroblastoma. *Radiology* 128:663, 1978.

64. DiChiro G, Schellinger D: Computed tomography of spinal cord after lumbar introduction of metrizamide (computer-assisted myelography). *Radiology* 120:101, 1976.

65. Harwood-Nash DC, Fitz CR: Computed tomography and the pediatric spine: Computed tomographic metrizamide myelography in children, in Post MJD (ed): *Radiologic Evaluation of the Spine.* New York, Mason Inc, 1980, p 4.

66. Resjo M, Harwood-Nash DC, Fitz CR, et al: CT metrizamide myelography for intraspinal and paraspinal neoplasms in infants and children. *AJR* 132:367, 1979.

67. Gilday DL, Ash JM, Reilly BJ: Radionuclide skeletal survey for pediatric neoplasms. *Radiology* 123:399, 1977.

68. Mall JC, Bekerman C, Hoffer A, et al: A unified radiological approach to the detection of skeletal metastases. *Radiology* 118:323, 1976.

69. Kaufman RA, Thral JH, Keyes JW Jr, et al: False negative bone scans in neuroblastoma metastatic to the ends of long bones. *AJR* 130:131, 1978.

70. Feldman JA, Norales JO: Gallium scanning for neuroblastoma. *J Pediatr Surg* 10:553, 1975.

71. McCartney W, Nusynowitz ML, et al: ^{99m}Tc-diphosphonate uptake in neuroblastoma. *AJR* 126:1077, 1976.

72. Dinmick NR, Castellina RA: Arteriographic manifestations of ganglioneuromas. *Radiology* 115:323, 1975.

73. Bolande RP: The neurocristopathies: A unifying concept of disease arising in neural crest maldevelopment. *Hum Pathol* 5:409, 1974.

74. Aterman K, Schneller EF: Maturation of neuroblastoma to ganglioneuroma. *Am J Dis Child* 120:217, 1970.

75. Sitary AL, Santulli TV, Wigger MJ, et al: Complete maturation of neuroblastoma with bone metastases in documented stages. *J Pediatr Surg* 10:533, 1975.

76. Schneider KM, Becker JM, Krasna IH: Neonatal neuroblastoma. *Pediatrics* 36:359, 1965.

Chapter 10

Tumors of the Heart and Pericardium

Tumors of the heart and pericardium are extremely rare; they have been found in 1 out of 10,000 routine autopsies.[1] Nevertheless, several significant reviews have been published.[2-4] Rhabdomyomas constitute approximately 80 percent of all cardiac neoplasms in children. Others include fibroma, myxoma, lymphangioma, hemangioma, mesothelioma, neurofibroma, pericardial cyst, teratoma, and fibrosarcoma.

Less than 10 percent of all childhood cardiac and pericardial tumors and cysts are malignant, and most of these are malignant teratomas, rhabdomyosarcomas, and fibrosarcomas. Malignant mesenchymoma, neurogenic sarcoma, and Anitschkow cell sarcoma are extremely rare. In spite of the histologic classification of these tumors, they must all be considered a threat to life because of their critical location. In one study, 11 of the 22 histologically benign tumors resulted in the death of the patients.[5]

The following lesions have been selected for discussion in this chapter:

1. Rhabdomyoma
2. Fibroma
3. Myxoma
4. Teratoma
5. Malignant tumors

Rhabdomyoma

Rhabdomyomas are either single or multiple and may involve the muscle or any other portion of the heart. Impingement on chambers and outflow tracts causes symptoms of obstructed blood flow, cardiac failure, conduction abnormalities, and/or murmur.[6] On occasion, rhabdomyoma may be confused with localized hypertrophy of cardiac muscle in the septum, walls, or outflow tracts.

Chest films are of some use when the enlarged heart assumes an unusual shape (Figure 10-1A and

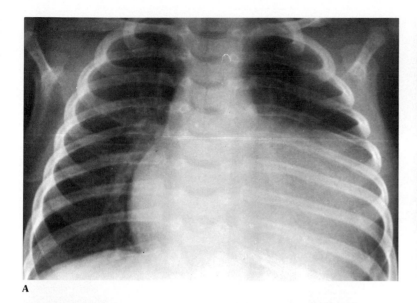

A

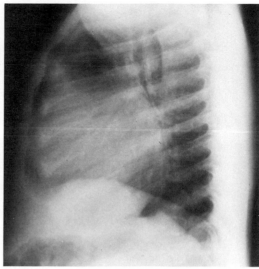

B

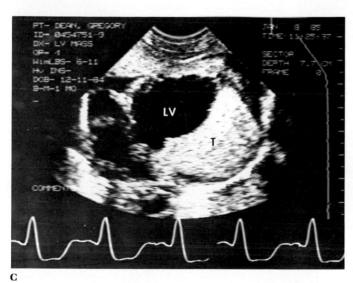

C

Figure 10-1 Myocardial tumor (rhabdomyoma?). This child has clinical stigmata of tuberous sclerosis. **A** and **B.** The chest films show marked cardiomegaly extending predominantly to the left. The lungs are clear and the vascularity is normal, suggesting a primary myocardial abnormality. **C.** The echocardiogram defines an echogenic mass (T) that involves most of the left ventricular wall (LV = left ventricular chamber). The child remains well on conservative therapy. The association of tuberous sclerosis and rhabdomyoma is suggestive but not diagnostic.

B). Most often the associated cardiomegaly is nonspecific, and the diagnosis (Figures 10-1C and 10-2) must be confirmed with echocardiography, angiography, or, in some cases, computed tomography (CT).[7]

Fifty percent of patients with rhabdomyoma have associated tuberous sclerosis, a generalized disease that may dominate the clinical picture.[8] On occasion, the tumor is discovered as an incidental finding at autopsy.

Surgical removal of rhabdomyoma has been accomplished successfully.[4]

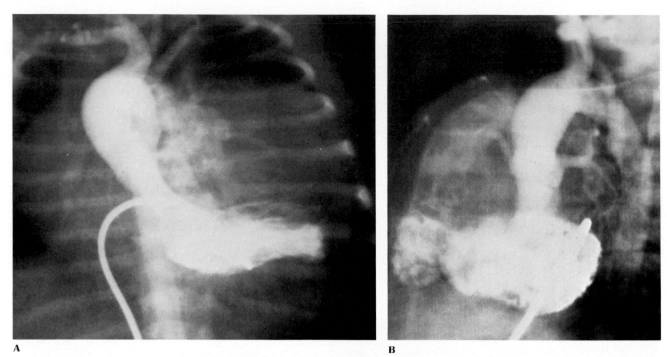

A

B

Figure 10-2   Rhabdomyoma. Cardiac angiography was performed because of unexplained cardiomegaly and signs of congestive heart failure. **A** and **B.** Left ventricular injection. Frontal and lateral projections show a relatively small left ventricular cavity displaced inferiorly by a large intramural mass. A small muscular ventricular septal defect is also present. The initial diagnosis was right and left wall hypertrophy, but a rhabdomyoma was found at surgery.

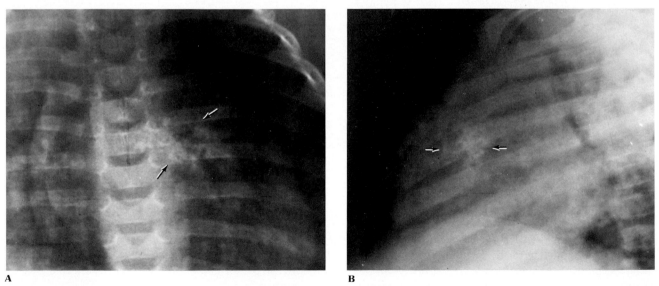

A

B

Figure 10-3   Fibrohamartoma. This 11-month-old child was referred because of a heart murmur first noted at 3 weeks of age. The patient was asymptomatic; growth and development had been normal. At surgery, a mass was removed from the right ventricle. **A** and **B.** Frontal and lateral projections demonstrate an irregularly calcified intracardiac lesion (arrows). The heart appears otherwise normal.

Fibroma

Cardiac fibromas include rhabdomyofibroma, congenital mesoblastic tumor, and fibrous hamartoma. These rare tumors are second in incidence to rhabdomyoma and constitute approximately 5 to 14 percent of cardiac tumors.[5,9–14] The lesions have been reported in patients from ages 42 h to 65 years.[12]

Most patients manifest sudden onset of congestive failure, but unexplained dysrhythmia and cardiomegaly are additional presenting symptoms. One-third of patients die suddenly of arrhythmia;[12] involvement of the conduction system is thought to be the responsible mechanism. Right ventricular outflow tract and tricuspid obstruction have also been observed.[5,13]

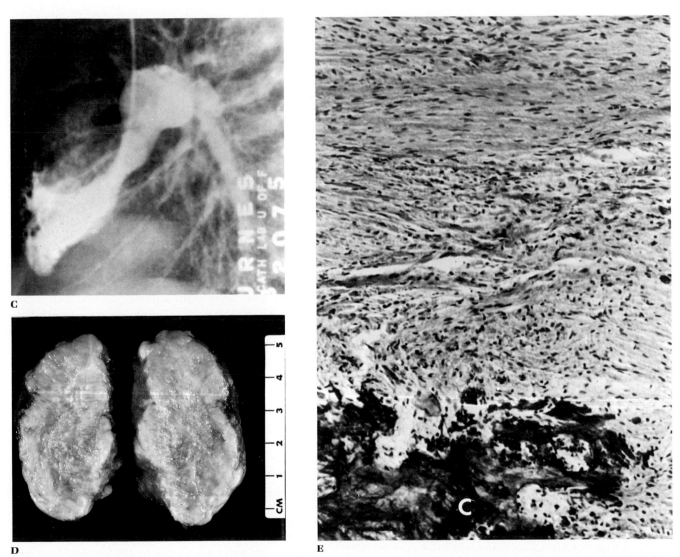

Figure 10-3 (*cont.*) **C.** The right ventriculogram shows a large, intramural mass indenting the right ventricular chamber. The right ventricular outflow tract is narrowed. **D.** The pathologic specimen is an ovoid, firm, gritty mass weighing 40 g; the coarse fibrotic character is evident from the surface appearance. **E.** The histologic section shows the fibroblastic character of the lesion with intermixed calcific foci (C).

The most commonly described radiographic finding of cardiac fibroma is cardiomegaly, often of unusual shape. Calcification, when present in fibromas, serves to differentiate them from rhabdomyoma, a tumor that does not calcify (Figure 10-3). Fluoroscopically, the calcific mass may be observed as a conglomerate density that moves with the cardiac muscle.[15] Echocardiography and CT are of value in defining the anatomy of these lesions (Figure 10-4). Angiocardiography may also help by revealing a filling defect in one of the ventricular chambers or outflow tracts (Figures 10-2A and B and 10-3C). Abnormalities that simulate fibroma radiographically include endocardial fibroelastosis, anomalous coronary artery circulation, hypertrophic subaortic stenosis, pulmonic stenosis, and other cardiac tumors.

On gross examination, fibromas exhibit a firm, gritty, gray-white appearance similar to dermoid tumors (Figure 10-3D). They are not encapsulated and usually extend into the surrounding cardiac muscle. Almost always located within the myocardium, fibromas are found most commonly in the ventricular septum, in the left ventricular wall, and less often in the right ventricular muscle.

Histologically, fibromas are composed mainly of hyalinized, fibrous tissue. Central calcification and

cystic degeneration probably result from poor blood supply (Figure 10-3E). Mitoses are rare, but increased cellularity commonly surrounds the lesion. Metastasis from this tumor has not been reported. Surgical removal has been accomplished in some cases.[4-6,12,14,15]

Myxoma

Cardiac myxomas, as a group, are classified as follows:

1. Angioreticuloma
2. Atrial myxoma
3. Endothelioma
4. Intracardiac endodermal heterotopia

Myxomas represent approximately 13 percent of cardiac tumors found in children, but are much more common in adults. The youngest patient with a cardiac myxoma in the series from the Armed Forces Institute of Pathology (AFIP) was 4 years old, although others report a large right ventricular myxoma in a child of 4 months.[1,6]

Myxomas arise from subendocardial mesenchymal cells and project as polypoid, often pedunculated masses into a cardiac chamber. Of all myxomas, 75 percent occur in the left atrium and usually arise from a pedicle near the fossa ovalis; 20 percent inhabit the right atrium; only 5 percent occupy the ventricles.[16] Approximately 75 percent of myxomas occur in women.

Symptomatology is protean and depends upon tumor size, morphology, and location. More than 50 percent of patients present with congestive failure that simulates mitral stenosis. Cardiac myxomas should be suspected in a patient with recent onset of cardiac symptoms and a dubious history of rheumatic fever. Constitutional symptoms of fatigue, fever, weight loss, and joint pain occur in patients with cardiac myxoma and tend to masquerade the underlying cardiac tumor. Hypertrophic osteoarthropathy is an additional complication in rare cases.

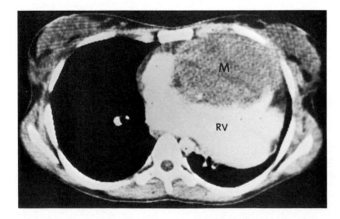

Figure 10-4 Cardiac hamartoma. Computed tomogram with contrast injection shows a large, soft tissue mass (M) that is replacing the wall and impinging upon the chamber of the right ventricle (RV). A cobblestone-like hamartoma was resected. (From Larrieu et al.,[3] with permission.)

Obstructed pulmonary venous return is a frequent finding in patients with left-sided myxomas. Other obstructing lesions that must be considered in the differential diagnosis of myxoma include cor triatriatum, anomalous pulmonary venous connection, and congenital mitral stenosis. These congenital lesions, however, manifest symptoms earlier in life, usually in infancy.

While most myxomas are smooth, some develop a papillary frondlike configuration which increases the probability of embolization. These usually originate from the left side of the heart, and alert the patient to their presence with sudden peripheral arterial and/or cerebral vascular occlusion. Right-sided tumors are more likely to produce signs and symptoms simulating pulmonic stenosis, tricuspid valve disease, or pericarditis. Pulmonary emboli from right-sided lesions may confuse the clinical picture of right-sided congestive failure.[17]

Plain chest film findings of myxoma depend upon the size and location of the tumor. The radiographic changes may show anything from normal heart and lungs to severe cardiomegaly and typical mitral configuration (enlarged left atrium, right ventricular hypertrophy). Left-sided tumors cause pulmonary venous obstruction (vascular redistribution, intralobular septal lymphatic engorgement, pulmonary edema, and pleural effusions). When these findings are present without cardiomegaly or left atrial appendage enlargement, the diagnosis of left atrial myxoma should be suspected.

Echocardiography is the diagnostic modality of choice (Figure 10-5) but angiography may add to the anatomic delineation (Figure 10-6). Vascularization of atrial myxomas is uncommon, but has been reported arising from coronary arteries.[16] The use of CT has also been reported.[18]

The site of origin within the heart does not alter the gross or microscopic appearances of myxomas. Grossly, myxomas are of two general types. Most common are polypoid, smooth, and pedunculated lesions that have a gelatinous, gray-white appearance (Figure 10-7A). Others assume a frondlike appearance (Figure 10-7B). They vary in diameter from 1 to 15 cm. Some may have a short, broad base, and rarely they may be sessile.

Histologically, myxomas are composed of an acid mucopolysaccharide myxoid matrix within which are embedded polygonal cells. They may be single and stellate-shaped and resemble multipotential mesenchymal cells. Reticular collagen, elastic fibers, and smooth muscle cells are scattered throughout the myxoid stroma. Large blood vessels are present in the base of these lesions, and foci of calcification and even bone formation may be noted. Considered as true neoplasms, they never arise from cardiac valves.

Myxomas can usually be removed with complete

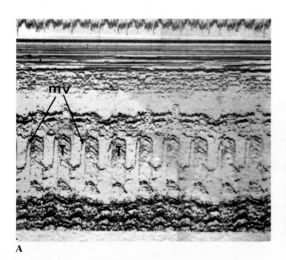

A

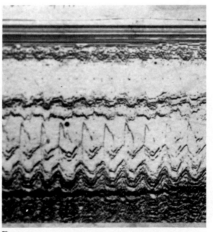

B

Figure 10-5 Cardiac myxoma. M-mode echocardiogram at the level of the mitral valve and left ventricle. **A.** The echodensity (T) represents a tumor that appears behind the anterior mitral valve leaflet (mv) during diastole. **B.** Repeat study, following surgery, shows the lesion is no longer present. (Courtesy of Dr. A. J. Larrieu, Philadelphia, Pennsylvania.)

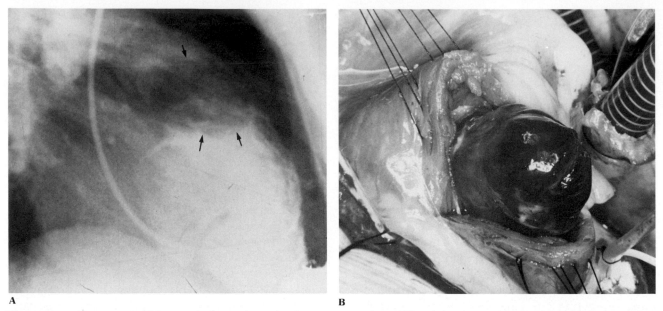

Figure 10-6 Myxoma. A. Right ventricular angiography demonstrates a large filling defect (arrows) in the right ventricular outflow tract. **B.** At surgery, a shiny mass is visible in the opened cardiac chamber. (Courtesy of Dr. James Scatliff, Chapel Hill, North Carolina.)

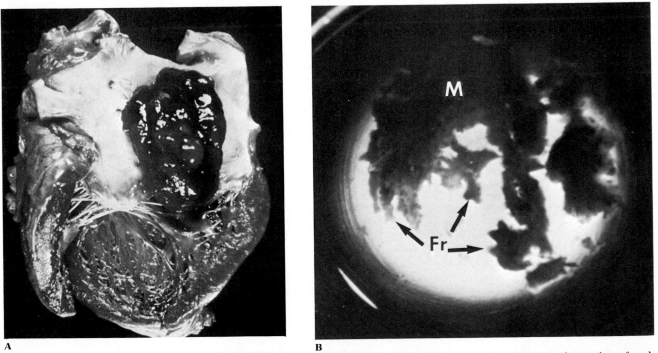

Figure 10-7 Cardiac myxoma. Two examples with different morphologic characteristics. **A.** A gross specimen of smooth surfaced, nodular, myxoid mass attached to the left atrial endocardium adjacent to the mitral valve. **B.** A photograph of the gross specimen myxoma (M) from a different patient. Note the many frondlike projections (Fr) that tend to separate and embolize. (Courtesy of Dr. A. J. Larrieu, Philadelphia, Pennsylvania.)

cure, but rare cases of recurrence and occasional metastatic spread are reported.[3,19,20] Histologic differentiation between benign and malignant varieties may be difficult, but when metastasis occurs, the tumor usually represents a myxosarcoma. Larrieu found a much higher incidence of malignancy in right atrial myxomas.[3]

Teratoma

Cardiac and pericardial teratomas are extremely rare; most have been reported in the pericardium and fewer in the heart.[21−23] They usually originate from the interventricular septum and grow into the right ventricle or atrium (Figure 10-8). Most cases of

Figure 10-8   Intracardiac teratoma. A. A two-dimensional echocardiogram along the cardiac axis. The tumor (T) is seen as a dense, echogenic, partially cystic 3- to 4-cm mass arising from the interventricular septum (ivs) and projecting into the right ventricle (rv). (lv = left ventricle, ao = aorta, la = left atrium.) **B.** The postoperative study discloses a thick endocardial flap protruding into the right ventricle (arrow). **C.** The gross specimen shows a well-encapsulated, multicystic tumor. **D.** Histologic sections reveal derivatives of three germ layers: bone (b), cartilage (c), fat (f), mucous glands (mg), neural tissue (n), and tracheobronchial epithelium (t). (From Maeta et al.,[23] with permission.)

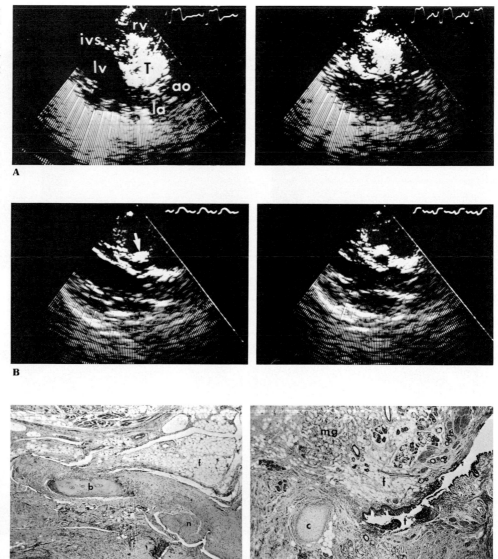

cardiac teratoma are diagnosed at postmortem, but rare patients have had successful excisions.[23,24] Echocardiography is the most successful diagnostic modality, but any of the usual cardiac imaging studies may be used (Figure 10-8A and B).

Intrapericardial teratomas often arise near the root of the great vessels, especially near the aorta, and carry a high risk of bleeding during extirpation (Figure 10-9).[25]

Malignant Tumors

Malignant cardiac fibrosarcomas consist of several histologic variants (fibromyxosarcomas, malignant xanthofibromas, and fibroxanthosarcomas). These malignant cardiac tumors are considered together because of their relative rarity and their common origin from fibroblasts. The AFIP reported on 14 pa-

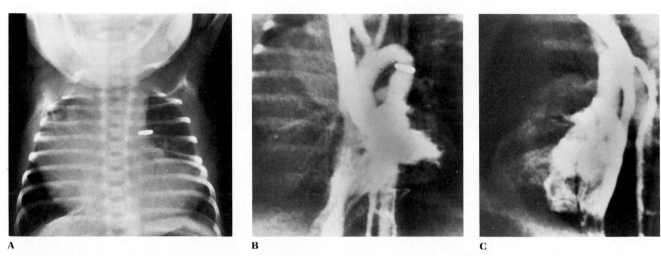

A   B   C

Figure 10-9   Pericardial teratoma. A. A large soft tissue mass is seen extending into the right hemithorax. The clip represents a previously closed patent ductus arteriosus. **B** and **C.** Cardiac angiography shows displacement of the heart to the left and posteriorly by what proved to be a teratoma of the pericardium. (From Sumner et al.,[21] with permission.)

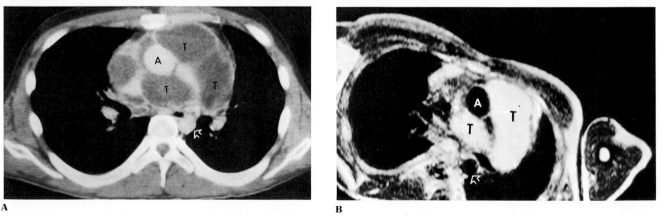

A   B

Figure 10-10   Cardiac angiosarcoma. A. Computed tomography shows normal cardiac anatomy replaced by large conglomerates of tumor masses (T) surrounding the ascending aorta (A) and aortic arch (the arrow indicates the descending aorta). **B.** Magnetic resonance imaging at approximately the same level shows the tumor tissue in white surrounding the black aorta. (Courtesy of Dr. David Turner, Chicago, Illinois.)

tients with lesions of this type, 12 of whom had primary involvement of various chambers of the heart.[2] Of the 14, 5 had pericardial lesions, although they did not necessarily originate in the pericardium. The age range was not reported.

Primary malignant tumors of the pericardium are extremely rare, and definitive conclusions are difficult to substantiate. The few examples reported are usually teratocarcinomas. Although accurate statistics are not available, metastasis to the pericardium occurs 20 to 40 times more often than primary neoplasia.[26]

The roentgenographic diagnosis of pericardial tumors is difficult from conventional film studies. The possibility of a cardiac or pericardial tumor might be suggested in the presence of unexplained cardiomegaly and/or pericardial effusion.[21,27,28] The use of a blood pool scan may be confusing but will often separate the cardiac and pericardial components.[29,30] Digital subtraction or conventional angiography is often relied upon to yield definitive information. Echocardiography, CT, and magnetic resonance imaging (Figure 10-10) are probably the most useful imaging modalities.[7]

References

1. Nadas HS, Ellison RC: Cardiac tumors in infancy. *Am J Cardiol* 21:363, 1968.
2. McAllister HA Jr, Fenoglio JJ Jr: Tumors of the cardiovascular system. *Atlas of Tumor Pathology*, 2d series, Fasciol 15. Washington, DC, AFIP, 1978.
3. Larrieu AJ, Jamieson WRE, Tyers GFO, et al: Primary cardiac tumors: Experience with 25 cases. *J Thorac Cardiovasc Surg* 83:339, 1982.
4. Reece IJ, Cooley DA, Frazier OH, et al: Cardiac tumors: Clinical spectrum and prognosis of lesions other than classical benign myxoma in 20 patients. *J Thorac Cardiovasc Surg* 83:439, 1984.
5. Van der Hauwaert LG: Cardiac tumors in infancy and childhood. *Br Heart J* 33:125, 1971.
6. Simcha A, Wells BG, Tynan MJ, et al: Primary cardiac tumours in childhood. *Arch Dis Child* 46:508, 1971.
7. Gross BH, Glazer GM, Francis IR: CT of intracardiac and intrapericardial masses. *AJR* 140:903, 1983.
8. Tsakraklides V, Burke B, Mastri A, et al: Rhabdomyomas of heart. *Am J Dis Child* 128:639, 1974.
9. Patterson D, Gibson D, Gomes R, et al: Idiopathic calcified myocardial mass. *Thorax* 29:589, 1974.
10. Wilson JB, Hood RH, Johnson HH Jr, et al: Primary myocardial fibroma: Report of 2 cases. *Radiology* 84:1976, 1965.
11. James U, Stanfield HM: A case of fibroma of the left ventricle in a child of 4 years. *Arch Dis Child* 30:187, 1955.
12. Geha AS, Weidman WH, Soule EH, et al: Intramural ventricular cardiac fibroma: Successful removal in 2 cases and review of the literature. *Circulation* 36:427, 1967.
13. Van der Hauwaert LG: Cardiac tumors in childhood, in Watson H (ed): *Pediatric Cardiology*. Lloyd-Luke, 1973, 1968.
14. Williams DB, Danielson GK, McGoon DC: Cardiac fibroma: Long term survival after excision. *J Thorac Cardiovasc Surg* 84:230, 1982.
15. Aryanpur I, Nazaraan I, et al: A calcified right ventricular fibroma causing outflow obstruction. *Am J Dis Child* 130:1265, 1976.
16. Rasmussen KK, Peeples TC, Nellen JR: Unusual variant in tumor vascularity associated with left atrial myxoma. *AJR* 141:927, 1983.
17. Gladden JR, Dreiling R, Gollub S, et al: Two-dimensional echocardiographic features of multiple right atrial myxomas. *Am J Cardiol* 52:1364, 1983.
18. Nordlindh T, Nyman U, Hellekant C: Left atrial myxoma demonstrated with CT. *AJR* 137:153, 1981.
19. Read RC, White HJ, Murphy ML, et al: The malignant potentiality of left atrial myxoma. *J Thorac Cardiovasc Surg* 68:857, 1974.
20. Dang CR, Hurley FJ: Contralateral recurrent myxoma of the heart. *Ann Thorac Surg* 21:59, 1976.
21. Sumner TE, Crowe JE, Klein A, et al: Intrapericardial teratoma in infancy. *Pediatr Radiol* 10:51, 1980.
22. Arciniegas E, Hakimi M, Farooki ZQ, et al: Intrapericardial teratoma in infancy. *J Thorac Cardiovasc Surg* 79:306, 1980.
23. Maeta H, Hiyama T, Okamura K, et al: Successful excision of an intracardiac teratoma. *J Thorac Cardiovasc Surg* 83:909, 1982.
24. Gerbode F, Kerth WJ, Hill JD: Surgical management of tumors of the heart. *Surgery* 61:94, 1967.
25. Yeoh CB, Harris PD, Leff E, et al: Intrapericardial teratoma. *NY State J Med* 76:708, 1976.
26. Prichard R: Tumors of the heart. Review of the subject and report of 150 cases. *Arch Pathol* 51:98, 1951.
27. Reynolds JL, Donahue JK, Pearce CW: Intrapericardial

teratoma: A cause of acute pericardial effusion in infancy. *Pediatrics* 43:71, 1969.

28. Zarella JT, Halpe DCE: Intrapericardial teratoma—neonatal cardiorespiratory distress amenable to surgery. *J Pediatr Surg* 15:961, 1980.

29. Wagner HN, McAfee JL, Mozley JM: Diagnosis of pericardial effusion by radioisotope scanning. *Arch Intern Med* 108:679, 1962.

30. Deland FH, Felman AH: Pericardial tumor compared with pericardial effusion. *Nucl Med* 13:697, 1972.

Chapter 11

Disorders of Lymphoid Tissue

1. Malignant disease
   a. Hodgkin's lymphoma
   b. Non-Hodgkin's lymphoma
2. Benign disease
   a. Pseudolymphoma
   b. Infectious mononucleosis
   c. Giant lymph node hyperplasia (Castleman's disease)[1]
   d. Sinus histiocytosis (Rosai-Dorfman disease)[2]

Malignant Disease

Hodgkin's Lymphoma

Hodgkin's and non-Hodgkin's lymphomas are the third most common malignancies of childhood. They rank behind leukemia and tumors of the central nervous system.[3] Hodgkin's disease alone accounts for slightly more than 4 percent of all child-

hood malignancies.[4] The disease is rare in infancy and uncommon under the age of 5; most cases affect young adults. In the first decade, boys outnumber girls by approximately 2 to 1; in adolescence, girls outnumber boys.[5] The classification, treatment, and prognosis of Hodgkin's disease have changed considerably. Once thought to be a universally fatal disease, it is now second only to Wilms's tumor in cure potential.[6]

Painless lymph node enlargement is the most common presenting complaint. In the majority of patients, adenopathy begins in the cervical region, and about half show associated mediastinal involvement. Primary mediastinal presentation is rare, as is initial axillary and inguinal adenopathy. Hepatosplenomegaly is a nonspecific finding, and its presence cannot be considered as evidence for Hodgkin's involvement of these organs. On occasion, the disease may complicate long-standing immunodeficient states (Figure 11-1).

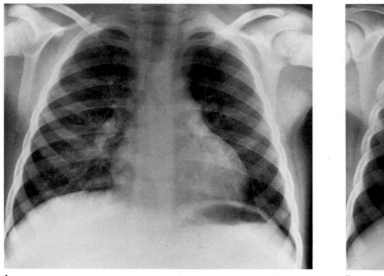

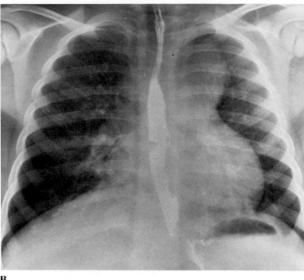

A   B

Figure 11-1   Hodgkin's lymphoma—Wiskott-Aldrich syndrome. A. Mild, diffuse peribronchial changes in the lungs are the result of chronic infection in this patient with Wiskott-Aldrich syndrome. The mediastinum is normal. **B.** One year later there is marked mediastinal adenopathy caused by Hodgkin's lymphoma.

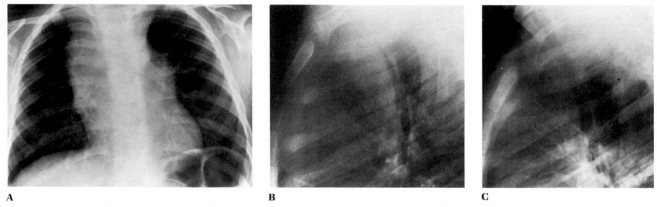

A   B   C

Figure 11-2   Hodgkin's lymphoma with tracheal compression. A. The initial frontal chest film shows mediastinal and hilar adenopathy. **B.** In the lateral projection, the trachea is markedly narrowed by pressure from the anterior mediastinal adenopathy. **C.** Five days after treatment of mediastinal lymphadenopathy with radiation therapy, the tracheal lumen has returned to normal.

The typical complex of presenting symptoms includes fever, anorexia, weight loss, and lassitude.[7,8] Night sweats, pruritis, and Pel-Ebstein fever are features of adult Hodgkin's but are uncommon in childhood. Most patients are aware of symptoms for less than 3 months, but no correlation is seen between the stage of disease and length of symptoms. Although tracheobronchial compression (Figure 11-2; see also Chapter 26, Figure 26-33) has not been considered a significant feature of Hodgkin's disease in the past, Mandell[9] and coworkers in Philadelphia found that over half of their patients with Hodgkin's disease had some degree of tracheal narrowing that caused symptoms in approximately one-third.

Hematologic and biochemical studies are often abnormal in patients with Hodgkin's disease. Anemia, leukopenia, leukocytosis, and elevated sedimentation rates may be present at some time during the course of illness. Correlation between liver function tests and liver involvement is poor. Elevated serum copper, a finding in active Hodgkin's disease, relates closely to clinical activity and is especially helpful in monitoring recurrent disease. Serum copper levels may be elevated before other tests become positive.[10,11]

One of the more important concepts in the treatment and prognosis of Hodgkin's disease relates to the mode of spread to contiguous organs through lymphatic channels. It is therefore necessary to accurately define the anatomic boundaries and organ involvement in order to predict the potential metastasis. Neighboring organs and anatomic regions that are at risk should be treated with prophylactic radiation therapy.[10,12]

The pathologic staging for Hodgkin's disease (Ann Arbor classification), originally devised by Carbone et al.,[13] is as follows:

Stage I. The disease is limited to one lymph node region or a single extralymphatic organ, exclusive of liver, bone marrow, skin, lung, etc. *Example*: cervical lymph nodes or extranodal thyroid.

Stage II. The disease is limited to one side of the diaphragm, but there is possible involvement of two or more lymph node regions. Direct invasion of an adjacent organ is present. *Example*: mediastinal lymph nodes and cervical lymph nodes, or mediastinal lymph nodes with direct extension into the lung, stomach, and paraaortic lymph nodes.

Stage III. The disease has progressed beyond stage II and involves lymph nodes on both sides of the diaphragm. *Example*: supraclavicular, mediastinal, and paraaortic.

Stage IV. There is diffuse involvement of other organs such as the lung, liver, bone marrow, and central nervous system.

Each of these stages is divided into two subcategories: (1) without systemic symptoms and (2) with systemic symptoms, such as fever, weight loss, and night sweats.

Diagnostic Evaluation

Radiographs of the chest are important instruments used to note and record the original extent of disease. They are also of use in the follow-up and monitoring of response to therapy and possible recurrence. Frontal and lateral films are usually obtained at the outset, but hilar tomography may be of help in visualizing small mediastinal masses and further defining the extent to which specific lymph node groups are implicated.

The presence of mediastinal involvement at the time of discovery of Hodgkin's disease will diminish the survival rate approximately 10 percent, according to North[14] and coworkers. They recommend computed tomography (CT) of the mediastinum in all patients with low neck or supraclavicular adenopathy in whom chest radiographs suggest mediastinal or lung extension (see Chapter 26, Figures 26-39 and 26-40). This information is of critical use to the radiation therapist for field planning. Treatment plans may have to be altered to include chemotherapy and low-dose irradiation to the lungs in those patients with mediastinal mass diameters of 7.5 cm or greater, regardless of stage.[14] Computed tomography may also add information in the detection of small masses and chest wall involvement (see Chapter 26, Figure 26-39).[15] Nuclear magnetic resonance is another method of diagnostic imaging in this condition (see Chapter 27, Figure 27-21).

Pulmonary parenchymal disease occurs in 10 to 14 percent of children with newly diagnosed Hodgkin's disease.[16,17] When the parenchyma is involved, mediastinal disease is invariably present. Contiguous pulmonary spread, thought to be extensions of disease in the hilar and mediastinal lymph nodes, does not affect the numerical staging; discrete lesions within the lung imply stage IV disease. Obscure pulmonary radiopacities on plain film may be resolved by whole lung tomography, but in the presence of normal chest films, further evaluation is not recommended.[16]

Differentiation of anterior mediastinal adenopathy from normal thymus gland is difficult, but Francis and coworkers[18] have reported success using CT in older children and adults. These authors placed considerable emphasis on the retention of the normal shape of the thymus in simple hyperplasia, compared with a lobular look of lymphadenopathy in leukemia and lymphoma. (See Chapter 8.)

Follow-up chest films may show persistent widening of the mediastinum, even in successfully treated patients. Calcification of mediastinal lymph nodes in children following radiation therapy is a rare observation, the significance of which is undetermined.[19-21] When recurrent disease involves the lung, it is usually nodular and infiltrative. Differentiating pulmonary Hodgkin's disease recurrence from superimposed infections or drug therapy reactions may be difficult or impossible with the roentgen ray. Thoracoscopy and biopsy constitute an excellent method of retrieving tissue for diagnosis.[22]

Pathologic Findings

The histologic examination of involved tissue shows the presence of Reed-Sternberg cells. They alone are not pathognomonic, however; similar-appearing structures have been described in infectious mononucleosis.[23] The four major histologic types of Hodgkin's lymphoma (Rye classification) and their approximate frequency are as follows:

Lymphocytic predominance	±12%
Nodular sclerosis	±55%
Mixed cellularity	±30%
Lymphocyte depletion	±3%

In children, the mixed cellularity and lymphocyte predominant types have the best prognosis, and lymphocyte depletion the worst.

Non-Hodgkin's Lymphoma

Non-Hodgkin's lymphoma consists of a heterogeneous group of entities with a variety of histopathologic terms and clinical presentations. The National Cancer Institute has divided these into (1) low grade, (2) intermediate grade, (3) high grade, and (4) miscellaneous (composite lymphoma, mycosis fungoides, histiocytic lymphoma extramedullary plasmacytoma). They are often more aggressive than the Hodgkin's group, with a greater tendency toward generalized dissemination.[24] The clinical symptoms from chest involvement are often related to tracheal compression.[25]

Mediastinal and hilar adenopathy in this disease cannot be distinguished radiographically from

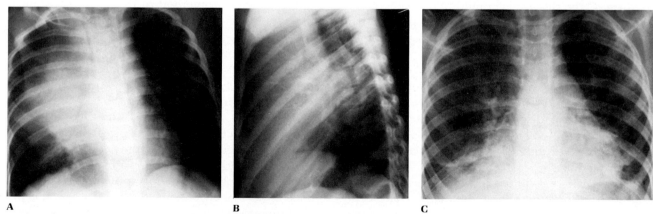

A   **B**   **C**

Figure 11-3 Acute T-cell lymphocytic leukemia. The patient is a 6-year-old-girl with a 6-week history of weight loss, anorexia, and decreased appetite. **A** and **B.** The initial frontal and lateral chest films show a large anterior mediastinal mass extending into the right lung with adjacent parenchymal infiltrate. The diagnosis of acute leukemia was made, and the patient was treated with chemotherapy and corticosteroids. **C.** The mass regressed, but the patient returned 2 months later with pulmonary symptoms. The chest film shows bilateral confluent infiltrates; *Pneumocystis carinii* was isolated from the lung.

Hodgkin's or other lymphomas or from other malignant or benign disease (Figure 11-3). Marked tracheal compression, however, favors the diagnosis of non-Hodgkin's lymphoma, and emergency radiation or chemotherapy may give rapid relief. Non-Hodgkin's lymphoma has a much higher incidence of pulmonary involvement than Hodgkin's disease. Pleural effusion is also more common, but the roentgen ray will fail to separate malignant pleural effusions from those caused by lymphatic or venous obstruction. Pericardial effusions occur in non-Hodgkin's as well as Hodgkin's disease (see Chapter 26, Figure 26-38; Chapter 27, Figure 27-29).

Benign Diseases

Pseudolymphoma

Saltzstein,[26] in 1963, first recognized pseudolymphoma as a benign tumor separate from lymphocytic lymphoma and other lymphoproliferative diseases. Since then, numerous additional reports of this tumor have appeared, and further define its radiologic and clinical features.[27–30] These are rare entities in all ages, particularly in childhood. Nevertheless, separating pseudolymphoma from other more serious grievances is important.

Clinical symptoms are usually nonexistent or very mild. Radiographically, pseudolymphoma presents as a dense mass lesion with indistinct borders, often cavitary or cystic in appearance and frequently containing air bronchograms. They localize at random throughout the lung and may involve contiguous lobes. The lesions tend to be smaller than those of lymphoma, measuring less than 4 to 6 cm in most cases. Pleural effusions are not common, but visceral pleural infiltration has been observed.[28] The presence of hilar adenopathy favors lymphoma rather than pseudolymphoma. However, rare cases of pseudolymphoma may have enlarged hilar lymph nodes, and lymphoma may occur without adenopathy.[29]

In contrast to pseudolymphoma, the pulmonary lesions of lymphomas tend to be larger, better marginated, and more centrally placed. Major bronchi are more often involved, but air bronchograms and inhomogeneous cystic lesions develop in both. Pleural effusion is more common in lymphomas.

Lesions other than lymphoma that are closely related in radiologic and histologic appearance include lymphocytic (lymphoid) interstitial pneumonitis, giant cell interstitial pneumonitis, and chronic relapsing alveolar pneumonitis. Some clinicians question the existence of any differentiation between these diseases.[31]

The prognosis for patients with pseudolymphoma is generally excellent; local surgical excision is usually curative.

Infectious Mononucleosis

While the etiology of infectious mononucleosis is, in all likelihood, a virus (Epstein-Barr), it is included with this group because roentgenographic changes simulate the lymphomatous diseases. Infectious mononucleosis may produce moderate to marked mediastinal adenopathy indistinguishable from that caused by lymphoma, leukemia, or Hodgkin's disease. Pulmonary infiltrates also result from the disease proper or from superimposed bacterial infections.

Giant Lymph Node Hyperplasia

Giant lymph node hyperplasia is also known as Castleman's disease and angiomatous-lymphoid hamartoma. First reported by Castleman,[1] this abnormality occurs most often in patients between the ages of 10 and 45. Affected individuals are usually asymptomatic but may complain of vague mediastinal pressure. The anterior mediastinum is most often involved and is widened unilaterally or bilaterally by enlarged lymph nodes.[30] Posteriorly situated masses and rib erosions that mimic neurogenic tumors have been described.[34] Calcification of the involved lymph nodes has also been reported,[35] but pulmonary infiltration does not occur.

Two varieties of giant lymph node hyperplasia have been recognized: (1) hyaline-vascular and (2) plasma cell.[36] While these tumor masses behave in a benign fashion, iron-refractory anemia, hypergammaglobulinemia, and retarded growth are occasionally disconcerting complications.[37–39]

Sinus Histiocytosis

Sinus histiocytosis (Rosai-Dorfman disease) is marked by painless cervical adenopathy.[2,40] It is a disease of youth; most patients are under 20 years of age, and the majority of them are between 7 months and 9 years. Mediastinal lymph nodes may enlarge in 30 percent of patients, but mediastinal mass development is rare.[41] Hilar and paratracheal adenopathy has also been observed (Figure 11-4),[42] but pulmonary involvement does not occur. More than one-fourth of patients manifest extranodal disease, consisting of mass lesions of the orbits, testicles, and subcutaneous tissue, as well as osteolytic defects of bone.

The microscopic appearance is that of markedly dilated sinusoids filled with histiocytes. In some cases, the histology suggests the plasma cell form of giant lymph node hyperplasia.

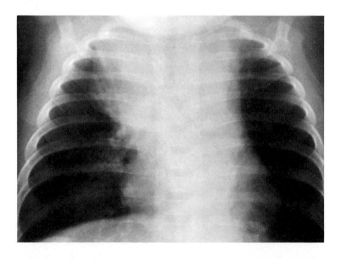

Figure 11-4 Sinus histiocytosis—Rosai-Dorfman syndrome. The patient is a 3-month-old black male with tachypnea since birth and recent respiratory infection and cough. The chest film shows bilateral mediastinal mass densities with partial volume loss of the right upper lobe. A mediastinal lymph node biopsy showed reactive hyperplasia with sinus histiocytosis. (Courtesy of Dr. Britt B. Gay, Jr., Atlanta, Georgia.)

Fever and leukocytosis may accompany the cervical swelling. Spontaneous recovery usually occurs, but the course may be protracted and recurrent.

References

1. Castleman B, Iverson L, Menendex VP: Localized mediastinal lymph node hyperplasia resembling thymoma. *Cancer* 9:822, 1956.
2. Rosai J, Dorfman RF: Sinus histiocytosis with massive lymphadenopathy: A pseudolymphomatous benign disorder. Analysis of 34 cases. *Cancer* 30:1174, 1970.
3. Young JL, Miller RW: Incidence of malignant tumors in United States children. *J Pediatr* 86:254, 2975.
4. Parker BR, Castellino RA: Hodgkin's disease, in Parker BR, Castellino RA (eds): *Pediatric Oncologic Radiology.* St Louis, CV Mosby, 1977, p 160.
5. Sullivan MP, Fuller LM, Butler JJ: Hodgkin's disease in children, in Sutow WW, Vietti TJ, Fernbach DJ (eds): *Clinical Pediatric Oncology.* St Louis, CV Mosby, 1977, p 410.
6. Donaldson SS, Glatstein E, Rosenberg SA, et al: Pediatric Hodgkin's disease II. Results of therapy. *Cancer* 37:2436, 1976.
7. Schnitzer B, Nashiyama RN, Heidelberger KP, et al: Hodgkin's disease in children. *Cancer* 31:560, 1973.
8. Evans HE, Nyhan WL: Hodgkin's disease in children. *Bull Johns Hopkins Hosp* 114:237, 1964.
9. Mandell GA, Lantieri R, Goodman LR: Tracheobronchial compression in Hodgkin lymphoma in children. *AJR* 139:1167, 1982.
10. Kaplan HS: *Hodgkin's Disease.* Cambridge, Harvard University Press, 1972.
11. Hrgovic M, Tessmer CF, Minckler TM, et al: Serum copper levels in lymphoma and leukemia: Special reference to Hodgkin's disease. *Cancer* 21:743, 1968.
12. Peters MV: Prophylactic treatment of adjacent areas in Hodgkin's disease. *Cancer Res* 26:1232, 1966.
13. Carbone PP, Kaplan HS, Mushoff K, et al: Report of the committee on Hodgkin's disease staging classification. *Cancer Res* 31:1860, 1971.
14. North LB, Fuller LM, Hagemeister FB, et al: Importance of initial mediastinal adenopathy in Hodgkin's disease. *AJR* 138:229, 1982.
15. Kirks DR, Korobkin M: Chest computed tomography in infants and children. An analysis of 50 patients. *Pediatr Radiol* 10:75, 1980.

16. Parker, BR, Castellino RA, Kaplan HS: Pediatric Hodgkin's disease I. Radiographic evaluation. *Cancer* 37:2430, 1976.

17. Kolygin BA, Vesnin AG: Hodgkin's disease in children: Clinicoroentgenologic features of the lesion in the chest. *Pediatr Radiol* 4:144, 1976.

18. Francis IR, Glazer GM, Bookstein FI, et al: The thymus: Reexamination of age-related changes in size and shape. *AJR* 145:249, 1985.

19. Rivero H, Gaisie G, Bender TM, et al: Calcified mediastinal lymph nodes in Hodgkin's disease. *Pediatric Radiol* 14:11, 1984.

20. Wyman, SM, Weber AL: Calcification of intrathoracic nodes in Hodgkin's disease. *Radiology* 93:1021, 1969.

21. DeGiuli E, DeGiuli G: Lymph node calcification in Hodgkin's disease following irradiation. *Acta Radiol Oncol Radiat Phys Biol* 16:305, 1977.

22. Rodgers BM, Talbert JL: Thoracoscopy for diagnosis of intrathoracic lesions in the chest. *Pediatr Surg* 5:703, 1976.

23. Saltzstein SL: Pulmonary malignant lymphomas and pseudolymphomas: Classification, therapy, and prognosis. *Cancer* 16:925, 1963.

24. Murphy SB, Frizzera G, Evans AE: A study of childhood non-Hodgkin's lymphoma. *Cancer* 36:212, 1975.

25. Castellino RA, Parker BR: Non-Hodgkin's lymphoma, in Parker BR, Castellino RA (eds): *Pediatric Oncologic Radiology*. St Louis, CV Mosby, 1977, p 183.

26. Saltzstein SL: Pulmonary malignant lymphomas and pseudolymphomas: Classification, therapy, and prognosis. *Cancer* 16:925, 1963.

27. Hutchinson WB, Friedenberg MJ, Saltzstein S: Primary pulmonary pseudolymphoma. *Radiology* 82:48, 1964.

28. Greenberg SD, Heisler JG, Gyorkey F, Jenkins DE: Pulmonary lymphoma versus pseudolymphoma: A perplexing problem. *South Med J* 65:775, 1972.

29. Julsrud PR, Brown LR, Chin-Yang L, et al: Pulmonary processes of mature appearing lymphocytes: Pseudolymphoma, well-differentiated lymphocytic lymphoma and lymphocytic interstitial pneumonitis. *Radiology* 127:289, 1978.

30. Feigin DS, Siegelman SS, Theros EG, et al: Nonmalignant lymphoid disorders of the chest. *AJR* 129:221, 1977.

31. Reich, NE, McCormack LJ, Van Ordstrand HS: Pseudolymphoma of lung. *Chest* 65:424, 1974.

32. Rosenthal T, Hertz M: Mediastinal lymphadenopathy in infectious mononucleosis. Report of two cases. *JAMA* 233:1300, 1975.

33. Fermaglich DR: Pulmonary involvement in infectious mononucleosis. *J Pediatr* 86:93, 1975.

34. Culver GJ, Choi BK: Benign lymphoid hyperplasia (Castleman's tumor) mimicking a posterior mediastinal neurogenic tumor. *Chest* 62:512, 1972.

35. Sang Oh K: Personal communication, 1981.

36. Keller AR, Hochkolzer L, Castleman B: Hyaline-vascular and plasma-cell types of giant lymph node hyperplasia of the mediastinum and other locations. *Cancer* 29:670, 1972.

37. Ballow M, Park BH, Dupont B, et al: Benign giant lymphoid hyperplasia of the mediastinum with associated abnormalities of the immune system. *J Pediatr* 84:418, 1974.

38. Boxer LA, Boxer GJ, Flair RC, et al: Angiomatous lymphoid hyperplasia associated with chronic anemia, hypoferrinemia, and hypergammaglobulinemia. *J Pediatr* 81:66, 1972.

39. Sethi G, Krepes JJ: Intrathoracic angiomatous lymphoid hamartomas: A report of three cases, one of iron refractory anemia and retarded growth. *J Thorac Cardiovasc Surg* 61:657, 1971.

40. Sanchez R, Rosai J, Dorfman RF: Sinus histiocytosis with massive lymphadenopathy: An analysis of 13 cases with special emphasis on its extranodal manifestations (abstract). *Lab Invest* 36:349, 1977.

41. Friedman MJ, Rossoff LJ, Aftalion B: Sinus histiocytosis presenting as a mediastinal mass. *Chest* 86:267, 1984.

42. Pickering LK, Phelan E: Sinus histiocytosis. *J Pediatr* 86:745, 1975.

Chapter 12

Vascular Tumors and Tumor-Like Conditions

This chapter will consider three groups of lesions that produce mass densities in and around the mediastinum: (1) vascular tumors, (2) vascular abnormalities (congenital and acquired), and (3) nonvascular congenital malformations.

1. Vascular tumors
   a. Lymphangioma, lymphangiosarcoma
   b. Hemangioma
2. Vascular abnormalities
   a. Dilation of the superior vena cava
   b. Cervical arch
   c. Aneurysm of the ductus arteriosus
   d. Total anomalous pulmonary venous return
   e. Anomalous left pulmonary artery (pulmonary or vascular sling)
   f. Aneurysm of the aorta and major vessels
   g. "Aberrant" innominate artery
3. Nonvascular congenital malformations
   a. Diaphragmatic hernia and eventration

Vascular Tumors

Lymphangioma, Lymphangiosarcoma

Of the two proliferative lesions of the lymphatic vascular space, lymphangioma is the more common. Lymphangiosarcoma, the malignant counterpart, is virtually nonexistent in childhood, but it may occur as a complication of lymphangioma.[1] Considerable difference of opinion exists regarding the etiology, classification, and terminology of these lesions.

In all likelihood, lymphangiomas are congenital anomalies, arising from localized lymphatic stasis secondary to congenital blockage of normal lymphatic drainage.[2] However, their ability to grow and proliferate gives them a true neoplastic character, and they probably should be considered as tumors.[3,4]

Lymphangiomas are classified into two major types:[2,4,5]

1. Simple lymphangioma: those lesions composed of microscopic or small lymph-filled channels
2. Cavernous lymphangioma (cystic hygroma): larger tumors containing lymph-filled cysts varying in size from a few millimeters to several centimeters[2,4]

Over 50 percent of lymphangiomas occur in the head, including the tongue, cheek, mouth, and neck; less than 10 percent occupy the mediastinum. The cavernous types often present as large, deforming, soft mass lesions, most often in the neck and head tissue. When found in the neck, axilla, and mediastinum, these tumors tend to be more cystic. Not uncommonly, features of both cavernous and simple lymphangioma exist within the same lesion. Tumors arising in the neck may extend into the mediastinum (see Chapter 27, Figure 27-30), but usually the mediastinal component is not removed during resection of the cervical portion.

Intrathoracic lymphangiomas characteristically occupy the anterior or superior mediastinum. Often asymptomatic, they are commonly discovered on chest films taken for other reasons (Figure 12-1). An uncommon but serious complication results when thoracic lymphangiomas infiltrate lung tissue, pleura, and chest wall structures. Chylothorax and extensive destruction of lung, chest walls, and ribs may cause severe disability and death.[6] Symptoms resulting from compression of adjacent structures and secondary infection have also been reported.[7]

Surgical resection is the recommended treatment for lymphangiomas of sufficient size. Well-circumscribed cystic hygromas are easier to remove than simple lymphangiomas which infiltrate into adjacent muscle and soft tissue. Multiple operations are often needed because of the lymphangioma's size and location. Even when most or all of the tumor can be removed, residual lymphatic drainage and secondary infection are troublesome sequelae.[6] In some cases, gross tumor left unresected may remain stable and not enlarge. Cervical lymphangiomas in infants may have a mediastinal component that on plain films is indistinguishable from a large thymus (see Chapter 27, Figure 27-30; also see Chapter 8).

When present in the peritoneal cavity, lymphan-

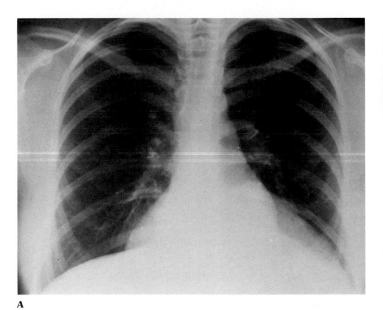 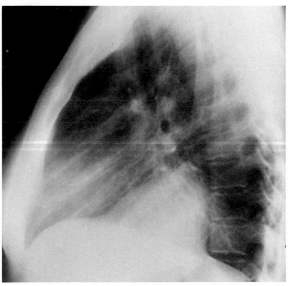

A   **B**

Figure 12-1 Lymphangioma. Lymphangioma discovered on a routine chest film in an asymptomatic patient. **A** and **B.** Frontal and lateral films disclose a soft tissue mass in the middle mediastinum posterior to the heart and crossing the midline. It blends imperceptibly into the diaphragm. The mass was removed surgically. (Courtesy of Dr. James Scatliff, Chapel Hill, North Carolina.)

giomas often take the form of mesenteric cysts, and may achieve considerable size. They may retain their clear lymphatic fluid or develop a milky chyle if in communication with the lymphatics of the gastrointestinal tract.

Disseminated lymphangiomatosis (see Chapter 26, Figure 26-53) is a rare variety of lymphangioma that is associated with well-defined lytic lesions of bone.[8,9] The osseous lesions may remain dormant or aggressively destroy bone and invade critical soft tissue structures. Chylothorax is an occasional complication that may be difficult or impossible to control.[6] Death or seriously disabling illness often results.

Differentiation of lymphangiomas from other mediastinal masses is often impossible from plain radiographs. They are usually anterior and superior in location. Calcification, a feature of extrathoracic lymphangiomas, is less common in mediastinal lesions (Figure 12-2). Computed tomography (CT) and magnetic resonance imaging are useful in the preoperative evaluation (see Chapter 26, Figure 26-53; Chapter 27, Figure 27-30). Sonography may help delineate those tumors that abut the chest wall.[7]

The histopathologic distinction between the various types of lymphangiomas is not well-defined. Both lymphangioma simplex and cystic or cavernous lymphangiomas consist of epithelium-lined concatenated cystic spaces and channels, separated by varying amounts of connective tissue. The spaces vary from capillary size to several centimeters in diameter. Lymphangioma simplex tends to be less encapsulated and more admixed with muscle and soft tissue. It is found predominantly in the region of the parotid gland, lips, nose, eyelids, scalp, preauricular skin, and larynx. In many cases, however, elements of cystic change are found.

Histologic features of both lymphangioma and hemangioma are sometimes present in the same tumor. Lymphangiography occasionally shows contrast entering the tumor, a finding that helps distinguish lymphangioma from hemangioma.[10,11]

Inflammation and hemorrhage may complicate

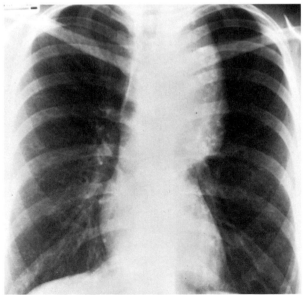

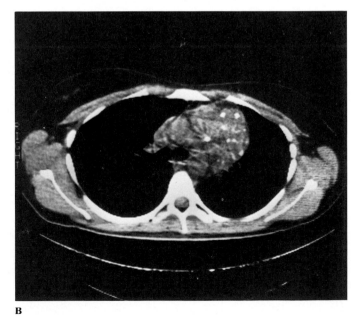

A   **B**

Figure 12-2   Lymphangioma—with calcification. A. The plain chest film demonstrates an anterosuperior mediastinal mass that displaces the trachea to the right. Multiple, discrete calcifications are visible. **B.** Computed tomography confirms the size and location of the mass as well as the calcific densities. Deviation of the trachea and stem bronchi is also noted, an unusual finding for these relatively soft tumors.

the treatment of lymphangioma.[12] Pressure on adjacent structures is not usually a problem, but large lesions may compromise the laryngeal and tracheal air columns, necessitating tracheostomy. Spontaneous regression of some tumors is to be expected, possibly because of the opening of collateral lymphatic channels.

Hemangioma

Mediastinal hemangiomas may exist as a segment of a lymphangioma (see the previous section), as an isolated tumor, or in association with generalized hemangiomas. Their traditional location is the anterior mediastinum, but they may appear in the middle or posterior mediastinum as well.[13]

Plain-film diagnosis is limited because of the nonspecific nature of the mass, although the finding of occasional phleboliths will indicate the diagnosis. The delineation of cavernous hemangioma by CT is possible;[14] but contrast enhancement should be performed (Figure 12-3). (See Chapters 26 and 27.)

Vascular Abnormalities

Dilatation of the Superior Vena Cava

Dilatation of the superior vena cava (SVC) usually produces a right superior paramediastinal density (Figure 12-4).[15–17] The cause of SVC dilatation is unknown but presumed to result from an inherent weakness in the vessel wall. Antecedent trauma has not been implicated.

The condition is benign, and most patients are asymptomatic. On occasion, other tributary veins in the lower neck are involved and become dilated and engorged with blood during valsalva maneuver (Figure 12-5). Only when complicated by superimposed disease has this condition been of any medical significance.[18,19] Spontaneous rupture has not been reported, the dilatation apparently does not progress, and surgical intervention is discouraged.

Superior vena cavography is a reliable method for the evaluation of this condition; CT with bolus contrast injection and magnetic resonance imaging are

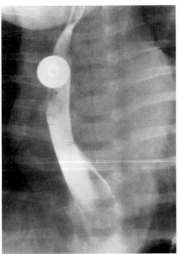
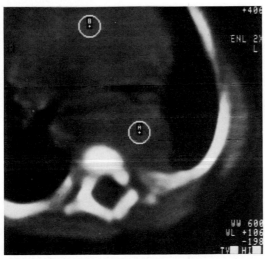
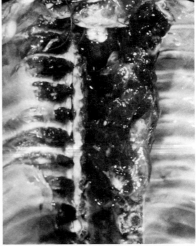

A   B   C

Figure 12-3 Hemangioma. This 6-week-old-child presented with multiple cutaneous hemangiomas, gastrointestinal hemorrhage, and clinical signs of coarctation of the aorta. Laparotomy disclosed multiple hemangiomas throughout the bowel wall. **A.** An elongated left posterior mediastinal mass is present, displacing the trachea and barium-filled esophagus to the right. The heart is enlarged. **B.** With contrast-enhanced CT, the mass measures 43 Hounsfield units (13 units before contrast). The heart measures 37 Hounsfield units. **C.** At autopsy a cavernous hemangioma is present. *Note:* Contrast-enhanced CT is needed to evaluate the vascular nature of these lesions.

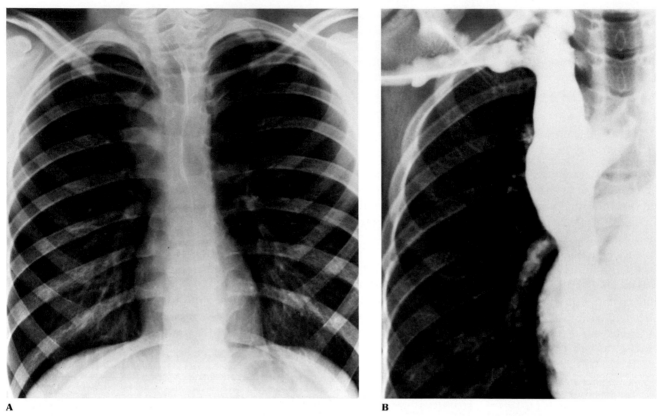

A   **B**

Figure 12-4   Idiopathic dilatation of the SVC. A. The frontal film demonstrates a right superior mediastinal density. **B.** The superior vena cavogram shows the density to be an aneurysmal dilatation of the SVC. Flow is not obstructed. (From Heil et al.[17])

also diagnostic (Figures 12-4 and 12-5). Digital subtraction angiography, another proven method for evaluation of vascular abnormalities in the chest, should provide diagnostic information.[20] (See Chapter 2.)

Cervical Arch

Cervical arch anomaly is a rare congenital malformation.[21–23] This anomaly results from cranial displacement of the aortic arch as it extends to the base of the neck before turning caudally to descend in the thorax. Approximately two-thirds occur on the right side and one-third on the left. Cervical arch anomaly was not associated with congenital cardiac anomalies in early reports,[24] but tetralogy of Fallot, pseu-

dotruncus arteriosus, double-outlet right ventricle, and ventricular septal defect have since been acknowledged.[21]

Cervical arch usually produces minimal symptoms; stridor, respiratory infections, and dyspnea on exertion are common complaints in children. Adults are more likely to complain of dysphagia and odynophagia, while headaches, dizziness, and hoarseness are less commonly experienced. The diagnosis is often suspected from palpation of a pulsatile mass at the base of the neck or medial supraclavicular region that may be confused with an aneurysm.

Cervical arch probably results from maldevelopment of the primitive aortic arches.[24,25] Normally, the third aortic arch involutes in fetal life, and the fourth persists as the aorta. Cervical arch deformity results

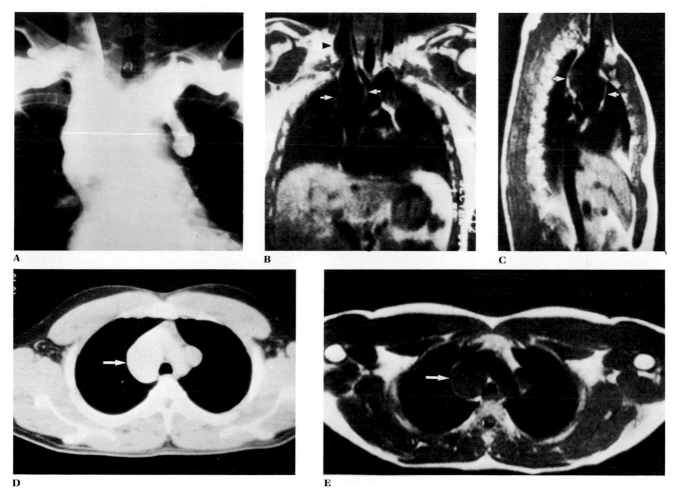

Figure 12-5   Idiopathic dilatation of the SVC. A. The contrast injection shows the dilated SVC and tributary veins. **B** and **C.** Magnetic resonance imaging in the frontal and lateral projections confirms the presence of a dilated SVC (arrows). *Note:* There is a dilated jugular vein (arrowhead). Computed tomography (**D**) and magnetic resonance imaging (**E**), at approximately the same levels, demonstrate the dilated SVC in cross section (arrows). (Courtesy of Dr. David Turner, Chicago, Illinois.)

when the third aortic arch persists and the fourth, or normal one, involutes.

The following outline depicts some of the potential vessel variations to be expected with this anomaly:

1. Right cervical arch (two-thirds of cases)
   a. Virtually always, the left-sided descending aorta crosses behind the esophagus (one case exception).
   b. The great vessel anatomy is always abnormal.

2. Left cervical arch (one-third cases)
   a. The descending aorta on the left side has normal takeoff and position of great vessels (elongated arch).
   b. The descending aorta on the right side has abnormal great vessel takeoff.

The roentgenographic findings of cervical arch depend upon the existing anatomy. Displacement of the trachea by an apical mediastinal mass is one clue to the diagnosis; poorly defined or nonvisible aortic knob is another. Lateral films may show anterior tracheal displacement, and a contrast esophogram will frequently disclose a large posterior vascular indentation on the barium column as the vessel crosses to the opposite side (Figure 12-6). This posterior indentation should not be confused with an aberrant subclavian artery, which is smaller and more cranial in position. Left-sided cervical arch and descending aorta are more difficult to appreciate; the cranial position of the aortic knob is the clue to this anomaly. Computed tomography and digital subtraction radiography are the diagnostic studies of choice.

Aneurysm of the Ductus Arteriosus

Aneurysmal dilatation of the ductus arteriosus may suggest the presence of a middle mediastinal mass. This abnormality is extremely rare; reports of preoperative diagnosis and successful surgical removal are sparse.[26–28] Enlargement of the normal ductus arteriosus is not uncommon in the neonate, but this should not persist after 72 h of age. Often referred to as the ductus bump, this dilatation may produce a rounded density adjacent to the normal aortic arch in the aorticopulmonary window.[29]

Aneurysmal dilatation of the ductus arteriosus usually presents in infancy or childhood with clinical signs of patency, thromboembolic phenomena, or infection.[30] Stretching of the recurrent laryngeal or phrenic nerve may lead to voice changes or diaphragmatic paralysis. Rupture or dissection is a rare complication in patients with Marfan's syndrome.[31]

Kirks et al.[28] have advanced two theories to explain the etiology of spontaneous aneurysms of the ductus arteriosus; (1) delay in closure of the aortic end of the ductus produces a diverticulum of the aorta which then undergoes myxoid degeneration and aneurysmal dilatation, and (2) primary myxoid degeneration occurs within the ductus wall with secondary aneurysmal dilatation. Traumatic injury

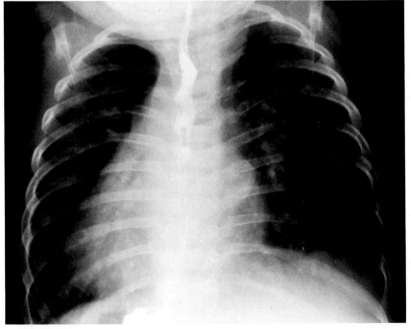

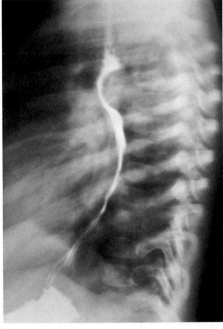

A

B

Figure 12-6 Cervical arch. A. The barium column is deviated by a right-sided cervical arch in the apex of the right chest. An intracardiac shunt to the lungs is present. **B.** The aortic arch produces a large posterior indentation on the barium-filled esophagus as it crosses to descend on the left.

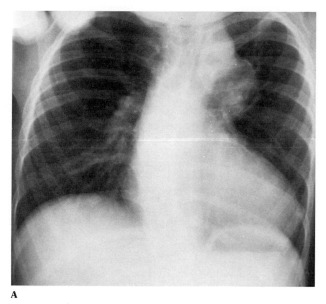

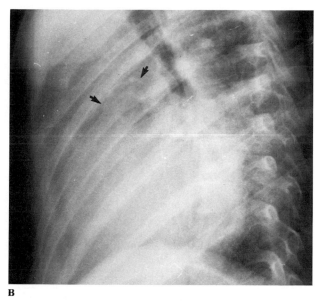

A   B

Figure 12-7   Aneurysm of the ductus arteriosus. A. A round mass density with peripheral curvilinear calcification occupies the aorticopulmonary window. **B.** The mass, outlined by faint calcification (arrows), is located anterior to the pulmonary arteries.

is another possible cause.[32] Mitcell and coworkers have reported success with surgical treatment in five consecutive patients.[33]

On frontal chest film, a ductus arteriosus aneurysm forms a rounded, soft tissue mass in the aorticopulmonary window (Figure 12-7A). In the lateral view, it may lie in front of or behind the trachea (Figure 12-7B). Calcifications frequently occur within the wall.[34] Differential diagnosis includes bronchogenic cyst, duplication, adenopathy, and other causes for aneurysm.

Diagnosis may be confirmed by CT or thoracic aortography. Pulmonary angiography usually shows normal lung vasculature and absent opacification of the aneurysm.

Total Anomalous Pulmonary Venous Return

In the early stages of normal pulmonary embryogenesis, venous return from the lung reaches the heart via the cardinal system (superior vena cava) and the umbilical-vitelline system (inferior vena cava) (Figure 12-8). As these primitive pathways obliterate, the common pulmonary vein (CPV) develops behind the heart, incorporates into the systemic atrium, and receives the pulmonary venous drainage. The CPV eventually becomes the left atrium; the atrial appendage represents residual cardiac tissue from the primitive systemic atrium.

Total anomalous pulmonary venous return (TAPVR) occurs when the CPV fails to develop normal communication with the left atrium. Pulmonary venous blood must return to the heart via alternative channels, either the cardinal or umbilical-vitelline drainage systems. The closure sequence of these primitive drainage systems (cardinal and umbilical-vitelline) determines the anatomy of anomalous venous return in any given patient. Total anomalous pulmonary venous return below the diaphragm develops when the cardinal vein obliterates first, and blood reaches the heart through the umbilical-vitelline system, below the diaphragm. When the umbilical-vitelline veins are the first to close, pulmonary venous blood returns to the heart via the cardinal vein, innominate vein, and SVC (snowman). On rare occasions, when both the cardinal and umbilical-vitelline collateral drainage systems obliterate and the CPV fails to connect to the systemic atrium, the only

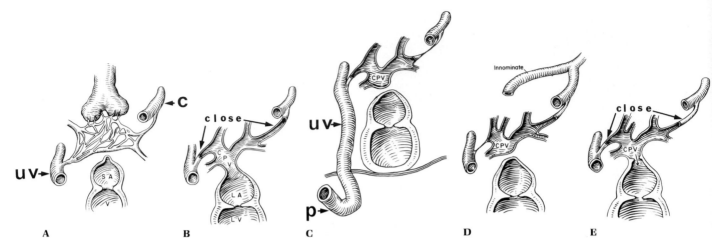

Figure 12-8   Total anomalous pulmonary venous return—embryology. A. In early embryologic development the splanchnic pulmonary vascular bed drains via the umbilical-vitelline (uv) and the cardinal (c) systems (SA = systemic atrium; V = ventricle). **B.** In normal development the CPV forms behind the heart and incorporates into the left atrium (LA). The connections to the umbilical-vitelline and cardinal systems close, allowing normal pulmonary blood return to the left atrium. **C.** Anomalous return below the diaphragm results when the CPV fails to incorporate into the left atrium, the connection to the cardinal system obliterates, and the umbilical-vitelline (uv) system remains patent (p = portal vein). **D.** Anomalous return above the diaphragm results when the CPV fails to incorporate into the LA, the umbilical-vitelline connection obliterates, and the cardinal system remains open. **E.** Cor triatriatum results when the connection between the CPV and left atrium remains stenotic. The anomalous connections above and below the diaphragm close. (Adapted from Lucas RV Jr, Anderson RC, Amplatz K, et al: Congenital causes of pulmonary venous obstruction. *Pediatr Clin North Am* X: 781, 1963.)

pulmonary venous return possible is through the bronchial artery–pulmonary vein collaterals.[35,36] This condition is rarely diagnosed antemortem and until recently has been uniformly fatal.[37] The unusual abnormality, cor triatriatum, occurs when the CPV fails to develop a complete connection with the systemic atrium, thus creating an obstruction to pulmonary venous return similar to that seen in mitral stenosis.

Anomalous pulmonary venous return above the diaphragm is often compatible with life if adequate communication between the atria is present. Obstructed TAPVR above the diaphragm is uncommon except when the vertical vein is compressed between the left pulmonary artery and left stem bronchus. The anomalous (snowman) vessels simulate a mediastinal mass on plain films (Figure 12-9). Mild cardiomegaly and shunt vascularity are common.

Total anomalous pulmonary venous return below the diaphragm usually connects to the portal vein, inferior vena cava, hepatic veins, or other venous channels. Obstruction to blood flow in TAPVR

below the diaphragm often results from constriction of the vessel as it traverses the diaphragm or, in portal vein connections, as blood passes through the liver.

The radiographic features of TAPVR depend largely upon the abnormal vascular anatomy and severity of pulmonary venous obstruction. Significant cardiomegaly does not usually develop early in life because intracardiac shunts (PDA and patent foramen ovale) protect the right ventricle from diastolic overload. Persistent elevated pulmonary artery pressure contributes to the right-left transductal blood flow, thus eliminating the expected radiographic changes of obstructed pulmonary venous return (Figure 12-10A).[38] After the ductus closes, the pulmonary alterations are characterized by increased numbers of linear, fine, parenchymal densities, by loss of vascular definition, and by thickening of fissures and subpleural lymphatics. Hilar unsharpness and pulmonary overaeration are associated features (Figure 12-10B).

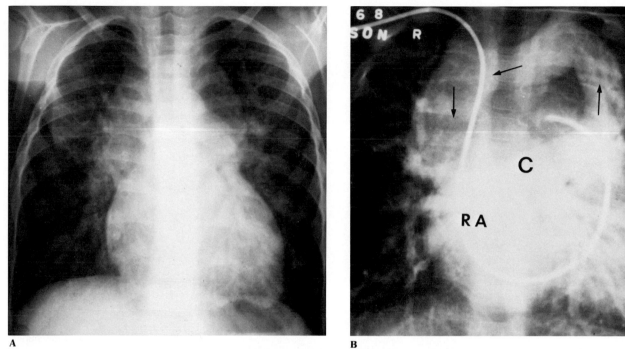

Figure 12-9   Total anomalous pulmonary venous return above the diaphragm (snowman). A. A large, well-defined superior midline density is present. The aortic and pulmonary artery silhouettes are preserved, but the density appears to merge into the right-sided vascular structures and heart border. There is mild cardiomegaly and increased flow to the lungs. **B.** Contrast, injected into the main pulmonary artery, opacifies the common pulmonary vein (C), persistent left SVC, innominate vein, and right SVC, as it returns to the right atrium (RA).

In TAPVR below the diaphragm, an anterior indentation on the barium-filled esophagus just above the diaphragm is occasionally produced by the venous confluence as it journeys to its destination. Ultrasonography may be useful in detecting partial anomalous pulmonary venous return[39] and has also been used to evaluate the presence of a common pulmonary vein behind the heart (Figure 12-10C). However, as indicated above, these channels may not dilate in the early days of life when the ductus remains open and shunts blood away from the lungs.

Anomalous Left Pulmonary Artery (Pulmonary or Vascular Sling)

This anomaly results when the left pulmonary artery arises from the right pulmonary artery, courses around the right stem bronchus, passes between the trachea and esophagus, and enters the hilum of the left lung (Figure 12-11). The trachea and right stem bronchus are narrowed by the adjacent aberrant artery. This anomaly is often associated with intrinsic deformities of the trachea in the region of the impinging vessel; other areas of stenosis and tracheo-bronchomalacia may occur distally.[40,41]

Children who suffer from this anomaly are often symptomatic at or shortly after birth. Wheezing, dyspnea, respiratory distress, and sudden death are associated clinical features.

Right lung overaeration is the most consistent roentgenographic feature of pulmonary sling (Figure 12-12A). However, the hyperaeration may be bilateral or confined to the left lung (Figure 12-13). Right-sided atelectasis is a less common but reported observation.[41–43] On well-exposed high-KVp films, the

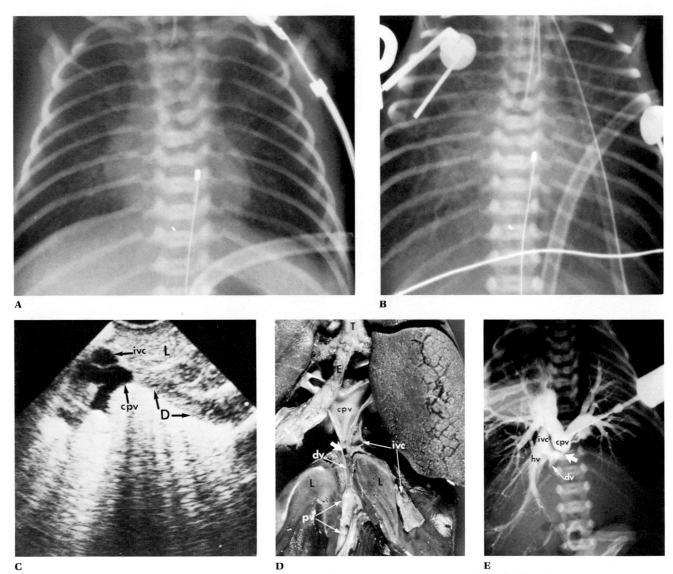

Figure 12-10   Total anomalous pulmonary venous return—below the diaphragm. A. This early film of the chest shows normal heart and indistinct vascularity. *Note:* There are vertebral anomalies. Esophageal atresia and tracheoesophageal fistula were known. **B.** Several days later the lungs have taken on a pattern of pulmonary venous obstruction with pulmonary edema and dilated pulmonary veins. **C.** Real time ultrasonography disclosed a V-shaped echolucent structure (cpv = common pulmonary vein) abutting the diaphragm (D). The inferior vena cava (ivc) lies anterior to the common pulmonary vein. (L = liver.) **D.** Gross dissection at autopsy from behind: The unroofed common pulmonary vein (cpv) receives solitary pulmonary veins from each lung and drains into a confluence (arrow) of the ductus venosus (dv) and hepatic vein. The portal vein (pv) drains into the ductus venosus. The inferior vena cava is seen passing through the right lobe of the liver coursing anteriorly to the common pulmonary vein. The lower esophageal segment (E) communicates with the trachea (T) at the carina. **E.** A radiograph of the injected gross specimen: The arrow denotes the strictured common pulmonary vein as it joins the hepatic vein (hv) and ductus venosus (dv).

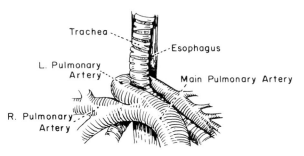

Figure 12-11 Vascular sling. This is a diagrammatic representation of a vascular sling. (Compare with Figures 12-12 and 12-13.)

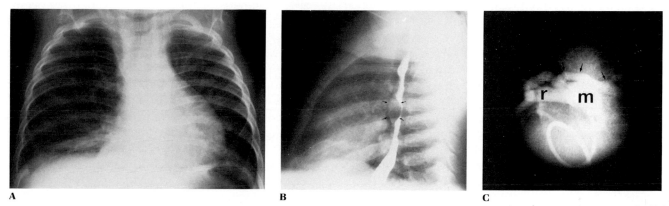

Figure 12-12 Aberrant left pulmonary artery (vascular sling). A. The frontal film shows overdistension of a portion of the right lung with compression of the medial basal segments. **B.** The lateral film shows a typical (almost pathognomonic) anterior, ovoid indentation (arrows) on the barium-filled esophagus produced by the left pulmonary artery as it passes between the esophagus and trachea. **C.** Contrast injection into the main pulmonary artery (m) confirms the takeoff of the aberrant left artery (arrows) from the right pulmonary artery (r). (Compare with Figures 12-11 and 12-13.)

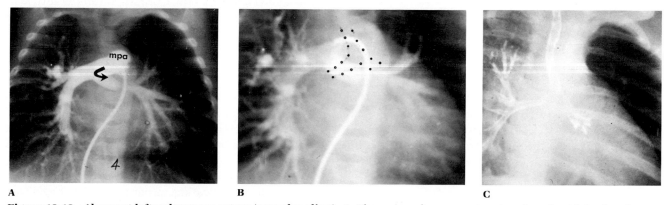

Figure 12-13 Aberrant left pulmonary artery (vascular sling). A. The main pulmonary artery (mpa) contrast injection demonstrates the origin (arrow) of the left pulmonary artery from the right. The left pulmonary hilum is lower than normal. **B** and **C.** Comparable films of the arterial injection and tracheobronchial opacification show deviation of the carina, elongation and narrowing of the right stem bronchus, and widening of the carina. *Note:* The right lung is smaller than the left; the narrowed bronchus has not produced air trapping.

carina may be displaced inferiorly and have a wider than normal angle. The left hilus may also be displaced inferiorly.

A valuable roentgenographic sign of vascular sling is an ovoid opacity occupying the tracheoesophageal septum, or "party wall" (Figure 12-12B). This "mass," representing the aberrant left pulmonary artery as it passes between the trachea and esophagus, produces an anterior indentation on the barium-filled esophagus.[44] Other abnormal vascular structures that cause anterior impressions on the esophagus include the common pulmonary vein in TAPVR below the diaphragm, and multiple bronchial collateral arteries that develop in cases of severe pulmonary stenosis or atresia.

Pulmonary angiography has served as the most reliable diagnostic method (Figures 12-12C and 12-13C). Digital subtraction angiography and CT are additional proven methods.[20,45,46] Tracheobronchography is useful in subtle cases and will delineate other areas of stenosis or bronchomalacia of the tracheobronchial tree distal to the major lesion (Figure 11-13B and C). The knowledge of these abnormalities is important for predicting postoperative symptoms.[41]

The results of operative repair of vascular sling may be inconstant; some patients take several years to recover. Conservative management is successful in others.[47]

Aneurysm of the Aorta and Major Vessels

Aneurysms are uncommon arterial lesions in children. Most are associated with cardiovascular malformations or connective tissue disease, including cystic medial necrosis. Mycotic aneurysms may occur following the use of intraluminal catheters.[31] Thompson et al.[32] have classified aneurysms in children and young adults; a partial list from their review follows:

1. Congenital or presumed congenital: aortic, cerebral, ductal, and/or coronary
2. Cardiovascular malformation: aortic stenosis and/or coarctation of the aorta

3. Syndrome-related: Marfan's, Ehlers-Danlos, tuberous sclerosis
4. Mycotic: bacterial, tuberculous, rubella, fungal
5. Arteritis-related: Takayasu's disease, periarteritis, mucocutaneous lymph node syndrome
6. Traumatic

The use of arterial catheters for monitoring the cardiopulmonary status of critically ill newborns and older children is an accepted procedure. Catheter injury to the endothelium of a vessel apparently sets the stage for secondary invasion, usually by bacteria or fungus.[48–50] In adults, mycotic aneurysms arising in the absence of trauma are usually associated with atherosclerosis.

Symptoms of mycotic aneurysm depend upon the location and size of the aneurysms. In the mediastinum, they may cause wheezing, respiratory distress, and sudden onset of tachypnea. Aneurysms occurring elsewhere may cause renal and hepatic failure, pulmonary hemorrhage, sepsis, rupture, and death.

The presence of mycotic aneurysm should be suspected in an infant with a history of previous umbilical artery catheter placement and sepsis. Plain films that disclose a well-defined mass density or densities should increase suspicion and call for definitive diagnostic studies (Figure 12-14A). Angiography is the traditional method for confirming the diagnosis (Figure 12-14B). Computed tomography with contrast enhancement,[51] digital subtraction radiography, and ultrasonography are additional useful diagnostic tools.[52]

Aneurysmal dilatation of an aberrant subclavian artery related to atherosclerosis has been reported primarily in adults.[53,54] Dysphagia is the usual presenting symptom in older patients. Rodgers et al.[55] reported a child with progressive aneurysmal dilatation of an aberrant right subclavian artery several years after cardiac catheterization through this vessel (Figure 12-15). The symptoms consisted of coughing while eating, progressive dysphagia, and Horner's syndrome. The aneurysm was resected successfully. Aneurysms of other vessels, including the superior mesenteric artery, have also been reported in children.[52]

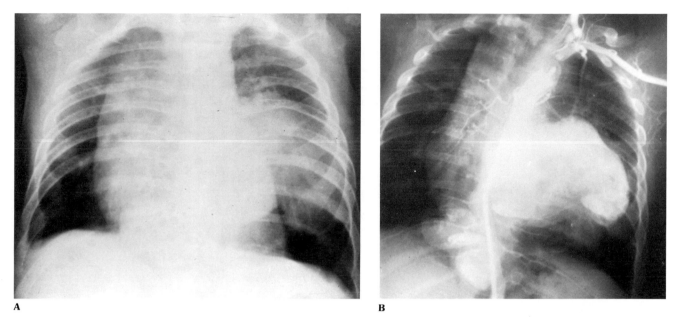

A   B

Figure 12-14   Mycotic aneurysm. An 8-month-old-boy had umbilical artery catheters placed during the first week of life. He was treated for staphylococcal sepsis and did well until 3 months of life, when chest films were obtained because of failure to thrive and a heart murmur. **A.** This frontal film discloses a large, rounded, homogeneous density in the left midlung field and a smaller one in the right cardiophrenic angle behind the heart. **B.** A thoracic angiogram confirms the presence of several large aortic aneurysms that were removed surgically. The patient is well to date. (Courtesy of Dr. Ehsan Afshani, Buffalo, New York.)

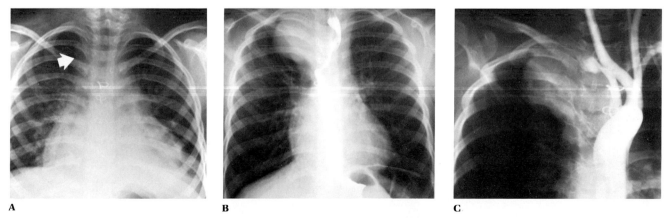

A   B   C

Figure 12-15   Aneurysm of the subclavian artery. This child underwent cardiac catheterization through the right subclavian artery at 1 year of age. **A.** The film study after closure of an atrial septal defect shows a small right superior paramediastinal mass (arrow). **B.** Films obtained 4 years later because of Horner's syndrome, cough while eating, and respiratory stridor show a large mass deviating the esophagus and compressing the trachea. **C.** Contrast injection shows the clot-filled mass contiguous with the aberrant right subclavian artery. Surgical removal was accomplished without difficulty. (From Rodgers et al.[55])

"Aberrant" Innominate Artery

The causal relationship between innominate artery compression of the trachea and clinically significant airway obstruction is not well-established. Rare patients with innominate artery–tracheal compression, who manifest symptoms of stridor, dyspnea, and intermittent apnea, will probably benefit from aorto-pexy.[56,57] Conservative management is acceptable in children with no apnea or significant respiratory symptoms.[56]

Angiography will define the relationship of the innominate artery to the trachea, but airway fluoroscopy may be needed to help determine the degree of narrowing (Figure 12-16). The trachea remains narrowed during all phases of respiration in patients

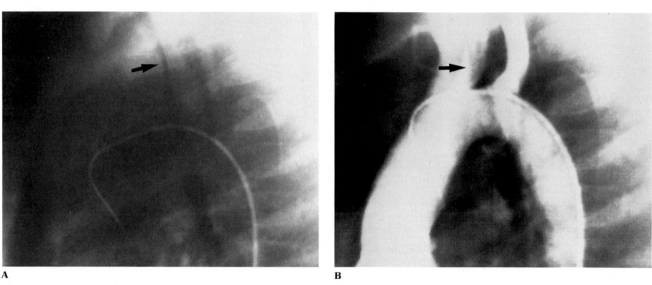

A   **B**

Figure 12-16   Innominate artery compression of the trachea. A. The tracheal air column is compressed anteriorly (arrow). **B.** The innominate artery is seen adjacent to the tracheal air column (arrow).

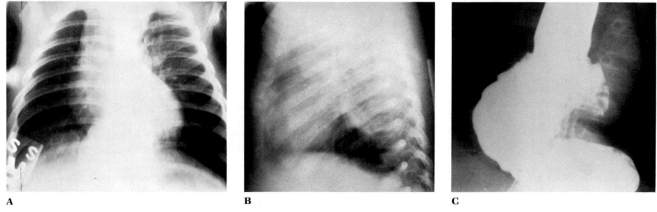

A   **B**   **C**

Figure 12-17   Hiatus hernia. A. A paramediastinal opacity occupies the right cardiophrenic sulcus. **B.** The lateral film discloses a poorly defined air-filled structure. **C.** A barium esophogram confirms hiatus hernia.

with significant innominate artery compression; the normal trachea in the area of the innominate artery narrows only during expiration.

Pulsations of the anterior tracheal wall, when observed bronchoscopically, constitute a helpful sign. If the pulse in the right arm loses amplitude with bronchoscopic compression of the pulsating anterior trachea, the diagnosis is much more secure.

Congenital Malformations

Diaphragmatic Hernia and Eventration

Diaphragmatic hernia and eventration (see Chapter 4) may on occasion be confused with mass lesions of the chest or mediastinum. Hiatus hernia usually is a straightforward roentgenographic diagnosis when air or air-fluid levels are present (Figure 12-17). Barium esophogram is the diagnostic procedure that confirms its presence (Figure 12-17C).

Eventration of the diaphragm is more subtle than herniation, but radiographic features are usually quite typical (Figures 12-18 and 12-19). Almost always anterior, the contour of eventration usually blends into the diaphragmatic silhouette. When a significant portion of liver is contained within the eventration, the lower hepatic edge is higher than normal. Hepatic nuclide scan is a reliable way to confirm the diagnosis, but ultrasonography is equally diagnostic (Figures 12-18C and 12-19C).[58]

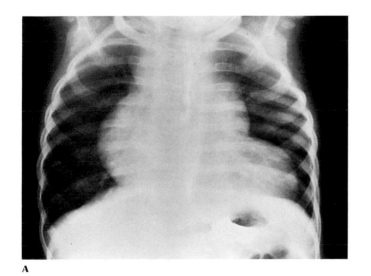

A

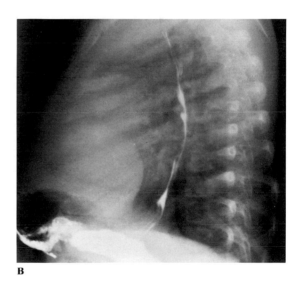

B

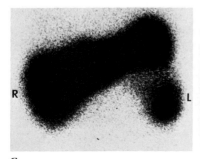

C

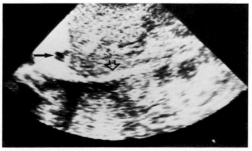

D

Figure 12-18 Diaphragmatic eventration. A. The frontal film shows a rounded density contiguous with the lower left border of the heart. The medial portion of the mass blends with the diaphragmatic shadow. **B.** The anterior location of the eventration is evident. **C.** A radionuclide liver scan shows the liver bulge under the left hemidiaphragm. **D.** Ultrasonography confirms the presence of liver adjacent to the cardiac chamber. The inferior vena cava (open arrow) can be seen entering the right atrium containing a cardiac valve (solid arrow).

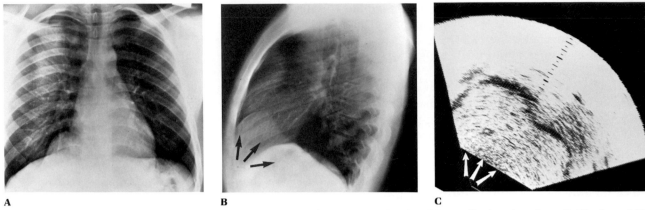

A   B   C

Figure 12-19   Diaphragmatic eventration. A. A soft tissue density occupies the right cardiophrenic sulcus. **B.** The lateral film reveals the anterior location and characteristic appearance of a diaphragmatic eventration. **C.** The longitudinal ultrasound study shows the bilobed contour of the diaphragm with the underlying liver. The arrows on **B** and **C** indicate the arc described by the ultrasound transducer.

References

1. Dehner LP: *Pediatric Surgical Pathology.* St Louis, CV Mosby, 1975, p 163.

2. Bell A Jr, Sumner DS: A unified concept of lymphangioma and cystic hygroma. *Surg Gynecol Obstet* 120:79, 1965.

3. Goetsch E: Hygroma colli cysticum and hygroma axillare; pathologic and clinical study and report of 12 cases. *Arch Surg* 36:394, 1938.

4. Potter EL, Craig JM: *Pathology of the Fetus and the Infant.* Chicago, Year Book Medical Publishers, 1975, p 185.

5. Landing B, Farber S: Tumors of the cardiovascular system. *Atlas of Tumor Pathology.* Washington, DC, AFIP, 1956.

6. Ducharme JC, Belanger R, Simard P: Chylothorax, chylopericardium with multiple lymphangioma of bone. *J Pediatr Surg* 17:365, 1982.

7. Sumner TE, Volberg FM, Kiscr PM et al: Mediastinal cystic hygroma in children. *Pediatr Radiol* 11:160, 1981.

8. Miller WT, Cornog JA Jr, Sullivan MA: Lymphangiomyomatosis. A clinical-radiologic-pathologic syndrome. *AJR* 3:565, 1971.

9. Najiman E, Sabadi F, Temmer B: Lymphangioma in the inguinal region with cystic lymphangiomatosis of bone. *J Pediatr* 71:561, 1967.

10. Lanning P, Suramo I, Heikkinen E, et al: General lymphangiomatosis in a child. *Pediatr Radiol* 7:49, 1978.

11. Kutarna A: Value of lymphangiography in the diagnosis and treatment of lymphangioma. *Neoplasm* 22:81, 1975.

12. Nink TN, Nink TX: Cystic hygroma in children: A report of 126 cases. *J Pediatr Surg* 9:191, 1974.

13. Kaliciński ZH, Joszt W, Perdzynski W, et al: Hemangioma of the superior vena caval vein. *J Pediatr Surg* 17:178, 1982.

14. Gindhart TD, Tucker WY, Choy SH: Cavernous hemangioma of the superior mediastinum. Report of a case with electron microscopy and computerized tomography. *Am J Surg Pathol* 3:353, 1979.

15. Polansky S, Gooding CA, Potter B: Idiopathic dilatation of the superior vena cava. *Pediatr Radiol* 2:167, l974.

16. Gabriele AR, North L, Pircher FJ, et al: Aneurysmal dilatation of the superior vena cava. *J Nucl Med* 13:227, 1972.

17. Heil BJ, Felman AH, Talbert JL, et al: Idiopathic dilatation of the superior vena cava. *J Pediatr Surg* 13:193, 1978.

18. Knight JA, Cancilla PA: Neurofibroma involving the superior vena cava with formation of an aneurysm. *Arch Pathol* 86:427, 1968.

19. Ream CR, Giardina A: Congenital superior vena cava aneurysm with complications caused by infectious mononucleosis. *Chest* 62:755, 1972.

20. Tonkin ILD, Gold RE, Moser D, et al: Evaluation of vascular rings with digital subtraction angiography. *AJR* 142:1287, 1984.

21. Moncade R, Shannon M, Miller R, et al: The cervical aortic arch. *AJR* 125:591, 1974.

22. Haughton VM, Fellow KE, Rosenbaum AE: The cervical aortic arches. *Radiology* 114:675, 1975.

23. Klinkhamer AC: *Esophagography in Anomalies of the Aortic Arch System*. Baltimore, Williams & Wilkins, 1969, p 83.

24. Shuford WH, Sybers RG: *The Aortic Arch and Its Malformations*. Springfield, Ill., Charles C Thomas, 1974, p 145.

25. Edwards JE: Anomalies of the aortic arch system. *Birth Defects* (original article series) XIII:47, 1977.

26. Rutishauser M, Rowen G, Wyler F: Aneurysm of the non-patent ductus arteriosus in the newborn. *Acta Paediatr Scand* 60:649, 1977.

27. Ferlic RM, Hobschire PJ, Mooring PK: Ruptured ductus arteriosus aneurysm in an infant: Report of a survivor. *Ann Thorac Surg* 20:456, 1975.

28. Kirks DR, McCook TA, Serwer GA, Oldham HN Jr: Aneurysm of the ductus arteriosus in the neonate. *AJR* 134:573, 1980.

29. Berdon WE, Baker DH, James LS: The ductus bump. *AJR* 95:91, 1965.

30. Mackler S, Graham EA: Aneurysm of the ductus Botalli as a surgical problem. *J Thorac Surg* 12:719, 1942.

31. Gillan MB, Costigan DC, Keeley FW, et al: Spontaneous dissecting aneurysm of the ductus arteriosus in an infant with Marfan's syndrome. *J Pediatr* 105:953, 1984.

32. Thompson TR, Tilleli J, Johnson DE, et al: Umbilical artery catheterization complicated by mycotic aortic aneurysm in neonates. *Adv Pediatr* 275, 1980.

33. Mitcell RS, Seifert FC, Miller DC, et al: Aneurysm of the diverticulum of the ductus arteriosus in the adult. *J Thorac Cardiovasc Surg* 86:400, 1983.

34. Kneidel JH: A case of aneurysm of the ductus arteriosus with post mortem roentgenographic study after instillation of barium paste. *AJR* 62:223, 1949.

35. De Lise CT, Schneider B, Blackman MS: Common pulmonary vein atresia without anomalous pulmonary venous connection. *Pediatr Radiol* 8:195, 1979.

36. Lucas RV Jr, Woolfrey BV, Anderson RC, et al: Atresia of the common pulmonary vein. *Pediatrics* 29:729, 1962.

37. Khonsari S, Saunders PW, Lees MH, et al: Common pulmonary vein atresia—Importance of immediate recognition and surgical intervention. *J Thorac Cardiovasc Surg* 83:443, 1982.

38. Strife J: *Proceedings of Society of Pediatric Radiology*. Boston, 1985.

39. Kangarloo H, Gold RH, Benson L, et al: Sonography of extrathoracic left-to-right shunts in infants and children. *AJR* 141:923, 1983.

40. Sade RM, Rosenthal A, Fellows K, et al: Pulmonary artery sling. *J Thorac Cardiovasc Surg* 69:333, 1975.

41. Siegel MJ, Shackelford GD, McAlister WH: Tracheobronchography in the evaluation of anomalous left pulmonary artery. *Pediatr Radiol* 12:235, 1982.

42. Capitanio, MA, Ramos R, Kirkpatrick JA Jr: Pulmonary sling—roentgen observations. *AJR* 112:28, 1971.

43. Williams RG, Jaffe RB, Condon VR: Unusual features of pulmonary sling. *AJR* 133:1065, 1979.

44. Wittenberg MH, Tantiwongse T, Rosenberg BF: Anomalous course of the left pulmonary artery with respiratory obstruction. *Radiology* 67:339, 1956.

45. Stone DN, Bein ME, Garris JB: Anomalous left pulmonary artery: Two new adult cases. *AJR* 135:1259, 1980.

46. Rheuban KS, Ayres N, Still JG: Pulmonary artery sling: A new diagnostic tool and clinical review. *Pediatrics* 69:472, 1982.

47. King D, Walker HA: Pulmonary artery sling. *Thorax* 39:462, 1984.

48. Faer MJ, Taybi H: Mycotic aortic aneurysm in premature infants. *Radiology* 125:177, 1977.

49. Malloy MH, Nichols MM: False abdominal aortic aneurysm: An unusual complication of umbilical arterial catheterization for exchange transfusion. *J Pediatr* 90:285, 1977.

50. Wind ES, Wisoff BG, Baron MG, et al: Mycotic aneurysm in infancy: A complication of umbilical artery catheterization. *J Pediatr Surg* 17:324, 1982.

51. Gomes MD, Schellinger D, Hufnagl CA: Abdominal aortic aneurysms. Diagnostic review and new technique. *Ann Thorac Surg* 27:249, 1979.

52. Cristophe C, Burniat MS, Cogaert C, et al: Ruptured mycotic aneurysm of the superior mesenteric artery secondary to bacterial endocarditis in a 6-year-old girl. *Pediatr Radiol* 15:202, 1985.

53. Hunter JA, Dye WS, Javid H, et al: Arteriosclerotic aneurysm of anomalous right subclavian artery. *J Thorac Cardiovasc Surg* 59:754, 1970.

54. Dickman SH, Baron M, Gordon AJ: Right aortic arch with ruptured aneurysm of anomalous left subclavian artery. *Am J Cardiol* 34:245, 1974.

55. Rodgers BM, Talbert JL, Hollenbeck JI: Aneurysm of the anomalous subclavian artery: An unusual cause of dysphagia lusoria in childhood. *Ann Surg* 187:158, 1977.

56. Berdon WE, Baker DH, Bordiuk J, et al: Innominate artery compression of the trachea in infants with stridor and apnea. *Radiology* 92:272, 1969.

57. Swischuck LE: Anterior tracheal indentation in infancy and early childhood: Normal or abnormal? *AJR* 112:12, 1971.

58. Moccia WA, Kaude JV, Felman AH: Congenital eventration of the diaphragm. Diagnosis by ultrasound. *Pediatr Radiol* 10:197, 1981.

Chapter 13

Infections

Infections of the mediastinum are caused by varieties of bacteria, viruses, and fungi that often originate in regional lymph nodes or adjacent structures (vertebrae, pericardium). Infectious processes may be self-contained, or they may assume life-threatening proportions as a result of regional spread to great vessels, respiratory airways, esophagus, and other contiguous areas.

It is difficult to make too many generalizations regarding mediastinal infections; many factors are responsible for the clinical, radiographic, and pathologic alterations that result. Among these are the nature of invading organisms, anatomic location, and duration of disease. Infections with *Histoplasma capsulatum* and mycoplasma tuberculosis frequently show specific patterns, usually involving lymph nodes.

This chapter will cover three types of mediastinitis: (1) suppurative infections, (2) histoplasmosis, and (3) tuberculosis.

Suppurative Mediastinal Infections

Primary suppurative mediastinitis is less of a problem than it has been in past years. Nevertheless, postoperative infections from thoracic surgical procedures are occasionally seen. Tracheal and esophageal perforations, sometimes related to the use of life-support systems, account for cases of acute suppurative mediastinitis.

Neonates are particularly susceptible to traumatic perforation of the esophagus and/or trachea with secondary mediastinal infection.[1-4] Reflex constriction of the cricopharyngeus muscle, which often accompanies nasopharyngeal intubation, probably contributes to esophageal perforation. The trachea is also susceptible to rupture from suction catheters.

On rare occasions, pyogenic mediastinitis may result from caudal extension of cervical and retropharyngeal abscesses (Figure 13-1).

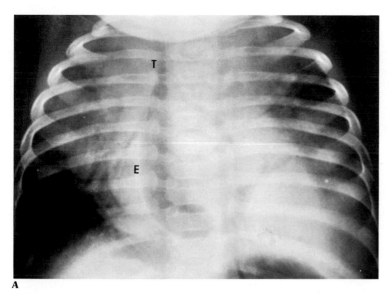
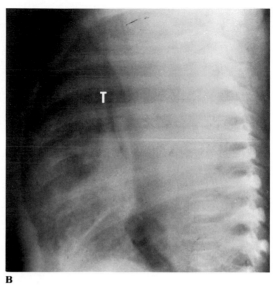

A   B

Figure 13-1   Retropharyngeal-posterior mediastinal abscess. A. Extensive opacities are present bilaterally. The trachea (T), carina, and air-filled esophagus (E) are deviated to the right. **B.** A large posterior mediastinal opacity extends from the retropharynx to the diaphragm. The tracheal air column (T) is attenuated and displaced anteriorly by the abscess. (Courtesy of Dr. Bernard Blumenthal, Jackson, Mississippi.)

Chronic suppurative mediastinitis occurs in association with lymph nodes that are infected with numerous organisms, notably tuberculosis or histoplasmosis. Vertebral infections may spread to involve the posterior medial thoracic region. Staphylococcus is the most frequent organism associated with vertebral osteomyelitis, but group B beta-hemolytic streptococci are additional agents responsible for bone and soft tissue infections in early years (Figure 13-2).[5,6]

Intervertebral disk infections (idiopathic diskitis or nonspecific spondylitis) are chronic, indolent, and usually self-limited; they are rarely in need of surgical drainage. Staphylococcus is the organism most often associated with these infections, but a cause-and-effect relationship is difficult to establish. Other organisms responsible for disk space infection include brucella, salmonella, and tuberculosis. These agents can usually be excluded by serum antibody examinations and skin tests in immunologically intact individuals. Antibiotic treatment of intervertebral disk infections is of questionable therapeutic value. Differentiation between intervertebral diskitis and vertebral osteomyelitis may be difficult or impossible; the separation will often hinge on the clinical presentation, response to therapy, and radiographic changes. Osteomyelitis of the spine should be drained when the symptoms are severe or when spinal cord compression is present. Diskitis usually responds to conservative management.

Vertebral tumors, both primary and metastatic, may produce paramediastinal masses that simulate infections. Vertebral collapse, a feature of primary and metastatic tumor, does not usually cause a visible mass density. Biopsy and histologic examination are necessary to identify these conditions.

Prompt and accurate diagnosis of acute suppurative mediastinitis is imperative. Surgical drainage of mediastinitis secondary to esophageal perforation has been the traditional mode of therapy, but more conservative treatment using antibiotics and central venous alimentation is acceptable in selected cases. Most upper esophageal perforations can be approached through a cervical incision.

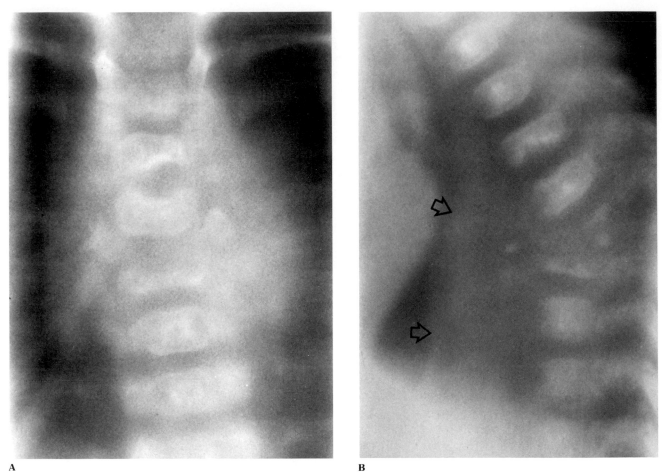

A   B

Figure 13-2   Group B beta-hemolytic streptococcal mediastinitis and osteomyelitis. This 6-week-old child had no symptoms. Minimal kyphosis was discovered on a "well-baby" visit, and films were obtained. **A.** Paramediastinal opacities have developed in association with extensive destruction of contiguous vertebral bodies and disks. **B.** The soft tissue mass (arrows) extends anteriorly from the point of infection. (From McCook T.A., Felman A.H., Ayoub E.: Streptococcal skeletal infections: Observations in 4 infants. *AJR* 130:465, 1978. © 1978, American Roentgen Ray Society.)

Radiologic Findings

The radiographic features of acute suppurative mediastinitis depend heavily upon the underlying cause. Postoperative mediastinitis is an uncommon but occasional complication of cardiac and other operations of the mediastinum. Roentgenographic changes of postoperative infection are often difficult to separate from those expected following surgery. Small lingering air pockets suggest postoperative in-

fection, but they will be overlooked unless films are taken with a horizontal beam, preferably in the lateral projection. Infectious changes in the sternum are difficult to identify, but persistent soft tissue swelling over the infected bone should arouse suspicion. In some cases, a portion of the bone may disappear.

Mediastinitis from esophageal perforation often produces pockets of air and sinuses that persist (Figures 13-3A and B and 13-4). Examination with con-

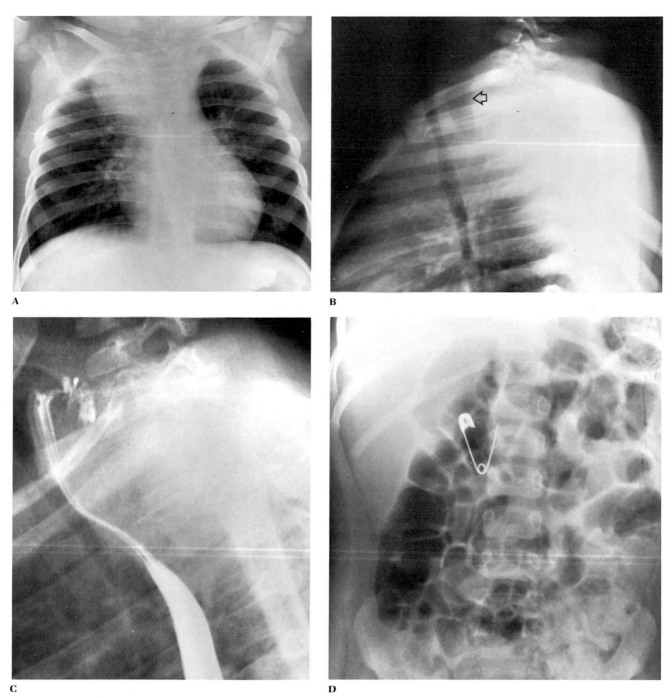

Figure 13-3   Mediastinal abscess—foreign body perforation. A. The upper right paramediastinal mass density is visible with symptoms of infection. The esophagus is deviated. **B.** The lateral projection shows a persistent air collection (arrow) behind the anteriorly displaced trachea. **C.** A barium collection extends into the substance of the mass through a fistula from the esophagus. **D.** This abdominal film obtained later shows an ingested pin.

trast material administered by mouth or through a soft, opaque, end-hole rubber catheter is usually necessary to confirm the diagnosis (Figure 13-3C). A traumatic diverticulum may simulate congenital esophageal atresia with tracheoesophageal fistula.[7,8] (See Chapter 24.)

When suppurative mediastinitis cannot be established with certainty from conventional films, addi-tional imaging procedures such as radionuclide scintigraphy and computed tomography (CT) may be of help.[9] Magnetic resonance imaging does not detect calcifications as well as CT, but is superior in assessing vascular patency.[10] Rholl and coworkers[11] found adenopathy associated with fibrosing medi-astinitis that they considered benign because of rel-atively low signal intensity on T_2-weighted images.

Combined vertebral body and disk infections often produce a paravertebral extrapleural radio-density. Early osseous changes may be very subtle or nonexistent, and on occasion the paraspinous soft tissue changes precede any bony alterations. Mini-mal mineral loss may be the only changes in the ad-jacent vertebral endplates. Narrowing of the disk space follows later, and is difficult to appreciate without careful comparison to the intervertebral disk spaces above and below. Progressive disk space narrowing and destructive changes of adjacent bone may be self-limited or continue on to complete fu-sion. Calcification of the disk space and kyphosco-liosis are known sequelae of these infections. Radio-nuclide bone scintigraphy may help locate bone infection that produces no recognizable change on conventional radiographs. This technique is some-what less reliable in young infants and may be falsely negative in cases of idiopathic diskitis.

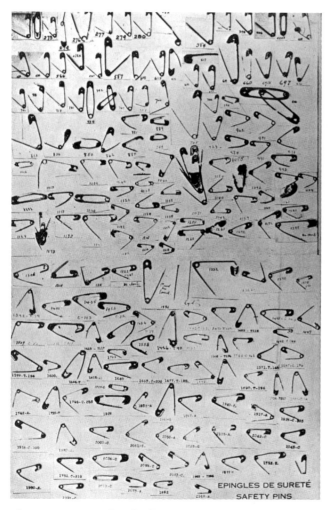

Figure 13-4 Foreign bodies. Examples of safety pins re-moved from the trachea and esophagus by Dr. Chevalier Jack-son, pioneer Philadelphia bronchoesophagoscopist. (From Brenneman and McQuarrie: *Practice of Pediatrics*. Philadelphia, JB Lippincott, 1952, vol. 2, with permission.)

Histoplasmosis (Darling's Disease, Reticuloendothelial Cytomycosis, Cave Sickness)

Histoplasmosis, first described by Darling in 1905,[12] occurs in two recognizable forms: (1) North Ameri-can and (2) African. In North America, the disease is caused by *Histoplasma capsulatum* and in Africa by *Histoplasma capsulatum* var. *duboisii*. Initially histo-plasmosis was thought to be a protozoan, but later work established it as a yeastlike fungus. However, strain differences exist, and the organism produces a complement-fixing and skin test antigen.[13] The his-toplasmosis organism is found in the soil and in an assortment of animals. Infection in humans occurs by inhalation or ingestion of organisms, but animal-to-human or interpersonal transmission has not been confirmed.

The geographic distribution of histoplasmosis is unusual in that more than half of the recorded cases occur west of the Appalachian Mountains, especially along the Ohio, Mississippi, and Missouri river basins. Other small endemic foci are located in eastern North Carolina, Montreal, and parts of New England.[14]

Histoplasma capsulatum is particularly prevalent in the highly nitrogenous soils of bird droppings found in abandoned barns, caves, and similar areas. Some years ago, in Cincinnati, Ohio, Dr. Ben Felson reported on a group of workers who developed a diffuse, miliary, granulomatous pneumonitis after cleaning pigeon dung that had accumulated for years in an abandoned water tower.[15] This disease was identified as histoplasmosis.[16]

Histoplasmosis presents in several clinical forms. Most citizens who contract the disease show few signs of illness.[17] Others develop fever, malaise, fatigue, and nonproductive cough. On chest radiograph, hilar adenopathy and pulmonary infiltrate may appear. The primary infection of *Histoplasma capsulatum* is usually benign and resolves spontaneously. However, progression with hematogenous dissemination may be a serious and life-threatening complication, especially in immunologically depleted infants or debilitated adults.

Features of disseminated disease include anemia; hepatosplenomegaly; and ulcers of the skin, mucous membranes, and occasionally the intestines.[13] Adrenal gland involvement may cause Addison's disease. Endocarditis, meningitis, and pericarditis are additional manifestations.[18]

Histoplasmosis of the mediastinum assumes two major clinical forms: (1) granulomatous mediastinitis and (2) fibrous mediastinitis.[19] Histoplasmosis and tuberculosis, in approximately equal numbers, are responsible for most cases of granulomatous mediastinitis. The exact cause of fibrous mediastinitis is rarely discovered, although histoplasmosis is thought to be the cause in most cases.[19]

Differentiation between granulomatous and fibrous mediastinitis is often impossible, and indeed, both may represent different manifestations of one disease process. Concomitant pulmonary lesions are found with each. They may involve adjacent structures, but superior vena caval obstruction is especially common in fibrous mediastinitis. Esophageal obstruction, tracheobronchial erosion (Figure 13-5), pulmonary artery and/or venous compression, thoracic duct obstruction, and recurrent laryngeal nerve involvement are additional complications.[20]

Radiologic Findings

Histoplasmosis and tuberculosis share many radiographic features, although most infections produce no roentgenographic abnormalities. When radiographic changes occur, both manifest parenchymal infiltrates and regional adenopathy, although histoplasmosis may occur as an isolated parenchymal process. In addition, the lymph nodes of histoplasmosis tend to be smaller. Fibrous scarring, calcification, and bronchial compression occur in both diseases. Calcified lymph nodes may erode into bronchi and be expectorated as broncholiths. In children particularly, histoplasmosis may simulate lymphoma when adenopathy and fever are the presenting signs.[21]

The primary infiltrate of histoplasmosis may enlarge and cause tissue destruction, necrosis, and fibrosis (histoplasmoma). Progressive enlargement of the primary infection may lead to a caseous form of granulomatous pneumonia with widespread consolidation but infrequent calcification. These complications are especially common in senior types.

Other complications include bronchopulmonary spread and bloodstream dissemination leading to calcified granulomas throughout the lung, spleen, liver, and adrenals.[22] Silverman[22] has highlighted the importance of geography when offering the diagnosis of histoplasmosis as opposed to other diseases, notably tuberculosis. He thought it to be a safe 10:1 that disseminated intrapulmonary calcifications in New York City are tuberculosis, but in Cincinnati and the Ohio Valley, the odds are no better than 4:1.

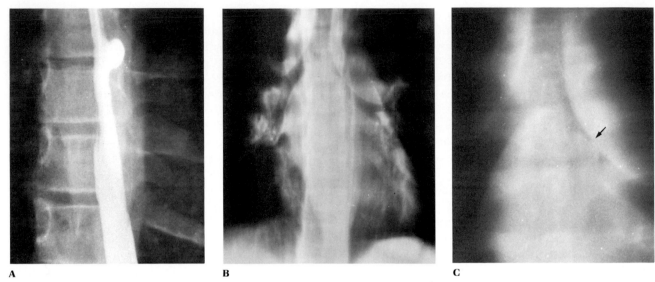

A   B   C

Figure 13-5   Histoplasmosis lymphadenopathy—granulomatous mediastinitis. A. An esophageal diverticulum has resulted from chronic mediastinal adenopathy and associated fibrosis. **B.** Mediastinal tomography shows bilateral, stippled, calcified hilar lymph nodes and subcarinal and paratracheal adenopathy. **C.** A granulomatous mass is visible extending into the lumen of the left stem bronchus (arrow) (the mass is also present in part B).

Granulomatous mediastinitis typically locates in the hila or the superior mediastinum, anterior to and near the bifurcation of the trachea.[19] Larger lesions may extend from the innominate vein to the root of the involved lung, with projection to the right of the superior mediastinum.

Subcarinal adenopathy and fibrosis may involve adjacent structures, depending upon the degree and direction of spread. Anterior extension may lead to pulmonary venous obstruction, lateral spread may envelop major bronchi and pulmonary arteries, while the esophagus is the victim of posterior encroachment. Any or all combinations of these are possible.[23]

In most instances, conventional radiographic methods will suffice to evaluate middle mediastinal and hilar processes.[24] Contrast esophogram will often help evaluate esophageal involvement. Tomography or high-kilovolt-magnification radiographs of the airway may disclose narrowing or erosion by adjacent lymph nodes, as well as calcifications not visible on plain films.

Chronic fibrous mediastinitis, in contrast to the granulomatous form, frequently creates mass densities near the bifurcation of the trachea or the hilum of the lung, often with extension to the right. Obstruction of the superior vena cava is the most common sequela. Pulmonary artery stenosis may occur and lead to attenuation of flow to a lung or portion thereof (Figure 13-6).[20]

In addition to the conventional radiographic studies, radionuclide perfusion scan and pulmonary arteriography may help in the delineation of vascular complications. Computed tomography, in addition to demonstrating the anatomy of the fibrous process, is useful in the primary diagnosis by showing calcification in the mass and other structures (see Chapter 26, Figure 26-46).[9] Magnetic resonance imaging is an additional method of evaluation (see Chapter 27, Figure 27-4).[10,11] This technique does not reveal calcific densities as well as conventional radiographic methods, but better defines vascular anatomy, and may help separate benign from malignant disease.[11]

Mediastinal adenopathy similar to that caused by histoplasmosis may occur with other chronic fungal infections, as well as tuberculosis (Figure 13-7).

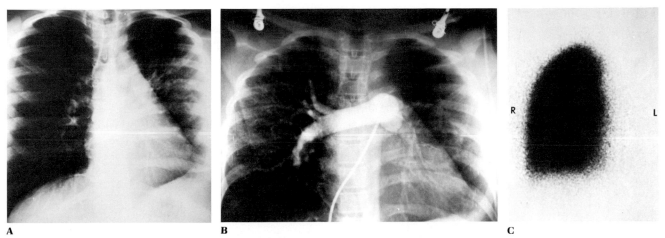

A   B   C

Figure 13-6   Histoplasmosis—fibrosing mediastinitis. This 12-year-old girl suffered a "flulike" illness 2 years previously. The chest film at that time was normal. She presented on this occasion with symptoms of shortness of breath, cough, and occasional blood-streaked sputum of 1 month's duration. The histoplasmin skin test was strongly positive (22 mm), and PPD (purified protein derivative) was negative. **A.** The present chest film shows a mediastinal shift to the left, left-sided volume loss, pleural fibrosis, and diminished blood flow to the left lung. **B.** The pulmonary arteriogram shows diminished blood flow to the left lung. **C.** The ^{99m}Tc perfusion scan shows absent perfusion to the left lung; washout was normal. (From Weider et al: Pulmonary artery occlusion due to histoplasmosis. *AJR* 138:243, 1982. © 1982, American Roentgen Ray Society. Courtesy of Dr. Ina Tonkin, Memphis, Tennessee.)

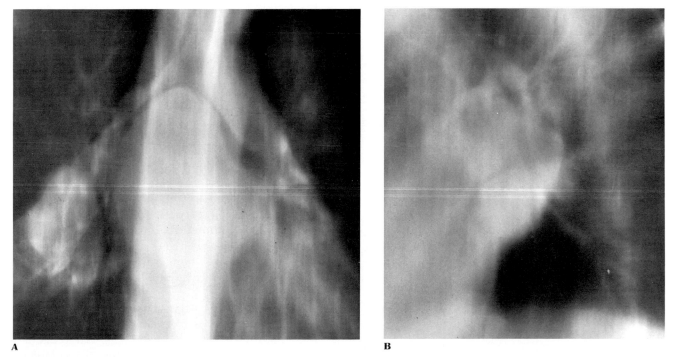

A   B

Figure 13-7   Nocardia adenopathy. A and **B.** Large subcarinal lymph nodes compressing both stem bronchi are visible. Nocardia was isolated from the nodes in this patient with chronic granulomatous disease of childhood (impotent white cell disease).

Tuberculosis

While a medical student of the University of Cincinnati and an intern at the Philadelphia General Hospital (Figure 13-8), I was exposed to the tail end of the tuberculosis era. Nevertheless, it is difficult, if not impossible, to convey the true impact of this disease on the history of mankind. For an intriguing and fascinating personal account of this dreaded affliction, the reader is referred to Dr. Benjamin Felson's "Letter from the Editor."[25] As Dr. Felson says, "Tuberculosis, though no longer a scourge, is still with us. It is not rare."

Mycobacterium tuberculosis is the causative agent of tuberculosis in humans. These organisms appear as refractile, slender, red rods approximately 4 by 0.5 μm in acid-fast stain. They may remain virulent for many months when kept in the dark, but they are killed by direct sunlight or ultraviolet rays.

The development of clinical tuberculosis depends upon many factors, including host resistance, virulence of organisms, and number of bacilli in the inoculum. Most infections result from inhalation of the bacillus in droplet form; 95 percent of cases start in the lung parenchyma. In a previously uninfected person, the initial infestation causes an inflammatory focus in the lung. This primary inflammatory focus appears histologically as a tubercle with polymorphonuclear leukocytes, epithelioid cells, giant cells, and surrounding lymphocytes. Most often, the primary tubercle is single, but two or more may develop simultaneously.

After establishing the primary infection in the lung parenchyma, the infectious bacilli travel to the hilar and mediastinal lymph nodes. As hypersensitivity develops, these regional lymph nodes enlarge. The combination of pulmonary focus, enlarged regional nodes, and interfocal zone is known as the *primary tuberculous complex.* Lymph node enlargement may be massive and compress or erode adjacent bronchi. While many children recover without sequelae,[26] areas of atelectasis may follow bronchial compression and develop secondary infection and bronchiectasis.[27] Erosion into adjacent bronchi, fistula formation, and endobronchial dissemination is an added threat. Invasion of the adjacent structures such as esophagus, pericardium, and blood vessels is an uncommon, but occasionally severe, complication.

As the lymph nodes heal, they regress in size, but some adenopathy may remain. Calcification occurs most often in untreated individuals. Viable bacteria may be recovered many years later; live organisms are reputed to have been found in Egyptian mummies.

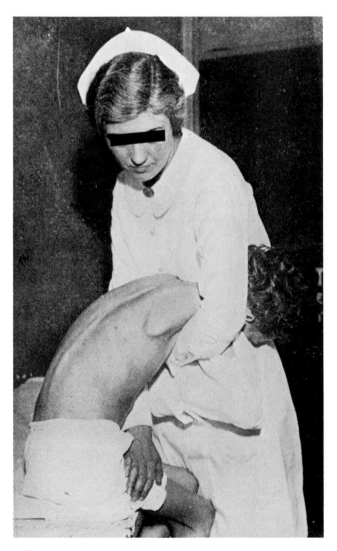

Figure 13-8   Preparation for thoracentesis, circa 1930. Patient's arms are restrained in the hospital gown.

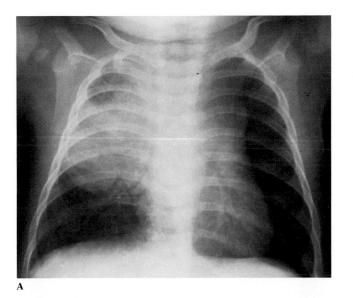

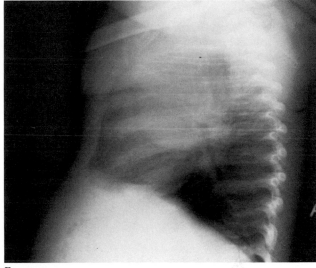

A

B

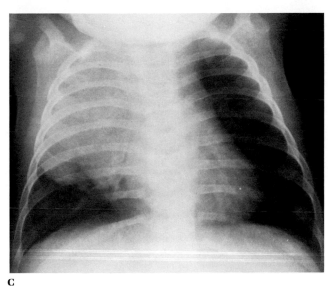

C

Figure 13-9 Tuberculosis. A and **B.** This child had minimal cough and fever. These initial films show an area of consolidation in the right lung field. The presence of lymphadenopathy is difficult to determine in the presence of adjacent pulmonary disease. **C.** This film, taken after several weeks of antituberculous treatment, shows progressive enlargement of the pneumonic infiltrate. This is not uncommon in the early course of treatment for tuberculosis. Tuberculosis should be considered when there is a discrepancy between the amount of infiltrate and the severity of the disease.

Reinfection, or chronic tuberculosis, may follow a primary tuberculous process. This complication is uncommon in children; it is seen most often in adolescent girls. Whether reinfection tuberculosis follows reactivation of endogenous disease, exogenous reinfection, or superinfection cannot always be determined. Mortality rates from infectious tuberculosis before isoniazide therapy was available were as high as 24 percent but are now less than 1 percent.[28]

Radiologic Findings

Most patients with primary tuberculosis infection manifest no radiographic changes. However, within 6 weeks, some will develop a small parenchymal lesion, usually less than 5 mm in diameter and more commonly in the right lung. On occasion, the opacity representing the primary focus may be large enough to occupy a considerable portion of the lung.[29] Regional lymphadenopathy is a consistent finding in children with clinical and radiographic evidence of primary tuberculosis.[25,28,30]

The lung lesion caseates and encapsulates in the ensuing weeks as the patient develops hypersensitivity to the tubercle bacillus. It is during this phase that clinical symptoms manifest.

The pulmonary focus remains unchanged for 3 to 4 months and gradually begins to regress; antimicrobial therapy does not hasten this resolution. Transient enlargement of the pulmonary nodule and regional lymph nodes may occur following the onset of treatment, and this apparent radiographic progression should not be taken as evidence of worsening disease (Figure 13-9). On rare occasions, the primary lesion continues to enlarge and involve large volumes of lung. Even with the development of hypersensitivity, this pneumonic process may progress and cause pleural reactions as well as bronchial erosions. This poorly understood adverse reaction usually affects young infants, but older patients are not spared.

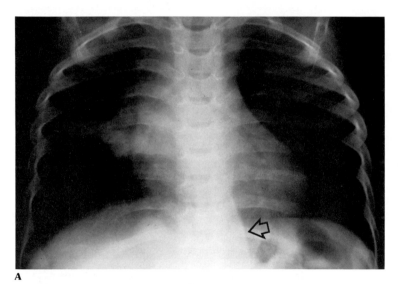

A

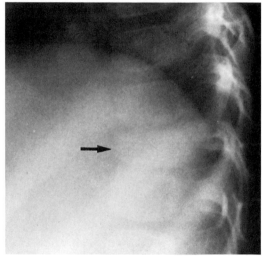

B

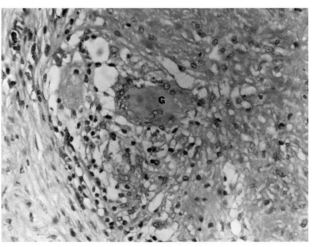

C

Figure 13-10   Tuberculous spondylitis. A. In addition to the right hilar and paratracheal adenopathy, a left paravertebral radiopacity is present (arrow). **B.** The lateral film, centered on T11–T12, demonstrates a partially collapsed vertebral body (arrow) with narrowed intervertebral disk spaces above and below. **C.** This histologic specimen from the biopsy of a cervical lymph node shows a tuberculoma. A typical giant cell (G) is surrounded by epithelioid histiocytes, scattered lymphocytes, and fibrous tissue.

Parenchymal lesions without hilar adenopathy are extremely rare, but the reverse is less true; approximately one-third of patients with enlarged hilar nodes have no visible lung changes. While most enlarged nodes are found in the hila, paratracheal adenopathy may accompany apical disease. When the complex exists in the right lung, adenopathy is usually more prominent and confined to that side; primary foci on the left regularly give rise to bilateral lymphadenopathy.

Secondary complications of pulmonary tuberculosis may remain local or become disseminated. Local pulmonary changes usually result when lymph nodes compress or erode adjacent bronchi. Pulmonary collapse, bronchiectasis, bronchial strictures, and fistulas are uncommon but reported complications. The proximity of the lymph nodes to the vertebrae (Figure 13-10) and/or pericardium is thought to be one avenue for spread of infection to these organs.

Acute hematogenous dissemination is possible at any time, but it usually manifests before the devel-opment of hypersensitivity. Miliary lesions in the lung probably result from bloodstream invasion by the organisms from the original focus or regional lymph nodes. The occurrence of isolated foci of infection in the eye, lung, bone, pericardium, and brain is additional heartache.

Chronic or "reactivation" tuberculosis is uncommon in childhood. It usually affects adolescents and manifests as small 2- to 3-cm-diameter, rounded shadows in the apices. These subtle lesions often escape attention on routine chest films, and apical lordotic views or frontal films centered on the lower cervical–upper thoracic level may be necessary. Cavitation, scarring, and retraction, all changes that indicate moderately or far advanced pulmonary tuberculosis, occur in children as well as adults.

Pleural effusions develop in approximately 8 percent of children with tuberculosis, most of whom have associated parenchymal infection.[30] However, effusions may occur on the contralateral side, probably as a result of hematogenous spread. Mostly seen in school-aged children, effusion occurs about twice

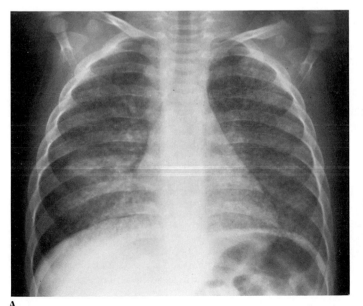

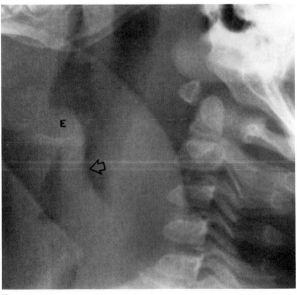

A   B

Figure 13-11 Miliary tuberculosis and scrofula. A. Diffuse miliary nodule densities give this chest film the appearance of a snowstorm. **B.** The airway study shows marked thickening of the epiglottis (E), aryepiglottic folds (arrow), and prevertebral soft tissues. These changes were secondary to extensive cervical tuberculous adenopathy, possibly on the basis of lymphatic blockage or compression of draining veins. Direct laryngoscopy showed no tuberculous involvement of the epiglottis.

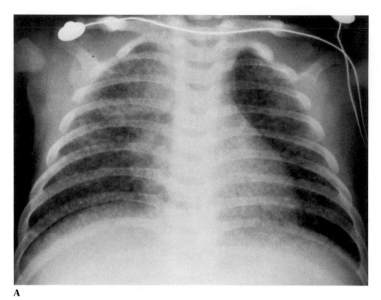
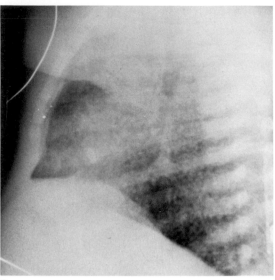

A

B

Figure 13-12   Miliary tuberculosis. A and **B.** Diffuse nodular lesions are spread throughout the lungs. Early coalescence is evident in the right upper lobe. The child also had tuberculous meningitis.

as often in boys as in girls. Tuberculous effusions have no characteristic radiographic features, but their prognosis in children is better than in adults.

Miliary tuberculosis results from generalized spread of tubercle bacilli through the bloodstream to the lung, a process that results in the production of multiple small densities (Figures 13-11 and 13-12). These minute opacities, 2 mm or less in diameter, are said to resemble millet seeds (see Chapter 27, Figure 27-23). This complication, usually occurring in the first 6 months of life, often causes little change in the chest roentgenogram other than overaeration for the first 7 to 14 days after the onset of the disease. Thereafter, the lungs take on a pattern characterized by diffuse, small nodular densities. These may coalesce into large lesions, but they gradually disappear with adequate treatment.

The radiographic differential diagnosis of miliary lung disease is extensive and includes other bacterial, viral, rickettsial, fungal, and parasitic infections, as well as noxious inhalants and other causes.[31] In infants, however, miliary tuberculosis is usually more specific, since few other diseases produce such a radiographic picture at that age.

References

1. Talbert JL, Rodgers BM, Felman AH, et al: Traumatic perforation of the hypopharynx in infants. *J Thorac Cardiovasc Surg* 74:152, 1977.
2. Eklof O, Lohr G, Okmian L: Submucosal perforation of the esophagus in neonates. *Acta Radiol* 8:187, 1969.
3. Lee SB, Kuhn JP: Esophageal perforation in the neonate. *Am J Dis Child* 130:325, 1976.
4. Shild JP, Wuilloud A, Kohlberg H, et al: Tracheal perforation as a result of nasotracheal intubation in a neonate. *J Pediatr* 88:631, 1976.
5. McCook TA, Felman AH, Ayoub E: Streptococcal skeletal infections: Observations in 4 infants. *AJR* 130:465, 1978.
6. Siskind B, Galliquez P, Wald ER: Group B beta-hemolytic streptococcal osteomyelitis/purulent arthritis in neonates: Report of three cases. *J Pediatr* 87:659, 1975.
7. Girdany BR, Sieber WK, Osman MZ: Pseudodiverticulum of the pharynx in newborn infants. *N Engl J Med* 280:237, 1969.
8. Ducharme JC, Bertrand R, Debie J: Perforation of pharynx in the newborn: A condition mimicking esophageal atresia. *Can Med Assoc J* 104:785, 1971.
9. Weinstein JB, Aronberg DS, Sagel SS: CT of fibrosing

mediastinitis: Findings and their utility. *AJR* 141:247, 1983.

10. Farmer DW, Moore E, Amparo E, et al: Calcific fibrosing mediastinitis: Demonstration of pulmonary vascular obstruction by magnetic resonance imaging. *AJR* 143:1189, 1984.

11. Rholl KS, Levitt RG, Glazer HS: Magnetic resonance imaging in fibrosing mediastinitis. *AJR* 145:255, 1985.

12. Darling ST: Protozoan general infection producing pseudotubercles in the lung and focal necrosis in the liver, spleen, and lymph nodes. *JAMA* 46:1283, 1905.

13. Christie A: Histoplasmosis, in Kendig EL Jr, Chernick V (eds): *Disorders of the Respiratory Tract in Children.* Philadelphia, WB Saunders, 1977, p 865.

14. Spender H: *Pathology of the Lung.* Philadelphia, WB Saunders, 1977, p 300.

15. Felson B, Jones GF, Ulrich RP: Roentgenologic aspects of diffuse miliary granulomatous pneumonia of unknown etiology. *AJR* 64:740, 1950.

16. Grayston JT, Furcolow ML: The occurrence of histoplasmosis in epidemics—Epidemiological studies. *Am J Public Health* 43:665, 1953.

17. Schwartz J, Baum GL: The history of histoplasmosis, 1906–1956. *N Engl J Med* 256:253, 1957.

18. Kirchner SG, Heller RM, Sell SH, et al: The radiological features of histoplasma pericarditis. *Pediatr Radiol* 7:7, 1978.

19. Schowengerdt CG, Suyemota R, Main FB: Granulomatous and fibrous mediastinitis. A review and analysis of 180 cases. *J Thorac Cardiovasc Surg* 57:365, 1965.

20. Weider S, White TJ III, Salazar J, et al: Pulmonary artery occlusion due to histoplasmosis. *AJR* 138:243, 1982.

21. Woods WG, Singher LJ, Krivit W, et al: Histoplasmosis simulating lymphoma in children. *J Pediatr Surg* 14:423, 1979.

22. Silverman FN: Pulmonary calcification—Tuberculosis? Histoplasmosis? *AJR 64:764, 1950.*

23. Goodwin RA, Michell JA, DesPrez RM: Mediastinal fibrosis complicating healed primary histoplasmosis and tuberculosis. *Medicine* 51:227, 1972.

24. Kirks DR, Korobkin M: Chest computed tomography in infants and children. An analysis of 50 patients. *Pediatr Radiol* 10:75, 1980.

25. Felson B: Letter from the editor. *Semin Roentgen* 14:173, 1979.

26. Giammona ST, Poole CA, Zelkowitz P, et al: Massive lymphadenopathy in primary pulmonary tuberculosis. *Am Rev Respir Dis* 100:480, 1969.

27. Forstad S: Segmental atelectasis in children with primary tuberculosis. *Am Rev Respir Dis* 79:597, 1959.

28. Kendig EL Jr, Chernick V: In *Disorders of the Respiratory Tract in Children.* Philadelphia, WB Saunders, 1977, p 792.

29. Bui HD, Keller MA, Yayich SA, et al: Radiological case of the month. *Am J Dis Child* 138:91, 1984.

30. Lincoln EM, Sewell EM: *Tuberculosis in Children.* New York, McGraw-Hill Book Co., 1963, p 81.

31. Felson B: Acute miliary diseases of the lung. *Radiology* 59:32, 1952.

Section IV

Roentgenographic Patterns in Pulmonary Disease

Pulmonary disease occasionally produces specific roentgenographic patterns on chest films. A recognizable pattern may suggest an underlying cause or group (gamut) of cases. Although pattern recognition and gamut methods are quite useful, certain pitfalls must be considered:

1. Roentgenographic patterns are not always typical and frequently evoke disagreement between observers.
2. Similar diseases may produce different patterns.
3. Similar patterns may result from different diseases.
4. Gamut lists are easily forgotten.

In spite of these reservations, four roentgenographic patterns seen in childhood lung diseases will be considered: (1) diffuse overaeration, (2) endobronchial pattern (bronchiectasis), (3) pulmonary edema pattern, and (4) major airway pattern. These four patterns are reasonably consistent and recognizable and provide reliable information regarding the underlying pathologic process. Since these patterns are instrumental to a harmonious conception of the underlying disease, they will be discussed in concert. However, recognition of roentgenographic patterns and knowledge of appropriate gamuts cannot substitute for a basic understanding of pulmonary anatomy, pathophysiology, and roentgenographic imagery. Unlike truth and beauty, patterns and gamuts are *not* "all ye know in life, and all ye need to know."

Chapter 14

Overaeration Pattern

Terms such as *diffuse overaeration, hyperaeration, hyperinflation, overexpanded lung,* and *overinflated lung* are used interchangeably to describe enlarged lungs. The term *emphysema* should not be used, as it implies the presence of alveolar wall distension and suggests a more destructive, chronic, and severe disease process.

Many diseases that produce generalized pulmonary overexpansion (bronchiolitis, asthma, cystic fibrosis) also manifest patterns of irregular, focal, asymmetrical hyperaeration. The salient roentgenographic features of generalized overaeration are listed below in decreasing order of reliability; the first six are most useful; the remaining three are less so.

1. Narrow cardiothymic silhouette
2. "Elevated" heart
3. Depressed diaphragm
4. Increased anteroposterior chest diameter
5. Clear retrosternal space
6. Consistent, unchanging finding
7. Horizontal, spread ribs
8. Separation of vessels
9. Disparity between lung volume and chest size

In addition to the foregoing radiographic criteria, several additional factors should be considered.

Age of patient. Overaeration in infants and young children (under 1½ years) is usually easier to identify than in older patients.

Position of patient. Supine chest films on infants tend to be expiratory because of upward pressure on the diaphragm. Therefore, overaeration on the supine chest study is a reliable indicator of air trapping.

Restraining devices. Deformity of the chest may be caused by some devices that constrict and thus alter the natural configuration of the chest. Supine films require a minimum of restraints such as sandbags over the arms and legs.

Bronchiolitis (peribronchial pneumonia, bronchiolytic inflammatory disease), chronic recurrent tracheobronchial aspiration, and bronchial asthma (reactive airway disease) are the diseases that will be discussed in this chapter. All produce a pattern of diffuse pulmonary hyperaeration.

Bronchiolitis

Bronchiolitis, a catarrhal disease of children under 2 years, is characterized by rapid respiration, chest retractions, and wheezing. It is usually a recognizable clinical syndrome, but cannot always be distinguished from other lower respiratory tract disorders that trigger wheezing.[1] It is often difficult or impossible to differentiate between wheezing caused by bronchiolitis, asthmatic bronchitis, bronchial asthma, bronchopneumonia, or laryngotracheobronchitis.[2] Henderson and coworkers[3] solved this dilemma by creating the term *wheezing associated respiratory infection* (WARI). Bronchiolitis is included in this group.

The histologic changes of bronchiolitis are characterized by inflammatory lesions that develop in small airways ranging from 75 to 300 μm in diameter. Cellular infiltration, edema of airway walls, sloughing of necrotic epithelial debris, and excess secretion of mucus all contribute to partial obstruction of the peripheral airways. These alterations in the peripheral airways account for the clinical symptoms of wheezing and air trapping seen in bronchiolitis.

Respiratory syncytial virus (RSV) is the most common etiologic agent implicated in bronchiolitis. Other responsible organisms include parainfluenza virus types 1 and 3, adenoviruses, rhinoviruses, and *Mycoplasma pneumoniae*. In one series, these organisms accounted for 87 percent of all infections.[3] Epidemics of RSV tend to occur between October and June and last approximately 5 months.[4]

Clinical Symptoms

Bronchiolitis begins with rhinorrhea and symptoms of mild upper respiratory tract infection. Fever is present in about one-half of patients, but rarely exceeds 102°F. Within a few days, the child develops labored, rapid respirations with prolonged expiration, typically accompanied by striking muscular effort as well as intercostal, suprasternal, and substernal retractions. Cyanosis may appear in severe cases.

Auscultation of the chest is dominated by a prolonged expiratory phase, rales, and rhonchi that are indistinguishable from those of bronchial asthma in older patients. Air trapping may be so severe that little air movement occurs, thus eliminating the typical auscultatory findings.

Although bronchiolitis is self-limited, recent work suggests that the condition may give rise to short-term and long-term sequelae. Abnormal blood gas values may not return to normal for 3 to 7 weeks.[5] Other authors have suggested that the return of blood gases to normal is delayed in children with secondary bacterial infection.[6] Of greater importance are the long-term sequelae. Gurwitz et al.[7] found a greater incidence of recurrent wheezing in children followed up to 10 years after an episode of bronchiolitis. Kattan et al.[8] reported residual pulmonary function abnormalities in 30 percent of patients up to 10 years after their initial episode of bronchiolitis. The authors suggest that bronchiolitis in infancy is not a benign disease and may produce irreversible small airway disease. More recent findings by McConnochie and colleagues have found no evidence of increased airway hyperactivity in patients 8 to 12 years of age after episodes of mild bronchiolitis in infancy.[9]

Airway hyperactivity, as manifested by wheezing, is difficult to categorize. Studies of patients with bronchiolitis show significantly higher levels of serum immunoglobulin E (IgE) levels in those with sporadic, presumably atopic, disease compared with those which occur in epidemics.[10] Serum IgE levels may be of value in predicting which bronchiolitic children are at risk for later development of asthma and other respiratory allergies. Other authors have found that cell-bound IgE in respiratory tract epithelium may persist for longer periods in children who contract bronchiolitis or asthma during an episode of RSV infection, compared with children who develop only pneumonia or upper respiratory infection.[11]

Radiologic Findings

Chest films exposed during the acute phase of bronchiolitis may include any or all of the following: (1) overaeration (Figure 14-1), (2) patchy radiopacities, (3) shifting atelectasis, (4) ill-defined pulmonary vessels, and (5) gradual thymic involution (Figure 14-2). The severity of overexpansion will depend upon the age of the patient and the duration of the illness. More severe overexpansion occurs in younger infants with prolonged illness.

Occasionally, irregular areas of focal emphysema and shifting atelectasis result from intermittent plugging of peripheral bronchi (Figure 14-2). Confluent conglomerations of segmental and subsegmental infiltrates may occupy the parenchyma. Intrapulmonary vascular shadows lose sharpness and definition as a result of adjacent bronchial inflammation and peribronchial edema.

The return of lung volume to normal may be the first radiographic sign of improvement, although the lung markings often become more numerous and patchy. Generalized nondescript opacities frequently remain for several weeks; abnormal chest films should be followed to complete clearing so that areas of atelectasis or residual pneumonia are not overlooked. Persistent overdistension beyond the period of acute illness should raise suspicion of other diseases responsible for pulmonary hyperaeration, such as cystic fibrosis, pertussis, chronic or recurrent aspiration, and immune deficiency syndromes. Recurrent attacks of wheezing often herald the onset of bronchial asthma.[12]

Hyperaeration may also occur with intracardiac shunts to the lung (Figure 14-3), metabolic acidosis, and tracheal obstruction.

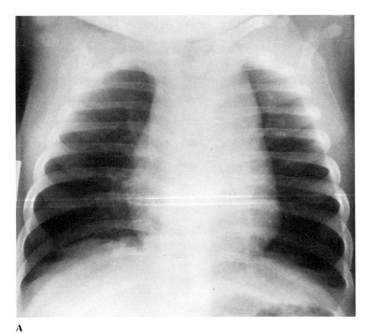
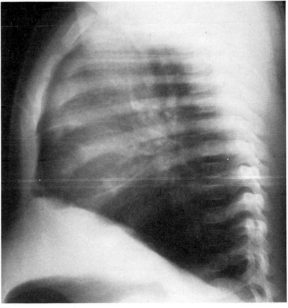

A   B

Figure 14-1 Bronchiolitis—clear lungs. A. The frontal film shows many features of overaeration: "elevated" heart, horizontal ribs, sparse vessels, and depressed diaphragm with scalloped costophrenic attachments. **B.** The lateral film shows additional findings of overaeration: horizontal ribs, flattened diaphragm, increased anteroposterior chest diameter, and increased retrosternal clear space. The relatively clear lungs should give no comfort to physician or patient in the presence of this degree of air trapping.

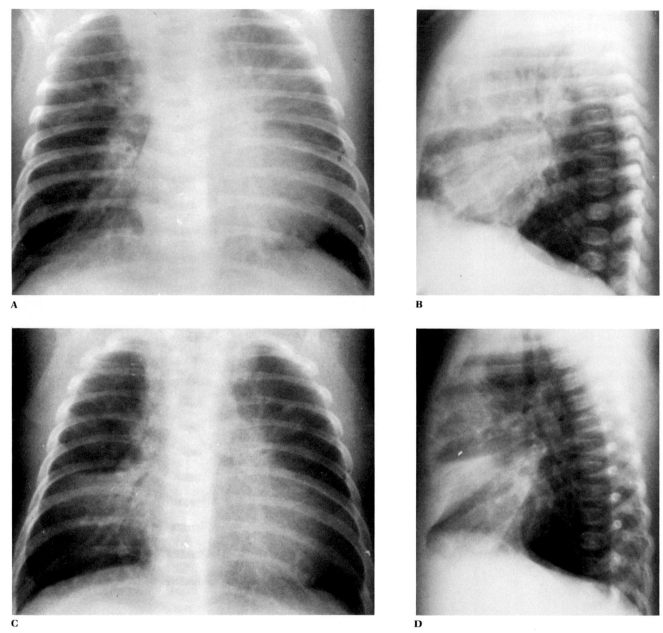

A

B

C

D

Figure 14-2   Bronchiolitis—atelectasis. A and B. Frontal and lateral films show overaeration as well as diffuse streaky opacities and selective overdistension of the right lower lobe. **C and D.** Follow-up studies 3 days later show persistent overaeration and right middle lobe atelectasis.

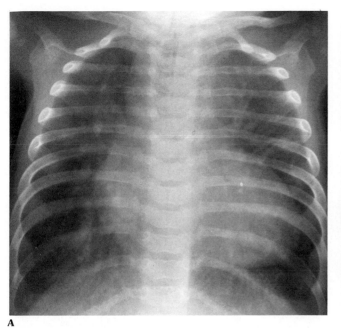

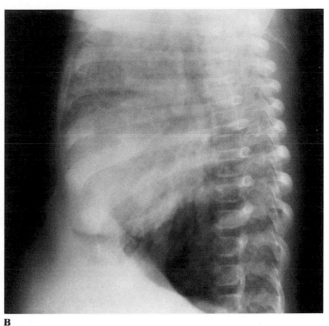

A

B

Figure 14-3   Overaeration—intracardiac shunt. A and B. Severe overaeration with cardiomegaly and intracardiac shunt to the lungs are present with no clinical symptoms of acute pulmonary infection. Because of the hyperaeration and plethoric pulmonary vasculature, it is often difficult or impossible to be definitive regarding a pulmonary infection on an isolated chest film. Previous studies and follow-up examinations are often necessary in making this determination.

Infants with lower respiratory tract infections develop generalized overaeration more often than older children and adults. To explain this difference, the following pathophysiologic mechanisms have been opined by Griscom and coworkers:[13]

1. Resistance to airflow is greater in young children (under 1½ years) because of anatomic differences in the airways. Studies comparing children and adults have shown that below the age of 5 years, the peripheral airways (beyond the tenth and fifteenth generations) are narrower in comparison with proximal airways.[14]
2. Inflammation, muscle spasm, and edema narrow the peripheral conducting channels and cause a relatively greater obstruction of airflow through the peripheral bronchi.
3. Increased air trapping and the susceptibility to atelectasis in young children are caused by less well developed pores of Kohn and canals of Lambert.[15]

4. Infants' peripheral airways contain greater numbers of mucous glands that elaborate secretions and contribute to airway obstruction.[16]
5. The airways of infants manifest greater collapsibility as intrathoracic pressure increases during forced expiration.[17]
6. Immunologic mechanisms peculiar to infants and young children render them more susceptible to severe lower respiratory infections.[18]

Chronic Recurrent Tracheobronchial Aspiration (Aspiration Pneumonia)

Pneumonia may result from an acute aspiration, or it may be associated with chronic, underlying inhalation of swallowed foodstuffs and/or regurgitated gastric contents. The clinicoradiographic pattern of aspiration pneumonia is determined by several factors: (1) the age of the patient, (2) the nature and amount of foreign materials aspirated, and (3) the chronicity of the insult.

An isolated episode of aspiration in an otherwise normal child often occurs during a period of somnolence or near unconsciousness. Patients are especially at risk during or after convulsions, in postanesthesia recovery, or when comatose for other reasons. Immobilization in restraining devices con-

tributes to aspiration. Severely retarded children represent another group at risk for developing pulmonary complications secondary to aspiration. Sondheimer et al.[19] studied 19 mentally and physically handicapped institutionalized children with 8 or more vomiting episodes per month. Of these, 6 had 1 or more episodes of aspiration pneumonia in the year before the study. Putrid lung abscesses are more likely to occur in this population.

Chronic, low-grade aspiration is often difficult to

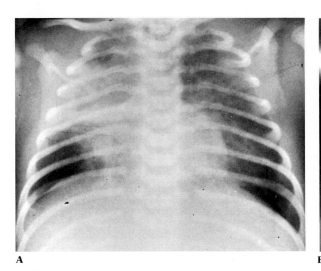

A

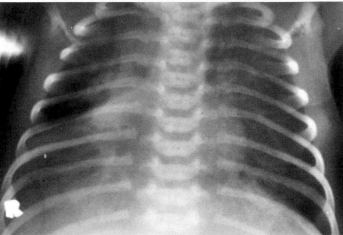

B

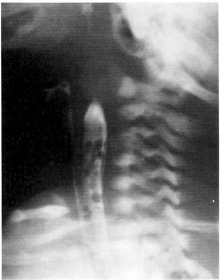

C

Figure 14-4 Chronic aspiration. A. The frontal film shows bilateral central radiopacities and right upper lobe segmental consolidation-atelectasis. **B.** Nine days later the right lower lobe is atelectatic and the right upper lobe has cleared. **C.** The barium swallow shows unequivocal tracheal aspiration.

document but should be suspected in children with chronic lung disease of unknown origin. The clinical symptoms and radiographic features are usually nonspecific. In suspicious cases, evaluation of the swallowing function, esophageal motility, gastroesophageal junction, gastric outlet, and gastrointestinal tract should be carried out to establish or exclude gastroesophageal reflux and/or aspiration (Figure 14-4).

Gastroesophageal Reflux

Gastroesophageal reflux (GER) and chronic pulmonary disease cannot be considered separately. While the association of GER and chronic nonspecific bronchopulmonary disease is well-recognized, the exact significance of this relationship is in dispute.[20–23] Theoretical considerations include microaspirations of gastric content[24,25] and vagus nerve reflex.[26,27]

The clinical pattern of patients with GER-associated respiratory disease has been defined in numerous reports.[21,22,28–31] The clinical features that should arouse suspicion of chronic aspiration include:

1. Chronic and recurrent episodes of nonseasonal wheezing, often beginning 1 to 3 h into sleep
2. Vomiting in infancy
3. Recurrent acute cough
4. Radiographically documented episodes of pneumonia several times per year
5. Failure to thrive
6. Anemia (hemoglobin less than 9 g)

Prolonged GER may produce esophageal stricture (see Chapter 15, Figure 15-9), achalasia, and odynophagia. Sandifer's syndrome (hiatus hernia, GER, and abnormal posturing of the head) is an uncommon but well-recognized complex of symptoms.

The radiographic findings that suggest chronic recurrent aspiration pneumonia are hyperaeration, consolidation, and/or collapse. Areas of collapse frequently shift about and often resist attempts at reinflation. Bronchiectasis and lung abscesses are infrequent. Small thymus, lines of growth arrest in the proximal humeri, and sparse soft tissue are secondary signs of chronic recurrent disease.

When GER is a suspected cause of chronic or recurrent lung disease, documentation of its presence becomes imperative. Two major questions arise in this regard: (1) What is the best method to diagnose GER? and (2) if GER occurs, what is its relationship to the patient's pulmonary disease?

Diagnosis and Documentation of GER

The choice of tests to confirm the presence of GER will depend largely upon local prejudice and expertise. At present, six recognized methods are used:

1. Laboratory
   a. Esophageal intraluminal pH probe test (Tuttle test)
   b. Acid perfusion test (Bernstein test)
   c. Esophageal manometry
   d. Esophagoscopy and biopsy
2. Radiographic imaging
   a. Barium esophogram
   b. Radionuclide scintigraphy (milk scan)

The pH probe test, barium esophogram, and radionuclide scintigraphy are the most frequently employed.

Esophageal Intraluminal pH Probe Test (Tuttle Test)

The Tuttle test is performed by placing a known quantity of 0.1 N hydrochloric acid in the stomach and a pH monitoring probe in the esophagus.[20,32] The presence of reflux is documented by the 24-h monitoring of changes in the pH of the distal esophagus.

The advantages of this test are:

1. It will determine the presence of reflux in some patients with otherwise negative tests.
2. It may have good correlation with the need for surgery to correct symptoms, especially when combined with abnormal lower esophageal sphincter pressure.[29]

The disadvantages are:

1. It is difficult to perform, especially in infants.
2. There is low sensitivity in infants, better sensitivity in older patients.

Barium Esophogram

The technique used to perform a barium esophogram may vary. One method is to feed the infant liquid barium in an amount approximately equivalent to a normal feeding. The child is then burped, and the gastrointestinal junction is observed with intermittent fluoroscopy for 5 min. During this time, care is taken not to give additional water. The child is kept supine and gently rolled from side to side at intervals of approximately 1 min. The number of reflux episodes that occur multiplied by 12 will give the approximate incidence of reflux that might be expected over the ensuing hour. The level to which the barium column rises, the ability of the esophagus to clear the refluxed barium, and any evidence of aspirated barium into the trachea are recorded (Figure 14-4C).

The advantages of the barium esophogram are:

1. It is easy to perform, readily available, and least traumatic.
2. It provides a good evaluation of deglutition and determines whether aspiration occurs during swallowing (Figure 14-4C).
3. It gives good assessment of function and anatomy (strictures, fistula, peristalsis).
4. It demonstrates the anatomy of the gastroesophageal junction and establishes the presence or absence of hiatus hernia.[33]
5. It reveals the presence or absence of gastric outlet obstruction.

The disadvantages are:

1. There is radiation exposure.
2. Reflux is revealed only during fluoroscopy.
3. Delayed reflux is missed.
4. It may be falsely negative.

Radionuclide Scintigraphy (Milk Scan)

This test is performed by adding ^{99m}Tc-labeled sulfur colloid to routine milk formula feedings.[34–38] Patients are monitored continuously for 1 h after feeding and sequentially for intervals up to 24 h. Reflux into the esophagus and aspiration into the lungs are recorded by the radionuclide camera and computer analysis.

The advantages of the milk scan are:

1. Milk is more physiologic than the barium-water mixture.
2. One is better able to observe for reflux over the immediate postfeeding hour and beyond.
3. Sensitivity is good (as much as 80 to 88 percent).
4. The radiation dose is lower.
5. Aspiration into the lung can be detected.

The disadvantages are:

1. It does not give information about the physiology of deglutition.
2. The anatomy of the esophagus, gastroesophageal junction, and gastric outlet is not revealed.
3. It is less available in departments not performing this study regularly.

Choice of Method

Accommodating the wide diversity of opinion is difficult if not impossible regarding (1) the most efficacious method for documenting GER, (2) the significance of GER in relation to chronic pulmonary disease, and (3) the necessary therapeutic measures. In addition, significant parochial bias is encountered when deciding upon the best method of evaluating GER.

Patients with chronic recurrent pulmonary disease and symptoms of GER should have a barium esophogram to evaluate not only reflux, but deglutition and tracheal aspiration during swallowing, esophageal motility, anatomy of the gastroesophageal junction, gastric outlet, and patency of the gastrointestinal tract. There is wide variation in the methods of performing contrast esophograms. The 5 min routine of McCauley et al.[33] and Condon,[39] described in the section "Barium Esophogram," has gained wide acceptance.

The acceptable number of reflux episodes in a 5-min period is summed up as follows:

Age-Related Criteria for Acceptable GER

Group	"Acceptable" Number of Reflux Episodes in 5 min
1 (birth to 6 weeks)	3
2 (7 weeks to 6 months)	2
3 (7 months to 1 year)	2
4 (1 year 1 month to 1½ years)	1
5 (1 year 7 months to 6 years)	1
6 and 7 (6 years 1 month to 18 years)	0–1

Source: Cleveland et al.[40]

However, in addition to the numbers of reflux episodes, the height of the barium column, the patency and configuration of the gastroesophageal junction,[33] and the rapidity with which barium is cleared from the esophagus are all qualitative and largely judgmental factors that must be included in the overall evaluation.

Complete studies of children suspected of having pulmonary disease secondary to GER should also include the radionuclide scan and probably the pH monitor for up to 24 h.[31,38] Lung biopsy in some cases is valuable and may reveal evidence of milk aspiration (fat-laden histiocytes).

Treatment should be directed toward prevention of reflux episodes. Orenstein and Whitington[41] advocate a prone, head-elevated position in a harness rather than the traditional infant seat. Surgical repair of the gastroesophageal junction has been advocated for children who cannot be controlled medically.[42]

Asthma

In the past, bronchial asthma was defined as a recurrent pulmonary disorder characterized by labored breathing, irritative tight cough, and wheezing. It affected children of all ages. Asthma could begin in infancy with repeated attacks of wheezing with or without associated respiratory infections. Increasing frequency of attacks, as well as prolongation of cough and chest congestion, alerted the physician to the possibility of asthma. As the child grew older, the respiratory symptoms often worsened and occurred without the usual preceding upper respiratory infection. The presence of infantile atopic eczema, as well as positive skin tests to allergens, especially in those infants with eczema, further increased the probability of asthma in later years.[43,44]

In older children, attacks frequently occurred at night with or without a preceding infection. Precipitating factors in an asthmatic attack included emotional upset, fatigue, exposure to larger than tolerable amounts of allergens (pollen, molds, and similar substances), excessive exercise, respiratory infections, and possibly changes in temperature or other climatic parameters. However, in many cases no precipitating event was apparent.

With prompt treatment, most attacks were self-limited, but some children experienced prolonged debilitating illness, weight loss, and dehydration. Death was a rare, but occasional, occurrence.[45] While typical allergic asthma usually did not result in chronic lung disease, repeated attacks were observed in patients with superimposed bronchial infections and progressive, irreversible lung damage characterized by extensive fibrosis and emphysema.

That was in the past. Today, some children still have asthma, to be sure, but others apparently have diseases with such euphemistic terminology as *reactive airway disease*[46] and *wheezing associated respiratory infection* (WARI).[3]

Radiologic Findings

Physicians caring for asthmatic children commonly seek help from the roentgen ray. Rather than review the already overexpanded radiographic literature on this disease, this material will be approached from the standpoint of the clinician. The "four questions of asthma," frequently asked of radiologists by clinicians caring for asthmatic children, are as follows:

Question 1

Does the patient have asthma? This question is put to radiologists with distressing frequency, causing some to respond with a bronchospasm of their own.

Asthma is a clinical diagnosis; the radiograph rarely reveals a pathognomonic pattern. However, in certain children, subtle, suggestive signs may be present.

Question 2

How do the radiographic findings in asthma differ from all other diseases? The lungs of asthmatic children appear tired—in need of a rest. Overaeration is the most consistent roentgen finding; it is reported in 36 to 70 percent of patients.[47–49] However, significant overaeration may be absent in more than 50 percent of patients, particularly older children. The hyperaeration in asthma and bronchiolitis has a similar radiographic appearance although the peak ages of each disease differ. In both diseases, bronchospasm, mucosal edema, and excess mucous production are the underlying pathophysiologic causes. As in bronchiolitis, the overaeration of asthma is often focal because of the tendency for mucous plugs to form and dislodge during the course of illness. The overaerated lungs of asthmatic children should return to normal after the attack is over.

Many other diseases may cause overaeration; among these are cystic fibrosis, chronic aspiration, immune deficiency syndromes, and left to right cardiac shunts. Tracheal obstruction, especially bronchial adenomas, constricting vascular rings, and foreign bodies, may cause overaeration (Figure 14-5). In most cases these conditions have sufficiently distinguishing clinical symptomatology.

The hilar shadows of patients with long-standing asthma often take on an appearance resembling a cobweb (Figure 14-6). Vascular structures lose their definition as they enter a conglomerate of hilar tissue opacity. Adenopathy in the hila may be associated with asthma, but it is difficult to define with certainty because of the surrounding densities. The cobweb appearance of the hila is not specific for asthma but can occur in a variety of acute and chronic infectious processes.

Scattered shifting atelectasis is a prominent feature of asthma, and results from mucus plugging, edema of bronchial mucosa, and extrinsic lymph node compression with resorption of air beyond. In most cases, the process clears with recovery, but occasional collapsed lobes fail to reexpand. The right middle lobe, by virtue of its location and bronchial anatomy, has a greater tendency to collapse and resist reexpansion (Figure 14-7). Dees and Spock[50]

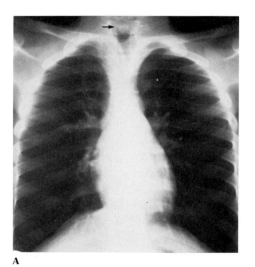

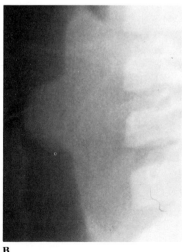

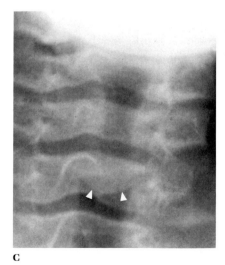

A

B

C

Figure 14-5 Tracheal tumor. This 7-year-old boy was treated for asthma over a 6-month period before referral. **A.** The representative frontal film shows diffuse hyperaeration. *Note:* There is interruption of the tracheal air column (arrow). **B.** The large mass almost occludes the trachea. **C.** The frontal view shows interruption of the tracheal air column and the well-defined inferior margin of the mass (arrowheads).

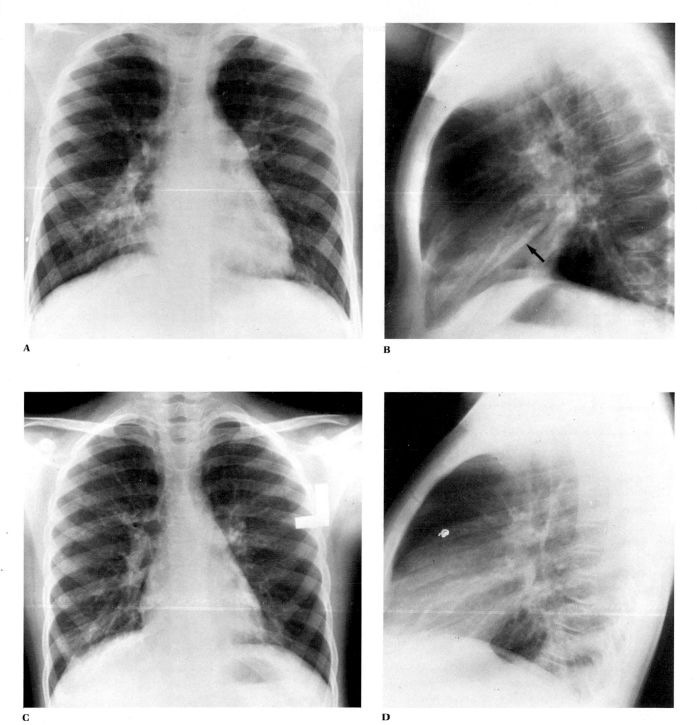

Figure 14-6 Asthma—hilar "cobweb" sign. A. The frontal film shows indistinct central pulmonary vessels (cobweb); diffuse, patchy, predominantly lower lung opacities; and obliteration of the right heart border by right middle lobe segmental atelectasis. **B.** The lateral film shows increased anteroposterior chest diameter, anterior bowing of the sternum with increased retrosternal clear space, patchy hilar densities, and a streaky opacity representing subsegmental right middle lobe atelectasis (arrow). **C.** Four days later, the lungs retain mild overaeration and generalized increased streaky, linear, and, in some areas, patchy markings. The right heart border is now well-defined. **D.** Corresponding lateral film shows less overaeration and a clear right middle lobe region.

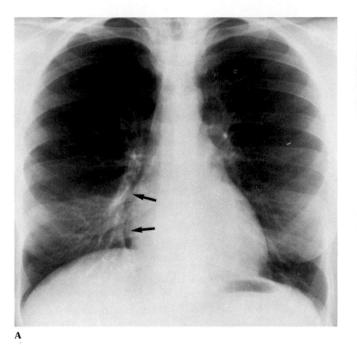

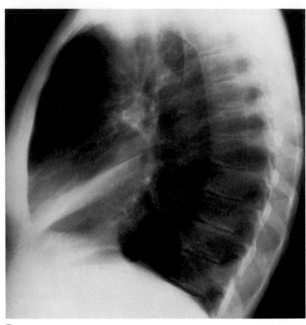

A   B

Figure 14-7   Right middle lobe collapse. A. The frontal film shows subtle changes: (1) increased opacity adjacent to the right heart border, (2) loss of the right heart border silhouette between arrows, (3) hyperlucent right upper lobe representing compensatory emphysema, and (4) depressed right hilum. **B.** The wedge-shaped opacity overlying the heart shadow represents the collapsed right middle lobe. Note the increased anteroposterior chest diameter and enlarged retrosternal clear space.

studied 30 children with chronic right middle lobe collapse, 23 of whom were atopic. These children had recurrent pneumonia localized to the right middle lobe. In 10, the lobe had been removed surgically. The authors stress the importance of defining this complication, since early recognition may allow for reexpansion and preservation of the lung.

Several notes of caution are in order when dealing with the right middle lobe. Careful attention should be paid to the right heart border, which may lose its normal silhouette when the adjacent middle lobe is infiltrated or collapsed (Figure 14-7A). The horizontal fissure will frequently be displaced downward. When the middle lobe collapses, the radiopacity visible on the frontal projection may disappear, giving the false impression of clearing. Lateral films or lordotic projections centered over the lower chest will often identify the collapsed lobe or segment (Figure 14-7B). Following right middle lobe disease with frontal films only is inadequate.

Mucoid impaction of bronchi, in addition to causing atelectasis and focal overaeration, may lead to a series of events that affect the lung beyond. A portion of lung may become infected and cause a well-defined radiopacity that is indistinguishable from a neoplasm. These shadows shift about or disappear spontaneously when the plug is coughed up. V-shaped or "gloved-hand" shadows represent bronchi that are filled with mucus or other debris. Shaw[51] reported on 10 asthmatic patients with this complication, 8 of whom had pulmonary resections. Rebuck[52] found this complication in 13 of 58 patients. These shadows also occur with generalized aspergillosis (see Chapter 20).

Asthma, if sufficiently prolonged and severe, may produce recognizable endobronchial changes on plain films. Hodson and Trickey[53] reported the presence of thickened bronchial walls in 121 of 190 patients and felt that superimposed infection was the major etiologic factor in their appearance. Robinson

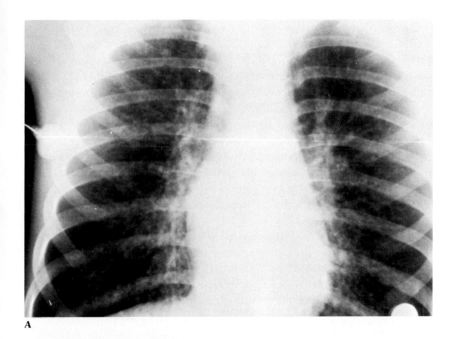

A

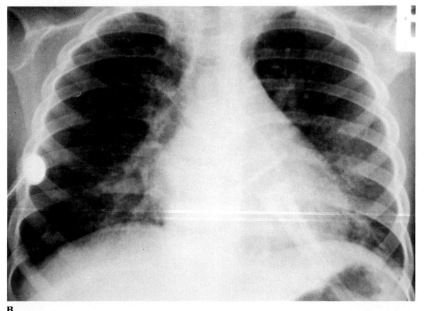

B

Figure 14-8 Status asthmaticus. A. This frontal study is representative of a series of films taken over several days while the patient was in status asthmaticus. Marked hyperaeration is present, and the central silhouette is significantly narrowed. The lungs show a myriad of small ringlike shadows representing thickened bronchi; these are more prominent in the central perihilar areas. **B.** After interruption of the asthmatic attack, the lung volume has returned to normal and contains scattered patchy opacities. This appearance commonly follows prolonged asthmatic attacks.

and Campbell[54] performed bronchograms on 57 asthmatic children aged 10 months to 13 years and observed the presence of widespread abnormalities that suggested bronchitis. The findings of peribronchial cuffing, interstitial thickening, and hyperaera-tion were present on plain films. Well-defined bronchial walls are often seen normally in the central regions of the lung; significant bronchial wall thickening should extend at least to the middle third of the lung. Truly abnormal bronchi are seen not only as thick circles on end but as irregular elongated densities ("railroad tracks"). As with bronchiolitis, the radiographic appearance of the asthmatic chest may look worse as the overaeration abates. This should not necessarily be taken as evidence of superimposed inflammatory disease.

These radiographic features seen in more severe asthmatics (bronchial thickening, mucus plugging, hyperaeration, and hilar enlargement) are quite similar and may at times be indistinguishable from the changes of cystic fibrosis or other causes of chronic endobronchial disease (Figure 14-8). In most cases, however, the peribronchial thickening in asthmatic lungs does not extend as far into the periphery as it does in fibrocystic disease. In addition, the hyperaeration of cystic fibrosis may come and go in the early stages, but eventually the lungs lose their ability to return to normal and the overaeration remains fixed. On occasion, separating cystic fibrosis (or immune deficiency syndromes) from asthma solely on the basis of chest radiographs is impossible. Careful analysis of all films is important in making this distinction.

Pneumothorax and pneumomediastinum occur infrequently in asthmatic patients (Figure 14-9).[48,52] When pneumomediastinum develops, however, it has a tendency to dissect into the soft tissues of the chest and neck, creating a typical radiographic pattern of soft tissue air that usually produces subcutaneous crepitation on palpation. Pneumothorax in asthmatics may develop tension, necessitating immediate evacuation.[46] Rare examples of arterial embolism in asthmatic patients have also been reported.[55]

Roentgenographic differentiation between asthma and pneumonia is occasionally difficult, if not impossible. Patchy, air space opacities that remain localized and gradually resolve probably represent pneumonia. Unfortunately, the evolution of these densities is helpful only in retrospect. Onset of pleural effusion in most cases signifies superimposed bacterial pneumonia.

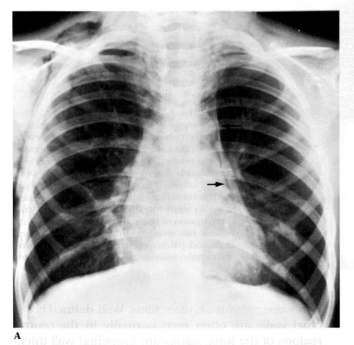
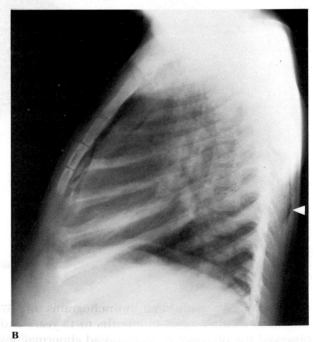

A   **B**

Figure 14-9   Pneumomediastinum. A. The lucent shadows outlining the aortic knob and upper mediastinal tissues (arrows) indicate the presence of mediastinal air. Subcutaneous emphysema is present in the right side of the chest and supraclavicular soft tissue. **B.** The substernal and posterior thoracic soft tissue lucencies (arrowhead) represent mediastinal and chest wall emphysema.

Question 3

Which asthmatic child needs a radiograph? No universal statement can answer this question, since the circumstances surrounding each case will differ. Several reviews of both emergency room and inpatient radiography of asthmatic children have been published. Zieverink and coworkers[56] recommend chest radiography in asthmatics treated in the emergency room when rales and rhonchi are present in addition to wheezing. Fife and coworkers[49] reported abnormal roentgen findings excluding peribronchial thickening and overaeration in 21 percent of 889 children. Brooks et al.[48] concluded that "routine chest roentgenograms may not have to be taken on all children hospitalized for acute asthma." However, these authors, and others, were unable to detect complications in their patients with the use of other clinical or laboratory parameters.[48,49]

Chest films should be obtained in any patient with an atypical clinical picture. A chest film is justified when wheezing is not generalized, when breath sounds are unequal, when no history of allergy exists, and when the attack is the patient's first.

Pain in the chest wall sometimes signifies a pneumothorax. If the patient is febrile, a superimposed or underlying pneumonia or atelectasis should be suspected and confirmed or excluded by chest film.

Failure of normal response to therapy should raise suspicion of an underlying complication and call for a radiographic examination. Certainly, chest films and contrast esophograms are mandatory when foreign body aspiration (or ingestion) or constricting vascular rings are considerations (Figure 14-10). Frequently, a history of foreign body ingestion is lacking, but any small child who develops sudden wheezing should be carefully scrutinized for this possibility (see Chapter 13). Vascular rings are well-known causes for chronic, recurrent wheezing, especially under 6 months of age.

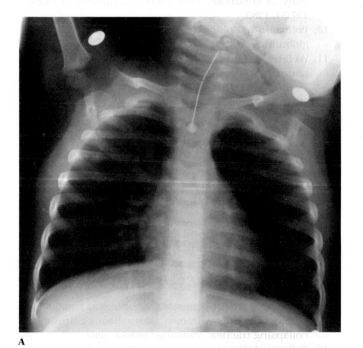
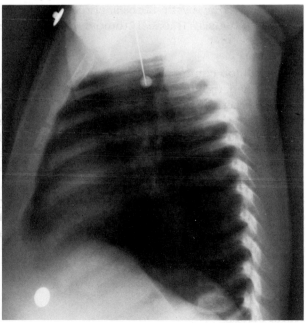

A   **B**

Figure 14-10 Tracheal foreign body. This child was treated over a 2-week period for asthma. Because of poor response, chest films were obtained. **A** and **B.** Frontal and lateral films demonstrate the presence of a hatpin in the trachea. "Rusty" sputum was not produced.

Question 4

How often should a child be radiographed during the course of an asthmatic attack? This question is often more troublesome than question 3, and there are no better answers available. Clinical judgment should always prevail, but this cliché may be rendered inoperative by future developments in the practice of medicine.

The debate over the filming of asthmatic children will probably never be solved. However, the most important points to be emphasized in relation to the child with asthma, or any other type of pulmonary disease, are as follows:

1. Collapse or localized emphysema, so common in asthma, should be followed until clear. Postasthmatic chronic collapse with secondary bronchiectasis is a preventable disease and should be recognized.
2. Hyperaeration should be followed until it resolves.[57] The physician must be concerned about other diseases in the face of chronic hyperaeration, including cystic fibrosis, chronic aspiration, foreign bodies, tracheal tumors, and vascular rings.

It is all too common for children with asthma to be examined, radiographed, treated, and discharged from emergency rooms, only to appear weeks or months later, see a different physician, and repeat the same routine. When examining the films in such a child's jacket, a normal study is often not available. This unhappy circumstance renders the distinction between recurrent acute illness and chronic disease difficult or impossible. Obviously, the two have very different prognostic and therapeutic implications. It is therefore important for films to be obtained at some time when the child is in normal health.

References

1. McConnochie KM: Bronchiolitis. What's in the name? *Am J Dis Child* 137:11, 1983.
2. Disney ME, Sandiford BR, Cragg J: Epidemic bronchiolitis in infants. *Br Med J* 1:1407, 1960.
3. Henderson FW, Clyde WA Jr, Collier AM, Denny FW: The etiologic and epidemiologic spectrum of bronchiolitis in pediatric practice. *J Pediatr* 95:183, 1979.
4. Glezen WP, Denny FW: Epidemiology of acute lower respiratory disease in children. *N Engl J Med* 288:498, 1973.
5. Hall CB, Hall WJ, Spurs DM: Clinical and physiological manifestations of bronchiolitis and pneumonia: Outcome of respiratory syncytial virus. *Am J Dis Child* 133:798, 1979.
6. Reynolds EOR: Recovery from bronchiolitis as judged by arterial blood gas tension measurements. *J Pediatr* 63:1182, 1963.
7. Gurwitz D, Mindorff C, Levison H: Increased incidence of bronchial reactivity in children with a history of bronchiolitis. *J Pediatr* 98:551, 1981.
8. Kattan M, Keens TG, Lapierre J, et al: Pulmonary function in symptom-free children after bronchiolitis. *Pediatrics* 59:683, 1977.
9. McConnochie KM, Mark JD, McBride JT, et al: Normal pulmonary function measurements and airway reactivity in childhood after mild bronchiolitis. *J Pediatr* 107:54, 1985.
10. Polmar SN, Robinson LD Jr, Minnefor AB: Immune globulin E in bronchiolitis. *Pediatrics* 50:279, 1972.
11. Welliver R, Kaul TN, Ogra PL: The appearance of cell-bound IgE in respiratory tract epithelium after RSV infection. *N Engl J Med* 303:1198, 1980.
12. High RH: Bronchiolitis. *Pediatr Clin North Am* 4:183, 1957.
13. Griscom NT, Wohl MEB, Kirkpatrick JA Jr: Lower respiratory infections: How infants differ from adults. *Radiol Clin North Am* 16:367, 1978.
14. Hogg JC, Williams J, Richardson JB, et al: Age as a factor in the distribution of lower airway conductance and in the pathologic anatomy of obstructive lung disease. *N Engl J Med* 282:1283, 1970.
15. Spencer H: *Pathology of the Lung*. New York, Macmillan Company, 1962, p 410.
16. Matsuba, K, Thurlbeck WM: A morphometric study of bronchial and bronchiolar wall in children. *Am Rev Respir Dis* 105:908, 1972.
17. Wittenborg MH, Gyepes MT, Crocker D: Tracheal dynamics in infants with respiratory distress, stridor, and collapsing trachea. *Radiology* 88:653, 1967.
18. Bellanti JA: Development of nonimmunologic, nonspecific mechanisms in resistance to airways and pulmonary infections in infants and children. *Pediatric Res* 11:224, 1977.

19. Sondheimer JH, Morris BA: Gastroesophageal reflux among severely retarded children. *J Pediatr* 94:710, 1979.

20. Euler AR, Byrne WJ: Twenty-four hour esophageal intraluminal pH probe testing: A comparative analysis. *Gastroenterology* 80:957, 1981.

21. Christie DL, O'Grady LR, Mach DV: Incompetent lower esophageal sphincter and gastroesophageal reflux in recurrent acute pulmonary disease of infancy and childhood. *J Pediatr* 93:23, 1978.

22. Fonkalsrud EW, Ament ME, Byrne WJ, et al: Gastroesophageal fundoplication for the management of reflux in infants and children. *J Thorac Cardiovasc Surg* 76:655, 1978.

23. Holyoux CL, Forget P, Lambrechts L, et al: Chronic bronchopulmonary disease and gastrointestinal reflux in children. *Pediatr Pulmonol* 1:149, 1985.

24. Mendelson CL: The aspiration of stomach contents into the lung during obstetric anesthesia. *Am J Obstet Gynecol* 52:151, 1946.

25. Barr RR, Notarangelo J, Smith VM: Wheezing: A clue to gastroesophageal reflux. *Am J Gastroenterol* 53:230, 1970.

26. Spaulding HS, Mansfield LE, Stein MR, Sellner JC, et al: Further investigation of the association between gastroesophageal reflux and bronchoconstriction. *J Allergy Clin Immunol* 69:516, 1982.

27. Mansfield LE, Stein MR: Gastroesophageal reflux and asthma. Demonstration of a possible reflux mechanism. *Am Rev Respir Dis* 117:72, 1978.

28. Berquist WE, Rachelefsky GS, Kadden M, et al: Gastroesophageal reflux-associated recurrent pneumonia and chronic asthma in children. *Pediatrics* 68:29, 1981.

29. Euler AR, Byrne WJ, Ament ME, et al: Recurrent pulmonary disease in children: A complication of gastroesophageal reflux. *Pediatrics* 63:47, 1979.

30. Herbst JJ: Diagnosis and treatment of gastroesophageal reflux in children. *Pediatr Rev* 5:75, 1983.

31. Leonidas JC: Gastroesophageal reflux in infants: Role of the upper gastrointestinal series. *AJR* 143:1350, 1984.

32. Tuttle SG, Grossman MI: Detection of gastroesophageal reflux by simultaneous measurement, intraluminal pressure and pH. *Soc Exp Biol Med* 98:225, 1958.

33. McCauley RGK, Darling DB, Leonidas JC, et al: Gastroesophageal reflux in infants and children: A useful classification and reliable radiologic technique for its demonstration. *AJR* 130:47, 1978.

34. Heyman S, Kirkpatrick JA, Winter HS: An improved radionuclide method for the diagnosis of gastroesophageal reflux and aspiration in children. *Radiology* 131:479, 1979.

35. Rudd TG, Christie DL: Demonstration of gastroesophageal reflux in children by radionuclide gastroesophagography. *Radiology* 131:483, 1979.

36. Boonyaprapa S, Alderson PO, Garfinkel DJ, et al: Detection of pulmonary aspiration in infants and children with respiratory disease: Concise communication. *J Nucl Med* 21:314, 1980.

37. Blumhagen JD, Rudd TG, Christie DL: Gastroesophageal reflux in children: Radionuclide gastroesophagography. *AJR* 135:101, 1980.

38. Seibert JJ, Byrne WJ, Euler AR, et al: Gastroesophageal reflux—The acid test: Scintigraphy or pH probe. *AJR* 141:53, 1983.

39. Condon VR: Panel on gastro-esophageal reflux, hiatus hernia, and respiratory disease. Presented at the Society for Pediatric Surgery, Denver, September 1978.

40. Cleveland RH, Kushner DC, Schwartz AN: Gastroesophageal reflux in children: Results of a standardized fluoroscopic approach. *AJR* 141:53, 1983.

41. Orenstein SR, Whitington PF: Position for prevention of infant gastroesophageal reflux. *J Pediatr* 103:534, 1983.

42. Harnsberger JK, Corey JJ, Johnson DG, et al: Long-term follow-up of surgery for gastroesophageal reflux in infants and children. *J Pediatr* 102:505, 1983.

43. Dees SC: Development and course of asthma in children. *Am J Dis Child* 93:228, 1957.

44. Buffum WP: Prognosis of asthma in infancy. *Pediatrics* 32:453, 1963.

45. Stableforth D: Death from asthma: Editorial. *Thorax* 38:801, 1983.

46. Rachelefsky GS, Katz RM, Siegel SC: Chronic sinus disease with associated reactive airway disease in children. *Pediatrics* 73:526, 1984.

47. Dees SC: Asthma, in Kendig EL Jr, Chernick V (eds): *Disorders of the Respiratory Tract in Children*, 3d ed. Philadelphia, WB Saunders, 1977, p 620.

48. Brooks LJ, Cloutier MM, Afshani E: Significance of roentgenographic abnormalities in children hospitalized for asthma. *Chest* 82:315, 1982.

49. Fife D, Twarog FJ, Geha RS: Evaluation of clinical data in childhood asthma. Application of a computer file system. *Am J Dis Child* 137:945, 1983.

50. Dees SC, Spock A: Right middle lobe syndrome in children. *JAMA* 197:78, 1966.

51. Shaw RR: Mucoid impaction of the bronchi. *J Thorac Surg* 22:149, 1951.

52. Rebuck AS: Radiologic aspects of severe asthma. *Aust Radiol* 14:264, 1970.

53. Hodson CJ, Trickey SE: Bronchial wall thickening in asthma. *Clin Radiol* 11:183, 1960.

54. Robinson AE, Campbell JB: Bronchography in childhood asthma. *AJR* 116:559, 1972.

55. Segal AJ, Wasserman M: Arterial air embolism: A cause of sudden death in status asthmaticus. *Radiology* 99:271, 1971.

56. Zieverink SE, Harper AP, Holden RW, et al: Emergency room radiography of asthma: An efficacy study. *Radiology* 145:27, 1982.

57. Kirkpatrick JA Jr: The problems of chronic and recurrent pulmonary disease. *Prog Pediatr Radiol* 1:294, 1967.

Chapter 15

Endobronchial Pattern (Bronchiectasis)

In children, as in adults, certain pulmonary diseases produce pathologic processes that primarily affect the tracheobronchial tree. Inflammation and infection lead to mucosal edema, increased secretions, destruction of bronchial endothelium, dilation of bronchial lumina, and peribronchial inflammatory reaction.

This chapter will emphasize the roentgenographic composition of bronchiectasis and review the clinicopathologic conditions characterized by this pulmonary pathosis.

1. Bronchiectasis
    a. Clinical signs and symptoms
    b. Radiologic findings
    c. Special imaging procedures
2. Acquired bronchiectasis
    a. Postinfectious bronchiectasis
    b. Postbronchial obstruction
    c. Postpulmonary edema

3. Host deficiencies
    a. Immune deficiency syndromes
    b. Immotile cilia syndrome
    c. Cystic fibrosis

Bronchiectasis

Bronchiectasis is defined in *Dorland's Illustrated Medical Dictionary* as a "chronic dilatation of the bronchi marked by fetid breath and paroxysmal coughing, with the expectoration of mucopurulent matter."[1] The definition is refined further, however, by the addition of several adjectives: *cylindric, sacculated, fusiform, capillary, cystic, dry,* and *follicular.*

Reid[2] has classified bronchiectasis into three groups:

1. Cylindrical. The bronchi are dilated but maintain a regular outline.
2. Varicose. The bronchi have irregular contours similar to varicose veins.
3. Cystic or saccular. Bronchial dilatation increases progressively toward the periphery of the lung and assumes a "ballooned" outline.

Bronchiectasis is less common than in the past because of a decrease in the occurrence of predisposing diseases. With the decline of tuberculosis, the development of vaccines to prevent measles and pertussis, and the use of antibiotics to limit the parenchymal destruction of bacterial pneumonia, bronchiectasis is now relatively uncommon. Better therapy for atelectasis and damaged lung, using postural drainage and physiotherapy, is an additional reason for the decline.[3] Fewer patients are operated on, and therefore pathologic verification is more difficult.[4]

Congenital bronchiectasis is rare in comparison with the acquired form, but may develop in portions of lung with abnormal bronchial connections, i.e., sequestration. Williams-Campbell syndrome, a congenital form of bronchiectasis, results from defective bronchial cartilage and has been reported in families (Figure 15-1).[5] It produces mild episodes of recurrent cough, wheezing, and respiratory infection. Tracheobronchomegaly (Mounier-Kuhn syndrome) is another condition with ectasia of the trachea, stem bronchi, and peripheral bronchi. Defective elastic tissue and muscle fibers of the tracheobronchial tree are contributing factors,[6] but some cases may result from acquired insult. (See Chapters 1, 18, and 19.)

Clinical Signs and Symptoms

Bronchiectasis is characterized by productive cough, intermittent fever, purulent sputum production, and other signs of pulmonary infections. Physical examination may be normal in the early stages, but rales over the affected areas develop later. Digital clubbing and osteoarthropathy (periosteal new bone) may complicate advanced cases.

Radiologic Findings

Plain-film radiographs may be diagnostic of bronchiectasis.[7] Pathologic alterations, characterized by thickened and distorted bronchial walls, mucous-plugged lumina, and volume loss, are responsible for the endobronchial-bronchiectasis pattern. Abscess formation and parenchymal destruction may develop in advanced cases.

The following are radiographic criteria of the endobronchial-bronchiectasis pattern:

1. Ringlike densities with clear centers represent thick-walled bronchi seen on end.
2. White, rounded densities are produced when the bronchial lumina become plugged with mucopurulent material.
3. Parallel lines (railroad tracks) represent thick-walled bronchi seen from the side; these often branch and may contain plugs of mucus. (See Chapter 20, "Aspergillosis.") They should not be confused with parallel blood vessels.
4. Irregular, ill-defined vascular markings result from distortion of the normal vessels by adjacent diseased bronchi.
5. Unequal aeration results from either partial or complete bronchial obstruction that produces areas of focal atelectasis and/or emphysema.

Well-exposed plain chest films usually demonstrate these features. Bronchial walls, seen only in

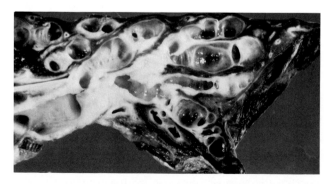

Figure 15-1 Congenital bronchiectasis. This is a pathologic specimen of severe congenital bronchiectasis. The bronchi are dilated, irregular in caliber, and filled with mucoid impactions.

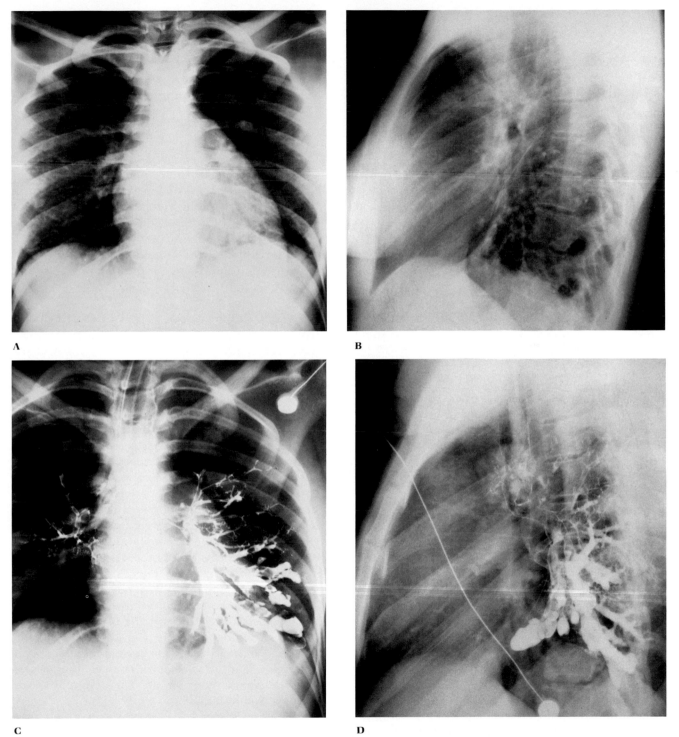

Figure 15-2 Bronchiectasis. A. Abnormal radiopacities and crowded markings are seen through the cardiac shadow. The left upper lobe shows mild compensatory emphysema. **B.** The lateral film shows ringlike shadows in the posterior basal lung. The major fissure is displaced minimally. **C** and **D.** The bronchogram shows left lower lobe fusiform and cystic bronchiectasis; partial volume loss is apparent.

the central and perihilar region on normal chest films, become apparent in the peripheral lung segments in the presence of bronchiectasis (Figure 15-2). Thus linear, circular, and ovoid shadows running in random directions in the midlung and peripheral lung fields suggest the possibility of bronchiectasis. In many cases, careful scrutiny will disclose the lucent bronchial lumina outlined by the thickened bronchial walls (Figure 15-2B). If the films are exposed at a time when bronchi are plugged with mucus, they appear as round, elongated, or sometimes branching (gloved-hand) opacities. A study of sequential films will often show intermittent bronchial plugging; unplugged, thick-walled bronchi frequently simulate railroad tracks.

The sharply defined margins and orderly tapering and branching of pulmonary vessels may be altered by adjacent diseased bronchi. Areas of volume loss and compensatory overaeration (Figure 15-2A) usually accompany this process. In most cases, a history of protracted illness is indicated by the heavy film jacket. Again, old studies must be evaluated if subtle changes (or lack of change) are to be appreciated. If only the most recent film is used for comparison, minor changes of bronchiectasis may be missed.

Old film studies may also disclose an area of preexisting pneumonia (Figure 15-3). The absence of any normal chest films should be viewed with great suspicion. Other signposts of chronicity should be noted, i.e., hilar adenopathy, lines of recurrent growth arrest in the proximal humeri, sparse soft tisssue, and diminished thymic tissue.

Special Imaging Procedures

1. Radionuclide scintigraphy. Lung perfusion scintigraphy with ^{99m}Tc has been advocated in the evaluation of bronchiectasis[8] since bronchiectatic lung will retain this radionuclide. While this method may add to the sensitivity, it does not increase the specificity since other infectious processes will do the same. The probability of bronchiectasis is remote in the presence of a normal chest film and a normal perfusion lung scan.

2. Computed tomography (CT). (See Chapter 26.) This is a noninvasive technique that may be used to evaluate bronchiectasis.[9] The method is most sensitive for the cystic type,[10] but is not as sensitive or specific as bronchography. Magnetic resonance imaging is helpful in the delineation of bronchial mucus plugging and other features of bronchiectasis in patients with cystic fibrosis.[11]

3. Positive-contrast bronchography. Positive-contrast bronchography remains the most reliable radiographic tool for the diagnosis of bronchiectasis. However, because the need for this procedure is infrequent, radiologic skill in the performance and interpretation of bronchography has suffered.

Bronchography is usually performed on patients who have a definite area of abnormality on plain films. The study should not be used to answer the oft-posed question, Does the child have bronchiectasis? If plain films and radionuclide scintigraphy are normal, bronchography is not likely to be positive.

The question of whether or not to perform bronchography usually arises with patients who demonstrate chronic or recurring parenchymal collapse after an adequate trial of therapy. Localized pulmonary damage may result from these conditions, and therefore the character and integrity of the bronchus leading to the diseased area must be evaluated. Questions about whether the bronchus is narrowed, collapsed, or extrinsically compressed should be answered before surgical resection.

The interpretation of bronchography must take into consideration the clinical history of the patient. Dilatation and irregular tapering of the bronchi are important bronchographic features of bronchiectasis (Figure 15-3). Videotape fluoroscopy helps evaluate areas of bronchomalacia that may otherwise escape detection. This finding can have important diagnostic and therapeutic implications.[12]

The total extent of disease within a collapsed lobe or segment is often not discernible. A collapsed segment is difficult to evaluate since lung that cannot exert the suction action necessary to pull contrast into the peripheral airways will often fail to

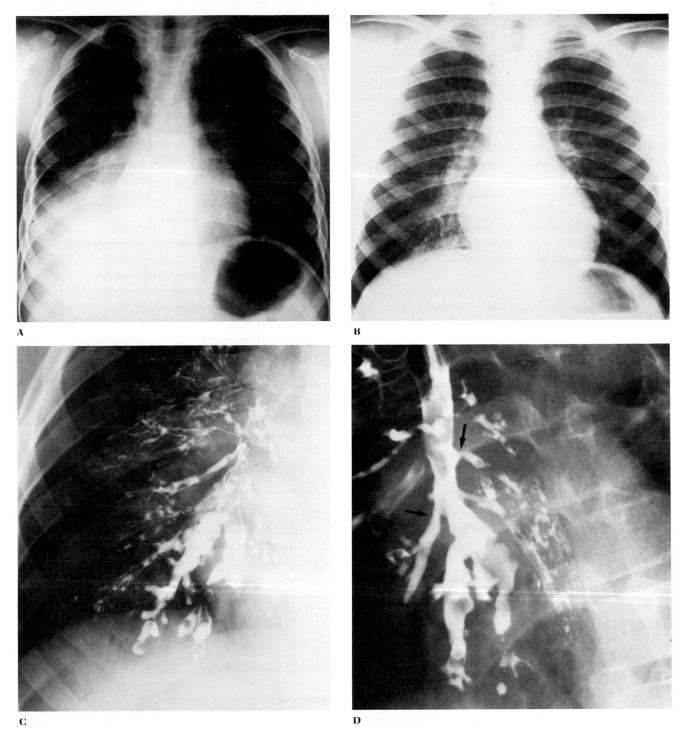

A

B

C

D

Figure 15-3 Bronchiectasis—postinfectious. A. The right lower lobe shows consolidation and volume loss during an episode of acute pneumonia. **B.** One year later, residual opacities in the same location suggest the presence of bronchiectasis. **C** and **D.** Bronchography shows a localized area of saccular bronchiectasis. Note the dilated, irregular, air-filled peripheral bronchi that do not accept contrast material. Note also the narrowed origins (arrows) of several abnormal bronchi. Numerous filling defects represent intraluminal mucoid plugs. (See Figure 15-1.)

opacify. Failure of bronchial opacification with contrast material also results from mucus plugging, but this finding cannot be used as the sole criterion for bronchiectasis.

Trapnell and Gregg[13] have called attention to the necessity of filling all peripheral bronchi. In children with bronchiectasis, the bronchographic changes are quite evident in the third- or fourth-generation bronchi, and a delayed film will often show retained contrast in diseased areas.

Fusiform and cylindrical bronchiectasis are both commonplace within collapsed lobes but frequently resolve with reexpansion. Occasionally, serial bronchograms are needed to evaluate therapeutic response.[14] Remarkable recovery with medical management is common; surgical solutions should be delayed as long as possible.

Acquired Bronchiectasis

Postinfectious Bronchiectasis

Antecedent infections, particularly measles, pertussis, and tuberculosis, have the capacity to damage bronchi and render them susceptible to secondary infection with bronchiectasis (Figure 15-3). Other bacterial pneumonias may do the same, although pinpointing exact etiologic agents is often quite difficult.[3,14,15] Bacterial infections of the lung have declined in incidence and severity, but viral infections, particularly adenovirus, may cause bronchiectasis, as well as its first cousin, obliterative bronchiolitis.[3,16,17] In some epidemics of obliterative bronchiolitis, type 21 virus has been isolated; several reports suggest that the problem of morbidity and mortality is worse in isolated populations as diverse as Eskimos and Polynesian islanders.[17] (See Chapter 19.)

The infectious origin of bronchiectasis may be difficult or impossible to pinpoint when the onset is insidious. Glauser and coworkers[15] documented an antecedent episode of pneumonia in 77 percent of cases; 12 percent were initiated by undocumented infections.

Asthma and sinusitis often accompany bronchiectasis, but causal relationships are difficult to substantiate.[3] In Glauser's patients,[15] 11 percent had both asthmatic bronchospasm and chronic bronchiectasis. Robinson and Campbell[7] studied 57 asthmatic children (10 months to 13 years of age) with bronchography and found "irregular bronchial dilatation" in 79 percent. They concluded that irreversible bronchiectasis is uncommon in asthmatics unless associated with lobar collapse.

Postbronchial Obstruction

Intraluminal obstruction may interfere with normal bronchial drainage and cause volume loss. Secondary dilatation of the obstructed bronchus further impairs removal of secretions. Superimposed infection compounds the problem and, if sufficiently protracted, destroys the bronchial mucosa or cartilage. Secondary fibrosis, stricture, and distortion may lead to irreversible bronchiectasis. Relief of obstruction before the occurrence of secondary scarring and bronchial wall damage will usually avoid permanent sequelae. Retained foreign bodies notoriously produce bronchiectasis through this mechanism, but in rare cases, the lung fills with fluid and other products of infection, with resulting bronchiectasis.

Postpulmonary Edema

The combination of heroin overdose, pulmonary edema, and bronchiectasis has been observed.[12,18,19] The exact pathophysiology of postedema bronchiectasis is unclear, and the association of other kinds of pulmonary edema with the development of bronchiectasis remains unknown.

Host Deficiencies

Immune Deficiency Syndromes

Diseases affecting the immunoglobulin defense mechanism, such as agammaglobulinemia, hypogamma-globulinemia, and Aldrich's syndrome, are uncommon but recognized causes for the endobronchial-bronchiectasis pattern.[15] Pulmonary involve-

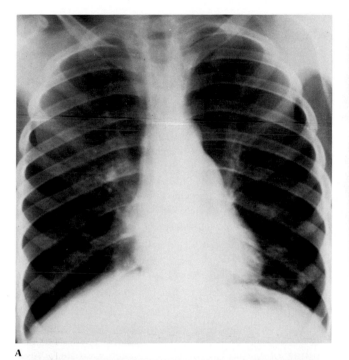

A

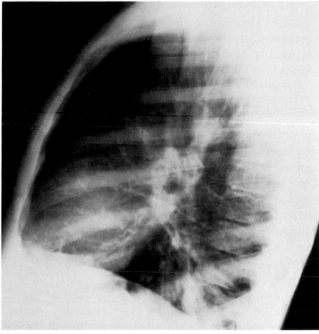

B

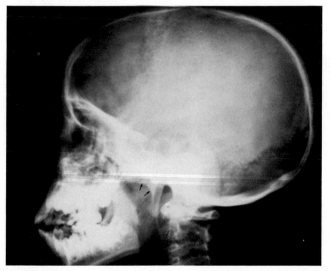

C

Figure 15-4 Congenital agammaglobulinemia. A. The frontal film shows diffuse overaeration and areas of thick-walled bronchi, especially in the basal segments. **B.** Thickened bronchial walls with luminal plugging are evident in the posterior costophrenic sulcus. Note the absence of hilar adenopathy in spite of chronic lung disease. **C.** The lateral skull and pharynx show no adenoidal tissue. The arrows indicate the interface of soft tissue and pharyngeal air, a region usually occupied by adenoids. The patient has not had an adenoidectomy. Note the opaque, unaerated mastoids; these structures, as well as the maxillary antra, are opaque on other films.

ment usually takes the form of bronchiectasis and may simulate cystic fibrosis, tuberculosis, or other forms of chronic lung disease (Figure 15-4). Unlike these, however, hilar adenopathy is usually absent. Patients with immunodeficiency syndromes are prone to lymphoma; thus the appearance of hilar or mediastinal adenopathy must be viewed with great suspicion. Aldrich's syndrome is one form of immune deficiency in which hilar adenopathy may occur in response to pulmonary suppuration.

Absent or depleted adenoidal lymphoid tissue (Figure 15-4C), on lateral films of the pharynx, and chronic sinus infection are additional radiographic features of patients with immune deficiency syndrome.

Immotile Cilia Syndrome

Immotile cilia syndrome (ICS) has been identified as a cause of chronic pulmonary disease.[20-22] It is characterized by genetically determined ciliary dysfunction; ciliated respiratory epithelium of the nasal mucosa, middle ear, and bronchi is immotile in these patients. Loss of the ability to clear secretions from the sinobronchial cavities leads to secondary infections including sinusitis, bronchiectasis, and otitis media. Sterility may result from decreased motility of spermatozoa tails.

In a study of 21 patients with ICS, Turner et al.[21] found that 100 percent of patients manifested symptoms of productive cough, sinusitis, and otitis. Of these, 48 percent had situs inversus, 29 percent

bronchiectasis, and 19 percent nasal polyps and digital clubbing. The relationship of this syndrome to Kartagener's syndrome (sinusitis, bronchiectasis, and situs inversus) is interesting in that many patients with ICS have situs inversus, but some do not. One report describes ICS in an 11-year-old girl whose older sibling had situs inversus.[23] Veerman and coworkers[24] examined four patients with Kartagener's syndrome and found no motile cilia. Two additional children of similar ages had chronic disease symptoms, immotile cilia, but normal situs. Immotile cilia are also reported in patients with polysplenia, with or without Kartagener's syndrome (Figure 15-5).[25,26] Kleinfelter's syndrome may also manifest chronic lung disease as a result of immotile cilia (Figure 15-6).

Radiographic findings in ICS depend upon the primary area of involvement. Sinusitis and otitis are regularly present. Pulmonary changes consist of bronchiectasis with accompanying areas of atelectasis, as well as focal and diffuse overaeration. As in other forms of chronic lung disease, middle lobe at-

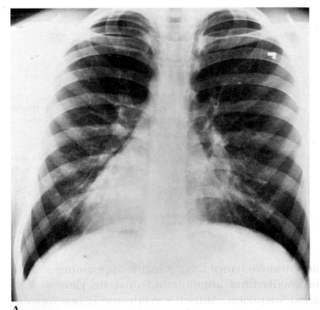
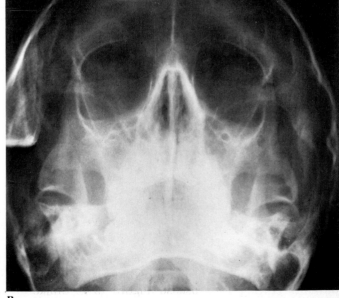

A   **B**

Figure 15-5   Kartagener's syndrome. A. Complete situs inversus is present, as well as basal peribronchial thickening suggestive of bronchiectasis. **B.** Maxillary and frontal sinuses are unaerated, a finding that suggests recurrent and/or chronic infection.

electasis is common. Radiographic features resemble cystic fibrosis but are usually less severe and not as progressive.[22]

Cystic Fibrosis

Cystic fibrosis is the term applied by Dorothy Anderson in 1938 to a disease state that she recognized as a clinical entity separate from celiac syndrome.[27] Many designations of this disease refer to the pancreatic involvement, although it was Farber in 1944[28] who first recognized cystic fibrosis as a systemic process involving many of the mucous-secreting glands.

In 1977, Shwachman[29] summarized the advances in our knowledge of the previous 25 years:

1. Cystic fibrosis may occur without evidence of pancreatic insufficiency.
2. The incidence is 1 per 1600 Caucasians and 1 per 17,000 blacks; it is less common in Asians.
3. Survival to adulthood and parenthood can be achieved, although 97 percent of males are sterile.
4. The diagnosis can be made in the neonatal period.
5. It is transmitted as a Mendelian recessive gene.
6. Respiratory system complications occur in nearly all cases.

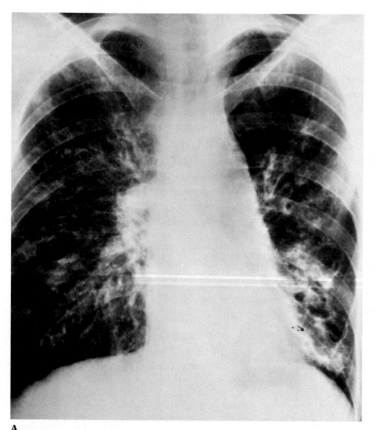

A

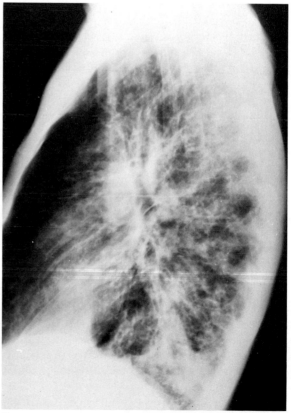

B

Figure 15-6 Bronchiectasis—Kleinfelter's syndrome. A 25-year-old man with gynecomastia, testicular atrophy, and XXY chromosomes. Iontophoresis and numerous sweat tests for cystic fibrosis were negative. **A** and **B.** Severe generalized bronchiectasis is evident. Partial atelectasis and mucoid bronchial plugging are present in the left lower lobe. (Courtesy of Dr. Joseph Smith, New Orleans, Louisiana.)

7. The cause of death is usually related to pulmonary involvement.

Clinical and radiographic manifestations of this disease are best appreciated by considering the effects of increased viscosity of secretions and small duct obstruction in numerous organ systems.

Respiratory Tract

The respiratory tract is invariably involved in cystic fibrosis. Except for neonatal deaths resulting from meconium ileus, pulmonary complications are responsible for most of the morbidity and virtually all the mortality associated with this disease.

The earliest histologic changes are hyperplasia and obstruction of the submucosal glands of the trachea and major bronchi. Obstruction of small bronchi and bronchioles causes scattered areas of collapse and overaeration.[29] Generalized air trapping is produced by several mechanisms which increase the resistance to airflow: (1) increased turbulence from irregular collections of mucus and exudates and (2) narrowed bronchial diameters caused by inflammation and/or fibrosis.[30] Destruction of alveolar septa does not occur except as a sequela of infection.

Advanced cases of cystic fibrosis demonstrate progressive changes of chronic pneumonia, bronchiectasis, and abscess formation. Bronchi suffer intermittent and chronic plugging with thick, tenacious mucoid secretions and inflammatory debris. Segmental and lobar collapse is a regular feature in association with bronchial stenosis and foci of interstitial fibrosis.

Superimposed infection complicates the entire picture. Staphylococci are the predominant invaders, but pseudomonas and coliform organisms are also plentiful.[31] The combination of staphylococcus and pseudomonas organisms makes the diagnosis of cystic fibrosis highly probable in a patient with chronic lung disease.

Pneumothorax, pleural effusions, and hemorrhage are potentially life-threatening complications that require immediate attention.[32] Fellows et al.[33] have reported the successful treatment of 12 of 13 cystic fibrosis patients with major bleeding by bron-

chial artery embolization. Emergency pulmonary resection has been advocated for life-threatening hemoptysis in cystic fibrosis.[34] Pulmonary involvement in cystic fibrosis may be quite localized, a feature that invites occasional surgical resection.[35,36]

Recurrent or refractory pneumothorax is occasionally difficult to control. In addition to conventional pneumothorax treatment, sclerosis of the pleura with 2 percent quinacrine has been successful.[37]

Gastrointestinal Tract

Meconium ileus occurs in 15 percent of neonates with cystic fibrosis; the exact cause of this complication is unclear. Obstruction results from impaction of viscid, sticky meconium at any site in the bowel, most frequently near the ileocecal valve. Associated anatomic anomalies, present in one-half of patients with meconium ileus, include ileal and jejunal stenosis and atresia, duplication, omphalocele, and mesenteric bands and defects.[38,39] Microcolon, Meckel's diverticulum, intestinal perforation, volvulus, and rectal prolapse are additional gastrointestinal abnormalities that accompany cystic fibrosis in early life. In older patients, right-sided colon obstruction (meconium ileus equivalent) is an occasional problem (Figure 15-7).[40,41] Benign pneumatosis intestinalis, pneumatosis coli, and intussusception are additional complications of cystic fibrosis.[30,42]

Some patients with cystic fibrosis show little or no evidence of pancreatic insufficiency. Others are more severely affected and manifest combinations of steatorrhea, growth failure, and nutritional deprivation. In general, as with other organs affected by this disease, the severity of involvement increases with age. In the liver, the increased viscosity of bile may lead to mucus plugging, distension, and proliferation of bile ducts. Secondary changes include liver cell atrophy, fatty metamorphosis, and periportal fibrosis. Early hepatic fatty infiltration may be recognized on abdominal film, but this finding is not specific for cystic fibrosis (Figure 15-8).[43,44] The fatty liver changes may also be imaged with ultrasonography and CT.

Total agreement on the exact pathogenesis of biliary cirrhosis in cystic fibrosis is lacking, but the incidence has been reported to be between 19 and 43 percent.[38,45] Periportal fibrosis may be extensive enough in some patients to distort the hepatic architecture and cause portal venous obstruction, esophageal varices, and hypersplenism. Jaundice, however, is not usually apparent, and the commonly used liver function tests are often normal.

Patients with cystic fibrosis are frequently the victims of gallbladder disease. L'Heureux et al.[46] found abnormal cholecystograms in 46.4 percent of 84 patients with cystic fibrosis who were examined consecutively. Of those whose gallbladders failed to visualize, 70.3 percent also had abnormal intravenous cholecystograms, and calculi were present in approximately 12 percent. Autopsy reports have shown abnormalities of the gallbladder in approximately one-third of patients who died of cystic fibrosis.[38]

The incidence of gallbladder disease increases with age.

Gastroesophageal reflux (GER) occurs more commonly in patients with cystic fibrosis than in the normal population (Figure 15-9).[47] The mechanical influence of a depressed diaphragm caused by hyperinflation, along with increased abdominal pressure from chronic coughing, may contribute to this complication.[48] The diagnosis of cystic fibrosis may be overlooked in patients with chronic lung disease that is incorrectly ascribed to GER.[49]

Other Organ Involvement

The male genital system is affected more severely than the female; most males are sterile. Sterility results from aspermia, hypoplastic and aplastic epididymal ducts, or complete absence of the sperm

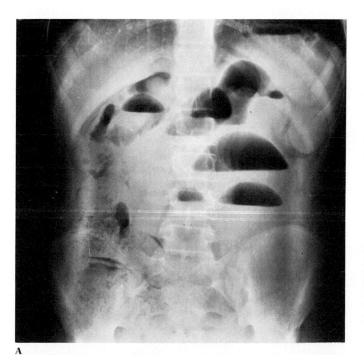
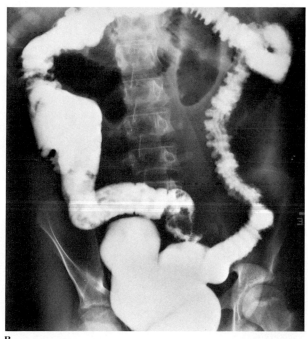

A   **B**

Figure 15-7   Meconium ileus equivalent. A 19-year-old boy with cystic fibrosis developed clinical signs of bowel obstruction. **A.** The supine abdominal film shows multiple loops of dilated, air-filled small bowel. The mottled density in the right lower quadrant represents inspissated fecal material and bowel content in the ascending colon. The transverse and descending colon is empty. **B.** A contrast enema outlines the collapsed, evacuated transverse and descending colon. The inspissated bowel content in the cecum and terminal ileum is outlined by the contrast material.

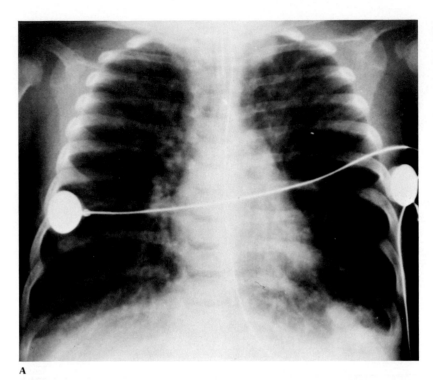

A

Figure 15-8 Cystic fibrosis—early fatty liver. A. The patient has overaerated lungs with diffuse peribronchial thickening. Note the absence of thymic tissue, sparse soft tissues, and proximal humeral growth arrest lines (poorly seen). **B.** This abdominal film taken at birth shows the relative lucency of the liver in comparison with the adjacent abdominal wall (arrows). **C.** The abdominal ultrasonography demonstrates the fatty, hyperechoic liver (L) compared with the normal kidney (K).

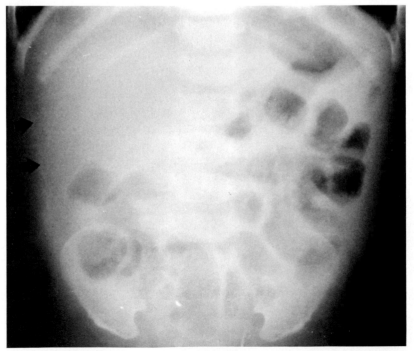

B

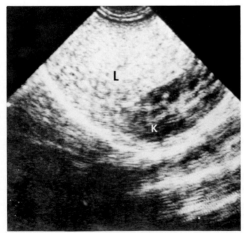

C

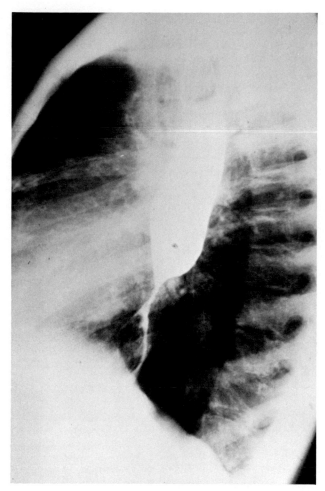

Figure 15-9 Cystic fibrosis—esophageal stricture. The esophageal stricture is probably secondary to long-standing GER. (Courtesy of Dr. Milton Wagner, Houston, Texas.)

transport system. Although sterility is a problem in females, some pregnancies have occurred.[50]

The kidneys are also affected by cystic fibrosis and may show calcifications and glomerular changes. Nasal polyps and salivary gland abnormalities are additional complications. Skin appendages secrete sweat with increased electrolyte concentrations leading to salt loss and systemic electrolyte depletion in hot weather. Episodes of arthritis have been reported in children with cystic fibrosis, and hypertrophic pulmonary osteoarthropathy occurs in approximately 5 percent of patients (Figure 15-10).[51,52]

Radiologic Findings

Chest roentgenograms are the most useful and frequently employed clinical tool in the diagnosis and treatment of cystic fibrosis. Comprehension of the pathologic changes that occur in the lung is important for a full understanding of the radiographic alterations.

Cystic fibrosis is a disease that affects the endobronchial structures of the lung. Thick, tenacious mucoid secretions collect in bronchi and are not cleared by normal ciliary action. As a result, persistent air trapping is an early manifestation of the disease. Atelectasis of segments or lobes may develop when bronchi are completely impacted. In the early stages of disease, reexpansion of atelectatic areas is often possible with aggressive therapy, but as the years pass, progressive, chronic, unyielding emphysema takes hold. Significant hilar adenopathy is a regular feature in older patients.

The overaerated lungs of infants and young children with cystic fibrosis may return to a relatively normal appearance between bouts of acute illness. This sometimes delays the diagnosis and may lead to confusion with recurrent bronchiolitis, asthmatic bronchitis, and aspiration pneumonia. Patients with cystic fibrosis who have significant GER are not uncommonly treated for recurrent aspiration pneumonia before the true cause is discovered. Eventually, the lungs lose their ability to contract and gradually take on an attitude of fixed overaeration (Figure 15-8). In older patients, the diaphragm may retain its curvature, even with advanced overaeration, but increased anteroposterior diameter and sternal protrusion are usually quite dramatic (Figures 15-10 and 15-11). As chronic endobronchial infection continues, the bronchial walls thicken and the lumina undergo irregular dilatation and become plugged with mucoid impactions. At this stage, the lungs take on the characteristic appearance of diffuse bronchiectasis (Figure 15-10). Recurrent and persistent areas of segmental and lobar atelectasis are often evident. Small cystlike lesions, representing extremely ectatic bronchi, and occasional larger bullae are additional findings in selected patients (Figure 15-10; see also Chapter 26, Figure 26-28; Chapter 27, Figure 27-14).

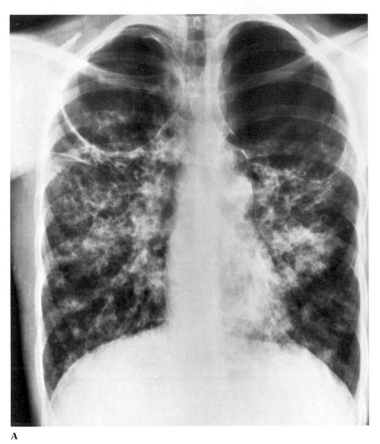

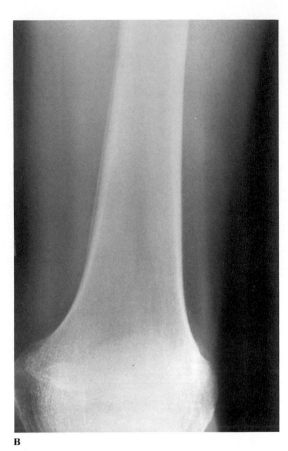

A

B

Figure 15-10   Cystic fibrosis—advanced. A. This representative film is characteristic of severe, diffuse, peribronchial disease. Note the numerous ringlike shadows that represent empty, thick-walled bronchi on end, and note the conglomerate opacities in the left lower lung representing mucoid-plugged bronchi. The large apical bullae are atypical of cystic fibrosis. **B.** The fine line of periosteal new bone along the medial shaft of the femur represents hypertrophic osteoarthropathy. This is not specific for cystic fibrosis and may occur in other chronic diseases.

Sequential films frequently show considerable variability as the bronchi are intermittently filled with or emptied of their mucous plugs. In spite of short-term variations in the appearance of chest films, inexorably the general pattern worsens. Hilar adenopathy develops in most patients, as abscess formation, fixed atelectasis, and focal emphysema all contribute to the deteriorating picture (Figure 15-11). For a better overall assessment of the patient's progress, it is mandatory that the film jacket be explored and old films be compared with recent studies.

Several scoring systems are available to quantitate and systematize the degree of pulmonary in-

volvement.[53–56] Meerman and coworkers[57] found the Crispin-Norman method of some advantage over the others.

Secondary changes of chronic and recurrent illness should be noted. Multiple lines of transverse growth arrest in the proximal humeral metaphyses, undermineralization of bone, and sparse soft tissue of the chest wall, best seen on the lateral film, are all signs of chronicity (Figures 15-8, 15-10, and 15-11). Like Cassius, these patients have a "lean and hungry look." The mediastinum may appear narrowed as a result of (1) depleted thymic tissue from chronic illness, (2) small cardiac shadow from poor nutrition,

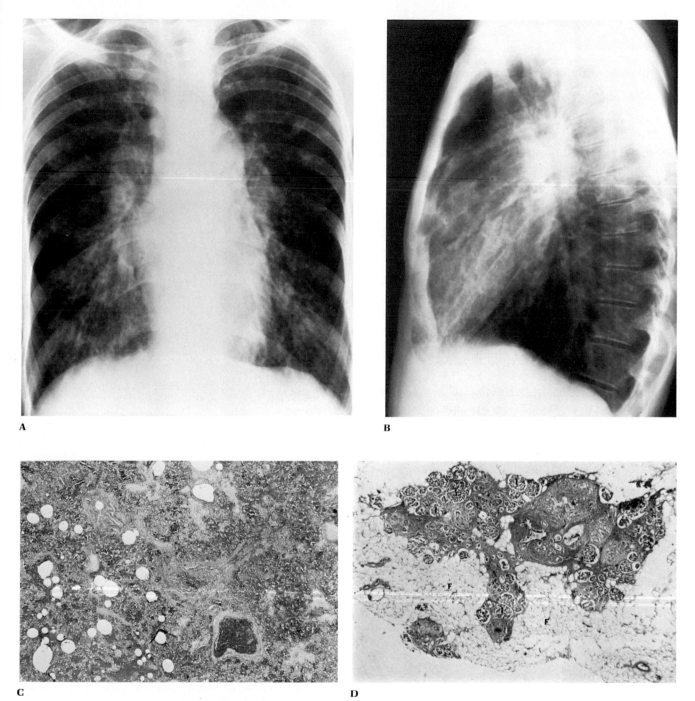

Figure 15-11 Cystic fibrosis—fatty infiltration of the pancreas. An 18-year-old-boy with cystic fibrosis was admitted to the hospital in cardiac and respiratory failure. His respiratory distress had been gradually increasing during the preceding 6 months, and he presented with cough, fever, weakness, cyanosis, and cor pulmonale. During the ensuing week his condition gradually improved, but he suffered an episode of massive hemoptysis and hematemesis, lapsed into coma, and died. **A** and **B.** The premortem chest films show severe changes of end-stage cystic fibrosis. The marked prominence of the central and main pulmonary arteries suggests the onset of pulmonary hypertension. **C.** The histologic sections of lung show the extent of hemorrhage with virtually all alveoli choked with erythrocytes. **D.** The pancreas has a striking reduction of acinar tissue. This island of fibrous tissue contains only scant ductular remnants; the majority of it consists of islets of Langerhans (I) and the surrounding adipose tissue (F).

and (3) elongation of the heart associated with over-aeration. Abnormal retrosternal lucency results from the overaeration and diminished thymic tissue.

Less common radiographic complications of cystic fibrosis include paranasal sinus opacification, esophageal varices, pancreatic calculi, cardiomegaly from cor pulmonale, and changes related to gastrointestinal abnormalities. Complications of pneumothorax are occasionally seen and may be quite refractory to treatment. Periosteal reaction (hypertrophic pulmonary osteoarthropathy) is an additional roentgen finding in rare cases (Figure 15-10B).

Nonpulmonary features that should be looked for on chest film include splenomegaly in patients with portal hypertension; dilated bowel and colon filled with excess, frothy-looking stool; and gallbladder calculi, if the upper part of the abdomen is included on the film. Pancreatic fibrosis is an additional feature (Figure 15-11).

The radiologist is often the first to recognize the possible existence of cystic fibrosis. This is especially true for patients who are seen repeatedly in emergency rooms and outpatient clinics. By reviewing previous film studies in sequence, a pattern of unremittent overaeration and increasing parenchymal involvement, never returning completely to normal, should suggest the diagnosis. Since there are no pathognomonic roentgenographic features of cystic fibrosis, verbal communication with the attending physician is better than placing the diagnosis of cystic fibrosis in the record based only on the radiographic interpretation.

References

1. *Dorland's Illustrated Medical Dictionary*, 26th ed. Philadelphia, WB Saunders, 1981, p 191.
2. Reid L: Reduction of bronchial subdivision in bronchiectasis. *Thorax* 5:233, 1950.
3. Nemir RL: Bronchiectasis, in Kendig EL Jr, Chernick V (eds): *Disorders of the Respiratory Tract in Children.* Philadelphia, WB Saunders, 1977, p 446.
4. Field CE: Bronchiectasis. Third report on a follow-up study of medical and surgical cases from childhood. *Arch Dis Child* 44:551, 1969.
5. Wayne KS, Taussig LM: Probable familial congenital bronchiectasis due to cartilage deficiency (Williams-Campbell syndrome). *Am Rev Resp Dis* 114:15, 1976.
6. Mounier-Kuhn P: Dilatation de la trachée. Constatations radiographiques et bronchoscopiques. *Lyon Med* 150:106, 1932.
7. Robinson AE, Campbell JB: Bronchography in childhood asthma. *AJR* 116:559, 1972.
8. Vandevivere J, Spehl M, Dab I, et al: Bronchiectasis in childhood. Comparison of chest roentgenograms, bronchograms and lung scintigraphy. *Pediatr Radiol* 9:193, 1980.
9. Müller NL, Bergin CJ, Ostrow DH: Role of computed tomography in recognition of bronchiectasis. *AJR* 143:971, 1984.
10. Naidich DP, McCauley DI, Khouri NF, et al: Computed tomography of bronchiectasis. *J Comput Assist Tomogr* 6:437, 1983.
11. Gooding CA, Lallemand DP, Brasca RC, et al: Magnetic resonance imaging in cystic fibrosis. *J Pediatr* 105:384, 1984.
12. Feist JH: Selective cinebronchography in obstructive and restrictive pulmonary disease. *AJR* 99:543, 1967.
13. Trapnell DH, Gregg I: Some principles of interpretations of bronchograms. *Br J Radiol* 42:125, 1969.
14. Avery ME, Riley MC, Weiss A: The course of bronchiectasis in childhood. *Bull Johns Hopkins Hosp* 109:20, 1961.
15. Glauser EM, Cook CD, Harris GBC: Bronchiectasis: A review of 187 cases in children with follow-up pulmonary function studies in 58. *Acta Paediatr Scand* 165:1 (Suppl), 1966.
16. Becroft DMO: Bronchiolitis obliterans. Bronchiectasis and other sequelae of adenovirus type 21 infection in young children. *J Clin Pathol* 24:72, 1971.
17. Gold R, Wilt JC, Adhihari PK, et al: Adenoviral pneumonia and its complications in infancy and childhood. *J Can Assoc Radiol* 20:218, 1969.
18. Banner AS, Muthuswamy P, Shah RS, et al: Bronchiectasis following heroin-induced pulmonary edema. *Chest* 69:552, 1976.
19. Shachter EW, Basta W: Bronchiectasis following heroin overdose: A report of 2 cases. *Chest* 63:363, 1973.
20. Eliasson R, Massberg B, Camner P, et al: The immotile-cilia syndrome. A congenital ciliary abnormality as an etiologic factor in chronic airway infections and male sterility. *N Engl J Med* 297:1, 1977.

21. Turner JAP, Corkey CWB, Lee JYC, et al: Clinical expressions of immotile cilia syndrome. *Pediatrics* 67:805, 1981.

22. Nadel HR, Stringer DA, Levison H, et al: The immotile cilia syndrome: Radiological manifestations. *Radiology* 154:651, 1985.

23. Sturgess JM, Chao J, Wong J, et al: Cilia defective radial spokes. A cause of human respiratory disease. *N Engl J Med* 300:53, 1979.

24. Veerman AJP, van Delden L, Feenstra L, et al: The immotile cilia syndrome: Phase contrast light microscopy, scanning and transmission electron microscopy. *Pediatrics* 65:698, 1980.

25. Teichberg S, Markowitz J, Silverberg M, et al: Abnormal cilia in a child with the polysplenia syndrome. *J Pediatr* 100:399, 1982.

26. Schnidlow DV, Katz SM, Turtz MG, et al: Polysplenia and Kartagener syndrome in a sibship: Association with abnormal respiratory cilia. *J Pediatr* 100:401, 1982.

27. Anderson DH: Cystic fibrosis of the pancreas and its relation to celiac disease. A clinical and pathological study. *Am J Dis Child* 56:344, 1938.

28. Farber S. Pancreatic function and disease in early life. V. Pathologic changes associated with pancreatic insufficiency in early life. *Arch Pathol* 37:238, 1944.

29. Shwachman H: Cystic fibrosis, in Kendig EL Jr, Chernick V (eds): *Disorders of the Respiratory Tract in Children.* Philadelphia, WB Saunders, 1977, p 760.

30. White H, Rowley WF: Cystic fibrosis of the pancreas: Clinical and roentgenographic manifestations. *Radiol Clin North Am* 3:539, 1963.

31. Esterly JR, Oppenheimer EH: Cystic fibrosis of the pancreas: Structural changes in the peripheral airways. *Thorax* 23:670, 1968.

32. Holsclaw DS, Grand RJ, Shwachman H: Massive hemoptysis in cystic fibrosis. *J Pediatr* 76:829, 1970.

33. Fellows KE, Khaw KT, Schuster S, et al: Bronchial artery embolization in cystic fibrosis: Technique and long-term results. *J Pediatr* 95:959, 1979.

34. Porter DK, Van Every MJ, Mack JW: Emergency lobectomy for massive hemoptysis in cystic fibrosis. *J Thorac Surg* 86:409, 1983.

35. Hodson CJ, Jackson ADM, Haworth EM, et al: Pulmonary resection in cystic fibrosis: Results in 23 cases 1950–1970. *Arch Dis Child* 47:499, 1972.

36. Marmon L, Schidlow D, Palmer J, et al: Pulmonary resection for complications in cystic fibrosis. *J Pediatr Surg* 18:811, 1983.

37. McLaughlin FJ, Matthews WJ, Strieder DJ, et al: Pneumothorax in cystic fibrosis: Management and outcome. *J Pediatr* 100:863, 1982.

38. Oppenheimer EH, Esterly JR: Pathology of cystic fibrosis: Review of the literature and comparison with 146 autopsied cases, in *Perspectives in Pediatric Pathology.* Chicago, Year Book Medical Publishers, 1975, vol 12, p 241.

39. Holsclaw DS, Eckstein HB, Mixon HH: Meconium ileus, a 20 year review of 109 cases. *Am J Dis Child* 109:101, 1965.

40. Jensen KG: Meconium-ileus equivalent in a 15 year old patient with mucoviscidosis. *Acta Paediatr* 51:344, 1962.

41. Berk RN, Lee FA: The late gastrointestinal manifestations of cystic fibrosis of the pancreas. *Radiology* 106:377, 1973.

42. Wood RE, Herman CJ, Johnson KW, et al: Pneumatosis coli in cystic fibrosis. Clinical, radiological and pathological features. *Am J Dis Child* 129:246, 1975.

43. Gibson B, Levin D, Currarino G, et al: Roentgenographically visible fatty liver in cystic fibrosis. *Pediatrics* 59:778, 1977.

44. Griscom NT, Capitanio MA, Wagnor NL, et al: Visible fatty liver. *Radiology* 117:385, 1975.

45. Landing B: Pathology of cystic fibrosis, "GAP" Conference Reports. Savannah, Ga, National Cystic Fibrosis Research Foundation, 1972.

46. L'Heureux PR, Isenberg JN, Sharp HL, et al: Gallbladder disease in cystic fibrosis. *AJR* 128:953, 1977.

47. Scott RB, O'Loughlin EV, Gall DG: Gastroesophageal reflux in patients with cystic fibrosis. *J Pediatr* 106:223, 1985.

48. Bendig DW, Seilheimer DK, Wagner ML, et al: Complications of gastrointestinal reflux in patients with cystic fibrosis. *J Pediatr* 100:536, 1982.

49. Thomas D, Rothberg RA, Lester LA: Cystic fibrosis and gastroesophageal reflux in infancy. *Am J Dis Child* 139:66, 1985.

50. Rosenow EC, Lee RA: Cystic fibrosis and pregnancy. *JAMA* 203:227, 1968.

51. Newman AJ, Ansell BM: Episodic arthritis in children with cystic fibrosis. *J Pediatr* 94:594, 1979.

52. Nathanson I, Riddlesberger MM: Pulmonary hypertrophic osteoarthropathy in cystic fibrosis. *Radiology* 135:649, 1980.

53. Brasfield D, Hicks G, Soong S, et al: The chest roentgenogram in cystic fibrosis. A new scoring system. *Pediatrics* 63:24, 1979.

54. Shwachman H, Kulczycki LL: Long term study of 105 patients with cystic fibrosis. *Am J. Dis Child* 96:6, 1958.

55. Reilly BJ, Featherby EA, Went TR, et al: The correlation of radiological changes with pulmonary function in cystic fibrosis. *Radiology* 98:281, 1971.

56. Crispin AR, Normal AP: The systematic evaluation of the chest radiograph in cystic fibrosis. *Pediatr Radiol* 2:101, 1974.

57. Meerman GJ, Dankert-Roelse J, Martijh A, et al: A comparison of the Shwachman, Crispin-Norman and Brasfield methods for scoring the chest radiographs of patients with cystic fibrosis. *Pediatr Radiol* 15:98, 1985.

Chapter 16

Pulmonary Edema Pattern (Interstitial, Alveolar-Air Space, Pleural)

Pulmonary edema occurs when an excess of fluid accumulates in the lung. For the lungs to remain "dry," the lymphatics must remove the fluid that normally extravasates into the interstitial spaces. Various disease processes may occur in which the lungs retain fluid and thus develop pulmonary edema. These diseases are grouped into three major categories:

1. Increased capillary permeability
2. Cardiogenic (elevated pulmonary venous pressure, congestive failure)
3. Renal overhydration

Blockage of lymphatic drainage is another mechanism that usually results from separate causes.

The excess lung fluid that constitutes pulmonary edema characteristically occupies one or more of three anatomic locations: (1) the interstitial tissue, (2) the alveoli, and (3) the pleural space.

The radiologic appearance of pulmonary edema depends upon several factors:

1. The etiologic disease (cardiogenic, increased capillary permeability, overhydration)
2. The major anatomic compartment in which the fluid has accumulated (interstitial, alveolar, pleural)
3. The age of the patient
4. The preexisting pathologic state of the lung
5. The position in which the patient has been placed
6. The rapidity of accumulation
7. Others

By the very nature of the pathophysiologic process, pulmonary edema tends to be transient and evanescent. Considerable overlap is to be expected in the clinicoradiologic presentation of pulmonary edema. Also, it is important to recognize at the outset that substances other than edema fluid, i.e., blood, purulence, and tumor, may and often do produce radiographic patterns that are indistinguishable from pulmonary edema. However, for the purpose of this chapter, the pulmonary edema pattern will be illustrated with diseases whose major radiographic manifestation is the accumulation of excess fluid in the lungs. Later chapters will review infections and other pulmonary conditions that produce a similar radiographic pattern.

Three major radiographic patterns result from pulmonary edema. The *interstitial* pattern is the first to appear and represents excess amounts of fluid within the interstitial septa. When the capacity of the interstitial space is exceeded, fluid overflows into the alveoli or air spaces, thus creating the *alveolar,* or *air space,* pattern. When fluid escapes from the confines of the parenchyma and leaks into the pleural space, the pattern of *pleural effusion* is created.

Milne and coworkers[1] have described specific roentgenographic criteria aimed at distinguishing cardiogenic from noncardiogenic pulmonary edema. Many of their recommendations pertain to children, but the age of the patient and the peculiarities of childhood illnesses must be considered when they are applied.

In the neonate, thickened fissures, subpleural density, indistinct vascularity, and generalized increased radiopacity are the most reliable roentgenographic signs of pulmonary edema (Figure 16-1). Less common changes include posterior gravitational fluid shifts in supine position,[2] soft tissue thickening with loss of normal skin creases and fat planes, and subtle alterations in cardiac size. (See Chapter 4.) These changes are often difficult to assess because of associated lung disease, which itself may be obscured by superimposed edema. Comparison with previous films is often necessary to fully appreciate the subtle fluid accumulation and the relationship of edema to the basic lung pathology.

Significant pulmonary edema in neonates and

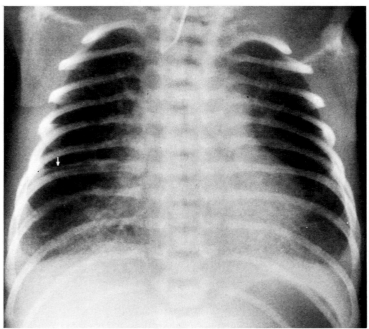
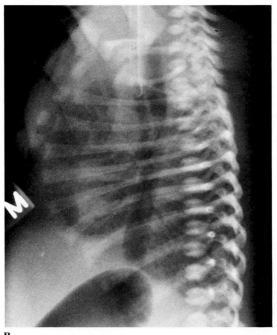

A   B

Figure 16-1   Neonatal pulmonary edema—retained fetal lung fluid.   A. Interstitial fluid has effaced the vascular shadows in the lower lung fields and blurred the heart margins, phrenic silhouettes, and costophrenic sulci. The horizontal fissure is thickened (arrow). **B.** The lateral exposure also shows vasculature effacement by intrapulmonary fluid, most of which has gravitated posteriorly. (See Chapter 4, Figure 4-7.)

young infants is commonly associated with congenital heart lesions such as obstructed anomalous pulmonary venous return, coarctation of the aorta, hypoplastic left heart syndrome, aberrant coronary arteries, and cor triatriatum. Additional cardiac lesions that may give rise to left-sided failure or pulmonary venous hypertension in later life include acute myocarditis, endocardial fibroelastosis, glycogen storage disease, pulmonary veno-occlusive disease, chronic pericarditis, atrial or ventricular myxomas, mitral or aortic stenosis, and chronic airway obstruction.

Older children and adolescents develop many of the same radiographic features of pulmonary edema as adults. The patterns that develop are influenced by several factors. Among these are the amount of fluid, the rapidity of accumulation, the status of the lungs,[3] and the primary cause of the pulmonary edema.[1] Although pulmonary edema is usually a complex and evanescent process, for simplicity, the radiographic findings are separated into those changes that result primarily from the collection of interstitial fluid and those that are produced when the fluid spills over into the alveoli and ultimately into the pleural space. To some extent, this distinction is an artificial one since these processes merge imperceptibly, one to another, and because the lungs are not affected in a uniform manner.

Interstitial Fluid Pattern

Although the recognition of interstitial lung disease is frequently hazardous on plain chest films,[4] excess interstitial fluid can usually be identified by the following criteria:

Loss of Vascular Silhouettes

With proper technique, the appearance of blood vessels can be a valuable clue to the early presence of interstitial fluid (Figure 16-2). Pulmonary vessels should have well-defined, sharp margins against adjacent lung.[5] Since the vessels lie in the same interstitial septa and tissue planes as the lymphatics and bronchi, they often lose their definition if excess fluid or inflammatory reaction occurs in the surrounding tissue.

Obscure, ill-defined hilar vessels are additional findings of early perivascular edema. Sometimes referred to as *hilar haze*, this change may be difficult to separate from adenopathy or enlarged pulmonary arteries. Lateral films are often helpful in the evaluation of hilar edema and other roentgenographic features of excess fluid[6] (Figure 16-2B and D) although there is a lack of agreement on this point.[7]

Swollen Interlobular Septa (Septal Lines)

Septal (Kerley) lines represent swollen interlobular septa that visualize on chest films when sufficiently engorged with fluid (Figure 16-3). Kerley lines are further classified as A, B, and C, depending upon their location and appearance. Kerley B lines, the most common, are fine, straight, horizontal shadows, several millimeters to 2 cm in length. They are most numerous in the lateral, basal segments of the lung. Kerley A lines are longer (2 to 6 cm) and radiate from the hila into the upper lobes. Kerley C lines, best seen in the lateral projection, are shorter and tend to form a reticulum in the central and basal portions of the lung. When correctly identified, Kerley lines are virtually pathognomonic of pulmonary edema in childhood but not necessarily in adults.

Kerley lines are more often seen in cardiogenic and renal-overhydration edema than in edema caused by increased capillary permeability.[1] They are less reliable indicators of pulmonary edema in neonates and small children.

Thickened Subpleural Lymphatics and Fissures

Thickened subpleural lymphatics and fissures are reliable signs of excess pulmonary fluid. Often changing from hour to hour, these swollen lymphatics are best seen between the underlying lung and the inner chest wall.

Peribronchial Cuffing

Peribronchial cuffing (Figure 16-3B) results from edema in the walls of bronchi and peribronchial tis-

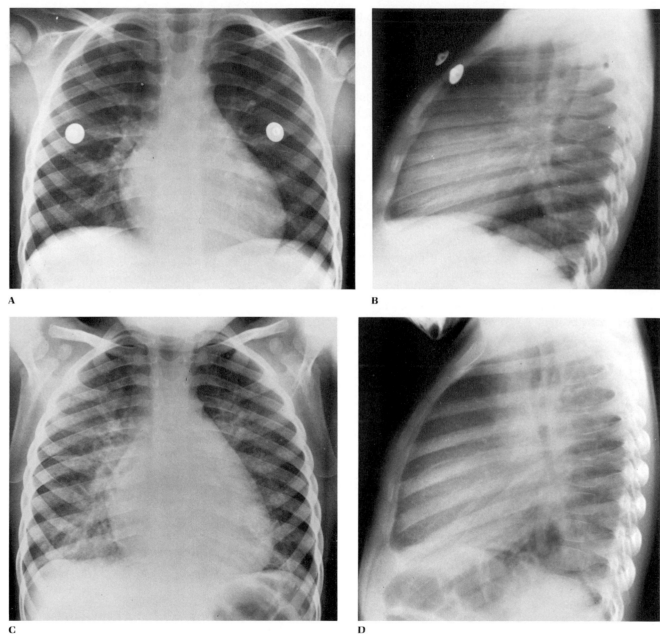

A

B

C

D

Figure 16-2   Pulmonary edema—acute rheumatic cardiopathy. A. The early study shows mild cardiomegaly, straightening of the left heart border, and indistinct lower lobe vessels. **B.** The hilar detail is altered by edema; vessels to the lower lobes are ill-defined; interlobar fissures are barely visible as thin white diagonal lines. **C.** Seven days later all but the most peripheral pulmonary vessels are obscured by perivascular edema. The left heart border is slightly convex. **D.** The lateral film, taken at the same time as part C, shows florid pulmonary edema; the hilar vessels are totally obliterated, fissures are thickened, and early alveolar coalescence has developed in the posterior costophrenic sulcus. *Note:* In this patient, the lateral film shows the edema to better advantage than does the frontal film.

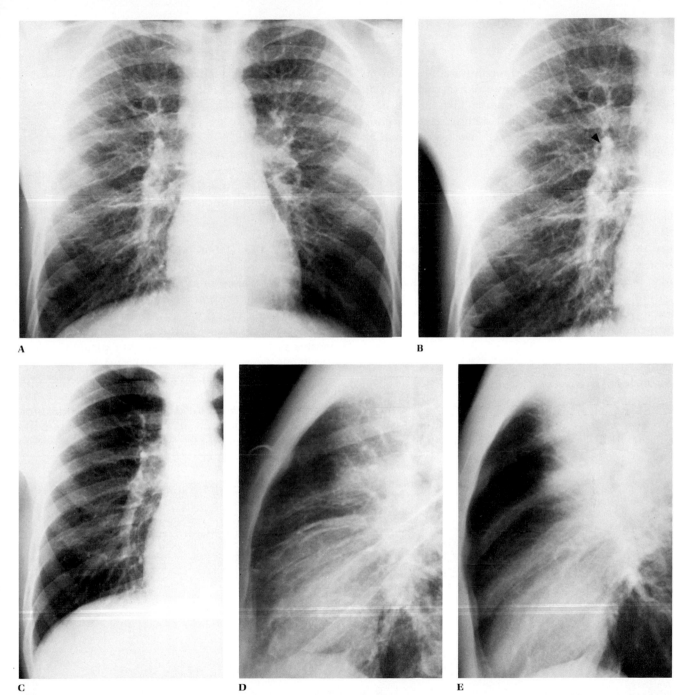

Figure 16-3 Interstitial pulmonary edema. This 14-year-old boy developed minimal symptoms of cough and low-grade fever. All clinical and laboratory tests were negative except for the presence of spermatozoa in the urine; eyesight was normal. **A.** Multiple, fine white lines represent swollen interlobular lymphatics (Kerley lines). **B.** In this close-up of the right side, the vascular detail is obscured. *Note:* The enlarged, ill-defined vessel adjacent to a bronchus with edematous walls and peribronchial cuffing (arrowhead) is present. **C.** The follow-up study, 24 h later, shows that many vessels have regained their definition and Kerley lines have resorbed. **D.** Initial lateral film with Kerley lines shows extensive interstitial edema. **E.** The follow-up lateral study shows resorption of the interstitial lymphatic fluid, but the hila remain edematous. The exact cause of this patient's pulmonary edema was never determined; feel free to draw your own conclusions.

sue. This sign frequently accompanies endobronchial inflammatory disease in children and is not always a reliable indicator of edema. Like the presence of septal lines, peribronchial cuffing is more common in cardiogenic and renal overhydration than capillary permeability edema.[1]

Comparison of Old Films

Comparison of old and new film studies is, by far, the most important of all radiologic procedures (Figure 16-2). Because of the evanescent character of pulmonary edema, previous examinations are of particular importance in the diagnosis, especially in patients with dyspnea of unknown cause. Previous films will often separate pulmonary edema from chronic interstitial lung disease.[8]

Alveolar-Air Space Pattern

Alveolar pattern was a term first popularized by Felson[4] to describe a specific radiographic appearance of the lung (Figure 16-4). He listed the following seven criteria that characterize this pattern:

1. Fluffy margins
2. Coalescence
3. Segmental and/or lobar distribution
4. Butterfly shadow
5. Air bronchograms or alveolograms
6. Peribronchial nodules
7. Rapid timing

Before the elaboration of this concept, acinar shadows were thought to represent the roentgenographic equivalent of intraalveolar lung disease.[9] Radiographically, the acinus casts a shadow with irregular borders of 0.5 to 1 cm in diameter. Rapid coalescence of these shadows into larger conglomerates is the rule, however, so that discrete acinar opacities are usually quite transient.[10]

While the alveolar opacities usually denote processes that involve the air space,[11] this pattern may be produced by histologically proven interstitial lung disease.[12] In a reappraisal of the entire concept of the relation of radiographic patterns to pulmonary his-

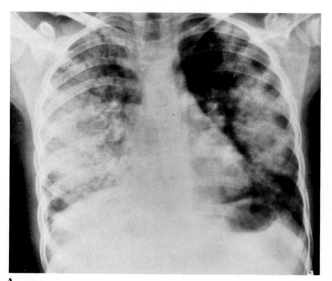
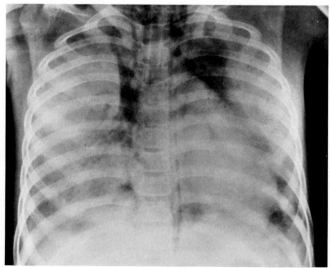

A   **B**

Figure 16-4   Alveolar-air space pattern–pulmonary hemorrhage. A. Diffuse radiopacities throughout both lungs illustrate several radiographic features of the alveolar-air space pattern: (1) fluffy, irregular margins, (2) coalescence, and (3) air bronchograms and air alveolograms. Minimal pleural reaction appears on the right. **B.** This film taken 24 h later, shows (4) lobar consolidation and (5) rapid timing. *Note:* There is extravasated air in the mediastinum and lower neck. The patient had chronic renal disease; severe pulmonary hemorrhage was found at autopsy.

topathology, Felson[13] recognized the difficulty of applying histologic terms to radiographs, but continued in his belief that the alveolar pattern is useful and can generally be relied upon to indicate the presence of air space pathology.

Differentiation between radiopacities that represent edema or infection is often impossible although some clues are helpful. Shifting of the opacities in response to positional change suggests edema rather than inflammation.[2] Sequential film studies are of inestimable value since edema tends to vary in its appearance from day to day or hour to hour, whereas inflammatory exudates remain localized or change slowly. Additional discussion of pulmonary infections may be found in subsequent chapters.

Several terms and concepts are commonly used in the discussion of pulmonary edema:

1. *Pulmonary venous hypertension.* This term is often used to denote increased pulmonary venous and capillary pressure. *Pulmonary conges-*

tion, passive congestion, and *pulmonary venous obstruction* (PVO) are synonymous terms. One early radiographic feature of pulmonary venous hypertension is redistribution or cephalization of blood flow (Figure 16-5A). Redistribution results from increased fluid in the lung, constriction of vessels to the lower lobes, and preferential flow to the upper lobes. Presumably, this phase precedes the development of overt pulmonary edema (Figure 16-5B). Redistribution of pulmonary blood flow in children almost always results from left heart failure. This sign is of limited value in small children who are often studied in the supine position.

2. *Pulmonary engorgement.* This term is used to describe excessive blood entering the lungs, usually in association with a left-to-right intracardiac shunt. States of increased blood volume, such as chronic anemia, polycythemia, and renal disease overhydration, also show engorged pulmonary vasculature. The radiographic appearance of vas-

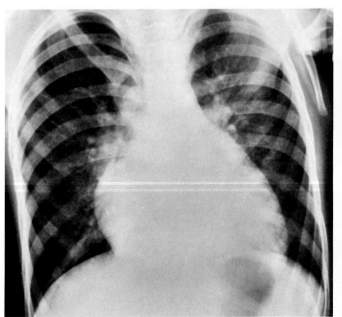 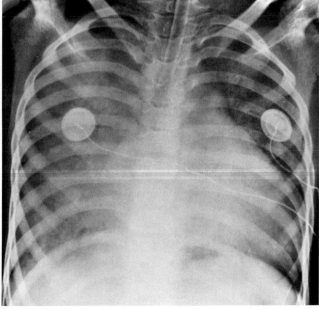

A   B

Figure 16-5   Pulmonary venous hypertension—vascular redistribution. A. Cardiomegaly is present. The lungs are clear, but hilar markings are ill-defined and the upper lobe vessels are as large as or larger than those in the lower lobes. This represents prepulmonary edema or pulmonary venous hypertension. **B.** Twenty-four hours later there is diffuse alveolar edema, more on the right. The child died of an acute myocardiopathy. *Note:* Films must be obtained in erect position to evaluate this sign.

cular engorgement differs from congestion or PVO. Pulmonary engorgement enlarges all vessels; with congestion or PVO, the upper lobe vessels are disproportionately enlarged. There are, unfortunately, no clear-cut divisions between these conditions; they frequently exist simultaneously. In this situation it may be difficult or impossible to differentiate between the two. Previous films are often of value, but in many cases the patient must be treated for congestive failure and reevaluated with follow-up radiographs.

To better illustrate the interstitial and/or alveolar-air space pattern, several diseases that characteristically manifest pulmonary edema will be reviewed.

Hydrocarbon Pneumonia

Hydrocarbon toxicity results from ingestion of petroleum products, including dry cleaning fluids, lighter fluids, gasoline, furniture polishes, kerosene, and similar products.[14] Although kerosene poisoning has decreased over the past 20 years, the ready availability of furniture polishes, cleaning fluids, and floor waxes within the home accounts for the persistence of hydrocarbon poisoning.[15] Poisoning from kerosene might increase as families turn to this fuel for home heaters in an effort to conserve electricity.

Lung injury is the most frequent and serious complication of hydrocarbon ingestion, but other organ systems may be involved. Weakness, confusion, coma, myocardiopathy, renal toxicity, and gastrointestinal symptoms are potential sequelae.

The mechanism whereby hydrocarbon injures the lungs is not completely understood. Considerable evidence supports the concept that pneumonia is caused by direct aspiration of hydrocarbon into the tracheobronchial tree; the theory of gastrointestinal absorption and excretion through the lungs has generally been abandoned.[16-19] Reports of individuals receiving petroleum distillate intravenously and developing generalized pneumonitis support the concept that when large quantities of hydrocarbon are ingested, enough may be absorbed from the gas-

trointestinal tract to produce pulmonary changes. However, oral intake of sufficient hydrocarbon to cause pneumonia solely from gastrointestinal absorption is unlikely in the usual clinical setting.[20,21]

Low surface tension and high volatility of hydrocarbons allow for the spread of irritants along the tracheobronchial tree into the alveolar spaces. This insult leads to necrosis of bronchiolar walls and alveolar tissue and edema of the interstitial and alveolar spaces, as well as vascular thrombosis and necrotizing bronchopneumonia. Alterations of surfactant predispose to alveolar instability, small airway closure, and atelectasis.[22] While these changes occur very rapidly and usually clear by 10 days, chronic proliferative disease may follow and take weeks to resolve.[23]

Secondary infection with bacterial agents is not a problem in most cases.[14] Antibiotics are not helpful, and corticosteroids may cause harm by promoting bacterial colonization in the lungs.[24] The clinical recognition of secondary infection is difficult because pyrexia and leukocytosis commonly accompany hydrocarbon aspiration and pulmonary defense mechanisms are impaired.

The clinical management of patients with hydrocarbon poisoning has for many years been plagued with the volatile controversy of whether gastric lavage is indicated, and whether this procedure causes more harm by enhancing pulmonary aspiration. No definitive data exist regarding the harm or efficacy of gastric lavage.

Radiologic Findings

Pulmonary complications may be expected from volatile hydrocarbon ingestion in 25 to 40 percent of patients.[14,25,26] Three-quarters of those with hydrocarbon ingestion will develop radiographic changes, but occasional patients with clinical findings have normal films.[27,28] The most severe pneumonias observed by Harris and Brown[26] were in patients who ingested furniture polish, while the least severe were seen with kerosene and turpentine. At least one lower lobe was involved in all patients except three.

Hydrocarbon pneumonia usually produces bilateral opacities in the mid and basal lung segments,

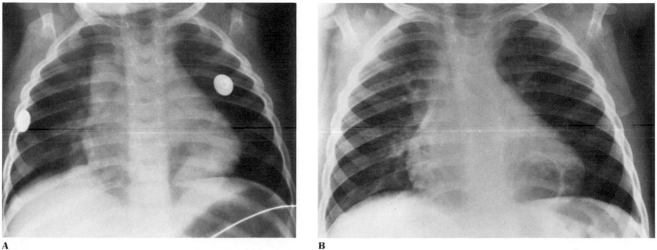

Figure 16-6 Hydrocarbon pneumonia. A. Bilateral, scattered, patchy opacities have developed in basal segments after ingestion and aspiration of kerosene. Confluent segmental infiltrate is present in the left lower lobe. **B.** Three weeks later pneumatoceles are present; the left lower lobe pneumatocele corresponds to the original consolidation. These eventually cleared.

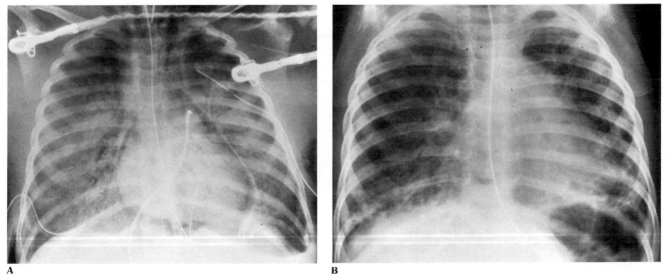

Figure 16-7 Hydrocarbon pneumonia—chronic lung disease. A. Diffuse pulmonary edema has developed following hydrocarbon ingestion. Air extravasation into the mediastinum, pericardium, and thorax is the result of positive ventilation therapy. **B.** Chronic changes of bronchiectasis remain several months after the original insult. (Courtesy of Dr. James Scatliff, Chapel Hill, North Carolina.)

often within the first hour or two of ingestion (Figure 16-6A). Pneumatocele formation is an occasional complication that follows lighter fluid and kerosene ingestion (Figure 16-6B).[26,29–31] Pneumothorax and mediastinal emphysema may further embellish pneumonias of furniture polish or other hydrocarbons. Infiltrates generally clear within 2 weeks; however, they may remain for several months. Pulmonary function abnormalities and abnormal lung patterns may persist (Figure 16-7).

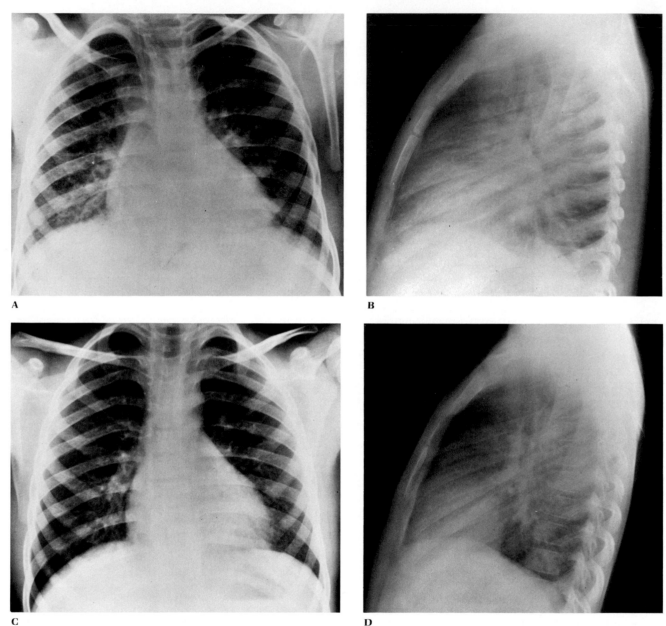

Figure 16-8   Acute glomerulonephritis. A. The initial film shows minimal cardiomegaly, blurred vessels, and chest wall edema. **B.** The lateral exposure, taken at same time as part A, shows obscured hilar vessels, thickened interlobar fissures, and soft tissue edema of the anterior and posterior chest. **C** and **D.** Films taken 5 days later have returned to near normal; the lateral film shows better hilar detail but residual edema (compare with part B).

Acute Glomerulonephritis

Acute glomerulonephritis (AGN), primarily a disease of childhood, is characterized by systemic hypertension, periorbital edema, elevated blood urea nitrogen, and urinary findings of blood, protein, and cellular casts. In many cases, a characteristic radiographic pattern of diffuse edema occurs early in the course of illness. Pulmonary edema of AGN probably results from increased capillary permeability, arterial hypertension, retention of sodium and water, some unknown factors, or any combination thereof.[32]

Holzel and Fawcitt[33] were among the first to recognize lung changes in AGN. More recently, Kirkpatrick and Fleisher[34] reported radiographic abnormalities on chest films (Figures 16-8 and 16-9) in 65 of 75 patients. They ranged in age from 16 months to 13 years; only two children were under 2 years of age. Their findings are summarized as follows:

1. *Cardiomegaly (62 percent).* The base of the heart was widened, a finding not always appreciated until follow-up films were obtained. In some patients the cardiac silhouette appeared normal, only to become distinctly smaller after the disease cleared.

2. *Pulmonary vascular changes (75 percent).* Changes included enlarged hilar vessels, loss of the normally sharp definition of intrapulmonary vessels, and an increase in the number of peripheral vessels that could not be traced to the hila (Figures 16-8 and 16-9).

3. *Pleural fluid (50 percent).* Pleural fluid tended to accumulate in the dependent portions of the pleural cavities and costophrenic sulci but often extended laterally along the lung margins. The appearance of two interlobar fissures was taken as evidence of fluid within.

4. *Pulmonary edema (33 percent).* Approximately one-third of patients manifested changes of diffuse (26 percent) or localized (7 percent) pulmo-

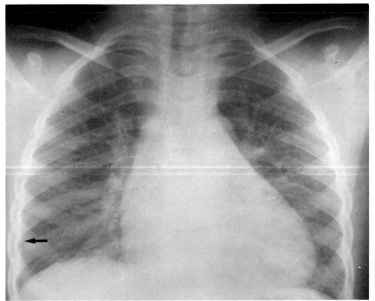
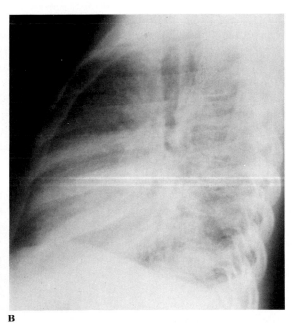

A   **B**

Figure 16-9   Acute glomerulonephritis. A. The heart is mildly enlarged, intrapulmonary vascularity is ill-defined, and there is minimal subpleural edema (arrow). Soft tissue edema has obliterated the normal fat-muscle plane along the lateral chest wall. **B.** The normal hilar anatomy is obscured by edema. Compare with patients in Figures 16-2 to 16-5, showing pulmonary edema and normal soft tissues.

nary edema. In some cases this assumed the appearance of inflammatory consolidation.

5. *Pulmonary consolidation (25 percent).* Pulmonary consolidation was felt to be inflammatory when it remained beyond the time of clearance of pleural fluid and return of normal pulmonary vascular shadows.

6. *Edema of the subcutaneous tissue (66 percent).* Subcutaneous edema manifested as a loss of sharp demarcation between the skin and subcutaneous soft tissues over the sternum, back, and sides of the chest (Figures 16-8 and 16-9).

The chest roentgenograms were normal in 14 percent of patients, all with mild clinical disease. No correlation between the presence of pulmonary edema, and the presence of hypertension or blood urea nitrogen levels was found.

Frequently, the diagnosis may be suggested from the chest radiograph. This is particularly important early in the disease, when neurologic symptoms often dominate the clinical picture and when neurogenic pulmonary edema is a consideration. In contrast to AGN, patients with neurogenic pulmonary edema rarely, if ever, develop pleural effusions; cardiac size usually remains normal, and soft tissue edema does not occur.[35] The nephrotic syndrome, an occasional differential consideration, usually produces more pleural effusion and soft tissue edema than does AGN. Unless there is pericardial effusion, the heart shadow is usually small in the nephrotic syndrome because of a contracted intravascular space, and the lungs remain clear. Patients with combined nephrotic-nephritic disease, those with chronic renal disease, and those on renal dialysis often have roentgenographic features that overlap; separation by history or response to treatment is usually necessary.

Congestive heart failure associated with acute rheumatic myocarditis may simulate the roentgen changes of AGN. In acute rheumatic fever, the heart size is usually greater than in AGN and the soft tissues are not swollen. Sequential films should be obtained to record a return of cardiac size to normal. Acute glomerulonephritis and pulmonary hemorrhage may coexist and produce extensive alveolar opacity.

Neurogenic Pulmonary Edema

Pulmonary edema occurs in association with a variety of central nervous system abnormalities including convulsions, trauma, hemorrhage, and neoplasms.[35–38] The lung changes similar to those that occur in humans have been produced experimentally in laboratory animals by artificial elevation of intracranial pressure, head trauma, and other central nervous system insults.[39–41] Sudden increases in intracranial pressure are most likely to produce secondary pulmonary edema, but insidious changes may have similar effects.

The pathophysiology of neurogenic pulmonary edema is incompletely understood but seems to be associated with massive sympathetic discharge resulting from hypothalamic dysfunction. Elevation of systemic pressures and lowered cardiac output tend to shift blood from the systemic to the pulmonary circulation. Extravasation of fluid results as the hydrostatic pressure across the pulmonary capillaries exceeds the intravascular oncotic pressure. The edema is often transient and may disappear within hours after the relief of the central nervous system abnormality. Patients with neurogenic pulmonary edema resulting from increased capillary permeability have also been reported.[42,43]

The radiographic appearance of neurogenic pulmonary edema is nonspecific but occasionally will demonstrate peculiar patterns. Both unilateral involvement and lobar distribution have been reported (Figure 16-10).[38,44] The upper lobes are most commonly affected; pleural effusion is rare or nonexistent.

Initial chest studies on patients with central nervous system insults may be normal, only to develop edema after administration of intravenous fluids (Figure 16-11). Fluid overload in patients with a compromised central nervous system occurs more readily than in normal subjects.

Aspiration pneumonia, congestive heart failure, acute glomerulonephritis, and other causes for pulmonary edema must be excluded. Aspiration pneumonia is frequently confused with pulmonary edema but is more likely to appear streaky and shaggy, with irregular overaeration. The condition is

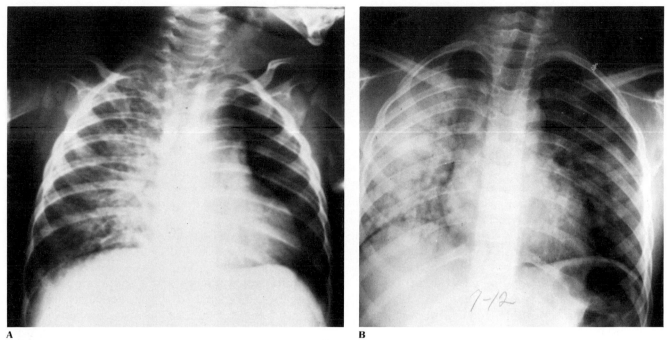

A   B

Figure 16-10   Neurogenic pulmonary edema—central nervous system leukemia.   A. Right-sided pulmonary edema involves the interstitial and air space compartments. **B.** Unilateral or lobar distribution of neurogenic pulmonary edema is not uncommon. (From Felman.[35])

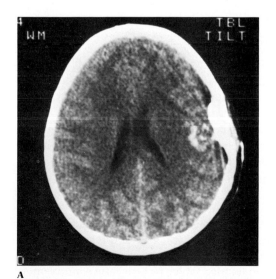
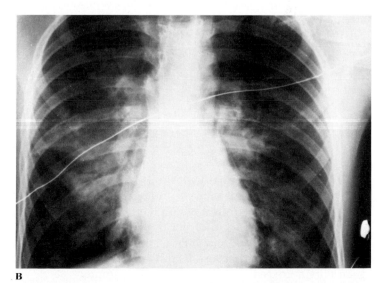

A   B

Figure 16-11   Neurogenic pulmonary edema—head trauma. This 13-year-old boy sustained head trauma from a fall. **A.** Computed tomography of the head shows a depressed left parietal fracture with underlying brain contusion and hemorrhage. The initial chest film was normal. **B.** Pulmonary edema developed in the ensuing 24 h. A small pneumomediastinum is present. The child died within several days.

generally stable, changing slowly over a period of days. Acute glomerulonephritis causes pleural edema or small amounts of free pleural fluid, a finding that almost never occurs in neurogenic pulmonary edema. Mild to moderate cardiomegaly and soft tissue edema of AGN are additional differentiating features. The symptoms of convulsions, somnolence, and hypertension seen with acute glomerulonephritis are often present in neurologic abnormalities as well, so care must be taken to differentiate between the two.

The pulmonary edema of congestive cardiac failure is usually associated with cardiomegaly or an abnormally contoured cardiopericardial silhouette. This must be differentiated from neurogenic pulmonary edema since conventional drugs used to treat congestive failure are contraindicated in patients with neurogenic pulmonary edema.

The treatment of patients with neurogenic pulmonary edema should be directed toward prevention and control of seizures and relief of intracranial pressure when present. Atropine as well as oxygen and positive end expiratory pressure may be of help in some cases.[36,40,45] However, care must be taken not to accentuate the increased intracranial pressure by the use of elevated positive end expiratory pressure. Not uncommonly, dramatic relief of the pulmonary edema will occur after minimal changes in the intracranial pressure. Restriction of fluid is often desirable, almost to the point of dehydration.

Near Drowning

Drowning, defined as death within 24 h of a submersion accident, is one of three leading causes of accidental death in the United States. The highest incidence occurs in the second decade of life,[25] and is a particularly catastrophic problem since it affects individuals who are otherwise healthy and usually engaged in a recreational activity. Approximately 65 percent of those who die in swimming pools in the United States are children under the age of 10.[46]

For subjects who survive submersion situations, the single most feared sequela is neurologic damage. Several reports suggest that certain circumstances surrounding the event may have prognostic significance. In addition to the obvious time of submersion, age and water temperature are important; young age and cold water are most favorable.[47,48]

A significant number of drownings also occur in bathtubs. With the increasing use of hot tubs and whirlpools, drownings in these receptacles are increasing in number. Warmer water temperature and the prevalence of *Pseudomonas aeruginosa* in this environment make these types of submersions much more dangerous.[49] The content of water (salt versus fresh) apparently has little prognostic significance.

Cerebral anoxia and ischemia, regularly associated with prolonged submersion, may be of greater importance in the production of pulmonary edema (neurogenic edema) than the actual aspiration of water.[50] Hypoxia caused by near-drowning may be followed by anoxic encephalopathy and other forms of neurologic sequelae in 5 to 20 percent (or more) of survivors.[51,52] The clinical status of the patient on admission to emergency facilities has been used to prognosticate the possible outcome of near-drowning victims, but Taylor and coworkers[53] found no correlation between these factors. These clinicians also found no relationship between the appearance of immediate computed tomography (CT) of the brain and the ultimate prognosis. However, they found that an abnormal CT within the first 24 h of admission was associated with a higher mortality. Severe neurologic sequelae were seen in most patients who developed an abnormal CT at some time during their illness. Basal ganglia lucencies, diffuse cerebral edema, and cerebral atrophy were all seen in decreasing frequency (Figure 16-12).

A. Ashley Weech, chairman of the Department of Pediatrics at the University of Cincinnati College of Medicine, was fond of delivering a lecture on neonatal hypoxia. He dropped newborn mice in water as he lectured. Toward the end of the hour he gradually withdrew them from the water and deposited them on the lecture table. To everyone's amazement but his, they were all crawling around the table at the end of the hour, seemingly no worse for the ex-

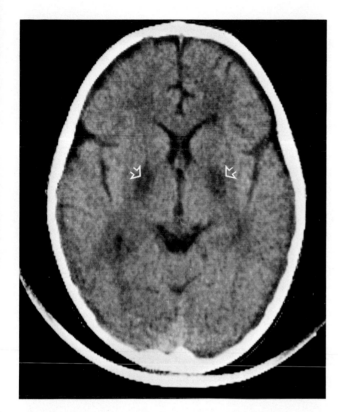

Figure 16-12 Near-drowning—central nervous system sequelae. Computed tomography of the head 8 days after near-drowning shows low densities bilaterally in the globus pallidi (arrows). This is a common finding in children with postimmersion neurologic sequelae. (Courtesy of Dr. Steven Taylor, Jacksonville, Florida.)

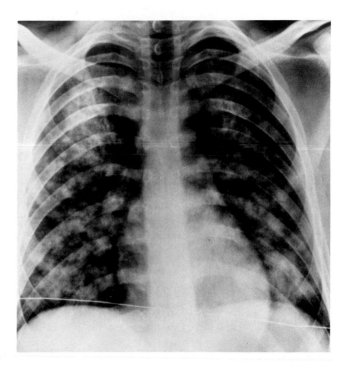

Figure 16-13 Near-drowning. The disseminated alveolar pattern is compatible with the pulmonary edema of near-drowning. This change may be the result of neurologic pulmonary edema rather than aspirated water.

perience, although we all figure they lose a step or two in the process.

Abnormal chest radiographs may be found in up to 60 percent of near-drowning victims.[51] The radiographic spectrum of near-drowning extends from normal to extensive amounts of disseminated alveolar infiltrates (Figure 16-13). These are undoubtedly caused by edema and superimposed hemorrhage.[51,54–56] The pulmonary involvement may manifest as perihilar hazy densities; ill-defined, fluffy shadows scattered throughout the lungs; or larger confluent alveolar opacities that often spare the apices, bases, and lateral lung fields. Scattered areas of atelectasis are not uncommon. Chest films are usually abnormal when first obtained and worsen over

the ensuing several days. However, there may be delays of 24 to 48 h before roentgen abnormalities develop.[56]

In general, some improvement is to be expected in the first 24 h, clearing should begin within 3 to 5 days, and complete return to normal may be expected within 7 to 10 days.[54,56] Secondary infection should be suspected when this gradual resolution is interrupted or the infiltrate begins to spread. Adult respiratory distress syndrome is a frequent complication of near-drowning and should be suspected when the lungs fail to clear normally. Pneumomediastinum and pneumothorax are additional complications, sometimes resulting from resuscitation. Severe necrotizing pneumonia, abscess, and/or atelectasis may result from aspiration of grossly contaminated water.

The association of pulmonary roentgenographic abnormalities with severity of disease and prognosis is not completely known. Some of this dilemma may relate to the altered circumstances of submersion included in the various reports. Putman and co-workers[56] found no correlation between the initial radiographic findings and the severity of illness but emphasized the possible late onset (24 to 48 h) of radiographic changes. Fuller[57] reported 16 of 57 cases with clinically overt pulmonary problems in which the radiographs were normal. Hunter and Whitehouse[56] found good correlation between the chest film and the severity of illness or length of hospitalization. Modell et al.[58] have emphasized that radiographic findings frequently lag behind the actual intrapulmonary status. They have not found it necessary to use endotracheal intubation in patients with normal chest films. While a normal chest radiograph on admission does not exclude significant intrapulmonary pathology, it is a good prognostic sign in an alert, conscious individual.

Croup, Epiglottitis, and Chronic Airway Obstruction

Croup, epiglottitis, and chronic airway obstruction are responsible for a variety of respiratory abnormalities, including pulmonary edema (Figure 16-14).[59] Chest films in these conditions may show, in addition to pulmonary edema, other signs of upper airway obstruction.[60] Among these are distension of the hypopharynx, underaeration of the lungs, and cardiac enlargement with or without pulmonary congestion.

Pulmonary edema may also occur following the sudden release of upper airway obstruction. The precise pathophysiologic mechanism for this phenomenon is in doubt, but has to do with alterations in intrathoracic pressures and the relationship of these factors to the drainage of lymphatic fluid and blood from the lung.[61,62]

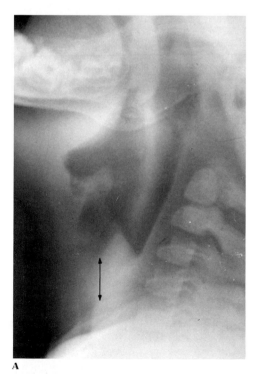

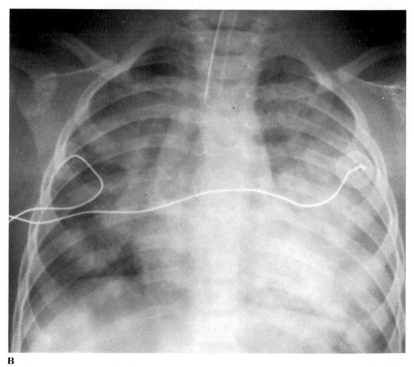

A   **B**

Figure 16-14   Pulmonary edema—upper airway obstruction. This patient developed sudden onset of croup. **A.** The tracheal walls are effaced by edema in the loose, areolar, subglottic tissues (arrows). The epiglottis is normal. Secondary contraction of the hypopharyngeal muscles with dilatation of the pharynx on inspiration frequently accompanies croup. **B.** Generalized pulmonary edema is secondary to the upper airway obstruction. This cleared rapidly after endotracheal intubation (see Figure 17-7).

Pulmonary hypertension from chronic hypoxemia is an additional mechanism contributing to cardiomegaly, right heart failure, and pulmonary edema. Unexplained pulmonary edema, with or without right heart failure, should suggest airflow obstruction. Enlarged tonsils and adenoids are well-known culprits in this scenario (Figure 16-15C).[63] Chest films may show subtle signs of interstitial edema, mild cardiomegaly, and enlarged pulmonary artery (Figure 16-15A and B). When these findings occur on chest films before tonsillectomy and adenoidectomy, the surgeon should be alerted to the possible development of postoperative pulmonary edema.[64]

In a study of children with cardiac failure, growth disturbance, and snoring, the obstructive symptoms occurred predominantly during sleep.[65] Periods of apnea, disturbed sleep, and noisy respirations were characteristic. In addition to cardiomegaly and, in some cases, pulmonary edema, these children were often hypersomnolent, small for their age, and enuretic, and they complained of headaches and other constitutional symptoms. Patients with this symptom complex usually had normal radiographic examination of the airway except for large adenoids and pharyngeal tonsils.

Video fluoroscopy of the airway during sleep is needed to define the obstruction in these patients.

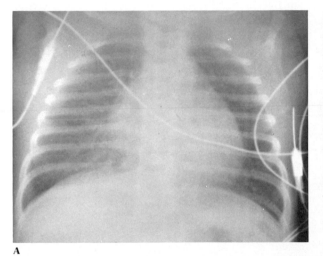

A

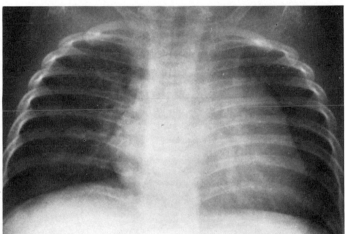

B

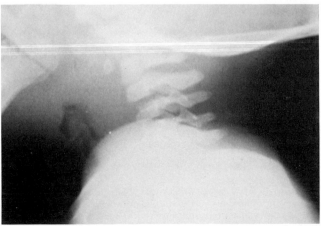

C

Figure 16-15 Chronic upper airway obstruction—cor pulmonale. This infant developed upper airway obstruction shortly after birth. **A.** The chest film in early life shows normal cardiac size but loss of vascular detail secondary to pulmonary edema. This pattern cleared following endotracheal intubation. **B.** This film, taken approximately 6 months later, reveals marked enlargement of the heart and main pulmonary artery segment. **C.** The nasopharyngeal airway is virtually obliterated.

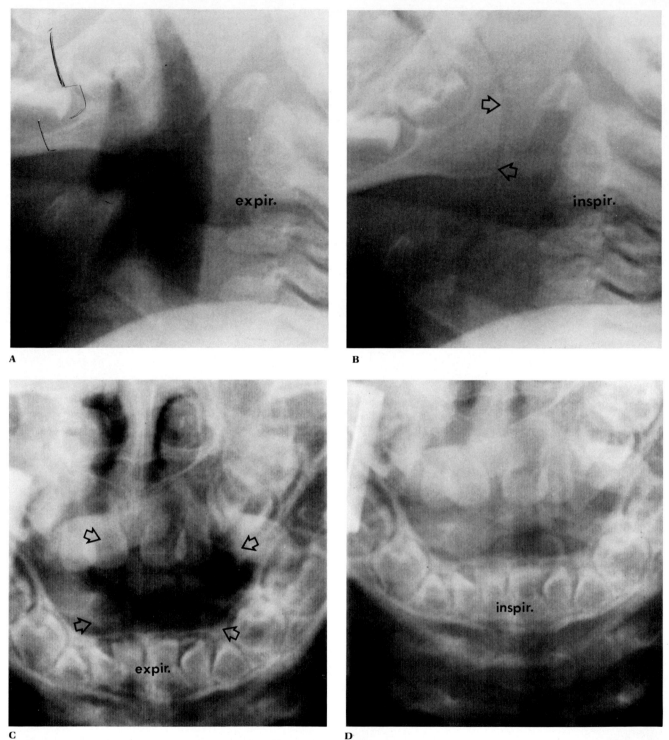

Figure 16-16   Chronic upper airway obstruction during sleep. A. The expiration airway film during sleep shows a widely patent pharynx. **B.** During inspiration the pharyngeal airway is reduced to a thin column (arrows) as the tongue and prevertebral soft tissues collapse inward. Obstruction of airflow by enlarged adenoids at the level of the nasopharynx leads to a negative pressure vacuum effect in the oropharynx during inspiration. This is accentuated during sleep when the muscles of the tongue and pharynx relax and the mouth is closed. **C** and **D.** The frontal projection shows similar changes during inspiration and expiration (arrows).

In affected individuals, fluoroscopic examination will show marked narrowing of the hypopharynx during inspiration with partial and/or complete obstruction of airflow (Figure 16-16). In most of these situations, a tonsillectomy and adenoidectomy will be curative, but occasionally patients require tracheostomy. Children with congenital or acquired abnormalities of the mandible and tongue, such as Pierre Robin syndrome, Treacher Collins syndrome, Down's syndrome, achondroplasia, and pyknodysostosis, are particularly susceptible to obstructive sleep apnea.

Heroin Overdose

The increased use of heroin by children, as well as adults, makes this an increasingly important cause of pulmonary edema. A triad of symptoms characterizes the acute intoxication syndrome: (1) an acutely ill patient in a stuporous or comatose state, (2) depressed respiration, and (3) constricted pupils.[66] Pulmonary edema after intravenous injections of the drug may be rapid in onset and often quite severe, with edema fluid filling the trachea and extruding from the nostrils and mouth.

The pathophysiologic mechanism for heroin-induced pulmonary edema is not completely understood. The problem is limited to acute overdose and is not a feature of chronic abuse. Theories used to explain the mechanism include physiologic reaction to vascular stress, trauma or high osmotic pressure gradient, cardiogenic abnormality, hypoxic reaction, neurogenic imbalance, potentiated localized histamine release, and hypersensitivity to injected material.[67] Seasonal variations have also been reported, with greater numbers occurring in April through July. Superimposed pneumonia or aspiration is an expected complication and should be suspected if the lungs are not clear after 24 h of treatment.

The radiographic appearance of heroin pulmonary edema is not specific; the changes may be much more extensive than expected from clinical symptoms. Improvement in the radiograph generally begins within hours after the start of treatment, and the lungs usually return to normal within 4 to 5 days.

Parathion Poisoning

Parathion is an organic phosphate derivative used extensively as an agricultural pesticide. The substance is rapidly absorbed through the skin and mucous membranes of the respiratory tract. A single drop in the eye may be fatal.[68] Death usually occurs from hypoxia due to interference with respiration by one or more of the following mechanisms: (1) bronchial constriction, (2) excessive respiratory tract secretions, (3) paralysis of muscles of respiration, and (4) failure of the respiratory center.[69]

High-Altitude Pulmonary Edema (Mountain Malady)

High-altitude pulmonary edema (HAPE), frequently seen in young patients, is not a well-known cause for pulmonary edema. Several reports have emphasized that children are more susceptible to this problem than adults.[70,71] As might be expected, this disease is largely dependent upon geographic location. It may occur at altitudes as low as 2200 m (approximately 7200 ft), but it is not usually seen under 3000 to 3600 m.

In susceptible individuals the onset of symptoms customarily begins within a few hours to a day or two after rapid ascent from low to high altitudes.[72] However, delays of weeks or months before the onset of HAPE are not unusual.[73] Cyanosis, pallor, dyspnea, cough, wheezing, chest pain, and occasional hemoptysis accompany the pulmonary edema. The prolonged expiration and wheezing may be mistaken for asthma. Rales may be asymmetrical, and signs of heart failure or infection are generally absent.

The precipitating causes of HAPE apparently relate to the development of pulmonary arterial hypertension and hypoxia. Exercise, cold exposure, and superimposed infections may contribute but are difficult to prove. Myocardial dysfunction is present in some patients. Other factors are no doubt operative, however, as symptoms are not completely relieved by administration of 100% oxygen.[70] Expiratory positive airway pressure may help in patients suffering from HAPE.

Radiographic findings in advanced cases include generalized, patchy, alveolar densities with areas of coalescence. A right-sided preponderance was observed in the patients reported by Menon.[73] Individuals with absent right pulmonary artery are more susceptible to HAPE.

Treatment consists of oxygen and bed rest in a semiupright position. Occasionally patients will benefit from cardiac support medication such as digoxin and morphine. Evacuation to lower altitudes is not always necessary, and patients may return to heights with only a slight risk that the pulmonary edema will recur. In addition to edema of the lungs, pulmonary hemorrhage is a recognized, but uncommon, complication.[74]

Salicylate Intoxication

Pulmonary edema in association with salicylate ingestion is extremely rare in patients under 16 years of age; however, young adults are susceptible. Factors that increase the probability of this complication include heavy cigarette smoking, metabolic acidosis, and neurologic disease.[75]

The mechanism of edema production probably relates to damage of the pulmonary vascular bed with escape of fluid into the interstitial and alveolar lung space.

Pleural Fluid Pattern

When the lung's capacity to hold fluid is exceeded, the excess may exude into the pleural space and collect as a pleural effusion. Purulent effusions are usually associated with underlying parenchymal inflammations; these are considered in Chapter 18.

Pleural effusions most often exist as either transudates or exudates and may be distinguished according to the following characteristics:[76]

Pleural Fluid	Transudate	Exudate
Liquid protein concentration	< 3 g/100 ml	> 3 g/100 g
Ratio of fluid to serum protein	< 0.5	> 0.5
LDH* concentration	< 200 IU	> 200 IU
Ratio of fluid to serum LDH	< 0.6	> 0.6

*LDH = lactic dehydrogenase.

In addition to transudates and exudates, chylous, hemorrhagic, and malignant effusions also occur in children. The term *pleural fluid* will be used generically to describe abnormal collections, although blood, pus, chyle, and other fluids may have a similar roentgenographic appearance.

The plain-film roentgen observations that signal the presence of pleural fluid depend upon several major conditions: (1) amount of fluid, (2) position of the patient, (3) condition of the underlying lung, (4) associated pleural fibroadhesive disease, and (5) physical characteristics of the fluid.

Anatomic and positional factors influence the radiographic configurations of pleural fluid.[77,78] When patients are radiographed in the supine position, pleural fluid gravitates to the dependent portion of the chest, rendering the involved hemithorax more opaque. In this position, fluid may also layer over the apex of the thorax (apical cap) and/or form a meniscus shadow in the costophrenic and cardiophrenic sulci. Decubitus films will usually confirm the presence of freely flowing pleural fluid; cross-table lateral films are also of diagnostic value with unilateral collections.

In the upright position, pleural fluid tends to collect in the subpulmonic potential space between the diaphragm and inferior surface of the lung. With sufficient collection of subphrenic fluid, several characteristic radiographic configurations are produced (Figure 16-17). A pseudodiaphragmatic shadow, representing the interface between lung and fluid, frequently has its apex or dome more lat-

Figure 16-17 Subpulmonic effusion. A. This upright film during remission shows no pleural effusion. **B1.** The right side shows a fluid-lung interface that is quite suggestive of subpulmonic effusion; the "dome" (open arrow—r) is more lateral than a normal hemidiaphragm. The medial-posterior edge of the hemidiaphragm is barely visible against the overlying lung (ar-

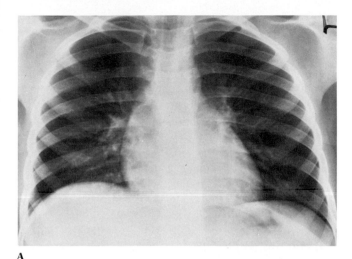

A

Figure 16-17 (*Continued*)
row). The left hemithorax is free of fluid. **B2.** This lateral film was taken at same time as B1; the right fluid-lung interface has a straight anterior edge up to the junction with the major fissure (open arrow—r). This is a typical configuration of subpulmonic effusion. The right posterior costophrenic sulcus is obliterated by a pleural fluid meniscus. The left hemidiaphragm (open arrow) is well visualized in its entirety; the anterior portion is adjacent to the air-filled splenic flexure. **C1.** On another occasion, a left subpulmonic effusion is present and is characterized by an elevated "dome-shaped" fluid-lung interface (open arrow) similar to that in B1. The distance between the lung and the stomach (S) usually confirms a left-sided subpulmonic effusion. The left paraspinous line (arrow) is obliterated by fluid in the posterior cardiophrenic sulcus (see the lateral film). **C2.** Left subpulmonic fluid is evident (open arrow), but some fluid has also formed a posterior meniscus between the lung and chest wall. A small right subpulmonic effusion is also present and shows the characteristic configuration seen in B2 (open arrow—r). Note the clear lung fields and normal heart size, which typify the nephrotic syndrome.

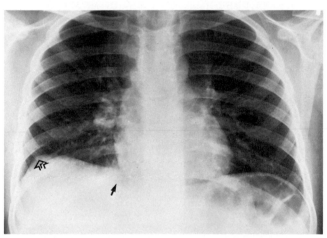

B1

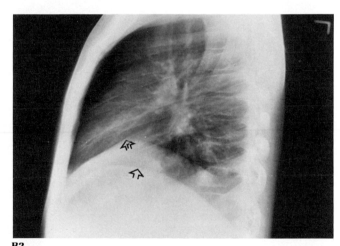

B2

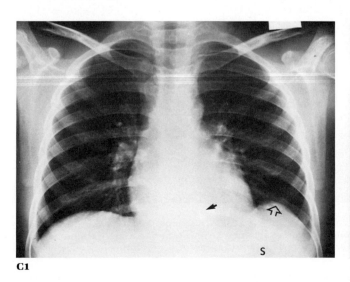

C1

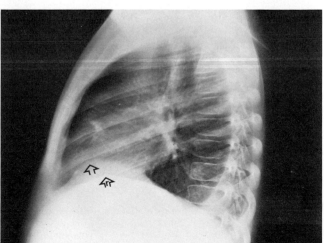

C2

eral than the apex of the normal diaphragm (Figure 16-17B1). This is accentuated in expiration. In the left chest, subpulmonic fluid is easier to recognize, as the pseudodiaphragmatic silhouette is separated from the stomach air bubble by subpulmonic fluid

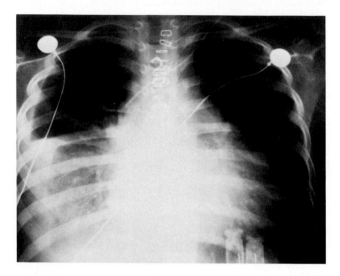

Figure 16-18   Pleural effusion—"middle lobe step" sign. A large amount of pleural effusion is seen between the chest wall and partially atelectatic right middle lobe, producing a steplike configuration.

(Figure 16-17C1). This finding must be interpreted with lateral films, since several centimeters between the stomach air bubble and the diaphragm may exist normally. On upright lateral films, subpulmonic fluid often produces a characteristic pseudodiaphragmatic contour (Figure 16-17B2). Even in the presence of subpulmonic effusions, fluid often escapes into lateral and posterior sulci.[77] Lateral upright films will often detect minimal collections in the posterior costophrenic sulcus (Figure 16-17C2).[79] The cardiophrenic angles also collect fluid with the patient in the upright position. A triangular opacity seen through the cardiac shadow is produced by fluid behind the pulmonary ligament or in the posterior paraspinal gutter (Figure 16-17C1). On the right, the normal curved shadow of the posterior costophrenic sulcus, as projected through the liver, is often distorted by small amounts of fluid in this recess.

While studies to confirm the presence of pleural fluid are usually requested in the upright position, the tendency for fluid to collect in the subpulmonic space often makes it difficult to detect. Fluid may be detected as well on supine films, but decubitus projections are most reliable.

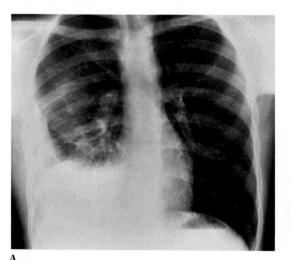

A

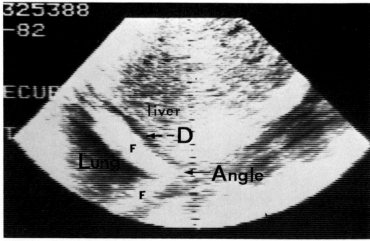

B

Figure 16-19   Pleuropneumonic disease—ultrasonography. **A.** This upright chest film shows a pleuropneumonic process in the right lower lung field that failed to change on decubitus positioning. **B.** Ultrasonography demonstrates an echo-free fluid collection (F) between the diaphragm (D) and the overlying, collapsed, infiltrated lung. Fluid is also present between the lung and chest wall (Angle = costophrenic angle).

Large amounts of subpulmonic fluid may accumulate without blunting the costophrenic angle or escaping between the chest wall and lung.[80] Massive effusions causing an entirely opaque hemithorax can make it virtually impossible to differentiate opacified lung from pleural fluid. In these situations, air bronchograms, which indicate the presence of atelectatic or consolidated lung, are helpful if present. Contralateral mediastinal shift favors the presence of a large effusion. Inversion of the left hemidiaphragm, recognized on upright films as an inferiorly displaced stomach, may result from massive left-sided effusions. When present, these patients may be intensely dyspneic.[81]

Additional roentgenographic features of pleural effusion include (1) visualization of fluid in major fissures, especially in the upright lateral film, (2) the "middle lobe step" (Figure 16-18),[77,78] (3) posterior layering on cross-table lateral film, and (4) layering along the inner chest wall on decubitus projections, among others.

The use of ultrasonography and CT can be very helpful when trying to determine the amount and location of fluid in the chest (Figure 16-19). Ultrasonography is of particular help in the separation of subphrenic from subpulmonic fluid and in directing thoracentesis in difficult cases.[82] This technique is also well suited to the separation of underlying

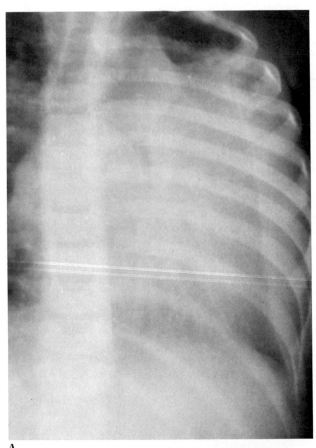

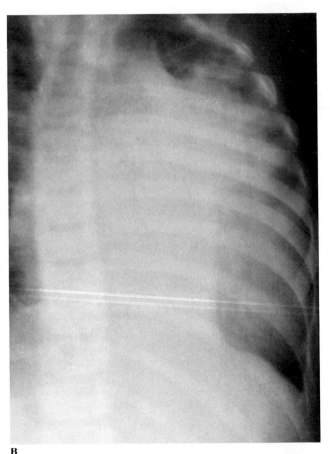

A   **B**

Figure 16-20   Lingular and upper lobe atelectasis.   A. The radiopacity along the left inner chest wall is caused by the lingula and left upper lobe that is collapsed between the enlarged heart and inner chest wall. The air–soft tissue interface represents the left major fissure and should not be confused with a pleural effusion. **B.** Later the same day, the left lower lobe is collapsed, and the left upper lobe and lingula are expanded. (From Felman.[83])

pneumonia or mass lesions that originate from the pleural surfaces, chest wall, or mediastinum from overlying pleural fluid. Computed tomography also makes this differentiation, but is more expensive, more cumbersome, and difficult to interpret.

Radiographic examination following thoracentesis still has value in ascertaining the presence of a mass or pneumonia underlying a pleural collection.

Lingular and left upper lobe atelectasis in patients with cardiomegaly should not be confused with pleural effusion (Figure 16-20).[83]

References

1. Milne ENC, Pistolesi M, Miniati M, et al: The radiologic distinction of cardiogenic and noncardiogenic edema. *AJR* 144:879, 1985.

2. Zimmerman JE, Goodman LR, St Andre AC, et al: Radiographic detection of mobilizable lung water: The gravitational shift list. *AJR* 138:59, 1982.

3. Hublitz UF, Shapiro JH: Atypical pulmonary patterns of congestive failure in chronic lung disease. The influence of preexisting disease on the appearance and distribution of pulmonary edema. *Radiology* 93:995, 1969.

4. Felson B: The roentgen diagnosis of disseminated pulmonary alveolar diseases. *Semin Roentgenol* 2:3, 1967.

5. Johnson TH Jr, Gajaraj A, Feist JH: Vascular key to diagnosis of pulmonary interstitial diseases. *AJR* 113:518, 1971.

6. Gleason DC, Steiner RE: The lateral roentgenograms in pulmonary edema. *AJR* 98:279, 1966.

7. Pistolesi M, Giuntini G: Assessment of extravascular lung water. *Radiol Clin North Am* 16:551, 1978.

8. Heitzman ER, Zitter FM Jr: Acute interstitial pulmonary edema. *AJR* 98:291, 1966.

9. Ziskind MM, Weill H, Payzant AR: The recognition and significance of acinus-filling processes of the lung. *Am Rev Resp Dis* 87:551, 1963.

10. Raskin SP: The pulmonary acinus. Historical notes. *Radiology* 144:31, 1982.

11. Recavarren S, Benton C, Gall EA: The pathology of acute alveolar disease of the lung. *Semin Roentgenol* 2:22, 1967.

12. Reed JC, Madewell JE: The air bronchogram in interstitial disease of the lungs. A radiological-pathological correlation. *Radiology* 116:1, 1975.

13. Felson B: A new look at pattern recognition in diffuse pulmonary disease. *AJR* 133:183, 1979.

14. Eade NR, Taussig LM, Marks MI: Hydrocarbon pneumonitis. *Pediatrics* 54:351, 1974.

15. Mellins RB: Lung injury from hydrocarbon aspiration and smoke inhalation, in Kendig EL Jr, Chernick V (eds): *Disorders of the Respiratory Tract in Infants and Children*, 3d ed. Philadelphia, WB Saunders, 1977, p 491.

16. Gerarde HW: Toxicological studies in hydrocarbons. V. Kerosene. *Toxicol Appl Pharmacol* 1:462, 1959.

17. Huxtable KA, Bolande RP, Klaus M: Experimental furniture polish pneumonia in rats. *Pediatrics* 34:228, 1964.

18. Wolfe BM, Brodeur AE, Shields JB: The role of gastrointestinal absorption of kerosene in producing pneumonitis in dogs. *J Pediatr* 76:867, 1970.

19. Wolfsdorf J: Kerosene intoxication: An experimental approach to the etiology of the CNS manifestations in primates. *J Pediatr* 88:1037, 1976.

20. Neeld EM, Limacher MC: Chemical pneumonitis after intravenous injection of hydrocarbon. *Radiology* 129:36, 1978.

21. Saulsbury FT, Chobanian MC, Wilson WG: Child abuse: Parenteral hydrocarbon administration. *Pediatrics* 73:720, 1984.

22. Giammona ST: Effects of furniture polish on pulmonary surfactant. *Am J Dis Child* 113:658, 1967.

23. Gross P, McNerney JM, Balyak MA: Kerosene pneumonitis: An experimental study with small doses. *Am Rev Respir Dis* 88:656, 1963.

24. Brown J, Burke B, Dajani AS: Experimental kerosene pneumonia: Evaluation of some therapeutic regimens. *J Pediatr* 84:396, 1974.

25. Press E: Co-operative kerosene poisoning study of the Sub-committee on Accidental Poisoning of the American Academy of Pediatrics. Evaluation of gastric lavage and other factors in the treatment of accidental ingestion of petroleum distillate products. *Pediatrics* 29:648, 1962.

26. Harris VJ, Brown R: Pneumatoceles as a complication of chemical pneumonia after hydrocarbon ingestion. *AJR* 125:531, 1975.

27. Shirkey HC: Treatment of petroleum distillate ingestion. *Mod Treatm* 4:697, 1967.

28. Daeschner CW Jr, Blattner RJ, Collins VP: Hydrocarbon pneumonitis. *Pediatr Clin North Am* 4:243, 1957.

29. Campbell JB: Pneumatocele formation following hydrocarbon ingestion. *Am Rev Respir Dis* 101:414, 1970.

30. Baghdassarian OM, Weiner S: Pneumatocele formation

complicating hydrocarbon pneumonitis. *AJR* 95:104, 1965.

31. Neuhauser EBD: Pneumatoceles following aspiration of hydrocarbons. *Postgrad Med* 49:57, 1971.

32. Farber SJ: Physiologic aspects of glomerulonephritis. *J Chronic Dis* 5:87, 1957.

33. Holzel A, Fawcitt J: Pulmonary changes in acute glomerulonephritis in childhood. *J Pediatr* 57:695, 1960.

34. Kirkpatrick JA Jr, Fleisher DS: The roentgen appearance of the chest in acute glomerulonephritis in children. *J Pediatr* 64:492, 1964.

35. Felman A: Neurogenic pulmonary edema. Observations in six patients. *AJR* 112:393, 1971.

36. Milley JR, Nugent SK, Rogers MC: Neurogenic pulmonary edema in childhood. *J Pediatr* 94:706, 1979.

37. Chang CH, Smith CA: Postictal pulmonary edema. *Radiology* 89:1087, 1967.

38. Richard P: Pulmonary edema and intracranial lesions. *Br Med J* 2:83, 1963.

39. Ducker TB, Simmons RL: Increased intracranial pressure and pulmonary edema. Part II. Hemodynamic response of dogs and monkeys to increased intracranial pressure. *J Neurosurg* 28:118, 1968.

40. Harrison W, Liebow AA: Effects of increased intracranial pressure on pulmonary circulation in relation to pulmonary edema. *Circulation* 5:824, 1952.

41. Reynolds RW: Pulmonary edema as a consequence of hypothalamic lesions in rats. *Science* 141:930, 1963.

42. Fein IA, Rackow EC: Neurogenic pulmonary edema. *Chest* 81:318, 1982.

43. Brigham KL: Factors affecting lung vascular permeability. *Am Rev Respir Dis* 115:165, 1977.

44. Rigler LG, Surprenant EL: Pulmonary edema. *Semin Roentgenol* 2:33, 1967.

45. Kosnik EJ, Paul SE, Rossel CW, et al: Central neurogenic pulmonary edema: With a review of its pathogenesis and treatment. *Childs Brain* 3:37, 1977.

46. Webster DP: Pool drownings and their prevention. *Public Health Rep* 82:587, 1967.

47. Frates RC: Analysis of predicted factors in the assessment of warm-water near-drowning in children. *Am J Dis Child* 135:1006, 1981.

48. Rogers MC: Near-drowning: Cold water on a hot topic. *J Pediatr* 106:603, 1985.

49. Tron VA, Baldwin VJ, Pirie GE: Hot tub drownings. *Pediatrics* 75:789, 1985.

50. Modell JH: Drowning and near-drowning, in Kendig EL Jr, Chernick V (eds): *Disorders of the Respiratory Tract in Children,* 3d ed. Philadelphia, WB Saunders, 1977, p 498.

51. Peterson B: Morbidity of childhood near-drowning. *Pediatrics* 59:364, 1977.

52. Pearn J: Neurologic and psychometric studies in children surviving fresh water immersion accidents. *Lancet* 1:7, 1977.

53. Taylor SB, Quencer RM, Holzman BH, et al: Central nervous system anoxic-ischemic insult in children due to near-drowning. *Radiology* 156:641, 1985.

54. Rosenbaum HT, Thompson WL, Fuller RH: Radiographic pulmonary changes in near-drowning. *Radiology* 83:306, 1964.

55. Hunter TB, Whitehouse WM: Fresh-water near-drowning: Radiological aspects. *Radiology* 112:51, 1974.

56. Putman CE, Tummillo AM, Myerson DA, et al: Drowning: Another plunge. *AJR* 125:543, 1975.

57. Fuller RH: The clinical pathology of human near-drowning. *Proc Soc Med* 56:33, 1963.

58. Modell JH, Graves SA, Ketova A: Clinical course of 91 consecutive near-drowning victims. *Chest* 70:231, 1976.

59. Travis KW, Todres D, Shannon DC: Pulmonary edema associated with croup and epiglottitis. *Pediatrics* 59:695, 1977.

60. Capitanio MA, Kirkpatrick JA Jr: Obstructions of the upper airway in children as reflected on the chest radiograph. *Radiology* 109:159, 1973.

61. Galves AG, Stool SE, Bluestone CS: Pulmonary edema following relief of acute upper airway obstruction. *Arch Otolaryngol* 80:112, 1980.

62. Sofer S, Bar-Ziv J, Scharf SM: Pulmonary edema following relief of upper airway obstruction. *Chest* 86:401, 1984.

63. Talaat AM, Nahhas MM: Cardiopulmonary changes secondary to chronic adenotonsillitis. *Arch Otolaryngol* 109:30, 1983.

64. Feinberg AN, Shabino CL: Acute pulmonary edema complicating tonsillectomy and adenoidectomy. *Pediatrics* 75:112, 1985.

65. Felman AH, Loughlin GM, Leftridge CA: Upper airway obstruction during sleep in children. *AJR* 133:212, 1979.

66. Stern WZ, Spear PW, Jacobson HG: The roentgen findings in acute heroin intoxication. *AJR* 103:522, 1968.

67. Morrison WJ, Wetherill S, Zyroff J: The acute pulmonary edema of heroin intoxication. *Radiology* 97:347, 1970.

68. Kopel FB, Starobin S, Gribetz I, et al: Acute parathion poisoning. Diagnosis and treatment. *J Pediatr* 61:898, 1962.

69. Hayes WJ Jr: Parathion poisoning and its treatment. *JAMA* 192:49, 1965.

70. Hultgren HN, Grover RF, Hartley LH: Abnormal circulatory responses to high altitude in subjects with a previous history of high altitude pulmonary edema. *Circulation* 44:759, 1971.

71. Frates RC, Harrison GM, Edwards GA: High altitude pulmonary edema in children. *Am J Dis Child* 131:687, 1977.

72. Marticorena E, Tapia F, Dyer J, et al: Pulmonary edema by ascending to high altitudes. *Dis Chest* 45:273, 1964.

73. Menon ND: High-altitude pulmonary edema. *N Engl J Med* 273: 66, 1965.

74. Dickenson J, Heath D, Gosney J, et al: Altitude-related death in trekkers in the Himalayas. *Thorax* 38:646, 1983.

75. Walters JS, Woodring JH, Stelling CB, et al: Salicylate-induced pulmonary edema. *Radiology* 146:289, 1983.

76. Pagtakhan RD, Chernick V: Liquid and air in the pleural space, in Kendig EL Jr, Chernick V (eds): *Diseases of the Respiratory Tract in Children* 3d ed. Philadelphia, WB Saunders, 1977, pp 475–487, 602.

77. Fleischner FG: Atypical arrangement of free pleural effusion. *Radiol Clin North Am* 1(2):347, 1963.

78. Raasch BN, Carsky EW, Lane EJ, et al: Pleural effusion: Explanation of some typical appearances. *AJR* 139:899, 1984.

79. Woodring JH: Recognition of pleural effusion on supine radiographs: How much fluid is required? *AJR* 142:59, 1984.

80. Rigby M, Zylak EJ, Wood LDH: The effect of lobar atelectasis on pleural fluid distribution in dogs. *Radiology* 136:603, 1980.

81. Mulvey RB: The effect of pleural effusion on the diaphragm. *Radiology* 84:1080, 1965.

82. Harnsberger HR, Lee G, Mukuno DH: Rapid, inexpensive real-time directed thoracentesis. *Radiology* 146:545, 1983.

83. Felman AH: Lingular and upper lobe atelectasis and cardiomegaly: An unusual pattern simulating pleural effusion. *Br J Radiol* 45:299, 1971.

Chapter 17

Patterns of Major Airway Disease

Respiratory distress resulting from disturbed airflow is a common problem of childhood. Proper radiographic evaluation will often define the nature and location of airway obstruction, but close clinicoradiologic coordination is of extreme importance in arriving at a correct diagnosis.

Loving care must be exercised when transporting these children to the x-ray department, and close monitoring during the radiographic procedure is absolutely essential. A radiologist should be on hand to tailor the examination and monitor all film studies.

This chapter is divided into three sections. The first part discusses various causes for clinical symptoms of stridor. The other two sections cover foreign bodies and tumors although these abnormalities frequently present with stridor.

Radiologic Evaluation of Upper Airway Obstruction

A large number of imaging modalities are available that are well suited for evaluation of the laryngotracheobronchial tree.

Anteroposterior and Lateral Plain Films of the Airway

Films of the airway should include the pharynx as well as the laryngotracheal air column (Figure 17-1A and B). Except in rare instances, the frontal projection should be obtained as well as the lateral. Frontal films may be taken in the conventional manner, but the high-kilovolt-magnification technique described by Joseph and coworkers is often of considerable benefit.[1]

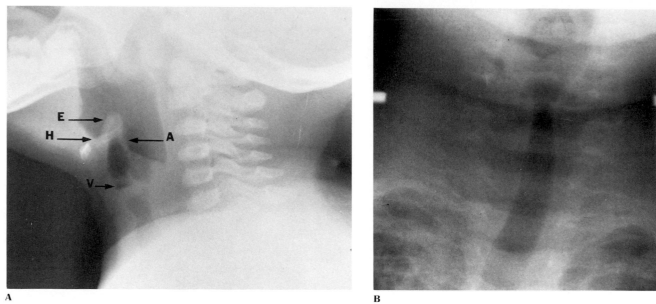

Figure 17-1   Normal airway. A. The lateral view demonstrates normal anatomy. The epiglottis (E) is a curved structure that is normal but appears slightly widened because of minimal obliquity. The aryepiglottic fold (A) is thin and curved. The hyoid bone (H) often overlaps the epiglottis. The ovoid lucency represents the laryngeal ventricle (V) between the false cords above and the true cords below. The inferior margin of the true cords is well-defined by the normal subglottic tracheal air. **B.** The high-kilovolt-magnification anteroposterior view outlines the laryngotracheal air column. The larynx is widely patent.

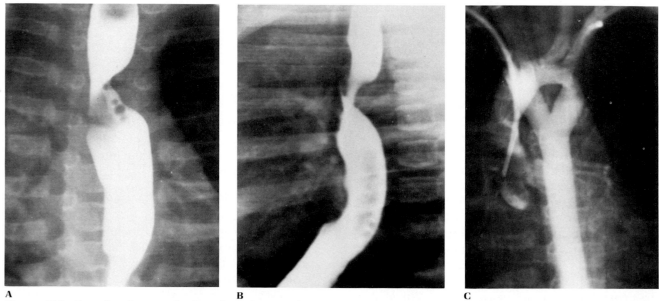

Figure 17-2   Vascular ring. A. The frontal esophogram shows marked constriction by the encircling vascular structures. The trachea, obscured by overlying barium, is midline, suggesting a right arch. The left arch produces the left-sided indentation of the esophagus. **B.** The lateral projection shows the esophagus and trachea markedly constricted by the vascular ring. **C.** The ascending aorta injection outlines the double-arch anatomy.

Fluoroscopy (Videotape)

Because of the marked malleability characteristic of the supporting soft tissues of the pediatric pharynx, plain films are often confusing or inconclusive. Frequently they show thickening of the prevertebral soft tissues, a finding that calls for definitive study. Fluoroscopic observation with videotape recording is the most helpful and easily performed procedure for evaluating this region.

Contrast Swallow and Esophogram

Barium swallow and esophogram provide an excellent way to define the pharynx and esophagus. Abnormal swallowing mechanism, congenital abnormalities, and vascular constrictions are best evaluated by this method since many lesions that constrict the trachea and stem bronchi also affect the esophageal lumen (Figure 17-2). When studying newborns and small infants, it is often safer to administer the contrast through an opaque, end-hole rubber catheter rather than by bottle.

Additional Studies

Xeroradiography should be employed in selected circumstances (Figure 17-3).[2] This technique is best suited for defining the tracheal air column and soft tissue detail and will occasionally show foreign bodies invisible on conventional radiographs. Edge enhancement characteristics of xeroradiography aid in the identification of small opacities such as foreign bodies and calcified normal cartilages.[3] Xeroradiography delivers more radiation than conventional radiography and is more difficult to use in children.

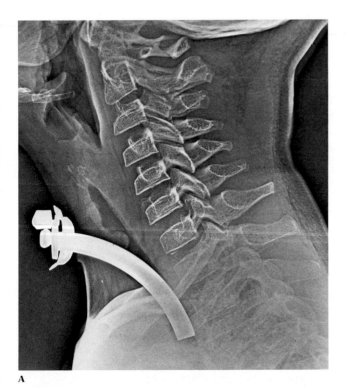
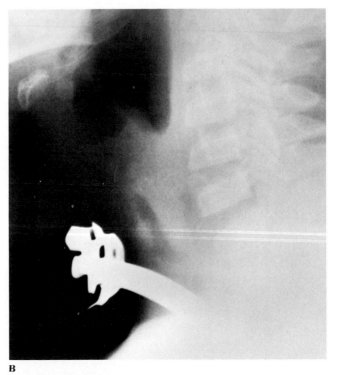

A   B

Figure 17-3 Xeroradiography. A. Lateral xeroradiography has the capacity to define the edges of structures very well. High-grade stenosis of the larynx is evident. A granuloma can be seen projecting into the trachea just above the tracheostomy. **B.** Conventional radiography defines the laryngeal stenosis but misses the tracheal granuloma.

Computed tomography (CT) is not generally used in acute situations but has value in defining causes of chronic stridor. This technique is helpful in defining the anatomy of choanal atresia and in differentiating bony from soft tissue obstruction.[4] Computed tomography is of proven worth in ascertaining the dimension of the tracheal lumen.[5-7] Stenotic lesions, with or without associated vascular compression, are nicely shown with this technique.[8] Computed tomography is also a valuable aid in the evaluation of tracheal compression caused by mediastinal masses.[9] According to Mandell et al.[10] the tracheal lumen must be narrowed by a third or more for symptoms to be manifest.

Magnetic resonance imaging is also of value in defining vascular lesions that affect the airway (Figure 17-4; see also Chapter 27).

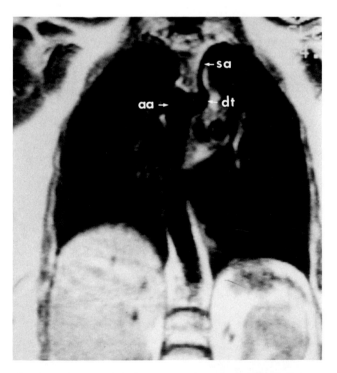

Figure 17-4   Magnetic resonance imaging. This study outlines a right aortic arch and right descending aorta with an aberrant left subclavian artery arising from a diverticulum of the aorta. This configuration produces a loose vascular ring, which is usually asymptomatic (aa = aortic arch, dt = diverticulum; sa = subclavian artery).

Stridor

The causes of stridor in children are largely age-dependent; the younger the child, the more likely the stridor results from congenital abnormalities. In a study of 219 children with stridor, whose ages were less than 2½ years, 87 percent had congenital anomalies; half of these had laryngotracheomalacia.[11] Less frequent in occurrence were subglottic stenosis (15 percent), vocal cord paralysis (9 percent), and vascular rings (8 percent). Approximately 25 percent of patients had an erroneous presumptive diagnosis of asthma, croup, or bronchiolitis, causing a delay in correct diagnosis for several months.

Congenital Anomalies

Nose

Associated congenital anomalies, occurring in as many as 50 percent of patients, include Treacher Collins syndrome and deformities of the face, nose, and palate; as well as congenital heart disease.[12] Choanal atresia is bony rather than membranous in 90 percent of cases. It is more common in females and is most often unilateral.

Choanal stenosis is less easily diagnosed and is not a clearly defined abnormality. Computed tomography may be of help in assessing choanal size but must be correlated with clinical symptoms.[4] Symptoms of chronic airway obstruction in the absence of another valid cause should raise suspicion of choanal stenosis. Several different types of mass lesions may account for nasal obstruction and include Tornwaldt's cyst, dermoid, encephalocele, glioma, and teratoma. A foreign body should always be suspect, especially with unilateral obstruction and nasal discharge.

Larynx and Supporting Structures (Vocal Cord Paralysis, Laryngeal Web, Laryngomalacia)

With the exception of laryngomalacia, obstructing lesions of the larynx are difficult to evaluate radiographically in infants and neonates. In vocal cord paralysis, unilateral involvement is more common than bilateral paralysis. This problem may not create symptoms until the infant is 3 to 4 days of age.[13] Radiographic diagnosis is difficult, but the lesion may be suspected when no vocal cord movement is evident on videofluoroscopy. An abnormal swallowing function manifested by nasopharyngeal reflux and tracheal aspiration may accompany this lesion.[14] Laryngoscopy is the diagnostic study of choice.

Laryngomalacia is the most common cause of infantile laryngeal obstruction.[15,16] The term was coined by Chevalier Jackson to emphasize the unusual laxity of laryngeal structures. The cry is usually normal, and the infant gains weight satisfactorily, but the condition produces inspiratory stridor along with crowing noises and substernal and intercostal retractions. The symptoms are usually exacerbated with crying or increased activity and lying in the supine position. In most cases the stridor is not recognized until the second or third week of life and usually subsides and disappears within 3 to 4 months.

The radiographic pattern of laryngomalacia is best appreciated with videotape fluoroscopy. Patients should be examined in the supine position with a horizontal fluoroscopic beam. This is best accomplished by positioning the fluoroscopic table vertically and placing the child on the table step. In the presence of laryngomalacia, the larynx will collapse on inspiration as the aryepiglottic folds and epiglottis fall inward. As the child inspires, the subglottic trachea will narrow. Many infants will manifest a certain amount of inspiratory crowing and laryngeal collapse with vigorous crying, but this should not be confused with laryngomalacia. There is considerable variation of normal laryngeal mobility depending upon the age and the individual.

Laryngeal web or stenosis (or both) usually produces symptoms of airway obstruction at birth.[17] Since most webs involve the vocal cords, the cry is usually hoarse or aphonic. Radiographic demonstration of a laryngeal web is difficult if not impossible because of the small, relatively featureless larynx. Videofluoroscopy will often demonstrate dynamic changes of laryngeal obstruction, such as dilatation

of the hypopharynx, narrowing of the subglottic trachea, and sternal retractions. In severe cases, cardiomegaly and pulmonary edema may ensue. When there is sufficient clinical suspicion of a laryngeal web, the child should be examined by direct visualization.

Trachea and Subglottis (See Chapters 1 and 27)

Symptoms from congenital cysts, subglottic stenosis, and related conditions may not present until several weeks of life or longer. They often masquerade as croup and are accentuated by upper respiratory infections. Stridor may be expiratory as well as inspiratory. These lesions are readily discernible on good-quality radiographs, but the technique should include anteroposterior as well as lateral projections. High-kilovolt-magnification films are often useful.[1] Xeroradiography and fluoroscopic examination may provide additional information. Confirmatory laryngoscopy and bronchoscopy are often diagnostic and may be therapeutic as well.

Symptoms of stridor from vascular compression usually do not present until several months of age. Most are caused by vascular rings; of these, double-arch anomalies are most likely to cause tracheal compression. Aberrant subclavian vessels rarely cause difficulty. Dilatation of great vessels (aorta) may also give rise to airway obstruction.[18]

Most infants and children with a double arch develop symptoms of airway obstruction, but some may remain asymptomatic. Later in life, the onset of dysphagia may bring the abnormality to attention.

Plain films of the chest often provide the first clue to the presence of a vascular ring. The trachea may appear more narrowed than normal and is often positioned in the midline rather than slightly to the right. Commonly, a dominant right aortic arch is present. A barium esophogram will confirm the presence of the abnormality and establish the correct nature of the anatomy in most cases, but a vascular study is usually obtained before definitive surgical correction (Figure 17-2C). Computed tomography with vascular enhancement[8] and magnetic resonance imaging are also able to define these lesions (Figure 17-4).

Acquired Abnormalities

Croup

The croup syndrome is a common cause of acute stridor in infants and young children. It is characterized by the acute onset of respiratory distress, stridor, and barking cough and usually occurs at night. It is partially or completely relieved by cold mist or vomiting. Children with croup are rarely studied radiographically because of the typical clinical symptomatology and usual prompt recovery. On occasion, symptoms not unlike croup occur in association with extreme toxicity, high fever, elevated white blood cell count, and general signs of severe illness. In some of these patients, extensive secretions that form in the larynx and trachea are visible on radiograph. Terms such as *bacterial tracheitis* and *laryngotracheobronchitis* have been used to describe this condition.[19-21] Nelson,[22] in a historical review, has

shed considerable light on this subject for the interested reader.

Patients with symptoms of croup and/or stridor usually are radiographed in an emergency manner, mostly to exclude other causes, such as epiglottitis and foreign body. The radiographic alterations of croup are produced by edema of the larynx and loose subglottic areolar tissue; the swelling obliterates the normal laryngeal and subglottic anatomy. Since the exclusion of epiglottitis is often the reason for obtaining the study, airway films are frequently taken only in the lateral projection. However, once the diagnosis of epiglottitis has been excluded, frontal studies should be performed.

In the frontal view, the subglottic soft tissue assumes a steeple-shaped rather than the normal "square-shoulder" appearance (Figure 17-5; see also Chapter 16, Figure 16-14). Secondary changes are best seen on lateral view and result from obstruction to airflow.[23] These include overdistension of the hy-

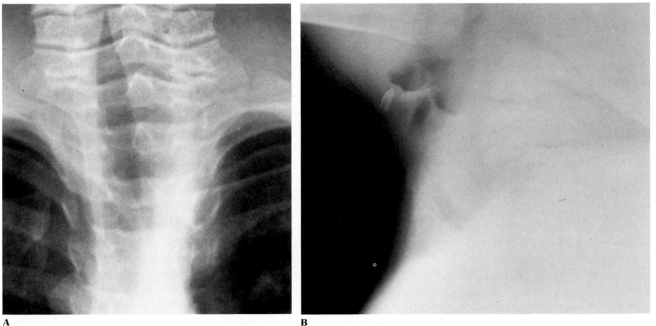

A   **B**

Figure 17-5   Croup. A. The frontal projection shows the narrowed subglottic air column, sometimes called *steepling*. This sign may be seen in normal patients. **B.** Edema of the larynx and subglottic tissues has obliterated the normal subglottic air column. Note the distended hypopharynx and widely patent laryngeal opening. The epiglottis and aryepiglottic folds are normal. In croup, listening to the patient breathe and cough is often very helpful when reading the film (see Figure 16-14).

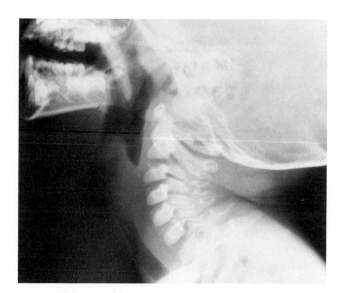

Figure 17-6 Supraglottitis. The epiglottis is swollen and resembles a thumb; the aryepiglottic folds are many times their normal thickness, and the subglottic air column is well defined.

popharynx, narrowing of the trachea on inspiration, substernal retractions, and occasional cardiomegaly and pulmonary edema. Children with membranous croup or bacterial tracheitis may develop collections of inspissated mucus in the tracheal lumen, which, on occasion, may simulate foreign bodies.[21]

Epiglottitis (Supraglottitis)

The clinical onset of epiglottitis usually is abrupt with symptoms of fever, toxicity, air hunger, difficulty swallowing, excess secretions, and anxiety. Stridor is an associated finding, but the barking cough of croup is usually absent. When the clinical circumstances are unclear, radiographic evaluation is diagnostic.

Radiographic changes of epiglottitis are usually limited to the epiglottis and aryepiglottic folds. The normal, thin, slightly curved epiglottis is replaced by a rounded thumblike structure, and the aryepiglottic folds are swollen and often ill-defined (Figures 17-6

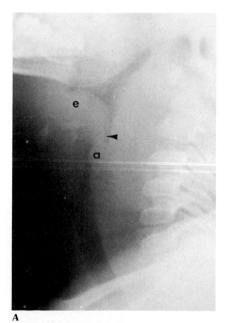

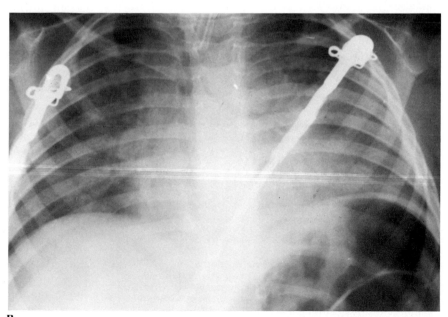

A   B

Figure 17-7 Supraglottitis—pulmonary edema. A. The lateral airway exposure shows swelling of the epiglottis (e) and aryepiglottic folds (arrowhead). (a = arytenoid cartilage.) **B.** The intrapulmonary vascular shadows and heart borders have lost their clear identity, signs of excess parenchymal fluid. This cleared following relief of upper airway obstruction (see Chapter 16).

and 17-7). The remaining laryngeal structures may also be swollen to a mild degree.

Extensive manipulation of patients suspected of epiglottitis and repeated attempts to obtain near-perfect films should be avoided. Needless to say, these patients must be closely observed throughout their radiographic studies and removed from the department as soon as diagnostic studies are obtained.

Enlargement of the epiglottic and aryepiglottic folds is not pathognomonic of acute epiglottitis. McCook et al.[24] emphasize close contact and coordination with the clinician. Normal variation, angioneurotic edema, tumors, and trauma are a few conditions which may simulate acute epiglottitis (Figure 17-8; see also Chapter 13, Figure 13-11).

Foreign Bodies

Children of all ages aspirate foreign bodies. The well-known "cafe coronary," in which chunks of food,

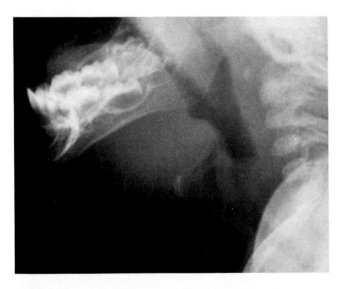

Figure 17-8 Lymphangioma. The epiglottis and submandibular soft tissues are invaded by a cavernous lymphangioma. The aryepiglottic folds are not markedly thickened. This dangerous-appearing radiograph was not associated with any respiratory distress, and the child has been followed for several years without progression. This patient and the one illustrated in Figure 13-11 suggest that the acuteness of the epiglottic swelling and associated inflammation must play a role in causing obstruction to airflow.

usually meat, lodge in the larynx or trachea, occasionally causes asphyxia in adults. Aspirated foreign bodies account for approximately 500 deaths per year in children under 5 years of age.[25] Peanuts are notorious unwanted inhabitants of the tracheobronchial tree. Figure 13-4, in Chapter 13, shows a few of the 3179 objects removed by the famous Philadelphia bronchoscopists, Chevalier Jackson and Chevalier L. Jackson, in a span of 45 years.[26]

A child's natural habit of placing objects in the mouth leads to the passage of these materials into the trachea and bronchial tree. Infants and toddlers are most prone to aspirate solid objects, but older children who habitually chew on weeds and similar vegetable matter are likely to have this matter enter the lungs. A history of sudden choking and cough followed by respiratory distress should suggest the possibility of an aspirated foreign object. In some cases a period of relative well-being may intervene, before the onset of wheezing, dyspnea, and occasional cyanosis.

Foreign bodies in the larynx may produce one or more of the following symptoms: hoarseness, croupy cough, aphonia, dysphagia, hemoptysis, wheezing, dyspnea, or cyanosis. Attempts at manual removal of aspirated foreign bodies are associated with significant risk of increased, occasionally fatal, airway obstruction.

Tracheal foreign bodies may produce several clinical signs: (1) "audible slap," (2) "palpable thud," and (3) "asthmatoid wheeze."[26] "Tracheal flutter" occasionally accompanies aspirated watermelon seed.

Careful auscultation of the chest is extremely important, since radiographic changes may be subtle or nonexistent. In cases where the object remains loose in the trachea or a major bronchus, the stethoscope may outperform the roentgen ray. Swallowed objects may become lodged in the esophagus, impinge on the trachea, and cause respiratory obstruction.[27] Occasionally, hemoptysis will be the presenting symptom, or a lesion may be discovered on chest film taken for other reasons. In most cases, the exact time of aspiration cannot be determined.

The majority of aspirated foreign bodies are nonopaque; radiographic changes result from various degrees of airway obstruction. With careful

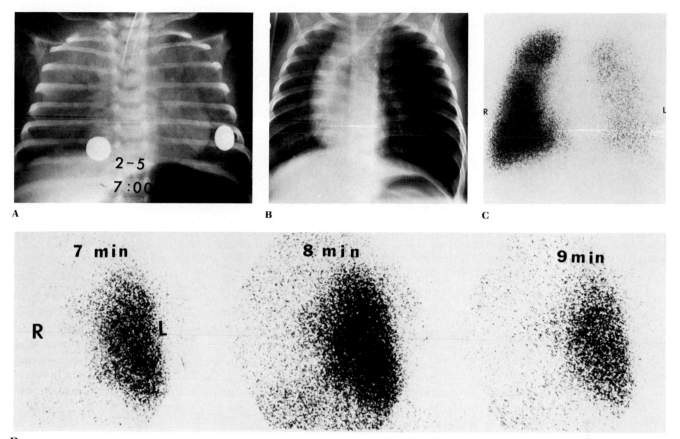

D

Figure 17-9   Foreign body—radionuclide evaluation. A. This 6-month-old child suffered a respiratory arrest at home in the early morning. The initial chest film shows a diffuse alveolar process, probably edema. **B.** After a prolonged hospitalization, including a negative bronchoscopy, she was discharged. Persistent overaeration of the left lung over the ensuing 6 months initiated repeat evaluation. **C.** The perfusion lung scan shows markedly diminished flow to the left lung. **D.** The xenon washout scan shows trapping in the left lung at 7, 8, and 9 min. A sandspur was removed from the left stem bronchus.

plain-film technique, using supplemental projections, fluoroscopy, and occasional xeroradiography, foreign bodies within the trachea and proximal stem bronchus may be identified.[28] Computed tomography is an additional method used to locate nonopaque objects.[29] Radionuclide perfusion and ventilation scans are of value in isolated cases but are probably unnecessary most of the time (Figure 17-9).[30]

Plain-film findings of foreign body aspiration are produced by airflow obstruction since most of the offending objects are nonopaque. The task of detecting these objects is compounded by the multiplicity

of potential radiographic configurations and by the transient changes that frequently occur.

Objects that partially obstruct a stem or major bronchus usually cause hyperaeration of the peripheral lung (spread ribs, depressed hemidiaphragm, and contralateral mediastinal shift; see Figures 17-9 and 17-10). These changes are exaggerated during expiration, a fact that justifies the use of inspiration-expiration films when there is suspicion of an aspirated foreign body.

Fluoroscopic evaluation of the diaphragmatic and mediastinal excursions is also helpful in troublesome cases. When fluoroscopy is not available,

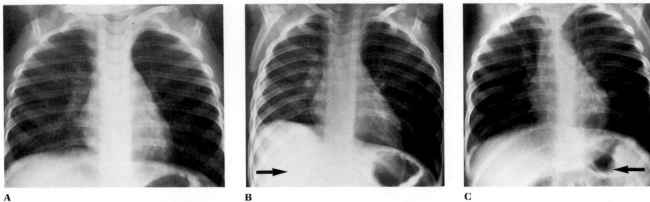

A   **B**   **C**

Figure 17-10   Foreign body—decubitus views. A. The left lung is hyperaerated following an episode suggesting foreign body aspiration. **B.** When placed in the right-side-down decubitus position, the dependent right hemidiaphragm elevates and the right lung empties normally. **C.** In the left-side-down position, the left hemidiaphragm remains depressed; the lung cannot empty normally because of a partial obstruction in the left stem bronchus. A foreign body was removed from the left stem bronchus.

decubitus chest films on a hard surface may be diagnostic (Figure 17-10).[31] With this technique, a normal dependent lung will empty its air as gravitational forces cause the abdominal contents to push against the hemidiaphragm. In the presence of partial bronchial obstruction, the hemidiaphragm on the affected side will not rise with the patient in the ipsilateral decubitus position. This method is not foolproof; the patient must be placed on a hard surface when the decubitus film is exposed.

Complete obstruction of a bronchus by a foreign body most often leads to collapse of the distal lung. Rarely, the distal parenchyma fills with fluid and presents as an overexpanded, opaque lobe. On occasion, a localized pneumothorax forms about a segment of lung that has collapsed from obstruction by a foreign body or mucous plug (Figure 17-11).[32] Air extravastion may also result from aspirated foreign bodies (Figure 17-12).

One consequence of chronic atelectasis from bronchial obstruction is secondary infection, with peripheral bronchiectasis and abscess formation. More often, the lung remains unaerated until the obstruction is removed, but permanent damage may result from inordinate delays (see Figure 15-3).

Bronchiectasis may occur following aspirated inert foreign objects that are not removed. Vegetal matter, especially peanuts, causes an intense inflamma-

tory reaction within the lung and bronchial mucosa in addition to changes of obstruction (Figure 17-13). Rapid development of purulent exudates and mucopus may become evident to the bronchoscopist trying to remove the foreign matter. Severe hemoptysis is an additional complication of vegetal bronchitis.

Tumors of the Laryngotracheobronchial Tree

Tumors of the laryngotracheobronchial tree are uncommon in childhood. Most are benign but may be life-threatening because of their size, location, and obstruction to airflow.

Included among benign tumors in children are the laryngeal papilloma, hemangioma, granular cell tumor (myoblastoma), neurogenic tumor, mucous gland adenoma, and chondromatous hamartoma. Usually located in the larynx, trachea, or major bronchi, they rarely cause problems in microscopic interpretation.[33] Neurogenic tumors are extremely rare solitary lesions found in the bronchus or parenchyma.[34] Mucous gland adenomas are pedunculated endobronchial tumors that consist of tightly packed

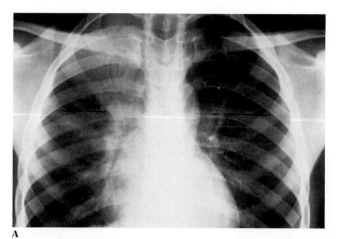
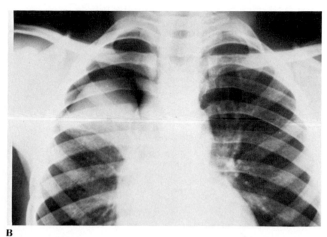

A   B

Figure 17-11   Bronchial obstruction—pneumothorax. **A.** The right upper lobe is partially collapsed in this child with bronchial asthma. **B.** The following day the collapsed right upper lobe is surrounded by a halo of air in the apex of the chest. Several days later, with conservative management, the lungs returned to normal and the pneumothorax resolved. The negative pressure created by the collapsed lung is probably responsible for the "leakage" of air into the thorax; this same phenomenon has been reported in association with bronchial obstruction—especially from a foreign body.[32]

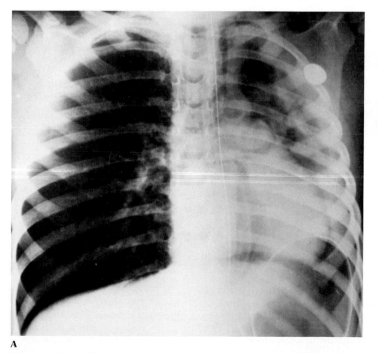
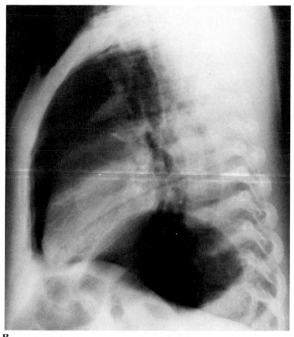

A   B

Figure 17-12   Foreign body—air leak. **A** and **B.** The pneumothorax and pneumomediastinum have developed following the aspiration of a foreign body. The presence of an extensive air leak and respiratory distress suggests asthma and similar diseases, but a foreign body should be considered in the differential diagnosis. (Courtesy of Dr. Webster Riggs, Memphis, Tennessee.)

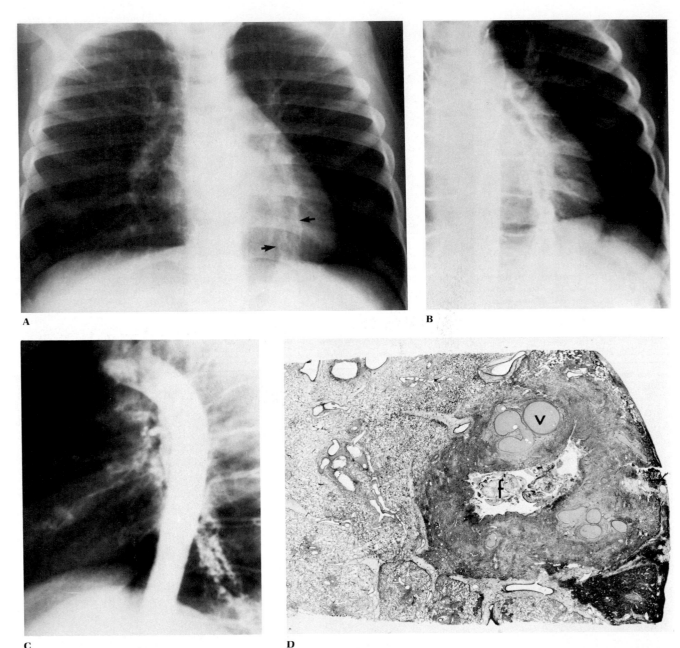

Figure 17-13 Vegetal bronchitis—hemoptysis. This 4-year-old girl with repeated hemoptysis, requiring up to two to three units of blood replacement, had no history of foreign body ingestion. **A.** Several linear opacities, extending from the hilum to the left hemidiaphragm, are visible through the cardiac shadow (arrows). **B** and **C.** Aortography shows these to be dilated, tortuous vessels arising from the descending aorta and supplying the posterior-medial lung. **D.** A lung wedge resection was performed. Barium perfusion of the specimen vessels shows distended, tortuous vessels (v) around and within the chronically inflamed, ectatic bronchus. Within the granulomatous reaction is a vegetal fragment (f).

mucin-producing glands.[35] Chondromatous hamartomas are also rare in children, but occasional cases have been reported.[36] Papilloma, hemangioma, granular cell myoblastoma, and several "bronchial adenoma" tumors will be considered in greater detail.

Juvenile Laryngeal Papilloma-Papillomatosis

Squamous papillomas are the most common laryngeal tumors in older infants and children.[37,38] Occasional adults have been reported with multiple lesions.[39] The cause of these tumors is not known, but the tendency for them to disappear at puberty suggests a hormonal relationship.[40] Other theories include inflammation, congenital malformation, trauma, and metaplasia.[36]

A viral etiology for papilloma has been advanced.[41,42] The majority of children with juvenile laryngeal papilloma-papillomatosis (JLP) have mothers with a history of genital warts (condylomata acuminata) during pregnancy.[43] Transmission of the virus from mother to child during delivery with development of the tumor after years of latency has been postulated.

Clinical presentation and symptoms depend on tumor location and extent. Hoarseness is the most common early complaint while the lesions remain localized to the laryngeal area. Squamous papillomas usually remain solitary or multiple within the larynx, but may spread to the trachea and beyond. Approximately 2 percent disseminate throughout the bronchial tree and pulmonary parenchyma.[44]

The onset of wheezing, stridor, and progressive dyspnea signals spread to the trachea and bronchi. Cough, at first dry and later productive, often accompanies the progress of the disease. Increasing obstruction of the major airways may cause terminal asphyxia in some patients unless a diversion can be accomplished. Spontaneous regression during adolescence usually occurs, although occasional malignant degeneration has been reported.[45]

The radiographic appearance of papillomatosis

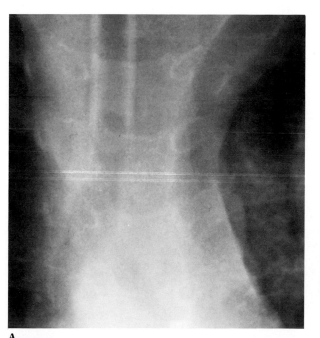 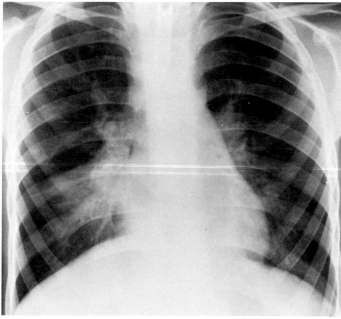

A   B

Figure 17-14   Juvenile laryngeal papillomatosis. A. The airway films show irregular margins of the trachea and stem bronchi. Papillomas are not evident. **B.** Dissemination into the lung has caused right middle lobe atelectasis and chronic changes in the left lower lobe.

depends upon the size and distribution of the lesions. They appear as irregular filling defects in the area of the larynx and trachea (Figure 17-14). Good-quality films of the trachea and stem bronchi, exposed for air column technique, will often show the intraluminal lesions.[1] Xeroradiography and tomography are also useful. Positive-contrast bronchography is unnecessary and should be avoided.

Secondary changes within the lung fields may result from lesions located in critical areas of the bronchial tree or parenchyma. Atelectasis, abscesses, localized aeration disturbances, bronchiectasis, and emphysema are all reported complications (Figure 17-14B).

Disseminated lesions may appear as diffuse nodular opacities. These frequently cavitate and show as cystic lesions (Figure 17-15).[37,46] These small cavities are usually not associated with systemic symptoms. Several studies advocate the use of CT for better delineation of the pulmonary dissemination of JLP.[43,47]

This technique may discover lesions not visible on plain films. (See Chapter 26, Figure 26-55.)

Histologic verification of papillomas cannot be made without biopsy. Microscopically, they consist of thin vascular stalks covered by layers of well-differentiated transitional or stratified squamous epithelium. Malignant change is rare in childhood but has occurred in 3 of 15 patients reported by Kawanami.[48]

Hemangioma

Hemangioma is the most common laryngeal and upper tracheal tumor in the newborn and young infant.[49] Females are affected more than males by about 2.5 to 1; and approximately one-half of all patients have associated cutaneous hemangiomas.

These lesions may cause respiratory distress in the immediate neonatal period, but symptoms are usually delayed for several weeks to months.[50] Re-

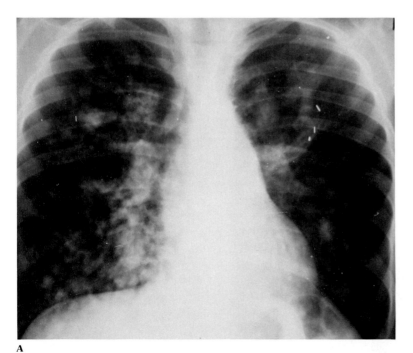
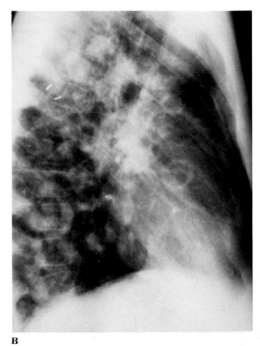

A   **B**

Figure 17-15   Juvenile papillomatosis—pulmonary spread. This 5-year-old boy had intermittent respiratory distress for 2 years. A laryngeal biopsy revealed JLP. He was treated on several occasions with local resection. The initial chest films were normal, **A** and **B**. Later films show the development of diffuse nodular and cystic lesions with both thick and thin walls. Lung biopsy revealed benign papillomatous tumor tissue identical to the laryngeal lesions. (Courtesy of Dr. Marvin S. Kogutt, New Orleans, Louisiana.)

spiratory difficulty and laryngeal stridor are the most troublesome symptoms; cyanosis, cough, dysphonia, and dysphagia are less common. Asphyxia and death may result from growth or engorgement of hemangiomas.[51] The presence of airway hemangiomas is not always apparent from the clinical picture, however; 12 of 24 patients in one series died of respiratory failure, and 9 were diagnosed post mortem.[48]

Subglottic hemangioma is frequently inaccessible to the bronchoscopist because of its position below the vocal cords. Good-quality radiographs of the airway are extremely important in the evaluation of patients suspected of hemangioma (Figure 17-16). Fluoroscopic studies should supplement plain films when the diagnosis is in doubt. Frontal projection views using high-voltage-magnification films are the most productive.

Tracheostomy may be necessary in these patients but should be undertaken with care lest a low-lying lesion be traumatized. In time, hemangiomas

usually resolve spontaneously, but steroid administration may help accelerate this process. Cryotherapy and carbon dioxide laser therapy have been used in the treatment of subglottic hemangiomas.[52]

Granular Cell Myoblastoma (Schwannoma)

This is a distinctive lesion that occurs as a discrete, firm, slow-growing mass in the dermis or beneath mucosal surfaces.[53] The lesions have been shown to arise from Schwann cells[54] and are most common in the tongue, upper respiratory tract, stomach, and biliary tree.

Symptoms usually result from impingement on the tracheal air column; wheezing, labored respiration, and dyspnea on exertion are presenting symptoms. The lesion may present as a rounded, sessile, or protuberant mass extending into the tracheal air column (Figure 17-17). Surgical excision of granular cell myoblastoma is usually curative.

Primary malignant tumors of the tracheobronchial tree are extremely rare in childhood. Most are metastatic,[55] but numerous primary carcinomas have been reported, including epidermoid, adenocarcinoma large cell, undifferentiated, and small cell carcinoma.[56]

Bronchial Carcinoid (Adenoma)

The term *bronchial adenoma* has been abandoned because of the recognition that these lesions are, in reality, low-grade malignant lesions. Bronchial carcinoid tumors account for approximately 4 percent of lung tumors in adults and are found even more often in children.[57,58] Carcinoids are related to the so-called amine precursor uptake decarboxylase group of tumors. These are malignant neuroectodermal tumors of the Kulchitsky cell, closely related to the oat cell.

Prognosis is largely dependent upon the location and extent of metastases at the time of discovery. Local resection is usually curative.[57,59]

Adenocystic Basal Cell Carcinoma (Cylindroma)

Adenocystic carcinoma is most aggressive. At the time of discovery, local invasion is present in 71 per-

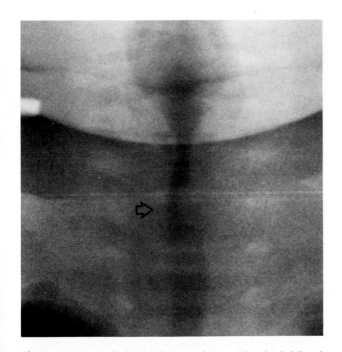

Figure 17-16 Subglottic hemangioma. This high-kilovolt-magnification frontal projection shows a left-sided ovoid density projecting into the subglottic tracheal lumen (arrow).

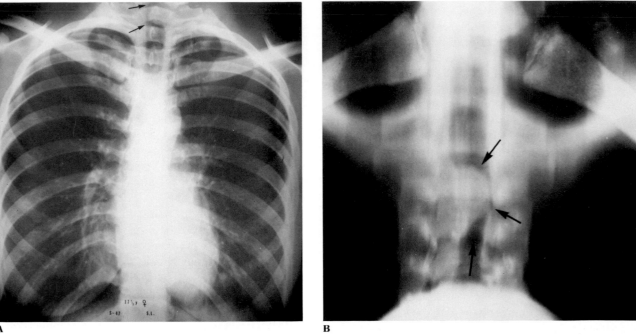

A **B**

Figure 17-17   Granular cell myoblastoma. A. The lungs are markedly hyperaerated as a result of the tracheal mass (arrows). **B.** A large, rounded mass is visible projecting into the tracheal lumen (arrows). (From Hicks GM: Two cases of tracheal abnormality in teenagers presenting as obstructive lung disease. *Ann Radiol* 19:7781, 1976.)

cent of cases, metastases to regional nodes is found in 47 percent, and distant lymphatic involvement is evident in 29 percent. In approximately 29 percent of the cases, the tumor will recur locally after resection, and the 5-year survival rate is only 25 percent.[60] There is debate in the literature regarding the commonest location of this tumor, but most are found in the right lung within reach of biopsy by bronchoscopy.

Mucoepidermoid Tumors

Mucoepidermoid tumors are extremely rare. They tend to occur in the trachea and are predominantly polypoid and intraluminal. Large mucin-secreting columnar cells form glands, ducts, and small cysts along with nonkeratinizing squamous epithelium. These tumors do not invade locally or metastasize via lymphatics. Survival is generally excellent with adequate surgical removal.[61,62]

The radiographic presentation of tracheal tumors will depend largely upon their size, location, and histologic character. While some patients with tracheobronchial tumors have normal radiographs, most develop changes resulting from partial or complete bronchial obstruction. Of 72 patients reported by Lawson et al., 53 presented with findings of atelectasis or consolidation, 13 had a discrete opacity, and 3 contained calcium.[63] Bronchiectasis beyond the point of obstruction was found in 25 patients.

Tracheal tumors may also present as well-defined, discrete opacities with little or no surrounding reaction.[64] Because of the proclivity of the tumors for the larger bronchi and trachea, bronchography may be necessary for the definitive localization of the lesion (Figure 17-18),[65] although CT and nuclear magnetic resonance are also capable of defining tracheal tumors. Peripheral bronchiectasis when present may also be defined with bronchography. A definite histologic diagnosis cannot be made from radio-

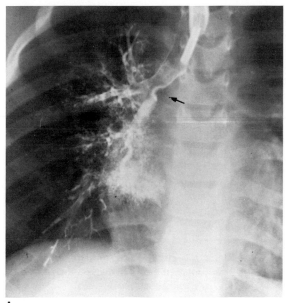

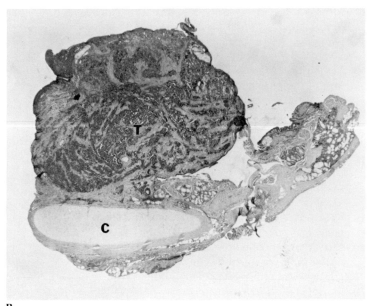

A   B

Figure 17-18   Bronchial adenoma. **A.** The bronchogram reveals the presence of a sessile mass in the right stem bronchus (arrow). **B.** The tumor was excised rather than biopsied. The tumor nodule (T) is firmly attached to the bronchial wall and adjacent cartilage (C).

graphic examination alone; thus bronchoscopy is usually the diagnostic method of choice when there is a suspicion of an endobronchial obstruction.

References

1. Joseph PM, Berdon WE, Baker DH, et al: Airway obstruction in infants and children. *Radiology* 121:143, 1976.

2. Wolfe JN: Xeroradiography: Image content and comparison with film roentgenograms. *AJR* 117:690, 1973.

3. Smith C, Ramsey RG: Xeroradiography of the lateral neck. *Radiographics* 2:306, 1982.

4. Slovis TL, Renfro B, Watts FB, et al: Choanal atresia: Precise CT evaluation. *Radiology* 155:345, 1985.

5. Griscom NT: Computed tomographic determination of tracheal dimensions in children and adolescents. *Radiology* 145:361, 1982.

6. Breatnach E, Abbott GC, Fraser RG: Dimensions of the normal human trachea. *Am J Radiol* 141:903, 1984.

7. Gamsu G, Webb RW: Computed tomography of the trachea: Normal and abnormal. *AJR* 139:321, 1982.

8. Berdon WE, Baker DH, Wung JT, et al: Complete cartilage-ring tracheal stenosis associated with anomalous left pulmonary artery: The ring-sling complex. *Radiology* 152:57, 1984.

9. Kirks DR, Fram EK, Vock P: Tracheal compression by mediastinal masses in children: CT evaluation. *AJR* 141:647, 1983.

10. Mandell GA, Lantieri R, Goodman LR: Tracheobronchial compression in Hodgkin's lymphoma in children. *AJR* 139:1167, 1982.

11. Holinger CD: The etiology of stridor in the neonate, infant, and child. *Ann Otol Rhinol Laryngol* 83:397, 1980.

12. Meyer CM, Cotton RT: Nasal obstruction in the pediatric patient. *Pediatrics* 72:766, 1983.

13. Ferguson C, Kendig E (eds): *Pediatric Otolaryngology* Philadelphia, WB Saunders, 1972, vol II, p 166.

14. Williams JL, Capitanio MA, Turtz MG: Vocal cord paralysis: Radiologic observations in 21 infants and young children. *AJR* 128:649, 1977.

15. Quinn-Bogard AL, Potsic WP: Stridor in the first year of life. *Clin Pediatr* 16:913, 1977.

16. Smith RJ, Catlin FL: Congenital abnormalities of the larynx. *Am J Dis Child* 138:35, 1984.

17. Benjamin B: Congenital laryngeal webs. *Ann Otol Rhinol Laryngol* 92:317, 1983.

18. Capitanio MA, Wolfson BJ, Faerber EN, et al: Obstruction of the airway by the aorta: An observation in infants with congenital heart disease. *AJR* 140:675, 1983.

19. Liston SL, Gehrz RC, Siegel LG: Bacterial tracheitis. *Am J Dis Child* 137:764, 1983.

20. Denny JC, Handler SD: Membranous laryngotracheobronchitis. *Pediatrics* 70:705, 1982.

21. Han BK, Dunbar JS, Striker TW: Membranous laryngotracheobronchitis (membranous croup). *AJR* 133:53, 1979.

22. Nelson WE: Bacterial croup: A historical perspective. *J Pediatr* 105:52, 1984.

23. Currarino G, William B: Lateral inspiration and expiration radiographs of the neck in children with laryngotracheitis (croup). *Radiology* 145:365, 1982.

24. McCook TA, Kirks DR: Epiglottic enlargement in infants and children: Another radiologic look. *Pediatr Radiol* 12:227, 1982.

25. *Accident Facts*. Chicago, National Safety Council, 1980, p 7.

26. Jackson C, Jackson CL: Foreign bodies in the air and food passages and vegetal bronchitis, in Brennemann and McQuarrie (eds): *Practice of Pediatrics*. Hagerstown, Md, WF Prior Inc, 1952, chap 56, p 1.

27. Smith PC, Swischuk LE, Fagan CJ: An elusive and often unsuspected cause of stridor or pneumonia (the esophageal foreign body). *AJR* 122:178, 1974.

28. Doust BD, Ying YM, Chuang VP: Detection of aspirated foreign bodies with xeroradiography. *Radiology* 111:725, 1974.

29. Berger PE, Kuhn JP, Kuhns LR: Computed tomography and the occult tracheobronchial foreign body. *Radiology* 134:133, 1980.

30. Leonidas JC, Stuber JL, Rudavsky AZ, et al: Radionuclide lung scanning of endobronchial foreign bodies in children. *J Pediatr* 83:678, 1973.

31. Capitanio MA, Kirkpatrick JA Jr: The lateral decubitus film. An aid in determining air-trapping in children. *Radiology* 103:460, 1972.

32. Berdon WE, Dee GJ, Abramson SJ, et al: Localized pneumothorax adjacent to a collapsed lobe: A sign of bronchial obstruction. *Radiology* 150:691, 1984.

33. Dehner LP, *Pediatric Surgical Pathology*, St Louis, CV Mosby, 1975, p 223.

34. Bartley TD, Arian VM: Intrapulmonary neurogenic tumors. *J Thorac Cardiovasc Surg* 50:14, 1965.

35. Emory WB, Mitchell WT Jr, Hotch HB Jr: Mucous gland adenoma of the bronchus. *Am Rev Respir Dis* 108:1408, 1973.

36. Poirer TJ, Van Oredstrand HS: Pulmonary chondromatous hamartomas. Report of seventeen cases and review of the literature. *Chest* 59:50, 1971.

37. Rosenbaum HD, Alavi SM, Bryant LR: Pulmonary parenchymal spread of juvenile laryngeal papillomatosis. *Radiology* 90:654, 1968.

38. Fagan CJ, Swischuk LE: Juvenile laryngeal papillomatosis with spread to the lung. *Am J Dis Child* 123:139, 1972.

39. Greenfield H, Herman PG: Papillomatosis of the trachea and bronchi in 3 adults. *AJR* 89:45, 1963.

40. Brooks JW: in Kendig EL Jr, Chernick V (eds): *Disorders of the Respiratory Tract in Children*. Philadelphia, WB Saunders, 1977, p 699.

41. Cohen SR, Geller KA, Seltzer S, et al: Papilloma of the larynx and tracheobronchial tree in children: A retrospective study. *Ann Otol* 89:497, 1980.

42. McCabe BF, Clark KF: Interferon and laryngeal papillomatosis: The Iowa experience. *Ann Otol Rhinol Laryngol* 92:2, 1983.

43. Borkowsky W, Martin D, Lawrence S: Juvenile laryngeal papillomatosis with pulmonary spread. *Am J Dis Child* 138:667, 1984.

44. Singer DB, Greenberg SD, Harrison GM: Papillomatosis of the lung. *Am Rev Respir Dis* 94:777, 1966.

45. Ogilvie OE: Multiple papillomas of the trachea with malignant degeneration—A report of 2 cases. *AMA Arch Otolaryngol* 58:10, 1953.

46. Smith A, Gooding CA: Pulmonary involvement in laryngeal papillomatosis. *Pediatr Radiol* 2:161, 1974.

47. Kramer SS, Wehunt WD, Stocker JT, et al: Pulmonary manifestations of juvenile laryngotracheal papillomatosis. *AJR* 144:687, 1985.

48. Kawanami T, Bowen A: Juvenile laryngeal papillomatosis with pulmonary parenchymal spread. A case report and review of the literature. *Pediatr Radiol* 15:102, 1985.

49. Swischuk LE, Smith PC, Fagan CJ: Abnormalities of the pharynx and larynx in childhood. *Semin Roentgenol* 9:283, 1974.

50. Christiaens L, Decroix G, Gaudier B, et al: Hemangiomas of the larynx and of the trachea in infants. *Arch Fr Pediatr* 22:513, 1965.

51. Askin FB: in Kissane JM (ed): *Pathology of Infancy and Childhood*, 2d ed. St Louis CV Mosby, 1975, p 463.

52. Adzik NS, Strome M, Gang D, et al: Cryotherapy in subglottic hemangioma. *J Pediatr Surg* 19:353, 1984.

53. Dehner LP: in Kissane JM (ed): *Pathology of Infancy and Childhood*, 2d ed. St Louis, CV Mosby, 1975, p 1167.

54. Bargle R Jr: An early granular-cell myoblastoma confined within a small peripheral myelinated nerve. *Cancer* 6:790, 1953.

55. Kilman JW, Kronenberg MW, O'Neill JA, et al: Surgical resections for pulmonary metastases in children. *Arch Surg* 99:158, 1969.

56. Niitu Y, Kubota H, Hasegawa S, et al: Lung cancer (squamous cell carcinoma) in adolescence. *Am J Dis Child* 127:108, 1974.

57. Hurt R, Bates M: Carcinoid tumours of the bronchus: A 33 year experience. *Thorax* 39:617, 1984.

58. Wellons HA, Eggleston P, Golden GT, et al: Bronchial adenoma in childhood. Two case reports and review of the literature. *Am J. Dis Child* 130:301, 1976.

59. McCaughan BC, Martini N, Bains MS: Bronchial carcinoids. Review of 124 cases. *J Thorac Cardiovasc Surg* 89:8, 1985.

60. Goldstraw P, Lauch D, McCormack RJM, et al: The malignancy of bronchial adenoma. *J Thorac Cardiovasc Surg* 72:309, 1976.

61. Markel SF, Abell MR, Haight C, et al: Neoplasms of the bronchus commonly designated as adenoma. *Cancer* 17:590, 1964.

62. Nakagawara A, Ikeda K, Ohgami H: Mucoepidermoid tumor of the bronchus in an infant. *J Pediatr Surg* 14:608, 1979.

63. Lawson RM, Ramanathan L, Hurley G, et al: Bronchial adenoma: Review of an 18 year experience at the Brompton Hospital. *Thorax* 31:245, 1976.

64. Knesevitch EM, McCormack LJ, Effler DB, et al: Bronchial adenoma: Clinicopathological study of 21 cases. *Clev Clin Q* 24:160, 1937.

65. Templeton AW, Moffat R, Nelson D: Bronchography and bronchial adenomas. *Chest* 59:59, 1971.

Pulmonary Infections and Infestations

Antibiotic treatment has altered the relationship of infectious agents that cause pneumonia. Mycoplasma and viruses have assumed the dominant roles in outpatient pneumonia;[1] bacteria and fungi remain significant in hospitalized patients. Secondary infections with a host of opportunistic organisms are gaining in importance as transplant and chemotherapeutic modalities develop.

Unlike the previous section where several different roentgenographic patterns of pulmonary disease were considered, this section will review lung infections according to their respective etiologies. In many, there is considerable overlap of the radiographic pictures.[2] Nevertheless, certain roentgenographic features often distinguish one infection from another, and their clinical and pathologic presentations are frequently characteristic.

References

1. Murphy TF, Henderson FW, Clyde WA Jr, et al: Pneumonia: An 11-year study in a pediatric practice. *Am J Epidemiol* 113:12, 1981.
2. McCarthy PL, Spiesel SZ, Stashwick CA, et al: Radiographic findings and etiologic diagnosis in ambulatory childhood pneumonias. *Clin Pediatr* 20:686, 1981.

Chapter 18

Bacterial Infections

This chapter will review the clinical and radiologic manifestations of several bacterial pneumonias that affect children. Staphylococcal pneumonia, along with complications of empyema, pneumatocele formation, and lung abscess, is considered in greater detail. Other bacterial pneumonias, i.e., pneumococcus and streptococcus, are not considered as extensively since their radiographic expressions are not unique and their distinguishing clinical and bacteriologic characteristics are well covered in textbooks on pediatric pulmonology and infectious disease. Space is devoted to some rare and obscure but occasionally bothersome pneumonias, i.e., tularemia, melioidosis, legionella, and *Pasteurella pestis.*

Staphylococcal Pneumonia

Staphylococcal pneumonia was quite prevalent in the preantibiotic era and recurred in epidemic form in the late 1950s and early 1960s. Since then, the incidence has diminished, but occasional cases continue to surface.

Staphylococcus aureus (Micrococcus pyogenes) is the most ubiquitous pathogen to which people are exposed. Most infections are superficial, but the organism has a tendency to develop resistance to antibiotic agents and cause debilitating and life-threatening disease. Staphylococcal pneumonia causes severe morbidity in children as well as adults, and significant mortality, particularly in newborn infants. In epidemics, antibiotic-resistant staphylococci may invade hospitals and nurseries and colonize both patients and hospital personnel.

Adults, especially postpartum mothers, develop abscesses in the breast and other areas of the body. Newborns are colonized in the nurseries from other infants or adults carrying the organism on nasal membranes and skin, and they, in turn, are victimized by skin infections and pneumonia. Eradication of the carrier state in both infants and adults is extremely difficult, if not impossible.

Primary staphylococcal pneumonia, while most threatening to the very young and very old, is more common in older children. The florid fastigium, so frequently fatal during epidemics, is now infrequent. However, complications such as empyema, abscess, and pyopneumothorax are not uncommon.

Secondary staphylococcal infections sometimes complicate other lung disease and are especially dangerous during epidemics of viral pneumonia.[1-3] Staphylococcal infections also complicate the course of illness in debilitated, immunosuppressed, and immunodeficient patients, as well as organ transplant recipients. Patients with cystic fibrosis and other forms of chronic and acute lung disease are notoriously susceptible to invasion by staphylococcus.[4]

The clinical presentation of staphylococcal pneumonia is often deceptive. Frequently, the pulmonary disease is overshadowed by systemic symptoms such as abdominal distension, paralytic ileus, vomiting, diarrhea, and generalized toxicity. Upper respiratory infection, followed by sudden onset of pallor and dyspnea, is a frequent history, particularly in infants with skin infections, and paronychias, and in homes of infected family members.

Radiologic Findings

The chest roentgenogram early in the course of staphylococcal pneumonia may appear deceptively benign; generalized overaeration may be the only significant feature. This is often followed by rapid progression to segmental, lobar, or multilobar consolidations, pleural effusion, pneumatocele formation, and pneumothorax (Figures 18-1 and 18-2).[5-7] In a series of 329 patients with staphylococcal pneumonia, Rebhan and Edwards[8] found infiltration in 83 percent, pleural effusion in 55 percent, pneumothorax in 21 percent, and pneumatocele in 13 percent of patients. An expanded discussion of staphylococcal pneumonia (empyema, infected pneumatoceles, and lung abscess) follows in the segment on empyema.

Systemic pulmonary emboli are occasionally associated with staphylococcal infections in other areas of the body, especially in the bones, joints, and soft tissues (Figure 18-3).[9] The primary source of infection and emboli may be overlooked in the face of the patient's general illness and extreme toxicity. The lungs characteristically develop multiple, poorly marginated, nodular lesions of 1- to 2-cm diameter. The nodules may remain discrete, or they may rapidly cavitate and coalesce into consolidations. Pleural effusion and empyema are additional roentgenographic features. The occurrence of this evolving pulmonary pattern in a septic child should initiate a search for a distant source of infection, often in a bone or joint.

Empyema, Lung Abscess, and Pneumatoceles

A discussion of pneumonia, especially staphylococcal pneumonia, would not be complete without a review of empyema and abscess. Empyema occurs almost invariably as a complication of underlying pulmonary inflammation, a condition that may be obscured by overlying fluid (Figure 18-4). Bacterial infections, both anaerobic and aerobic, are the most likely generators of pleural infection. Bartlett and Finegold,[10] in a study of 143 cases of anaerobic infection, found empyema as a complication in 47, lung abscess in 45, and one or the other in 69 cases. Among anaerobic organisms responsible for empyema are:

Microaerophilic streptococcus
Fusobacterium nucleatum
Bacteroides melaninogenicus
Bacteroides fragilis
Peptococcus
Peptostreptococcus
Gram-positive bacilli

Staphylococcus is the most common etiologic agent in primary empyema, although streptococcus has assumed a greater role and now accounts for more cases than pneumococcus.[11] In addition to staphylococcus, aerobic empyema-producing organisms include:

Hemophilus influenzae type B
Streptococcus pneumoniae
Pseudomonas aeruginosa
Klebsiella
Escherichia coli

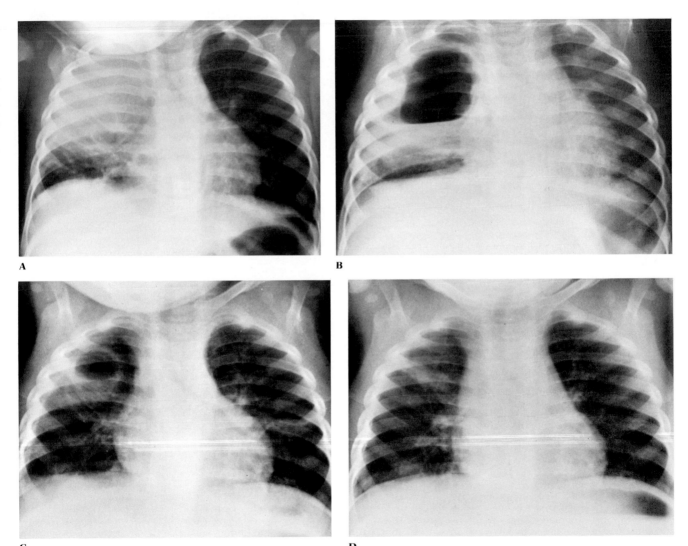

A   B

C   D

Figure 18-1   Staphylococcal pneumonia. A. The initial film shows a large, homogeneous, right upper lobe consolidation with patchy infiltrates elsewhere. The lobe appears expanded, but no pleural reaction is apparent. **B.** Two weeks later the process has been replaced by a large cavitary lesion with pleural reaction. This does not necessarily represent a lung abscess but is more likely an infected pneumatocele. **C.** Three weeks later, with no surgical drainage, there is marked improvement. **D.** One month later, the lung is almost normal.

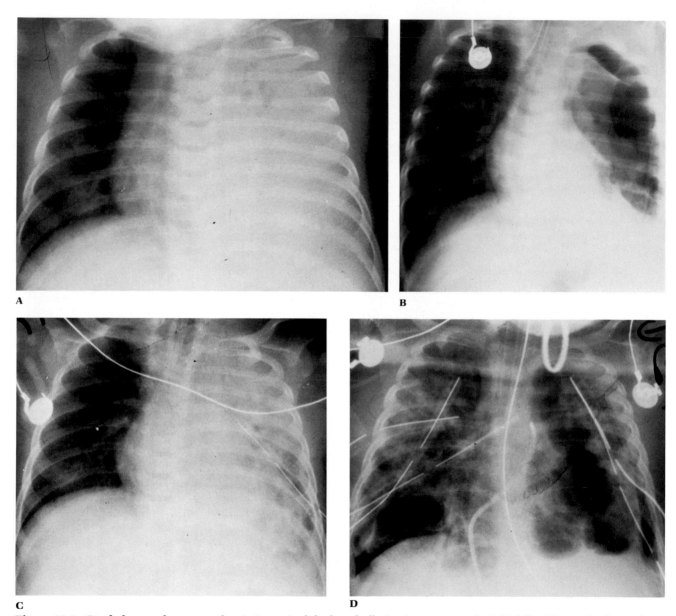

A

B

C

D

Figure 18-2   Staphylococcal pneumonia. A. A massive left pleural effusion is present on the initial film. The tracheal air column is shifted to the right, and the lucencies in the left upper hemithorax may represent early pneumothorax. Pleural effusion of this degree will mask the underlying pneumonic process. (*Note:* A decubitus projection is of no use in this case. Ultrasonography is the diagnostic study of choice.) **B.** A tension pyopneumothorax is now apparent several hours later. **C.** Tube drainage was established 4 h later. **D.** Twenty-nine days later a film shows diffuse lung destruction with pneumatoceles, pneumothoraxes, and 9 tubes of varying types. The child died shortly thereafter.

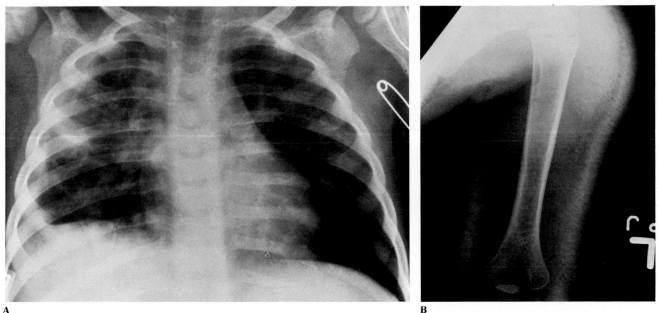

A   **B**

Figure 18-3 Sepsis and osteomyelitis. A. This film shows a right pleural effusion and coalescent opacities throughout the right lung. Thin-walled circular structures represent residua of preexisting nodular lesions and most likely represent subpleural pneumatoceles. All changes subsequently disappear, and the lungs return to normal. **B.** Extensive soft tissue swelling is evident; the underlying bone is normal. Osteomyelitis was proved on bone biopsy. (From Felman and Shulman,[9] with permission.)

The clinical symptoms of empyema depend upon several factors: (1) etiologic agent, (2) severity and extent of disease, (3) age of patient, and (4) speed of accumulation. In most cases the symptoms of pulmonary infection (cough, fever, tachypnea, and toxicity) are not sufficiently specific to differentiate between a limited pulmonic infection and a complicated pneumonia or a pleuro-pneumonic process. Sudden deterioration of the patient's clinical condition suggests a pneumothorax or other complication, i.e., mediastinitis, pericarditis, and bronchopleural fistula.

Empyema complicating retropharyngeal abscesses may also occur as a direct extension of pus caudally through the visceral compartment of the cervical fascia, a pathway with direct connection to the mediastinum (see Chapter 13, Figure 13-1).[12] Traumatic perforation of the esophagus, often from ingested foreign bodies, is an additional source of empyema (Figure 18-5).

In many ways, the diagnosis and therapy of empyema and lung abscess go hand in hand; treatment procedures are usually tailored to the evolving radiographic picture. In order to better appreciate the radiologic evolution of pleural infection, general therapeutic principles will be discussed before considering the radiographic aspects.

The treatment of empyema is controversial and will depend largely upon the radiographic patterns, clinical presentation, therapeutic response, and individual preference. As a general rule, the accumulation of pleural fluid justifies diagnostic thoracentesis, especially in the presence of an underlying infiltrate. The material obtained will often disclose the offending organism and help select appropriate therapy. In addition to the diagnostic advantage of thoracentesis, the extent and character of underlying lung disease are better seen following fluid removal. Thoracentesis also reduces respiratory distress when large volumes of fluid are present and

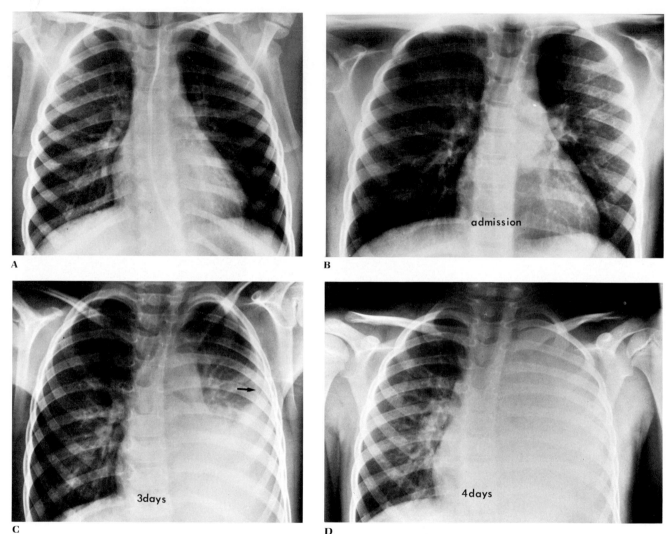

Figure 18-4   Pneumonia with empyema. A. This film, taken 1 year earlier, is normal. **B.** The child presented with consolidated pneumonia superimposed upon the left hilar region. **C.** Three days later the left lower hemithorax is opaque. Several features suggest fluid accumulation in addition to an underlying pneumonia: (1) absence of air bronchograms, (2) obliteration of the costophrenic sulcus, and (3) a line of demarcation (arrow) between the lung and the pleura. **D.** Massive effusion has accumulated over the next 24 h.

decreases the amount of material that must eventually be absorbed and removed (Figure 18-6). The decision to retap is highly individual and will depend upon the clinical progress and rapidity of fluid reaccumulation.

Tube drainage should be started when response is poor, when fluid reaccumulates rapidly, and when pneumothorax supervenes. Pagtakhan and

Chernick[13] suggest the use of intercostal tube drainage when faced with the need for repeated thoracenteses. Stiles et al.[14] performed intercostal tube drainage in almost half of their patients before 1962, but the need dropped to approximately 15 percent since that date. They recommend intercostal tube drainage for the first 24 h, particularly in the very young infant, but advise strongly against open tube

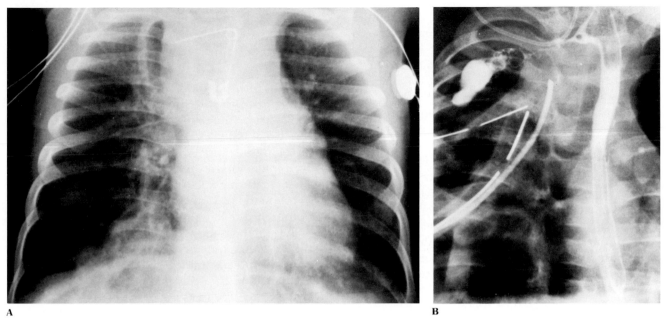

A   **B**

Figure 18-5   Empyema—esophageal perforation.   A. An open safety pin, lodged in the esophagus, has created an adjacent abscess cavity. Extensive pyopneumothorax followed, necessitating numerous drainage procedures. **B.** The contrast esophogram shows a fistulous tract from the esophagus to the pleural cavity.

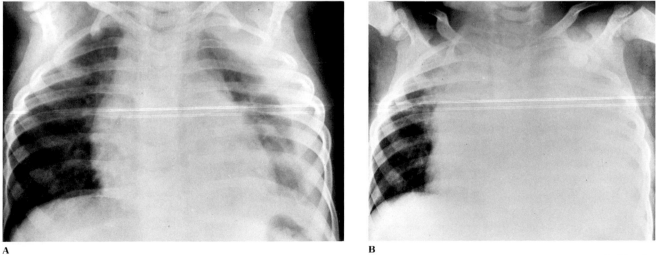

A   **B**

Figure 18-6   Empyema—pneumococcus.   A. Left lower lobe pneumonia and moderate pleural reaction are present. **B.** Massive pleural effusion with contralateral mediastinal shift has developed over the next 48 h. *Note:* Early aspiration and/or tube drainage would have prevented this sequence.

drainage and decortication. Burford,[15] commenting on the publication by Stiles et al., makes similar recommendations and cautions that "if there is any moral in this business of treating empyema, particularly in children, it is to remain fast on your feet and respond to any challenge." Bechamps and coworkers[11] prefer an initial management of multiple thoracenteses and appropriate systemic antibiotic coverage. For fluid that is thick and difficult to evacuate, closed underwater-seal drainage of the pleural space by an intercostal tube (inserted under local anesthesia) may be necessary. Of the twenty-one patients reported by Smith and Gerald,[16] nine were treated with repeat thoracenteses, nine with closed chest drainage, and three with open drainage. McLaughlin and coworkers[17] found that most of their patients could be treated successfully with antibiotics and tube drainage. They recommend prompt removal of nondraining chest tubes and placement of a second tube only if fever and respiratory distress persist.

Pleural effusion also complicates pneumonia caused by viral and mycoplasma organisms.[18-22] Children with sickle cell disease tend to develop more severe infiltrates and pleural effusion with mycoplasmal infections.[23] Differentiation between the causes for pleural reactions in the presence of infection is virtually impossible from roentgenographic studies.[24]

In summarizing the preceding review, the following conclusions may be drawn:

1. Any pleural fluid, the nature of which is in question, should be removed for diagnostic purposes.
2. Empyema may be safely treated with repeat aspiration, but tube drainage should be considered in the following circumstances or combinations thereof:
   a. A very young child
   b. Rapid reaccumulation necessitating numerous thoracenteses
   c. Large amounts of fluid contributing to respiratory distress
   d. Pyopneumothorax, especially with tension
   e. Failure to achieve prompt clinical response to appropriate antibiotics

Radiologic Findings

The radiographic features of empyema, especially in the early stages, are quite similar to those of nonpurulent pleural fluid (Figure 18-4C; also see Chapter 16). However, with the passage of time, loculation develops, and the patterns may change and become more fixed and irregular (Figure 18-7).

The development of free air within the thorax is not infrequent, and when present, it creates additional diagnostic and therapeutic problems. Leakage of air into the pleural space presumably occurs from rupture of subpleural pneumatoceles.

Boisett[6] has shown, in clinical and pathologic studies, that staphylococcal and other pneumonias produce air leaks into the parenchyma of the lung. Air, dissecting in a centrifugal manner along interlobular spaces, or "air corridors," collects in the subpleural spaces between the lung and visceral pleura (subpleural pneumatoceles). If rupture occurs, pneumothorax or pyopneumothorax results; tension within the thoracic cavity is a not infrequent sequela (Figure 18-2B). Loculations of air and purulent material may then occur and produce air-fluid levels

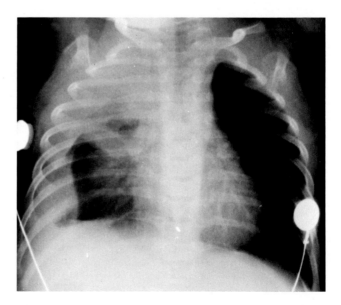

Figure 18-7 Empyema. This nondescript, unchanging, pleural reaction represents organized empyema secondary to bacterial pneumonia.

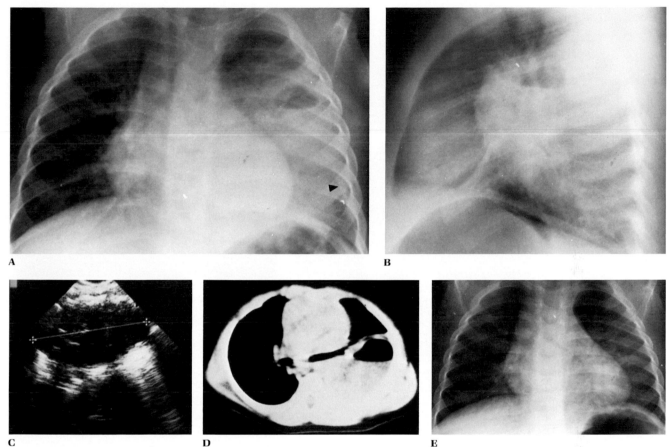

Figure 18-8   Loculated empyema—abscess. A and **B.** A large opacity with an air-fluid level occupies the left posterior chest. The pleural reaction is apparent on the frontal film (arrowhead). The mediastinum is shifted slightly to the right. The large size, location, and pleural reaction suggest a predominant component of empyema. **C.** Ultrasonography of the left chest shows a 15-cm, well-demarcated collection of mixed echogenic material abutting the chest wall. **D.** Computed tomography confirms the process to be well demarcated against the inner chest wall and in close proximity to the left stem bronchus. The mediastinal shift to the right also supports the presence of a large pleural component. **E.** This process was drained externally, and follow-up film shows normal lung.

within the pleural space. When adjacent to infected lung, these collections may be misinterpreted as lung abscesses (Figures 18-1 and 18-8).[25,26]

The patient whose films are illustrated in Figure 18-9 is a retarded child who presented with mild clinical symptoms of fever and cough. Her admission films show a thick-walled cavitary process located within a segment of lung (axillary subsegment), with a well-defined pulmonary interface and little if any pleural reaction. This probably represents a lung ab-

scess, but because of the proximity to the inner chest wall and the need for diagnostic material, the cavity was drained with a single aspiration. The child recovered with antibiotic therapy, and the lung returned to normal.

Lung abscess in the absence of aspirated foreign body or congenital abnormality is extremely rare in childhood. Patients with severe mental and physical retardation, however, show a higher incidence. The differentiation between lung abscess, infected pneu-

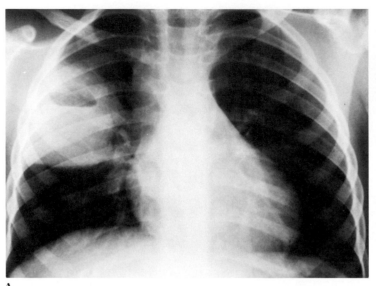
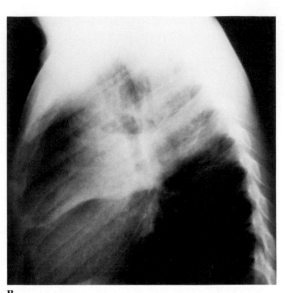

A   B

Figure 18-9   Lung abscess. A and B. A thick-walled, round, expansile opacity containing an air-fluid level occupies the axillary subsegment of the right upper lobe. No pleural reaction is apparent.

matocele, and various configurations of loculated empyema is not always straightforward (Figures 18-8 and 18-9). Plain films, if obtained in the early stages of disease, are usually sufficient to determine the changes that occur in pleuropneumonic processes. However, with the development of large amounts of fluid, the underlying parenchymal disease is often obscured.

Several imaging modalities are useful in the separation of pleural fluid from diseased lung. Ultrasonography is easiest to use and usually furnishes the most useful information (Figure 18-8; see also Chapter 16, Figure 16-19). This technique has the added advantage of portability and can be very helpful in guiding the thoracentesis aspiration.

Computed tomography (CT) is also of value but has the disadvantage of axial geometry and inconvenience, especially for patients who are difficult to transport (Figure 18-8; see also Chapter 27, Figures 27-10 and 27-17). Magnetic resonance imaging shares these disadvantages with CT but has the ability to image the pathologic process in the sagittal and co-

ronal projections (see Chapter 27, Figures 27-8 to 27-10, 27-12, 27-15, and 27-17). Stark and coworkers[27] have used CT to help distinguish between abscess and empyema, and offer the following differential criteria:

	Abscess	Empyema
Wall characteristic	Thick	Thin
Pleural separation	Absent	Positive
Lung compression	Absent	Positive
Chest wall angle	Acute	Obtuse
Shape	Round	Lenticular

The following criteria were of no help in differentiation: (1) air in the lesion, (2) lung consolidation, (3) free pleural fluid, (4) septation, and (5) multiple lesions. Rubin and coworkers[28] reported similar findings.

As indicated previously, old films are extremely important; when the pleuropneumonic process has been followed from the outset, the differentiation between abscess and empyema is usually straightforward. Subpleural pneumatoceles may also become infected and be confused with lung abscess.

Although the differentiation between lung abscess, infected pneumatoceles, and loculated empyema has been an important consideration in the past, external drainage of peripheral lesions that are associated with empyema and pleural reaction is now acceptable (Figures 18-8 and 18-9).[29-33] Lobectomies have been performed in some patients.[34] Antibiotic treatment is usually successful and has markedly decreased the need for operative intervention in most cases.[35]

The association of empyema with staphylococcal pneumonia is well known. All 21 patients with staphylococcal pneumonia studied by Smith and Gerald[16] developed empyema. In another series, half of the patients had disease limited to the parenchyma, while the other half had extensive and severe pleural disease, including pneumothorax and pyopneumothorax.[25] The combination of rapidly progressive unilateral lobar pneumonia with pleural effusion and pneumothorax is strongly suggestive of staphylococcal pneumonia. Pneumatoceles may form and remain for long periods of time but are not specific for this disease.

Other pleuropneumonic processes have few distinguishing roentgenographic characteristics except those involving the chest wall (actinomycosis) or those associated with mass lesions of the pericardium, mediastinum, or lung (see Chapter 20). In most cases, diagnostic thoracentesis is needed for a definitive diagnosis. Juvenile rheumatoid arthritis and other collagen vascular complexes also cause pleuropneumonic processes and pericardial fluid.[36,37]

Unresolved lung abscesses, postinflammatory bronchiectasis, chronic pleural thickening, and permanent lung damage are uncommon sequelae of empyema in childhood.[16,38] Extensive decortication procedures are rarely indicated; the worst-appearing radiographs will return to normal or near normal if the infection can be controlled (Figures 18-1D and 18-8E).

Chlamydia Pneumonia

Chlamydia trachomatis is an inclusion-forming, intracellularly growing organism that is transferred by direct contact. Although the organism is not a bacterium, the disease so resembles bacterial pneumonia that it is included in this section.

A common inhabitant of the genital tract, the chlamydia organism causes urethritis in men and cervicitis in women. It has been recognized as the causative agent for inclusion blennorrhea, a neonatal conjunctivitis contracted during passage through an infected birth canal.

From 25 to 50 percent of infected infants develop conjunctivitis in the first week of life. Chlamydia myocarditis may accompany this infection.

Chronic pneumonitis develops in 10 to 20 percent of patients infected by chlamydia organisms in the perinatal period.[39-45] Onset of disease is often delayed from 2 to 14 weeks. Symptoms begin with nasal obstruction and/or discharge, cough, and tachypnea. They may be mild for several weeks but then increase in severity with sudden onset of respiratory distress, pertussus-like coughing paroxysms, and apnea.[43]

On physical examination, patients are generally afebrile and remain so during the course of illness. A history of conjunctivitis is present in about 50 percent of patients. Crepitant rales are often present, but distinct wheezing is unusual in spite of chest overaeration. Absolute blood eosinophil levels are often elevated (≥ 300 mm^3), as is the serum level for immunoglobulin G and M.

Organisms may be cultured from appropriate nasopharyngeal secretion, and recovery of the lung by biopsy has also been reported.[40,46] Direct fluorescent monoclonal antibody stain is useful in confirming the diagnosis of chlamydial conjunctivitis and nasal pharyngitis.[47] This test is untried in chlamydia pneumonia, but it may well be diagnostic.

The radiographic findings of chlamydia pneumonia were first described in 1976 by K. J. Kranzler, a Chicago pediatric radiologist who died at the beginning of a very promising career. Radkowski and coworkers[45] added 125 new cases observed from 1975 to 1978. The major radiographic features were generalized hyperaeration, peribronchial thickening, and bilateral interstitial-type infiltrates. Scattered areas of atelectasis and alveolar pleural effusion were not observed in any of the 125 cases of Radkowski and coworkers, but sporadic examples of chlamydia pneumonias with effusion have been reported (Figure 18-10).[48,49] While the radiographic findings are not specific for this infection, a definitive diagnosis should be possible with the appropriate clinical history and laboratory data.

Cytomegalovirus not uncommonly accompanies infections with chlamydia. Other nonbacterial etiologic agents that may account for pneumonia in the first months of life and that may present similar radiographic features include pneumocystis and ureaplasma.[50]

Treatment with antibiotics including sulfisoxazole (150 mg/kg per 24 hours) or erythromycin (50 mg/kg per 24 hours) for 14 days usually results in negative cultures after the fourth day of treatment. The expected course is improvement of respiratory symptoms in 5 days and radiographic clearing in 3 weeks.[51]

Psittacosis (Ornithosis)

Psittacosis (ornithosis) is an acute infectious pneumonia caused by a member of the chlamydiae, antigenically related organisms that are intermediate between viruses and rickettsiae. While the exact nature of the psittacosis organism is unclear, it can be grown in tissue cultures and on the yolk sacs of embryonated egg. This disease should not be confused with bird-fancier or pigeon-breeder's lung, a form of hypersensitivity pneumonitis (see Chapter 22).

Humans acquire the infection by handling sick or well birds or their droppings or feathers. The clinical manifestations vary from a mild influenza-type illness to a severe pneumonia (Figure 18-11). The radiographic findings are similar to other generalized pneumonia patterns and cannot be considered specific. Acute and convalescent serum studies may confirm the diagnosis but are of little help in the acute care. A history of bird handling should be obtained to substantiate the diagnosis. Treatment with tetracyclines is usually curative.

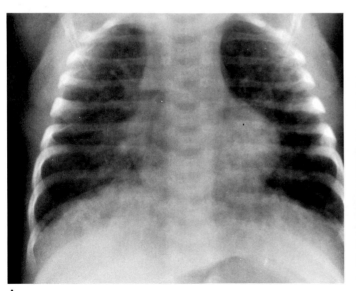

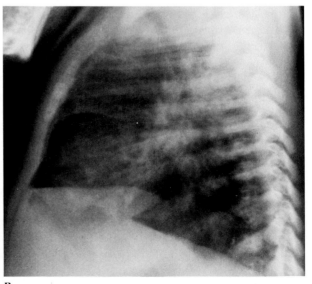

A   **B**

Figure 18-10   Chlamydia pneumonia. A and **B.** Diffuse, patchy, scattered infiltrates are present, along with moderate hyperaeration of the lung fields. The radiographic appearance is nonspecific but suggests chlamydia pneumonia in a patient with appropriate clinical and laboratory findings. (Courtesy of Dr. Mary Ann Radkowski, Chicago, Illinois.)

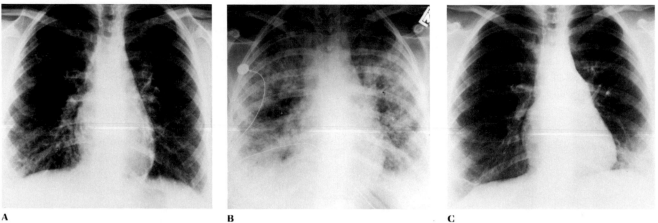

A   **B**   **C**

Figure 18-11 Psittacosis. This 16-year-old girl developed symptoms of respiratory infection that rapidly progressed to severe pneumonia. A lung biopsy during the course of treatment revealed evidence of adult respiratory distress syndrome, and cultures grew psittacosis organism. The girl's history disclosed contact with parrots. **A.** The initial film shows minimal, increased markings, mostly in the lower lobes. **B.** In 24 h, a disseminated alveolar pattern is present. **C.** After 1 month of intensive therapy, the lungs are near normal. (See Chapter 25.)

Legionella Pneumonia

In 1976, an epidemic of pneumonia occurred among American Legion conventioneers in Philadelphia.[52] The organism that caused the epidemic, *Legionella pneumophila*, was identified as a gram-negative bacterium. It has since been responsible for numerous outbreaks, sporadic infections, and secondary invasions of compromised hosts.[53,54] Other varieties of legionella organisms (i.e., Pittsburgh pneumonia agent) have been discovered and found to cause similar respiratory infections.[55] Most cases are seen in men between the ages of 50 and 55, but the disease may attack during any of the seven stages of man.

Since the disclosure of early Legionnaire's disease (LD) epidemics, numerous reports have appeared in which children are involved.[56,57] This disease rarely affects healthy children; it more commonly attacks those with systemic illness, i.e., leukemia and chronic granulomatous disease.[58,59]

The onset of legionella pneumonia is indistinguishable from other forms of pneumonia. Acute attack of high fever, cough, tachypnea, and pleuritic pain is typical. Depressed sensorium is common.

Rales are frequently present, as in other pneumonic processes.

The roentgenographic manifestations of legionella pneumonia are nonspecific; multilobar homogeneous shadows, often beginning as large nodules, are frequently seen. Hilar adenopathy, pleural effusions, atelectasis, and abscess may complicate the picture.[60] Progression of pulmonary opacities in spite of antibiotic therapy is typical. Slow resolution with delayed clearance of pulmonary infiltrates is to be expected.

Legionella pneumophila organisms may be grown on special media and can be stained in tissue using a special silver stain. Fluorescent antibody assay tests for LD constitute an additional diagnostic method.[61] Acute and convalescent serum antibody titers are also of value in confirming the diagnosis.[62]

Pertussis Pneumonia

Pertussis, a contagious disease caused by the organism *Bordetella pertussis*, may progress to pneumonia in approximately 10 percent of cases.[63] The old contagious wards were populated with children who had whooping cough, diarrhea, and polio. These diseases have been largely contained, but occasional cases of whooping cough still surface.

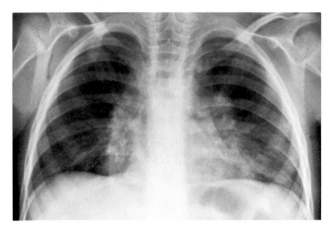

Figure 18-12 Pertussis pneumonia—"shaggy heart" sign. The lungs contain bilateral parenchymal infiltrates that obscure the cardiac silhouettes and extend into the left lower lung field. This pattern did not change over several weeks and, while not specific for pertussis, is compatible with the diagnosis.

Pertussis is often atypical in vaccinated children and adults and may not be suspected until transmitted to a susceptible infant, who in turn develops a classic and often serious form of the disease.[63] The characteristic "whoop" is limited to young infants and usually develops late in the course of the disease. *Bordetella pertussis* is difficult to culture, especially when obtained from older, vaccinated children. However, the development of enzyme-linked immunosorbent assay (ELISA) enables the diagnosis to be made, even in patients with negative cultures and atypical symptoms.[64]

In most patients, abnormal roentgenographic findings develop at some time during the course of illness. Moderate to severe pulmonary overaeration is a regular feature, especially in children less than 1 year. The so-called shaggy heart or Christmas tree heart is produced by irregular areas of infiltrate and atelectasis adjacent to the cardiac and mediastinal silhouette (Figure 18-12).[65] Scattered atelectasis, consolidations, and hilar adenopathy are additional manifestations.[66] Similar patterns are seen with a variety of other conditions, e.g., chronic aspiration, cystic fibrosis, immune deficiency syndromes, and

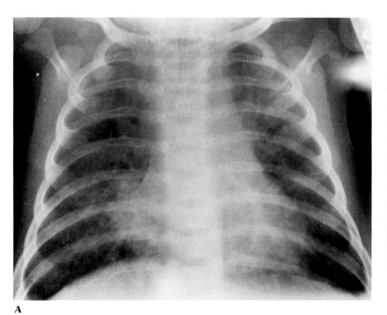

A

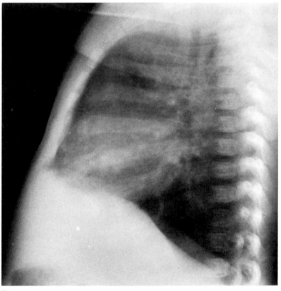

B

Figure 18-13   Pertussis pneumonia. A and **B.** Frontal and lateral studies are characteristic of diffuse peribronchial inflammatory disease of infancy. They are indistinguishable from bronchiolitis, chlamydia, cystic fibrosis, chronic aspiration, and like processes. Severe illness, paroxysmal cough, and apneic episodes complicated this child's life and supported the diagnosis of pertussis.

pneumonias caused by other infectious agents such as chlamydia, adenovirus, pneumocystis, and ureovirus (Figure 18-13).

Permanent lung damage from pertussis pneumonia is uncommon. Bronchiectasis, once thought to be a regular sequela of pertussis, is no longer considered significant.[63,67]

Whooping cough "syndrome" and pertussoid eosinophilic pneumonia are produced by viral and adenoviral agents. Patients with these diseases develop clinical, hematologic, and radiologic findings virtually identical to those caused by the pertussis organism.[68] Chlamydia, and possibly other organisms, may cause similar clinical syndromes with or without eosinophilia.[69] While these conditions simulate pertussis infection, the pertussis organism still remains a leading cause for the whooping cough syndrome.[70]

Tularemia Pneumonia

Tularemia is a disease caused by a gram-negative coccoid bacillus, *Pasteurella tularensis*. Humans acquire the infection from rodents and other animals by contact with infected material or by the bite of certain insect vectors, notably the tick. Hunters and others who handle wild game, especially rabbits and hares, as well as deer, squirrel, and fox, are at particular risk of infection.

The disease is more prevalent during the fall and winter hunting seasons. Characteristic clinical symptoms include abrupt onset of fever to 105–106° F, headache, chills, and vomiting. Glandular infection of the skin with regional lymphadenopathy is an inconsistent occurrence. Oropharyngeal, oculoglandular, and intestinal (typhoidal) infections are additional manifestations. Pulmonary symptoms consist of cough, dyspnea, and occasional pleuritic pain.

Roentgenographic patterns produced by tularemia are quite variable but frequently show hilar adenopathy and single or multiple oval densities with areas of consolidation.[71] The distribution may be localized, lobar, diffuse, unilateral, or bilateral. Less common changes include pleural effusion, medias-

tinal mass, miliary pattern, abscess, calcification, and bronchopleural fistula.[72,73] Tularemia occurs in children, but the pulmonary complications are distinctly uncommon.[74]

Melioidosis

Military personnel, especially during the war in Vietnam, and others who live in southeast Asia are occasionally infected with *Pseudomonas pseudomallei*, a saprophytic organism ubiquitous to the damp soil of that region. Melioidosis is derived from the Greek words *melis*, "a distemper of asses," and *eidos*, "resemblance," because of the disease's similarity to glanders, a disease of equines caused by *Pseudomonas mallei*.[75]

The clinical presentations of melioidosis include (1) acute, septicemic, overwhelming illness, fatal in approximately 30 percent, (2) subacute melioidosis, lasting from weeks to months, (3) chronic suppurative disease, (4) latent melioidosis, in which the disease may remain dormant for months to years, and (5) asymptomatic melioidosis, common in endemic areas.[75–78] With the immigration of southeast Asians to the United States, the disease must be considered in the differential diagnosis of obscure pneumonia.

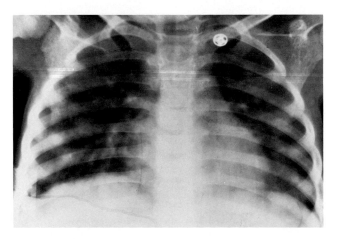

Figure 18-14 Melioidosis. This is the only film available of a Vietnamese child who died of infection with *Pseudomonas pseudomallei.*

The radiographic findings of melioidosis simulate any acute or chronic lung infection.[79] The following changes have been reported: (1) atelectasis, indistinguishable from other conditions, (2) disseminated nodular shadows, sometimes resembling metastatic abscesses, (3) small, miliary shadows, (4) cavitations, similar to tuberculosis, and (5) consolidations.[80] Pleural effusion also occurs (Figure 18-14).

The disease is uncommon in children but has been observed.[75] Treatment is not well-defined, but chloramphenicol, in addition to other drugs, seems most efficacious.

Plague

Pasteurella pestis, an organism discovered in 1894, has been responsible for widespread illness. While still a very unusual form of pneumonia, increasing numbers of cases are being reported in the southwestern United States, especially among American Indians (Custer's revenge). Several varieties of the disease exist: primary septicemic plague, pneumonic plague, and bubonic plague. All have roentgenologic changes that consist predominantly of nonspecific alveolar infiltrates. Pleural effusions are common (Figure 18-15).[81]

References

1. Oseasohn R, Adelson L, Kaja M: Clinicopathologic study of 33 fatal cases of Asian influenza. *N Engl J Med* 260:509, 1959.
2. Schwartzman SW, Adler JL, Sullivan RJ, et al: Bacterial pneumonia during the Hong Kong influenza epidemic of 1968–1969. *Arch Intern Med* 127:1037, 1971
3. Masterson J: Respiratory complications of epidemic influenza. *J Ir Med Assoc* 62:37, 1969.

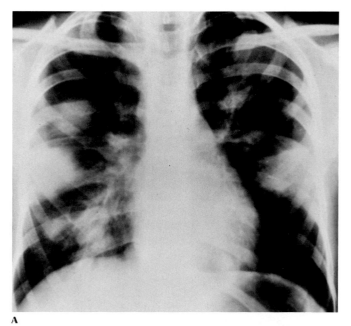

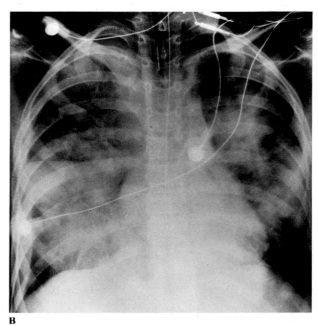

A

B

Figure 18-15   Pneumonic plague (*Pasteurella pestis*). A. Disseminated alveolar infiltrates are scattered throughout the lungs. **B.** This film, taken 10 h later, shows rapid progression with early right pleural effusion. The patient expired shortly thereafter. Examples of this disease are occasionally seen among the Indian population of the southwestern United States. (Courtesy of Dr. James Scatliff, Chapel Hill, North Carolina.)

4. Mausbach TW, Chao CT: Pneumonia and pleural effusion. Association with influenza A virus and *Staphylococcus aureus*. *Am J Dis Child* 130:1005, 1976.

5. Huxtable KA, Tucher AS, Wedgewood RJ: Staphylococcal pneumonia in childhood. Long term follow-up. *Am J Dis Child* 108:262, 1964.

6. Boissett GF: Subpleural emphysema complicating staphylococcal and other pneumonia. *J Pediatr* 81:259, 1972.

7. Ceruti E, Contreras J, Neira M: Staphylococcal pneumonia in childhood. Long-term follow-up including pulmonary function studies. *Am J Dis Child* 122:386, 1971.

8. Rebhan AW, Edwards HE: Staphylococcal pneumonia, review of 329 cases. *Can Med Assoc J* 82:513, 1960.

9. Felman AH, Shulman ST: Staphylococcal osteomyelitis, sepsis, and pulmonary disease. Observations of 10 patients with combined osseous and pulmonary infections. *Radiology* 117:649, 1975.

10. Bartlett JG, Finegold SM: Anaerobic infections of the lung and pleural space. *Am Rev Respir Dis* 110:56, 1974.

11. Bechamps GJ, Lynn HB, Wenge JE: Empyema in children: Review of Mayo Clinic experience. *Mayo Clin Proc* 45:43, 1970.

12. Ramilo J, Harris VJ, White H: Empyema as a complication of retropharyngeal and neck abscesses in children. *Radiology* 126:743, 1978.

13. Pagtakhan RD, Chernick V: Liquid and air in the pleural space, in Kendig EL Jr, Chernick V (eds): *Diseases of the Respiratory Tract in Children*, 3d ed. Philadelphia, WB Saunders, 1977, pp 475–487, 602.

14. Stiles QR, Lindesmith GG, Tucker BL, et al: Pleural empyema in children. *Ann Thorac Surg* 10:37, 1970.

15. Burford TH: Discussion of pleural empyema in children. *Ann Thorac Surg* 10:43, 1970.

16. Smith PI, Gerald B: Empyema in childhood followed roentgenographically: Decortication seldom needed. *AJR* 106:114, 1969.

17. McLaughlin FJ, Goldmann DA, Rosenbaum DM, et al: Empyema in children: Clinical course and long-term follow-up. *Pediatrics* 73:578, 1984.

18. Herbert DH: The roentgen features of Eaton agent pneumonia. *AJR* 98:300, 1966.

19. Bryant RE, Rhoades ER: Clinical features of adenoviral pneumonia in Air Force recruits. *Am Rev Respir Dis* 96:717, 1967.

20. Grix A, Giammona ST: Pneumonitis with pleural effusion in children due to *Mycoplasma pneumoniae*. *Am Rev Respir Dis* 109:666, 1974.

21. Fine NL, Smith LR, Sheedy PF: Frequency of pleural effusions in mycoplasma and viral pneumonias. *N Engl J Med* 283:790, 1970.

22. Simila S, Ylikorkala O, Wasz-Ho Chert O: Type 7 adenovirus pneumonia. *J Pediatr* 79:605, 1971.

23. Shulman ST, Bartlett J, Clyde WA, et al: The unusual severity of mycoplasma pneumonia in children with sickle-cell disease. *N Engl J Med* 287:164, 1972.

24. Tew J, Calenoff L, Berlin BS: Bacterial and non-bacterial pneumonia: Accuracy of radiologic diagnosis. *Radiology* 124:607, 1977.

25. Highman JH: Staphylococcal pneumonia and empyema in childhood. *Radiology* 106:103, 1969.

26. Caffey J: On the natural regression of pulmonary cysts during infancy. *Pediatrics* 11:48, 1953.

27. Stark DD, Federle MP, Goodman PC, et al: Differentiating lung abscesses and empyema. Radiography and computed tomography. *AJR* 141:163, 1983.

28. Rubin SB, Silbergleit A, Ruskin R, et al: Empyema or abscess? *Chest* 87:385, 1985.

29. Baker PR: The treatment of lung abscess—Current concepts. *Chest* 87:709, 1985.

30. Snow N, Lucas A, Horrigan TP: Utility of pneumonotomy in the treatment of cavitary lung disease. *Chest* 87:731, 1985.

31. Lacey SR, Kosloske AM: Pneumostomy in the management of pediatric lung abscess. *J Pediatr Surg* 18:625, 1983.

32. Lorenzo RL, Bradford BF, Black J, et al: Lung abscesses in children: Diagnostic and therapeutic aspiration. *Radiology* 157:79, 1985.

33. Towbin RB, Strife JL: Percutaneous aspiration, drainage, and biopsies in children. *Radiology* 157:81, 1985.

34. Nonoyama A, Tanaka K, Oskko T, et al: Surgical treatment of pulmonary abscess in children under ten years of age. *Chest* 85:358, 1984.

35. Asher MI, Spier S, Beland M, et al: Primary lung abscess in childhood: Long-term outcome of conservative management. *Am J Dis Child* 136:491, 1982.

36. Yancey CL, Doughty RA, Cohlan, BA: Pericarditis and cardiac tamponade in juvenile rheumatoid arthritis. *Pediatrics* 68:369, 1981.

37. Yousefzadeh DK, Fishman PA: The triad of pneumonitis, pleuritis, and pericarditis in juvenile rheumatoid arthritis. *Pediatr Radiol* 8:147, 1979.

38. Wise MB, Beaudry PH, Bates DV: Long term follow-up of staphylococcal pneumonia. *Pediatrics* 38:398, 1966.

39. Schackter J, Lum L, Gooding CA, et al: Pneumonitis inclusion blennorrhea. *J Pediatr* 87:779, 1975.

40. Frommell GT, Bruhn FW, Schwartzman JD: Isolation of

Chlamydia trachomatis from infant lung tissue. *N Engl J Med* 296:1150, 1977.

41. Kranzler KJ: Chlamydia pneumonia. *Proceeding of the Society for Pediatric Radiology,* Washington, DC, 1976.

42. Stickney RN, Bjelland JC, Capp MP, et al: *Chlamydia trachomatis:* A cause of an infantile pneumonia syndrome. *AJR* 131:914, 1978.

43. Tipple MA, Beem MD, Saxon EM: Clinical characteristics of the afebrile pneumonia associated with *Chlamydia trachomatis* infections in infants less than 6 months of age. *Pediatrics* 63:192, 1979.

44. Schaefer C, Harrison HR, Boyce WT, et al: Illnesses in infants born to women with *Chlamydia trachomatis* infection. A prospective study. *Am J Dis Child* 139:127, 1985.

45. Radkowski MA, Kranzler JK, Beem MO, et al: Chlamydia pneumonia in infants. Radiography in 125 cases. *AJR* 137:703, 1981.

46. Beem MD, Saxon EM: Respiratory tract colonization and a distinctive pneumonia syndrome in infants infected with *Chlamydia trachomatis. N Engl J Med* 296:306, 1977.

47. Bell TA, Kuo C, Stamm WE, et al: Direct fluorescent monoclonal antibody stain for rapid detection of infant chlamydial trachomatis infections. *Pediatrics* 74:224, 1984.

48. Marrie TJ, Haldane EV, Noble MA, et al: Causes of atypical pneumonia: Results of a 1-year prospective study. *Can Med Assoc J* 125:1118, 1981.

49. Stutman HR, Rettig PJ, Reyes S: *Chlamydia trachomatis* as a cause of pneumonitis and pleural effusion. *J Pediatr* 104:588, 1984.

50. Stagno S, Brasfield DM, Brown MB, et al: Infant pneumonitis associated with cytomegalovirus, chlamydia, pneumocystis, and ureaplasma. *Pediatrics* 68:322, 1981.

51. Lumicao GG, Heggie AD: Chlamydial infections. *Pediatr Clin North Am* 2:269, 1979.

52. Fraser DW, Tsai TF, Orenstein W, et al: Legionnaires' disease: Description of an epidemic of pneumonia. *N Engl J Med* 297:1189, 1977.

53. Broome CV, Fraser DW: Epidemiologic aspects of legionellosis. *Epidemiol Rev* 1:1, 1979.

54. Center for Disease Control: Legionnaires' Disease— United States. *Morbid Mortal Weekly Rep* 27:439, 1978.

55. Pope TL Jr, Armstrong P, Thompson R, et al: Pittsburgh pneumonia agent: Chest film manifestations. *Am J Radiol* 138:237, 1982.

56. Muldoon RL, Jaecker MS, Kiefer HK: Legionnaires' disease in children. *Pediatrics* 67:329, 1981.

57. Orenstein WA, Overturf GD, Leedom JM, et al: The frequency of Legionella infection prospectively determined in children hospitalized with pneumonia. *J Pediatr* 99:403, 1981.

58. Kovatch AL, Jardine DS, Dowling JN, et al: Legionellosis in children with leukemia in relapse. *Pediatrics* 73:811, 1984.

59. Peerless AG, Liebhaber M, Anderson S, et al: Legionella pneumonia in chronic granulomatous disease. *J Pediatr* 106:783, 1985.

60. MacFarlane J, Miller AC, Roderick Smith WH, et al: Comparative radiographic features of community acquired Legionnaires' disease, pneumococcal pneumonia, mycoplasma pneumonia, and psittacosis. *Thorax* 39:28, 1984.

61. Center for Disease Control: Legionnaires' disease in direct fluorescent antibody research reagents: Revised instructions. Center for Disease Control, Atlanta, December 1978.

62. Swartz MN: Clinical aspects of Legionnaires' disease. *Ann Intern Med* 90:492, 1979.

63. Jernelius H: Pertussis with pulmonary complications—A follow-up study. *Acta Paediatr* 53:247, 1964.

64. Mertsola J, Ruuskanen O, Eerola E, et al: Intrafamilial spread of pertussis. *J Pediatr* 103:359, 1983.

65. Barnhard HJ, Kniker WT: Roentgenologic findings in pertussis with particular emphasis on the "shaggy heart" sign. *AJR* 84:445, 1960.

66. Fawcitt J, Parry HE: Lung changes in pertussis and measles in childhood. *Br J Radiol* 30:76, 1957.

67. Bierling A: Childhood pneumonia, including pertussis pneumonia and bronchiectasis. A follow-up study of 151 patients. *Acta Paediatr* 45:348, 1956.

68. Collier AM, Connor JD, Irving WR Jr: Generalized type 5 adenovirus infection associated with pertussis syndrome. *J Pediatr* 69:1073, 1966.

69. Nemir RL: Pertussoid eosinophilic pneumonia, in Kendig EL Jr, Chernick V (eds): *Disorders of the Respiratory Tract in Children,* 3d ed. Philadelphia, WB Saunders, 1977, p 994.

70. Islur J, Anglin CS, Middleton PJ: The whooping cough syndrome: A continuing problem. *Clin Pediatr* 14:171, 1975.

71. Avery FW, Barnett TB: Pulmonary tularemia. A report of five cases and consideration of pathogenesis and terminology. *Am Rev Respir Dis* 95:584, 1967.

72. Miller RP, Bates JH: Pleuropulmonary tularemia. A review of 29 patients. *Am Rev Respir Dis* 99:31, 1969.

73. Overholt EL, Tigertt WD: Roentgenographic manifestations of pulmonary tularemia. *Radiology* 74:758, 1960.

74. Hughes WT: Tularemia in children. *J Pediatr* 62:495, 1963.

75. Patamasucon P, Schaad UB, Nelson JD: Melioidosis. *J Pediatr* 100:175, 1982.

76. Spotritz M, Rudnitzky J, Rambaud JJ: Melioidosis pneumonitis: Analysis of nine cases of a benign form of melioidosis. *JAMA* 202:126, 1967.

77. Prevatt AL, Hunt JS: Chronic systemic melioidosis: Review of literature and report of a case with a note on visual disturbance due to chloramphenicol. *Am J Med* 23:810, 1957.

78. Sanford JP, Moore WL: Recrudescent melioidosis: A Southeast Asia legacy, *Am Rev Respir Dis* 104:452, 1971.

79. Poe RH, Vassallo CL, Domm, BM: Melioidosis: The remarkable imitator. *Am Rev Respir Dis* 104:427, 1971.

80. Bateson EM, Webling DA: Radiologic appearances of pulmonary melioidosis: Report of twenty-three cases. *Australas Radiol* 25:239, 1981.

81. Alsofrom DJ, Mettler FA, Mann JM: Radiographic manifestations of plague in New Mexico. *Radiology* 139:561, 1981.

Chapter 19

Viral Infections

This chapter will focus on viral infections of the lung that usually affect children and young adults. Viral pneumonias of infancy (respiratory syncytial virus) are covered in Chapter 14 along with other agents that produce pulmonary overaeration.

The following viral pneumonias will be discussed:

1. Rubeola (measles) pneumonia
   a. Atypical measles pneumonia
   b. Giant cell pneumonia
   c. Superimposed bacterial pneumonia
2. Mycoplasma pneumonia
3. Adenoviral pneumonia (bronchiolitis obliterans)
4. Varicella (chicken pox) pneumonia
5. Other viral pneumonias
   a. Herpes simplex pneumonia
   b. Epstein-Barr pneumonia

Rubeola (Measles) Pneumonia

The usual course of measles (rubeola) has been altered by the development of preventive vaccines, but pulmonary involvement continues to be a serious complication in both children and adults.[1] Patients with measles regularly develop laryngotracheobronchitis, but more extensive infection of the peripheral bronchi, bronchioles, and alveoli by the measles virus is infrequent. Measles pneumonia is an especially ominous threat to malnourished, immunologically incompetent, debilitated, or otherwise compromised hosts.

The onset of measles pneumonia is often not apparent from clinical findings since moderate to severe cough is an expected feature of measles prodrome, fastigium, and convalescence. As a rule, measles pneumonia begins early in the course of the disease and is characterized by diffuse, mild to moderate parenchymal infiltrates that coalesce but rarely progress to lobar consolidation. Hilar adenopathy, atelectasis, and aeration abnormalities are frequently present.[2,3]

Pulmonary sequelae of measles pneumonia are not found in large numbers, but residual atelectasis has been reported in 25 percent of patients.[3] Bronchiolitis fibrosis obliterans, similar to that following other viral diseases, is an additional complication capable of producing considerable pulmonary insufficiency in later life (Figures 19-1 and 19-2). (See the section "Adenoviral Pneumonia.")

Atypical Measles Pneumonia

Killed virus vaccine was the first method used to immunize against measles and is still given on rare occasions. A form of atypical measles has been recognized in children who received this vaccine and were later exposed to the wild virus.[4] Severe lung disease with lobar consolidation, pleural effusions, and

hilar adenopathy are commonplace.[5-7] Residual nodules may remain for several years after the pneumonia of atypical measles has cleared; these may be confused in later life with pulmonary mass lesions.[6]

Giant Cell Pneumonia

Giant cell interstitial pneumonia, first described by Hecht in 1910,[8] is an interstitial pneumonitis virtually identical to measles pneumonia that develops in patients who do not manifest the clinical signs, or rash, of measles. The etiology of Hecht's giant cell pneumonia was obscure until the measles virus was isolated from the lungs of affected individuals.[9,10]

Hecht's pneumonia is characterized by the presence of multinuclear giant cells with intranuclear and intracytoplasmic inclusion bodies. While the disease was originally thought to occur only in children, giant cell interstitial pneumonia has been observed in adults.[11-13] Whether this represents the same disease as that seen in children is unclear.

Giant cell pneumonia may occur in previously normal patients, but it is more often seen in com-

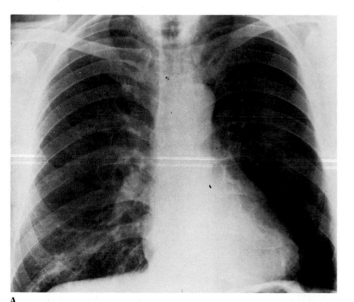

A

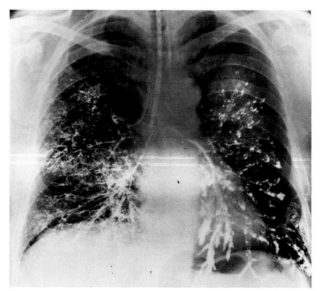

B

Figure 19-1 Postmeasles bronchiolitis obliterans (hyperlucent lung). A. The left lung is virtually devoid of vascularity except in the medial lower lobe. These changes followed measles pneumonia 2 years earlier. **B.** Bronchography reveals markedly dilated bronchi proximal to the obliterated segments beyond which no contrast passes. The bronchi to the medial lower lobe show fusiform bronchiectasis. The right lung is normal. (Courtesy of Dr. James Scatliff, Chapel Hill, North Carolina.)

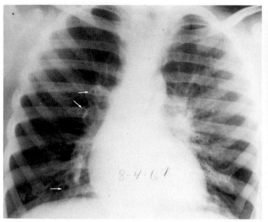
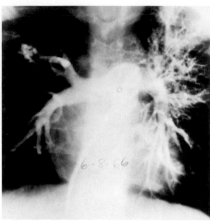
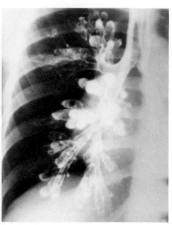

A   B   C

Figure 19-2   Postmeasles bronchiolitis obliterans. A. This representative chest film was taken several years after measles pneumonia. Only the left upper lobe retains normal vascular markings and normal radiopacity; the left lower lung and entire right lung are hyperlucent. *Note:* the attenuated vessels in the right hilum compared with the left and the ringlike shadows that represent dilated proximal bronchi (arrows). (Compare with part C.) The original pneumonia was concentrated mostly in the areas of hyperlucency. **B.** The pulmonary angiogram confirms the severe attenuation of the right pulmonary arteries and similar, less prominent, changes in the left lower lobe. The vascular supply to the left upper lobe is all that remains normal. **C.** The bronchogram of the right lung reveals complete obliteration of the bronchi at the third or fourth generation along with gross dilatation proximally during inspiration. (Courtesy of Dr. Marie Capitanio, Philadelphia, Pennsylvania.)

promised hosts. Patients taking antimetabolite therapy or those with histiocytosis X, leukemia, immune deficiency states, and other debilitating diseases are at greater risk of contracting the disease and of succumbing.

Documentation of the radiographic pattern of giant cell pneumonia is not well reported, but it differs little from that of measles. Hilar adenopathy is a prominent feature.

Superimposed Bacterial Pneumonia

Secondary infection superimposed upon measles is mainly due to bacteria, but may occur from a number of different organisms including fungi and other opportunistic invaders. In contrast to the early onset of Hecht's pneumonia, secondary bacterial infection usually causes symptoms later in the course of the illness. A sudden increase in temperature, leukocytosis, and increased respiratory symptoms herald this complication in a patient with an otherwise "normal" clinical course of measles.

Radiographs of superimposed bacterial pneumonia are more likely to show a consolidated area of lung with or without associated pleural effusion. Se-

quential films following therapy for bacterial infection may offer a retrospective diagnosis and help differentiate this secondary bacterial pneumonia from postmeasles atelectasis.

Mycoplasma Pneumonia

Mycoplasma pneumoniae, an organism that has the capacity to infect humans as well as animals, is a major cause of pneumonia in school-aged children and young adults. Also known by the terms *Eaton agent, pleuropneumonia-like organism (PPLO)*, and *primary atypical pneumonia*, this organism was originally thought to be a virus, but has since been identified as a mycoplasma. Nevertheless, since the clinical and radiologic presentation of this pneumonia simulates viral etiologies, it is considered in this chapter.

This organism most often attacks adolescents. However, young children and older patients are not immune to this infection; almost one-third of 60 patients reported by Finnegan and coworkers[14] were more than 35 years of age. Approximately 10 to 20 percent of adult pneumonias are caused by this organism. Patients less than 5 years old tend to be less ill.

The lung is the primary site of infection in humans, but the nasopharynx, throat, and trachea may also be involved, as well as extrapulmonary sites such as skin, central nervous system, blood, heart, and joints.[15] The pneumonia of mycoplasma is not highly communicable but tends to spread in families, schools, and other communal situations.[16,17] Epidemics usually begin in late summer or early fall and occur throughout the winter months.

The clinical onset of pneumonia, after an incubation period of 2 to 3 weeks, is characterized by headache, malaise, fever, and cough. Pharyngitis, laryngotracheobronchitis, otitis media, and bullous myringitis are additional miseries. Severity of symptoms often exceeds physical signs of illness. The diagnosis may be confirmed by culture of organisms from the sputum. Acute and convalescent serum for cold hemagglutinin titers will show a rise in 10 days to 3 weeks after the onset of illness. This test is not specific for mycoplasma and has been shown to be positive in other diseases.[15] A complement fixation test is also available that renders a diagnosis within several days. Hematologic parameters are generally normal.

The radiographic appearance of mycoplasmal pneumonia is not specific. Putman et al.[18] described three distinct clinicoradiologic presentations. Approximately one-half began with acute symptoms and developed roentgenographic changes of lobar or segmental consolidations (Figure 19-3) and occasional atelectasis. In this group, unilateral involvement occurred in three-fourths and pleural effusions in about one-fifth of patients. The lungs cleared in 5 to 14 days. Patients with sickle cell disease had prolonged and complicated disease, an observation reported by others.[19]

Approximately one-fourth of Putman's patients with mycoplasmal pneumonia had clinical symptoms of longer duration, including malaise, lethargy, and several weeks of shortness of breath. They were usually afebrile and free of cough. Chest roentgenograms in this group showed diffuse reticular-nodular infiltrates extending from the hila to the periphery with occasional Kerley B lines. Pleural effusions and consolidation were rare or nonexistent in this group, and the clinical symptoms and radiographic findings were unchanged by antibiotics.

The third group of patients in Putman's series developed features of both previous groups and, in effect, represented an overlap of clinical roentgenographic disease (Figure 19-3).

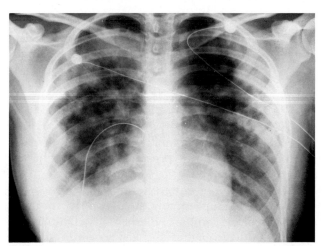

A   B

Figure 19-3 *Mycoplasma pneumoniae* **pneumonia. A.** The initial film study shows a generalized pattern that suggests increased interstitial fluid. (See Chapter 16, Figure 16-3.) This is characterized by ill-defined vessels and fine, randomly scattered markings that resemble Kerley lines. **B.** A disseminated alveolar pattern has developed in the ensuing 24 h.

Finnegan and coworkers[14] found four types of patterns in approximately equal numbers:

Confluent consolidation	28 percent
Patchy consolidation	25 percent
Nodular opacities	23 percent
Mixed nodular, patchy, or confluent	23 percent

Small pleural effusions were evident in only 4 of 60 patients. Others have shown a higher incidence, especially in compromised hosts, such as patients with sickle cell disease.[18,20,21] Aggressive progression into fulminant diffuse interstitial fibrosis has also been reported.[22]

Mycoplasma pneumonia is usually self-limited, postpneumonic sequelae are rare, but patients tend to complain for weeks thereafter.

Adenoviral Pneumonia (Bronchiolitis Obliterans)

Adenoviruses are responsible for approximately 5 percent of all respiratory tract disease in infants and children.[23,24] They may involve any portion of the respiratory tract, but pneumonia and its sequelae are most troublesome. Types 3, 4, and 7 are the most common serotypes responsible for respiratory tract disease, but more recently type 21 has been reported in localized epidemics.[25–28]

Some cases manifest pharyngoconjunctival fever, characterized by infection of the palpebral and bulbar conjunctivae, erythematous exudative tonsillitis, coryza, and fever. In the presence of pneumonia, the symptoms tend to be quite severe. In addition to the usual symptoms of cough, fever and dyspnea, patients may develop anemia, heart failure, vomiting, diarrhea, meningismus, and severe general toxicity.[29] Fevers tend to be higher and last longer than bacterial infections. Recently developed immunoassay for detection of adenovirus hexon antigen permits diagnosis within 24 to 30 h.[30,31] A syndrome similar to the infantile bronchiolitis caused by respiratory syn-cytial virus is also seen with frequency in infants (Figure 19-4).[28]

The radiographic features of adenoviral pneumonia are nonspecific. Most reports indicate a diffuse pattern of disease characterized by thickening of bronchial walls; peribronchial densities; and patchy, confluent, mixed infiltrates.[28] Air trapping is quite common, whereas hilar adenopathy and pleural effusions occur infrequently.[25,32]

Of particular interest is the capacity of adenoviral infections to produce both short- and long-term pulmonary sequelae. In an epidemic involving native Indians from Manitoba, Wenman and coworkers[28] found that more than half of their patients who were followed with radiologic examinations developed repeated episodes of pneumonia, and another 12 percent showed chronic structural damage, including bronchiectasis and chronic atelectasis. Adenoviral pneumonia also has a peculiar tendency to initiate a series of histologic changes leading to the complex of bronchial destruction, bronchiolitis obliterans, and hyperlucent lung.[25,33,34] This derives, in part, from the destructive and invasive character of the adenoviral organism (Figure 19-4C).

Considerable interest, and not a little confusion, surrounds the terminology of hyperlucent lung, bronchiolitis obliterans, Swyer-James syndrome, and McCleod's syndrome. Much of this confusion results from the histopathologic descriptions of what, in all likelihood, represent several different diseases with variable etiologies.[35]

The confusion is sometimes perpetuated when an attempt is made to correlate the radiographic pattern of abnormal pulmonary lucency with an underlying disease process. The radiolucency of bronchiolitis obliterans derives from several factors; chief among these is diminished vascularity that results from the obliteration of bronchioles and their adjacent blood vessels. Overaeration of the affected lobe, from dilated, cystic bronchi, contributes to the lucent appearance. These dilated, "cystic" bronchi are often visible in good-quality film studies. Old radiographs that match areas of previous pneumonia or atelectasis to the lucent lung region are of great help. Perfusion-ventilation lung scintigraphy is valuable, but bronchography is the definitive study (Figures 19-1 and 19-2).

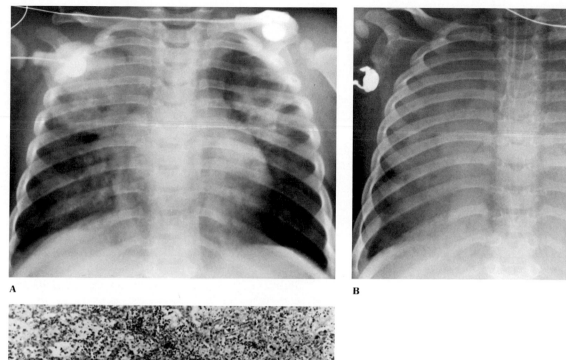

C

Figure 19-4 Adenoviral pneumonia. This 13-month-old child with trisomy 21 syndrome developed fever and cough for 6 days. **A.** A disseminated alveolar pattern is present with early right upper lobe confluence. **B.** Three days later, the lungs are totally consolidated, with minimal pleural reaction on the right. Death of this previously healthy girl followed soon after this film. **C.** A histologic examination of the lung reveals a severe, necrotizing pneumonia with extensive transmural inflammation and necrosis of the bronchial walls (acute bronchiolitis). The arrows indicate inclusion-bearing "smudge" cells, typical of adenoviral infection.

The syndrome of bronchiolitis obliterans has also been reported following other lung infections (measles, pertussis, tuberculosis), but in a review of 17 children referred for investigation of "unilateral hyperlucent lung," McKenzie and coworkers[36] could document previous viral pneumonia in only 2. Additional insults to the lung that may cause bronchiolitis obliterans include noxious agents and gas inhalation, connective and collagen vascular diseases, pulmonary alveolar proteinosis, lymphoma, and bone marrow transplantation.[37,38]

While the syndrome of bronchiolitis obliterans is a well-accepted underlying cause of pulmonary "hyperlucency," it should not be confused with differential "opacity" of lung. Several conditions may cause one side or a portion of the thorax to appear more lucent (or more opaque) than the opposite side. Among these are atelectasis and compensatory emphysema, differential thickness of the overlying chest wall, pleural effusion in the contralateral hemithorax, and decreased pulmonary blood flow from congenital or acquired processes. (See Section I and Chapter 13.)

Varicella (Chicken Pox) Pneumonia

Varicella, or chicken pox, is a highly contagious viral disease of childhood. Pulmonary complications are more common and of greater severity when adults are infected.[39-41] Adults with chicken pox stand a greater chance of contracting pneumonia (up to 16 percent in two series) and of dying as a result.[42,43] The outcome of varicella pneumonia is particularly grave in pregnant women.

Varicella pneumonia complicates chicken pox in 1 percent of children, most often occurring in neonates and in patients with immune deficiencies, leukemia, and nephrotic syndrome. The pneumonic process usually parallels the clinical symptoms. Cough, dyspnea, and occasional cyanosis appear between the second and fifth day of illness. Blood expectoration may occur.

Clinical findings are scarce when compared with the radiographic changes. The lungs typically develop diffuse, patchy infiltrates extending outward from the hila and scattered randomly throughout the lungs (Figures 19-5 and 19-6). Occasional sterile pleural effusions and hilar adenopathy are present. In milder cases, the disease is limited to the laryngotracheobronchial tree and produces few if any radiographic signs.

Pulmonary changes resolve as the rash clears.

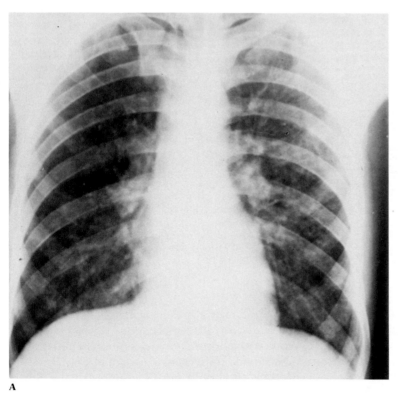
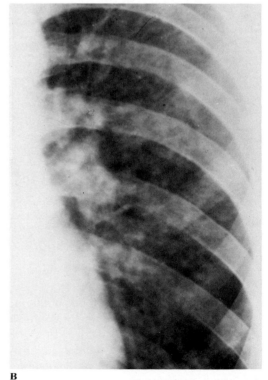

A   B

Figure 19-5   Varicella (chicken pox) pneumonia. These films were obtained on a teenage Puerto Rican girl in Philadelphia who contracted varicella. **A.** There are diffuse, nodular, ill-defined densities throughout the lung. The hila are prominent. **B.** This view shows a close-up of the left lung and hilum.

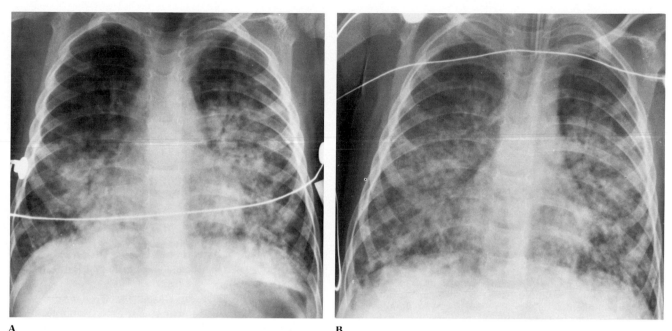

Figure 19-6   Varicella (chicken pox) pneumonia. This 18-month-old child developed varicella with pulmonary involvement. **A.** The central lung fields are involved with a confluent infiltrate; ill-defined, rounded, nodular densities are evident in the peripheral portions. **B.** Twenty four hours later, there has been rapid progression, but the individual nodular character is still apparent. Later films showed complete opacification.

Complete roentgenographic clearing is the rule, but calcifications in the lung parenchyma have been reported.[44,45] These usually appear within 2 years of the illness and often persist throughout life. Calcifications are characteristically 1 to 3 mm in diameter; are irregular, multiple, and bilateral; and prefer the basal segments.[46] Abnormalities of pulmonary function that follow varicella pneumonia suggest the development of secondary fibrosis.[47,48]

Occasional cardiac and pericardial disease may accompany varicella.[49,50] Pericarditis has not been a serious problem in childhood chicken pox, but fatal carditis has been reported.[51] Sargent et al.[52] reported 6 deaths among 20 patients with varicella pneumonia; 4 were children, and 2 were adults. Superimposed bacterial infection, particularly with staphylococcus, and associated sepsis are dreaded complications that contribute to fatalities.

Other Viral Pneumonias

The causes of most pneumonias are difficult or impossible to determine during the first hours or days of illness.[53] Two pneumonias that are uncommon but occasionally seen are caused by herpes simplex and Epstein-Barr viruses.[54-56] These usually attack neonates and debilitated or immune compromised hosts. Epstein-Barr virus pneumonia has been reported in children suffering from the childhood counterpart of acquired immunodeficiency syndrome.[57] On occasion, however, these organisms may attack otherwise normal individuals.

The radiographic patterns produced by these viruses are nonspecific. Patchy, fluffy, irregular opacities are frequent; central distribution is common early, but usually progresses rapidly to generalized involvement (Figure 19-7).

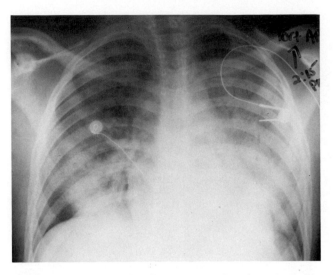

Figure 19-7 Herpes simplex pneumonia. There is a disseminated alveolar infiltrate with normal heart size and no pleural reaction. Herpes simplex infection was identified by lung biopsy in this leukemic patient. This organism is being recovered from immunologically compromised hosts with increasing frequency by using special immunofluorescent staining techniques.

References

1. Quinn JL: Measles pneumonia in an adult. *AJR* 91:560, 1964.

2. Kohn JL, Koiransky H: Further roentgenographic studies of chests in children during measles. *Am J Dis Child* 46:40, 1933.

3. Fawcitt J, Parry HE: Lung changes in pertussis and measles in childhood. A review of 1894 cases with a follow-up study of the pulmonary complications. *Br J Radiol* 30:76, 1957.

4. Rauh LW, Schmidt R: Measles immunization with killed virus. *Am J Dis Child* 109:232, 1965.

5. Fulginiti VA, Eller JJ, Downie AW, et al: Altered reactivity to measles virus. Atypical measles in children previously immunized with inactivated measles virus vaccine. *JAMA* 202:1075, 1967.

6. Young LW, Smith DI, Glasgow LA: Pneumonia of atypical measles. Residual nodular lesions. *AJR* 110:439, 1970.

7. Margolin FR, Gandy TK: Pneumonia of atypical measles. *Radiology* 131:653, 1979.

8. Hecht V: Die Riesenzellenpneumonia in Kindsalter, einehistorische-experimentelle Studie. *Beitr Pathol Anat Allg Pathol* 48:263, 1910.

9. McCarthy K, Mitus A, Cheatham W, et al: Isolation of virus of measles from three fatal cases of giant-cell pneumonia. *Am J Dis Child* 96:500, 1958.

10. Enders JF, McCarthy K, Mitus A, et al: Isolation of measles virus at autopsy in cases of giant-cell pneumonia without rash. *N Engl J Med* 261:875, 1959.

11. McConnell EM: Giant-cell pneumonia in an adult. *Br Med J* 2:289, 1961.

12. Liebow AA: New concepts and entities in pulmonary disease in the lung, in Liebow AA, Smith DD (eds): *The Lung.* Baltimore, Williams & Wilkins, 1968, p 332.

13. Reddy PA, Goulick DF, Christianson CS: Giant cell interstitial pneumonia (GIP). *Chest* 58:319, 1970.

14. Finnegan OC, Fowles SJ, White RJ: Radiographic appearance of mycoplasma pneumonia. *Thorax* 36:469, 1981.

15. Denny F, Clyde WA Jr, Gezen WP: *Mycoplasma pneumoniae* disease: Clinical spectrum, pathophysiology, epidemiology, and control. *J Infect Dis* 123:74, 1971.

16. Foy FM, Grayston JT, Kenny GE, et al: Epidemiology of *Mycoplasma pneumoniae* infection in families. *JAMA* 197:859, 1966.

17. Azimi PH, Koranyi KI: *Mycoplasma pneumoniae* infections in a family. A description with comments. *Clin Pediatr* 16:1138, 1977.

18. Putman CE, Curtis AM, Simeone JF, et al: Mycoplasma pneumonia. Clinical and roentgenographic patterns. *AJR* 124:417, 1975.

19. Shulman ST, Bartlett J, Clyde WA Jr, et al: The unusual severity of mycoplasmal pneumonia in children with sickle-cell disease. *N Engl J Med* 287:164, 1972.

20. Fine HL, Smith LR, Sheedy PF: Frequency of pleural effusions in mycoplasma and viral pneumonias. *N Engl J Med* 283:790, 1970.

21. Grix A, Giammona ST: Pneumonitis with pleural effusion in children due to *Mycoplasma pneumoniae. Am Rev Respir Dis* 109:665, 1974.

22. Kaufman JM, Cuvelier CA, Van der Straeten M: Mycoplasma pneumonia with fulminant evolution into diffuse interstitial fibrosis. *Thorax* 35:140, 1980.

23. Hamparian UV, Cramblett HG: Viral etiology of respiratory illness, in Kendig EL Jr, Chernick V (eds): *Disorders of the Respiratory Tract in Children,* 3d ed. Philadelphia, WB Saunders, 1977, p 416.

24. Fox JP, Hall CE, Cooney MK: The Seattle virus watch. VII. Observations on adenoviral infections. *Am J Epidemiol* 105:362, 1977.

25. Osborne D, White P: Radiology of epidemic adenovirus 21 infection of the lower respiratory tract in infants and young children. *AJR* 133:379, 1979.

26. James AG, Lang WR, Liang AY, et al: Adenovirus type 21 bronchopneumonia in infants and young children. *J Pediatr* 95:530, 1979.

27. Lang WR, Howden CW, Laws J, et al: Bronchopneumonia with serious sequelae in children with evidence of adenovirus type 21 infection. *Br Med J* 1:73, 1969.

28. Wenman WM, Pagtakhan RD, Reed MH, et al: Adenovirus bronchiolitis in Manitoba. Epidemiological, clinical, and radiologic features. *Chest* 81:605, 1982.

29. Bryant RE, Rhoades ER: Clinical features of adenoviral pneumonia in Air Force recruits. *Am Rev Respir Dis* 96:717, 1967.

30. Ruuskanen O, Sarkkinen H, Meurman O, et al: Rapid diagnosis of adenoviral tonsillitis. A prospective clinical study. *J Pediatr* 104:745, 1984.

31. Ruuskanen O, Meurman O, Sarkkinen H: Adenoviral diseases in children: A study of 105 hospital cases. *Pediatrics* 76:79: 1985.

32. Osborne D: Radiologic appearance of the lower respiratory tract in infants and children. *AJR* 130:29, 1978.

33. Becroft DMO: Histopathology of fatal adenovirus infection of the respiratory tract in children. *J Clin Pathol* 20:561, 1967.

34. Reid L, Simon G: Unilateral lung transradiancy. *Thorax* 17:230, 1962.

35. Epler GR, Colby TV: The spectrum of bronchiolitis obliterans. *Chest* 83:161, 1983.

36. McKenzie SA, Allison DJ, Singh MP, et al: Unilateral hyperlucent lung: Case or investigation. *Thorax* 35:745, 1980.

37. Macpherson RI, Cumming GR, Chernick V: Unilateral hyperlucent lung: A complication of viral pneumonia. *J Can Assoc Radiol* 20:225, 1969.

38. Seggev JS, Mason VG, Worthen S, et al: Bronchiolitis obliterans. Report of three cases with detailed physiologic studies. *Chest* 83:169, 1983.

39. Eisenklam EJ: Primary varicella pneumonia in a 3 year old girl. *J Pediatr* 69:452, 1966

40. Nakao T: Primary varicella pneumonia. *Tohoku J Exp Med* 72:249, 1960.

41. Knyvett AF: Complicated chickenpox. *Med J Aust* 2:91, 1957.

42. Ramey EK, Normane MG, Silver MD: Varicella pneumonitis. *Can Med Assoc J* 96:445, 1967.

43. Weber DM, Pellicchia JA: Varicella pneumonia: Study of prevalence in adult men. *JAMA* 192:572, 1965.

44. MacKay JB, Cairney P: Pulmonary calcification following varicella. *NZ Med J* 59:453, 1960.

45. Abrahams EW, Evans C, Knyvett AF, et al: Varicella pneumonia: A possible cause of subsequent pulmonary calcification. *Med J Aust* 2:781, 1964.

46. Nemir RL: Varicella pneumonia, in Kendig EL Jr, Chernick V (eds): *Disorders of the Respiratory Tract in Children*, 3d ed. Philadelphia, WB Saunders, 1977, p 955.

47. Bocles JS, Ehrenkranz NJ, Marks A: Abnormalities of respiratory function in varicella pneumonia. *Ann Intern Med* 60:183, 1964.

48. Dahlstrom G, Hillerdal O, Nordbring F, Uusitalo A: Pulmonary calcification following varicella and their effects on respiratory function. *Scand J Respir Dis* 48:249, 1969.

49. Helmly RB, Smith JO Jr, Eisen B: Chickenpox with pneumonia and pericarditis. *JAMA* 186:870, 1963.

50. Mandelbaum T, Terk BH: Pericarditis in association with chickenpox. *JAMA* 170:191, 1959.

51. Tatter D, Gerard PW, Silverman AH, et al: Fatal varicella pericarditis in a child. *Am J Dis Child* 108:88, 1964.

52. Sargent EN, Carson MJ, Reilly ED: Varicella pneumonia. A report of 20 cases, with post mortem examination in six. *Calif Med* 107:141, 1967.

53. Murphy TF, Henderson FW, Clyde WA, et al: Pneumonia: An eleven-year study in pediatric practice. *Am J Epidemiol* 113:12, 1981.

54. Hull HF, Blumhagen JD, Benjamin D, et al: Herpes simplex viral pneumonitis in childhood. *J Pediatr* 104:211, 1984.

55. Offit PA, Fleisher GR, Koven NL, et al: Severe Epstein-Barr virus pulmonary involvement. *J Adolesc Health Care* 2:121:1981.

56. Andiman WA, McCarthy P, Markowitz RI, et al: Clinical, virologic, and serologic evidence of Epstein-Barr virus infection in association with childhood pneumonia. *J Pediatr* 99:880, 1981.

57. Fackler JC, Nagel JE, Adler WH, et al: Epstein-Barr virus infection in a child with acquired immunodeficiency syndrome. *Am J Dis Child* 139:1000, 1985.

Chapter 20

Fungal Infections

Fungal infections of the thorax are frequently diagnosed with difficulty and after considerable delay. The roentgenographic alterations share many common features, and hence considerable overlapping is to be expected. Nevertheless, because of the characteristically indolent and protracted course of pulmonary fungal disease, radiographic observations are significant in establishing the extent of disease, in helping to guide diagnostic procedures, and in monitoring disease progress. Diagnostic imaging is also of importance when deciding upon a course of therapy. Most fungal disease is responsive to antibiotic therapy; however, in selected situations, surgical resection is sometimes the sole solution.[1]

The following radiographic findings are characteristic of pulmonary mycoses:

1. Infiltration
2. Cavitation
3. Cavitation with fungus ball
4. Solitary pulmonary nodule
5. Mediastinal mass
6. Great vessel obstruction
7. Pericarditis
8. Intraluminal mass
9. Pneumothorax
10. Effusion, empyema, bronchopleural, and/or chest wall fistula

Aspergillosis

Pulmonary aspergillosis, an uncommon infection in humans, is caused by several different species of the *Aspergillus* fungus. A ubiquitous organism, its airborne spores are frequently found as contaminants on the skin and in the sputum. Pulmonary infection with aspergillus organisms usually takes one of three clinicoroentgenographic configurations: (1) allergic, (2) intercavitary, or (3) invasive parenchymal.[2]

Allergic Bronchopulmonary Aspergillosis

First described by Hinson and coworkers,[3] allergic bronchopulmonary aspergillosis (ABPA) has subsequently been reported by additional authors.[4-7] It is uncommon in children, but has been reported.[4] This type of aspergillus infection probably results when atopic or asthmatic individuals inhale the fungal spores. Symptoms of asthma, bronchial wall damage (bronchiectasis), and bronchial mucus plugging probably result from host sensitivity to the fungal antigen. Individuals with cystic fibrosis are also affected, as are occasional persons with no antecedent pulmonary disease.

The significance of early diagnosis centers primarily on the use of corticosteroid therapy. In the presence of ABPA, small doses of steroids, often used to treat asthmatic patients, may cause progressive pulmonary destruction. Large steroid dosage, on the other hand, is usually curative. The following clinicoradiographic features suggest the presence of ABPA:[8,9]

1. Most common
   a. Asthma
   b. Blood eosinophilia (> 1000 per cubic millimeter)
   c. Immediate skin reactivity to aspergillus
   d. Precipitating antibodies against aspergillus antigen
   e. Elevated serum immunoglobulin E levels
   f. Central bronchiectasis (plain film or bronchogram)
   g. History of pulmonary infiltrates (transient or fixed)
2. Less common
   a. Mycelia or aspergillus in sputum culture
   b. Expectoration of brown plugs or specks in sputum
   c. Late skin reactivity to aspergillus antigen

Either form may progress to pulmonary fibrosis or chronic pulmonary insufficiency.[5]

Radiographic studies in patients with ABPA are strategic to the initial diagnosis. Central and upper lobe bronchiectasis with sparing of the peripheral bronchi is the definitive feature of the diagnosis of active ABPA in the absence of cystic fibrosis.[7] This distribution differs from other forms of bronchiectasis characteristically located in the periphery of lower lobe segments.

Perihilar pseudoadenopathy that represents central infiltrates, dilated bronchi filled with fluid and debris, and air-fluid levels in partially filled dilated cystic spaces are specific features of ABPA.[7-9] "Tramline" shadows (representing bronchial walls of normal width) and parallel line shadows (dilated tramlines) result from bronchial wall thickening and bronchiectasis. Mucoid intraluminal impactions appear as "gloved-finger" and/or "toothpaste" (Y-V) shadows that may shift about and disappear after cough.

The evaluation of the central bronchial anatomy and the delineation of "tramlines," mucoid bronchial plugging, and cystic changes are enhanced by the use of linear tomography[9] and possibly computed tomography (CT).

Large consolidations may accompany bronchial occlusion and lead to permanent lung damage. The typical Y- or V-shaped mucoid impactions may occur without sensitivity to aspergillus.[10]

Inhalation of thermophilic actinomycetes in moldy hay is another method whereby *Aspergillus* fungus may evoke a pulmonary reaction. This so-called extrinsic allergic alveolitis is not well understood and is probably related to entities, such as farmer's lung, pigeon-breeder's disease, bagassosis, mushroom-worker's disease, and others (see Chapter 22).

Intercavitary Aspergillosis (Pulmonary Mycetoma, "Fungus Ball")

Intercavitary mycetoma is a familiar manifestation of pulmonary aspergillosis. The fungus grows noninvasively as a saprophyte within previously existing pulmonary cavities. In adults, residual tuberculous cavities are most commonly involved, but mycetomas have been observed in association with sarcoidosis, emphysema, bronchiectasis, bullae or lung cysts, cavitated bronchogenic carcinoma, and pulmonary infarction.[11,12] Other fungal disease cavities (coccidioidomycosis, histoplasmosis, cryptococcosis, nocardiosis, blastomycosis), and apical fibrosis of ankylosing spondylitis may also house mycetomas.[13] Aspergilloma and ABPA may coexist.[5,10,14] Immunocompromised patients and those taking steroids and antimetabolites are at particular risk for this complication.[1]

The fungus hyphae of mycetomas grow on the wall, fall into the cavity, and, together with blood products and cellular debris, form a mass or fungus ball. Clinical diagnosis is difficult as sputum cultures are often negative. Since aspergillus is a common laboratory contaminant, repeated positive cultures are needed for definite diagnosis.[15]

Residual bronchopleural fistula and empyema are serious complications of aspergilloma. Life-threatening hemoptysis necessitates surgical resection in selected patients,[12,16] but removal of aspergillomas for other causes is unnecessary.[16] Steroid and antifungal therapies probably do not alter the natural course of the disease, but troublesome cough and hemoptysis may be relieved.[17] New antifungal agents such as ketoconazole hold some promise, at least for reducing life-threatening hemorrhage.

The characteristic radiographic appearance of aspergilloma is a well-defined, round, intercavitary structure, with an "air crescent" sign. The air crescent sign is inconstant and not specific for aspergilloma. Lung abscess, carcinoma, resolving hematoma, sclerosing hemangioma, Rasmussen's aneurysm, and other fungi, such as candida, may produce a similar configuration.[18] Air-fluid levels, poorly defined intracavitary masses, and the absence of a recognizable cavity are all to be expected. Pleural thickening adjacent to a previously empty cavity may herald the appearance of a fungus ball.[19] Fungus balls exist bilaterally, and one cavity may contain several.

The upper lobes are most commonly involved because of the predilection for tuberculous cavities; the middle and lower lobes are not spared. Tomography is sometimes necessary to identify the mass lesions with adjacent crescents of air. The development of a progressive parenchymal opacity around a cavity may be the first indication of invasive aspergilloma.[16]

Invasive Aspergillosis

Invasive aspergillosis is a progressive disease and carries a high mortality if not recognized and treated promptly. Normal individuals, especially inhabitants of farms, may develop this form of aspergillosis,[20,21] but debilitated, immunologically compromised patients, as well as those with leukemia and lymphoma, are most susceptible.[16,22] Others at risk are patients with solid neoplasms, connective tissue disorders, organ transplants, chronic granulomatosis, and recent bacterial infections, as well as those receiving immunosuppressants, cytoxic chemotherapy, corticosteroids, and antibiotics. Granulocytopenia contributes to this complication.

Pulmonary infection is seen in more than 90 percent of patients with invasive aspergillosis, but dissemination to visceral organs may occur in up to one-half. The gastrointestinal tract, brain, liver, kidney, thyroid, paranasal sinuses, heart, and skin are all potential sites of involvement.

The radiographic features of invasive aspergillosis are not always specific; one-third of patients may have negative chest films at the onset of disease.[23] Multiple and solitary nodular opacities, with or without cavitations; diffuse and focal consolidations; and diffuse interstitial disease have all been observed.

The air crescent sign may be caused by invasive aspergillosis, but unlike the pulmonary mycetoma, it occurs in the absence of a preexisting cavity. Air crescents are late features of invasive aspergillosis and cannot be relied upon as early evidence of disease (Figure 20-1).[24] Using CT, Kuhlman and coworkers[25] have shown that a low attenuation halo about a pulmonary lesion precedes the radiographic appearance of the air crescent. While this sign is not specific for aspergillosis, in the appropriate clinical setting, it should make the diagnosis highly suspect. The development of the air crescent probably results from vasoinvasion, vascular thrombosis, and infarction of the central inflammatory focus. Curtis and coworkers[18] reported four leukemic patients who de-

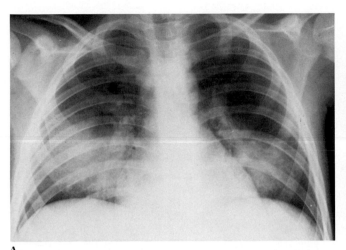
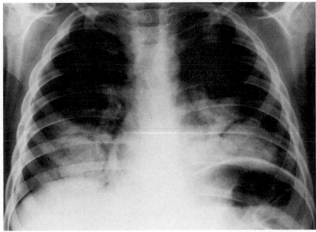

A   B

Figure 20-1 Invasive aspergillosis. A. Bilateral infiltrates have developed in this patient with leukemia. **B.** Several days later, there are bilateral lesions with central, rounded densities surrounded by air crescents. The lungs cleared on antifungal medications.

veloped air crescents within areas of pulmonary infiltration, and caution against the labeling of this pattern as a cavity containing a mycetoma.

Aspergillosis, confined mostly to the pleura, is found in patients with chronic granulomatosis, tuberculosis, bacterial empyemas, indwelling chest tubes, and bronchopleural-bronchocutaneous fistulas.[26 – 28]

Actinomycosis

Pulmonary actinomycosis is caused by the bacterial organism *Actinomyces israelii*.[20] However, the clinical and radiographic countenance of actinomycosis so resembles fungal disease, that it is included in this chapter.

The disease is uncommon in children; peak age periods for occurrence are reported from 11 to 20 years and 30 to 50 years.[29] Men are affected more than women, and the incidence is higher in rural areas.

The actinomycosis organism frequently attacks the face, neck, thoracic, and abdominal regions. Re-

tarded individuals, especially those with poor dental hygiene, are at greater risk. Primary pulmonary infections probably begin with aspiration of organisms into the lung.

Clinical symptoms of thoracic actinomycosis manifest late in the course of the disease because of low virulence. Cough, smoldering fever, weight loss, and pain are salient features. Chest wall swelling and draining sinuses are infrequent, but well-documented, complications.

The radiographic findings of actinomycosis feature chronic pulmonary infiltrates and empyema.[30] Lower lobes are most often involved. Chronic consolidations with the formation of fistulas crossing natural anatomic planes and fissures are characteristic. Pleural disease is common, occurring in 80 percent of patients reported by Flynn and Felson.[31] Extension of pleural infections through the chest wall (empyema necessitans) is a peculiar characteristic of actinomycosis (Figures 20-2 and 20-3), but invasive aspergillosis, nocardiosis, tuberculosis, and rare bacterial empyema may behave in a similar manner.[28]

Wavelike periosteal thickening of ribs is an additional feature of actinomycosis (Figure 20-4). Erosions into the trachea, esophagus, cardiovascular

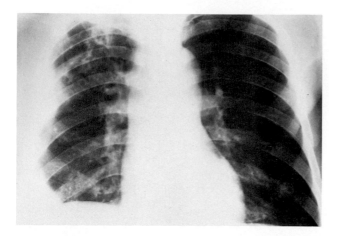

Figure 20-2   Actinomycosis—empyema necessitans. Pleural reaction and adjacent infiltrates are evident in the right lung along with cavitary lesions in the right upper lobe. Considerable soft tissue swelling of the right chest wall is present but not well produced on this print. The patient had an external draining sinus from the chest wall.

structure, and mediastinum are serious complications. Adjacent vertebrae may be destroyed, but unlike tuberculosis, the disk spaces are usually preserved.

While plain films are usually sufficiently diagnostic, CT is of value for better delineating the extent of disease. Ultrasonography is also a useful modality, especially in the presence of pleural reaction.[32]

Mucormycosis (Phycomycosis)

Mucormycosis is an extremely lethal fungus infection.[33] Factors that increase host susceptibility include acidosis, diabetes, ingestion of corticosteroids, cytotoxic agents, and antibiotics, as well as leukopenia and states of depressed phagocytosis. More than 75 percent of patients with pulmonary mucormycosis have leukemia or lymphoma,[34,35] but previously healthy individuals have contracted fatal cases of mucormycosis.[36]

Chest roentgenograms are not specific and usually do not help in the diagnosis of mucormycosis.

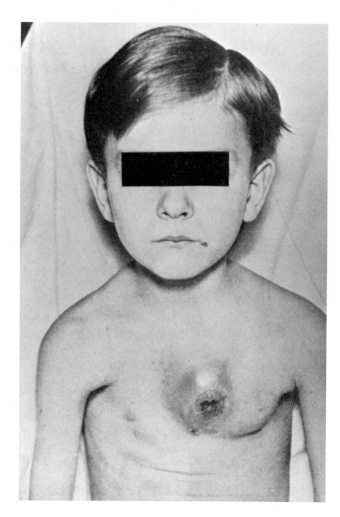

Figure 20-3   Empyema necessitans. This boy developed a chronic chest wall sinus as a result of pulmonary actinomycosis. The lesion drained "sulfur granules"; the sinus cleared following antifungal therapy. (From Brenneman and McQuarrie, *Practice of Pediatrics*, Philadelphia, Lippincott/Harper & Row, 1952. With permission.)

However, the appearance of diffuse nonhomogeneous infiltrates and/or consolidations in a compromised host should always raise the possibility of a secondary or opportunistic invader (Figures 20-5 and 20-6).[37] Cavitation is an occasional finding, and pleural effusion may occur in rare cases. Coin lesions and fungus balls have also been observed.

The presence of multiple consolidations with or without cavitations should suggest the possibility of

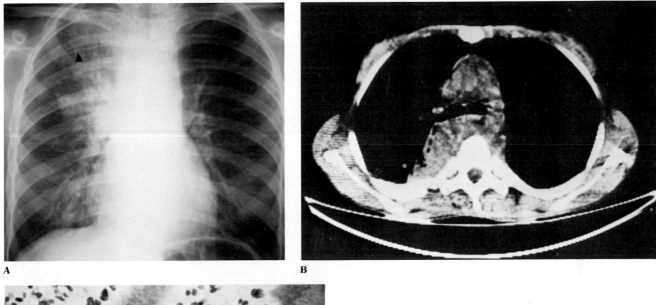

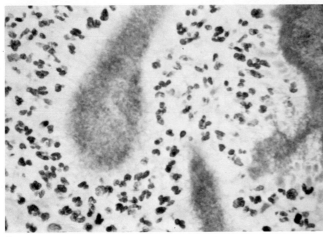

Figure 20-4 **Actinomycosis—empyema necessitans.** A 14-year-old girl with chronic pulmonary process; draining "boil" over the right scapula had drained 6 months earlier. **A.** The frontal film shows a posterior paramediastinal mass with heavy, wavy periosteal new bone (arrowhead) of the right upper ribs. **B.** Computed tomography confirms the presence of the paramediastinal inflammatory process; the adjacent rib is thickened and has an irregular surface. **C.** This biopsy specimen obtained from the posterior paramediastinal mass demonstrates hyphae consistent with *Actinomyces israelii* (hematoxylin-eosin, ×1000). (From Seibert JJ, et al: Radiological case of the month. *Am J Dis Child* 139:101, 1985. Copyright 1985, American Medical Association. With permission.)

a fungal rather than bacterial origin and call for specific culture or biopsy to affirm the correct diagnosis.[37] Lung biopsy is probably the most efficacious method for diagnosis and should be carried out soon after the onset of pulmonary symptoms and radiographic changes.

Coccidioidomycosis

Coccidioidomycosis, caused by the organism *Coccidioides immitis*, is a fungal disease endemic to the desert regions of the southwestern United States and the San Joaquin Valley of California. Due presumably to increased population mobility, the disease is being recognized with greater frequency beyond these endemic areas.[38] Sixty percent of infected children remain asymptomatic. Those with symptomatic disease may develop (1) pneumonitis (valley fever), (2) primary coccidioidal granuloma from direct inoculation or trauma, or (3) a chronic disseminated process that carries a poor prognosis.[39] Multiple systems including bone, skin, and meninges are also susceptible to infection with this organism.

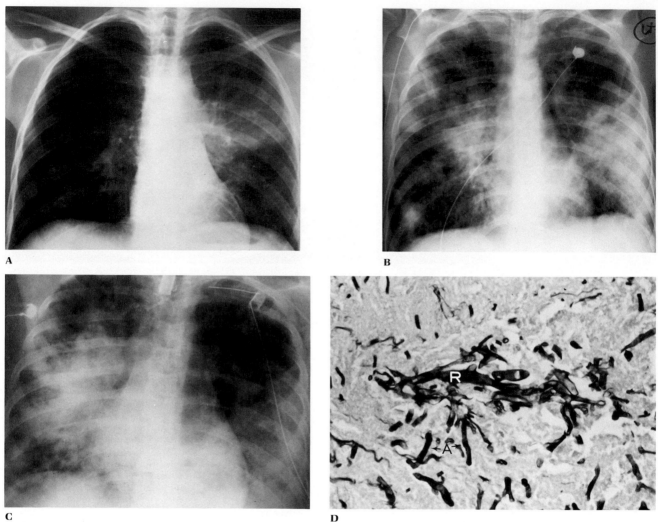

A

B

C

D

Figure 20-5   Mucormycosis. This 15-year-old diabetic girl developed a streptococcal throat infection followed by chills, cough, left chest pain, and tachypnea. These symptoms increased over a 10-day period, when a chest film disclosed a pneumonic infiltrate in the left lung. Because of her rapid clinical deterioration and progressive pulmonary infiltrates requiring ventilatory assistance, bronchoscopic examination was undertaken and returned histologic material, which was diagnostic. She expired approximately 1 week later. **A.** The initial chest film shows an alveolar infiltrate confined to the left midlung. **B.** Seven days later the pneumonic process has extended to involve most of the left lung as well as the perihilar portion of the right. **C.** This film was exposed just before death. A disseminated confluent alveolar infiltrate is apparent bilaterally with some sparing of the apices. **D.** The bronchial biopsy specimen consists of multiple, soft, gray-white fragments in which two types of hyphal structures are evident. The broader hyphae are typical of the nonseptate phycomycete *Rhizopus* (R), which was cultured from this tissue. The narrower hyphae represent an unidentified septate fungus, possibly *Aspergillus* (A). (Grocott silver methenamine.)

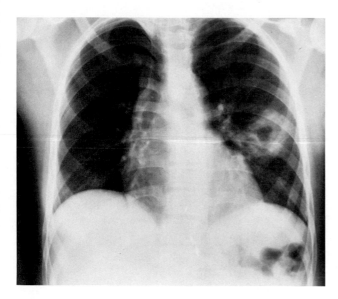

Figure 20-6 Mucormycosis. A thick-walled cavity is present in the left midlung in this post-renal transplant patient. The child died and was found to have widely disseminated phycomycosis with pulmonary infarction and fungal abscess in the left lower lobe.

Valley fever presents with influenza-like symptoms and may be accompanied by pruritis, maculopapular rash, cough, and pleuritic pain. In most cases, the disease is mild and self-limited, but in neonates and young infants, it is potentially devastating and lethal.[40]

The chest film changes are not unlike those of other mycoses. Consolidated parenchymal opacity with regional lymphadenopathy is a classic presentation that may simulate tuberculosis. Calcifications of the original lung lesion and regional lymph nodes are not uncommon. Pleural effusions are usually insignificant, but may be massive. Thin-walled cavities develop in limited cases and usually heal by fibrosis or calcification. Spontaneous rupture of coccidioidal cavities with pneumothorax is a recognized complication and frequently necessitates surgical intervention and pulmonary resection.[41]

Generalized pulmonary overaeration, focal consolidations, and diffuse nodular densities are peculiar radiographic changes of coccidioidomycosis in infants and neonates.[40] Pleural effusion and cavita-

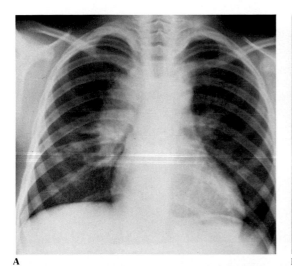
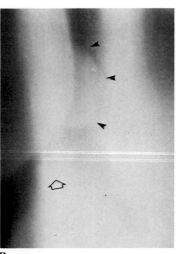
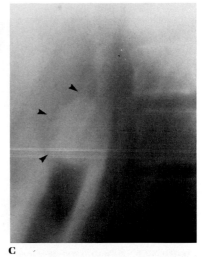

A   B   C

Figure 20-7 Coccidioidomycosis—upper airway obstruction. This 10-year-old boy with disseminated coccidioidomycosis developed cough, lethargy, and progressively severe stridor and wheezing. **A.** The frontal study shows mediastinal and right hilar lymphadenopathy. The distal trachea is narrowed above the carina. The frontal (**B**) and lateral (**C**) tomograms were taken at the level of tracheal bifurcation. In addition to extrinsic tracheal compression, the discrete endobronchial mass narrows the lumen of the distal trachea (arrowheads). A second, less well defined endobronchial mass narrows the lumen of the right stem bronchus (open arrow). (See Chapter 13.) (From Moskowitz PS, et al: Tracheal coccidioidomycosis causing upper airway obstruction in children. *AJR* 139:596, 1982. Copyright © 1982, American Roentgen Ray Society. With permission.)

tions are uncommon; hilar adenopathy may be a delayed feature. This roentgenographic appearance is not specific for coccidioidomycosis and may be seen in congenital tuberculosis, as well as bacterial and viral pneumonia.

Invasion of the airways is an uncommon but recognized complication of fungal disease (see Chapter 13, Figure 13-5, histoplasmosis). Moskowitz and coworkers[39] described the occurrence of upper airway obstruction by coccidioidal granulomas of the trachea (Figure 20-7).

Blastomycosis

North American blastomycosis is endemic to Ohio, Missouri, Mississippi, Kentucky, North Carolina, and Arkansas. The causative organism, *Blastomyces dermatiditis*, is a dimorphic fungus with worldwide distribution. This organism invades the respiratory system, and pneumonic disease is by far the most common manifestation. Other organ systems, however, are also involved, including the skeleton and brain.

The radiographic features of pulmonary blastomycosis are not specific but have been traditionally associated with inordinate hilar adenopathy. Halvorsen and coworkers[42] described four roentgen patterns: (1) air space disease, (2) nodular masses, (3) interstitial disease, and (4) cavitation (Figures 20-8 and 20-9). Others have emphasized the occurrence of miliary lesions in this disease.[43]

While treatment with antifungal agents is usually curative, delayed complications, especially in the brain, must be anticipated.

Cryptococcosis

Cryptococcus neoformans, the etiologic agent of cryptococcosis (torulosis), may produce significant lung disease. The pulmonary lesions are pleo-

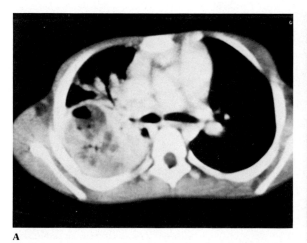
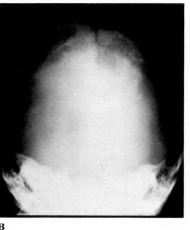
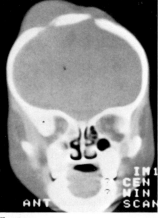

A   B   C

Figure 20-8   Blastomycosis—osseous involvement. A 3-year-old boy with progressive pneumonia unresponsive to antibiotics; *Blastomyces dermatitidis* was isolated from bronchial washings. **A.** Computed tomography shows a complex process in the right posterior lung with cavitation. This cleared after 27 days of amphotericin B. Nine months later he presented with a draining scalp abscess, destructive skull lesions, and a right frontal brain abscess caused by the same organism. The skull film (**B**) and CT scan (**C**) show destructive lesions of the calvarium with associated soft tissue masses. The child was treated with amphotericin B, rifampin, and surgical resection on this occasion and has remained free of disease. *Note:* This case emphasizes the need for close monitoring of the central nervous system in patients with pulmonary infection and/or malignancy. (Courtesy of Dr. James Scatliff, Chapel Hill, North Carolina.)

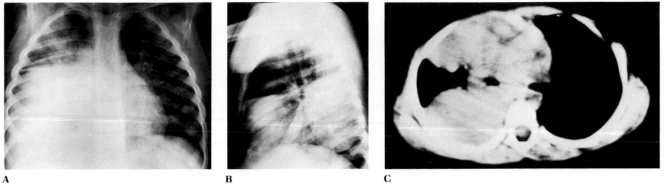

A   B   C

Figure 20-9 Blastomycosis. A and **B.** These studies show extensive air space consolidation of the right middle and right lower lung fields. **C.** Computed tomography confirms the confluent consolidation and absent cavitation. (Courtesy of Dr. Godfrey Gaise, Chapel Hill, North Carolina.)

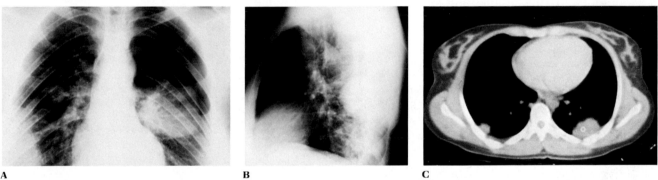

A   B   C

Figure 20-10 Cryptococcosis (torulosis). The patient is a 22-year-old woman. **A.** The lesions have the appearance of infiltrative lesions with irregular, poorly defined borders. **B.** In the lateral projection they are pleural-based and sharply defined and appear more "masslike." **C.** Computed tomography confirms the location against the inner chest wall and relatively sharp margination, making differentiation from malignancy hazardous or impossible.

morphic, but generally manifest as poorly defined masses or consolidative infiltrates that may be patchy, sharply confluent, or circumscribed. Feigin[44] has applied the term *infiltrative mass* because in one view the lesions resemble infiltration with ill-defined borders and segmental distribution (Figure 20-10A), while in the 90° view, the lesions appear as mass opacities with well-defined borders and nonsegmental localization (Figure 20-10B). Lymphadenopathy is a regular feature, but hilar retraction, scarring, volume loss, cavitation, and pleural reactions are uncommon. The diagnosis of cryptococcosis should be considered in a young individual with an infiltrative mass lesion and associated hilar adenopathy, especially when accompanied with minimal

or mild respiratory symptoms. In older patients, of course, the diagnosis of malignancy must be excluded.

Cryptococci may invade other organs, particularly bone. Central nervous system involvement is a particular problem for animals, especially in captivity.

Candidiasis

Candida albicans pneumonia, like so many other fungal infections, is usually seen in patients with other primary diseases, such as leukemia or lymphoma. No roentgenographic pattern is diagnostic, but candidiasis should be considered in debilitated patients with pneumonia. Unilateral, bilateral, lobar, nonlobar, and segmental consolidations are produced and resemble other fungal and bacterial pneumonias. However, candida pneumonia differs somewhat from other fungal disease in that it fails to produce adenopathy, cavitation, masslike opacities, or miliary patterns.[45] Correlation of candida pneumonia with histologic lung changes has been inconclusive.[46]

The increased use of parenteral alimentation, especially in small infants and neonates, is responsible for more candida infections. While many of these involve the lung, particular attention must be paid to other organs, i.e., kidney, liver, spleen, and central nervous system.

References

1. Newsom BD, Hardy JD: Pulmonary fungal infections—Survey of 159 cases with surgical implications. *J Thorac Cardiovasc Surg* 83:218, 1982.

2. Seabury JH: The mycosis (excluding histoplasmosis), in Kendig EL Jr, Chernick V (eds): *Disorders of the Respiratory Tract in Children*, 3d ed. Philadelphia, WB Saunders, 1977, p 897.

3. Hinson KFW, Moon AJ, Plummer N: Bronchopulmonary aspergillosis. *Thorax* 7:318, 1952.

4. Wang JLF, Patterson R, Mintzer R, et al: Allergic bronchopulmonary aspergillosis in pediatric practice. *J Pediatr* 94:376, 1979.

5. Saferstein BH, D'Souza JP, Simon G, et al: Five year follow-up of allergic bronchopulmonary aspergillosis. *Am Rev Respir Dis* 108:450, 1973.

6. Ricketti AJ, Greenberger PA, Mintzer RA, et al: Allergic bronchopulmonary aspergillosis. *Chest* 86:773, 1984.

7. Mendelson EB, Fisher MR, Mintzer RA, et al: Roentgenographic and clinical staging of allergic bronchopulmonary aspergillosis. *Chest* 87:385, 1985.

8. Mintzer RA, Rogers LF, Kruglik GD, et al: The spectrum of radiologic findings in allergic bronchopulmonary aspergillosis. *Radiology* 127:301, 1978.

9. Fisher MR, Mendelson EB, Mintzer RA: Allergic bronchopulmonary aspergillosis: A pictorial essay. *Radiographics* 4:445, 1984.

10. Klein DL, Gamsu G: Thoracic manifestations of aspergillosis. *AJR* 134:543, 1980.

11. Davis D: Aspergillosis and residual tuberculous cavities—The result of a resurvey. A report from the research committee of the British Thoracic and Tuberculosis Association. *Tubercle* 51:227, 1970.

12. Garvey J, Crastnopol P, Weisz D, et al: The surgical treatment of pulmonary aspergillomas. *J Thorac Cardiovasc Surg* 74:542, 1977.

13. Aspergilloma, editorial. *Lancet* 1:637, 1977.

14. McCarthy DS, Pepys J: Pulmonary aspergilloma—Clinical immunology. *Clin Allergy* 3:57, 1973.

15. Campbell MJ, Clayton YM: Bronchopulmonary aspergillosis: A correlation of clinical and laboratory findings in 272 patients investigated for bronchopulmonary aspergillosis. *Am Rev Respir Dis* 89:186, 1964.

16. Rafferty P, Biggs B, Crompton GK, et al: What happens to patients with pulmonary aspergilloma? Analysis of 23 cases. *Thorax* 38:579, 1983.

17. Hammerman KJ, Christianson CS, Huntington I, et al: Spontaneous lysis of aspergillomata. *Chest* 64:697, 1973.

18. Curtis AM, Walker Smith GJ, Ravin CE: Air crescent of invasive aspergillosis. *Radiology* 133:19, 1979.

19. Libshitz HI, Atkinson GW, Israel HL: Pleural thickening as a manifestation of aspergillus superinfection. *AJR* 120:883, 1974.

20. Hertzig AJ, Smith TS, Goblin M: Acute pulmonary aspergillosis. *Pediatrics* 4:331, 1949.

21. Allan GW, Anderson DH: Generalized aspergillosis in an infant 18 days of age. *Pediatrics* 26:432, 1960.

22. Meyer RD, Young LS, Armstrong D, et al: Aspergillosis complicating neoplastic disease. *Am J Med* 54:6, 1973.

23. Young RC, Bennett JE, Vogel CL, et al: Aspergillosis: The spectrum of disease in 98 patients. *Medicine* 49:147, 1970.

24. Gefter WB, Albelda SM, Talbot GN, et al: Invasive pulmonary aspergillosis and acute leukemia. Limitation in the diagnostic utility of the air crescent sign. *Radiology* 157:605, 1985.

25. Kuhlman JE, Fishman EK, Siegelman SS: Invasive pulmonary aspergillosis in acute leukemia: Characteristic findings on CT, the CT halo sign, and the role of CT in early diagnosis. *Radiology* 157:611, 1985.

26. Meredith HC, Cogan BM, McLaulin B: Pleural aspergillosis. *AJR* 130:164, 1978.

27. Gaisie G, Bowen AD, Quattromani FL: Chest wall inva-

sion by aspergillus in chronic granulomatous disease. *Pediatr Radiol* 11:203, 1981.

28. Altman AR: Thoracic wall invasion secondary to pulmonary aspergillosis: A complication of chronic granulomatous disease of childhood. *AJR* 129:140, 1977.

29. Bates M, Cruickshank G: Thoracic actinomycosis. *Thorax* 12:99, 1957.

30. James R, Heneghan MA, Lipkansky V: Thoracic actinomycosis. *Chest* 87:536, 1985.

31. Flynn MW, Felson B: The roentgen manifestations of thoracic actinomycosis. *AJR* 110:107, 1970.

32. Dershaw DD: Actinomycosis of the chest wall—Ultrasound findings in empyema necessitans. *Chest* 86:779, 1984.

33. Murray HW: Pulmonary mucormycosis: One hundred years later. *Chest* 72:1, 1977.

34. Meyer RD, Armstrong D: Mucormycosis: Changing status. *CRC Crit Rev Clin Lab Sci* 4:421, 1974.

35. Meyer RD, Rosen P, Armstrong D: Phycomycosis complicating leukemia and lymphoma. *Ann Intern Med* 77:871, 1972.

36. Record NB, Ginder DR: Pulmonary phycomycosis without obvious predisposing factors. *JAMA* 235:1256, 1976.

37. Bartrum RJ, Watnick M, Herman PG: Roentgenographic findings in pulmonary mucormycosis. *AJR* 117:810, 1973.

38. Fulginiti VA: Coccidioidomycosis in children: A persistent, difficult problem. *Infect Dis Newsletter (Tucson)* 6:3, 1980.

39. Moskowitz PA, Sue JY, Gooding CA: Tracheal coccidioidomycosis causing upper airway obstruction in children. *AJR* 139:596, 1982.

40. Child DD, Newell JD, Bjelland JC, et al: Radiographic findings of pulmonary coccidioidomycosis in neonates and infants. *AJR* 145:261, 1985.

41. Cunningham RT, Einstein H: Coccidioidal pulmonary cavities with rupture. *Chest* 84:172, 1982.

42. Halvorsen RA, Duncan JD, Merten DF, et al: Pulmonary blastomycosis: Radiologic manifestations. *Radiology* 150:1, 1984.

43. Stelling CB, Woodring JH, Rehm SR, et al: Miliary pulmonary blastomycosis. *Radiology* 150:7, 1984.

44. Feigin DS: Pulmonary cryptococcosis: Radiologic-pathologic correlates of its three forms. *AJR* 141:1263, 1983.

45. Buff SJ, McLelland R, Gallis HA, et al: *Candida albicans* pneumonia: Radiographic appearance. *AJR* 138:645, 1982.

46. Kassner EG, Kaufman SL, Yoon JJ, et al: Pulmonary candidiasis in infants. Clinical, radiological, and pathological features. *AJR* 137:707, 1981.

Chapter 21

Pulmonary Infestations

This chapter will consider pulmonary diseases that result from opportunistic organisms and parasites. Acquired immunodeficiency syndrome (AIDS) will be reviewed since children and adults with this condition are particularly susceptible to opportunistic pulmonary infections. *Pneumocystis carinii* pneumonia, one of the most ubiquitous and aggravating secondary invaders of host-compromised patients, is also discussed in detail. Because of the need for early and accurate diagnosis in these individuals, several methods used to obtain lung tissue are examined.

Parasitic pulmonary infestations are not common in the so-called developed countries, but occasionally these organisms may appear and cause significant illness. Toxocariasis and echinococcosis occur in selected geographic areas of the United States. Paragonimiasis is largely confined to far eastern countries but is increasing in incidence in the United States as a result of greater international travel.

Acquired Immunodeficiency Syndrome

Acquired immunodeficiency syndrome is caused by a virus that is transmitted through semen and blood inoculation. First discovered in the United States in homosexual males,[1] the disease has since been found among intravenous drug users, hemophiliacs, recipients of blood products, and otherwise normal individuals with exposure to the virus. The recognized complications of AIDS include certain malignancies such as Kaposi's sarcoma, non-Hodgkin's lymphoma, and life-threatening opportunistic infections, most commonly from *P. carinii* and cytomyelovirus.[2,3]

Infants and children are also victims of an AIDS-like illness that resembles genetic T-cell depletion syndrome.[4] The manifestations of pulmonary infections in AIDS, characterized by hilar adenopathy and inflammatory lung lesions, are not specific, and when present, usually herald serious disease.[5,6]

Pneumocystis carinii Pneumonia

Pneumocystis carinii pneumonia occurs most often in immunodeficient or seriously debilitated patients. Epidemics in normal neonates and infants occur sporadically in the United States, while in Europe the disease exists in endemic form. The organism may inhabit the lungs of healthy individuals, producing clinical disease only when defense mechanisms are impaired. It occurs most often in patients with chronic debilitating diseases, organ transplant recipients, and those under therapy for tumors, leukemia, and lymphoma. The odds of contracting the disease increase with the intensity of immunotherapy. However, prophylactic administration of trimethoprim and sulfamethoxazole (Septra) to susceptible individuals has decreased the incidence of clinically significant pneumocystis infections.

Two general clinical patterns of pneumocystis pneumonia are defined.[7] The first, or infantile type, is slow in onset, with nonspecific signs of poor feeding, lassitude, or restless behavior. Tachypnea and cyanosis herald pulmonary involvement, but cough and fever are not present. The disease worsens progressively in the ensuing 4 to 6 weeks and is fatal if untreated.[8]

The second pattern, usually confined to susceptible older children and adults, has a more abrupt clinical onset, with sudden fever, tachypnea, cough, cyanosis, and nasal flaring. Auscultatory chest signs are often subtle or normal. Blood gas studies usually reveal a marked decrease in arterial oxygen tension (Pa_{O_2}) with normal P_{CO_2}.

Pneumocystis infections are now being recognized with increasing frequency in patients with AIDS.[9-11] Wollschlager and coworkers[12] reported that of 15 patients with AIDS 14 had pneumocystis pneumonia at the time of initial evaluation. In some AIDS patients the roentgenographic features of pneumocystis pneumonia may be atypical and less obvious.[11] Differentiation from cytomegalic inclusion disease and other secondary invaders may be difficult or impossible from roentgen features alone.

The radiographic patterns of pneumocystis pneumonia have been the subject of many reports, but most describe the findings in advanced disease.[13-15] Chest films taken very early in the course of the disease may appear surprisingly normal, but subtle changes are usually present (Figures 21-1A and 21-2A). Most significant are indistinct, poorly defined, and tortuous vessels; enlarged and ill-defined hila; nonspecific increase in lung markings; and a diffuse "hazy" quality of the lungs. Generalized confluent radiopacities usually occur only after 2 to 3 days of symptoms when the disease is well advanced (Figure 21-2B).[14] Lobar distribution is found on occasion but is atypical (Figure 21-3). In most cases, the lungs have normal to decreased volume; pleural effusions and pneumothorax are rare or nonexistent. Cavitary lesions are distinctly unusual, but when present, the possibility of secondary fungus infection should be considered (Figure 21-4).

The radiographic findings of pneumocystis are nonspecific and overlap with other opportunistic invaders, such as cytomegalic inclusion disease and bacterial organisms. On occasion, drug reaction and irradiation may produce radiographic changes in the lung that resemble those of pneumocystis and other organisms. Since early diagnosis is of the utmost importance, treatment should not be delayed while awaiting the development of advanced radiographic abnormalities.

Diagnostic Methods

Opportunistic or superimposed pulmonary infections in immunologically compromised or debilitated individuals demand immediate diagnosis and therapy. Since radiologic and clinical findings are usually not definitive, several methods of obtaining diagnostic material from the lung have been developed. The choice in any given case will depend upon several factors: (1) the suspected etiologic agent that is most likely from clinical, laboratory, and radiologic assessment, (2) the condition of the patient, and (3) the expertise and capability of the individual physicians and laboratories.

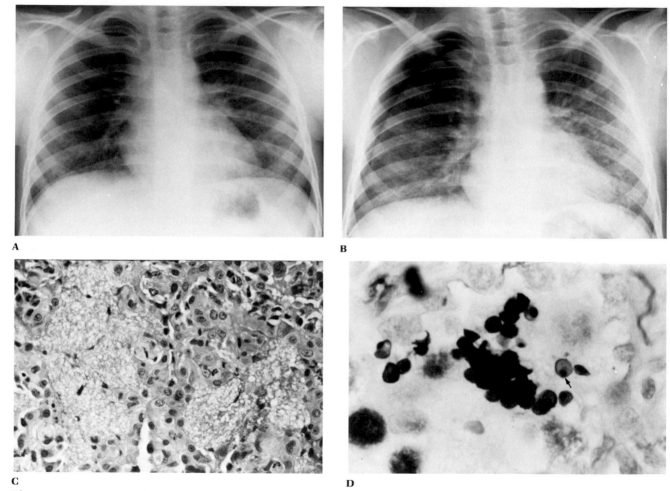

Figure 21-1 *Pneumocystis carinii* pneumonia. This 16-year-old boy, with a history of systemic lupus erythematosus and nephritis, developed a cough and a low-grade fever. **A.** The initial film shows changes in the periphery of the lungs that obscure the normal pulmonary vascularity and create confluent radiopacities bilaterally. The central lung fields and hilar vascular shadows are preserved. **B.** Twenty-four hours later, the pulmonary changes have progressed and obscure the central vascular shadows. The right-sided pneumothorax is secondary to lung biopsy. **C.** Low power: The histologic examination shows hypertrophied and hyperplastic alveolar lining cells. These lining cells become vacuolated during the infection, and the alveolar spaces fill with a foamy material. **D.** High power: The silver methenamine stain distinguishes the bowl-shaped, darkly stained, encysted forms of *P. carinii* within the foamy material. The smaller structures occasionally visible within the cysts are trophozoites (arrow).

The following are established techniques used to obtain diagnostic material from the lungs:

1. Sputum examination[16,17]
2. Tracheobronchial lavage and aspiration[18]
3. Endobronchial brush biopsy[1,19,20]
4. Transbronchial lung biopsy[21,22]
5. Percutaneous needle aspiration/biopsy[23-25] with sonographic guidance[26]
6. Thoracoscopy and lung biopsy[27,28]
7. Open lung biopsy[29-32]

The list of procedures available for making an etiologic diagnosis in patients with AIDS is quite long,

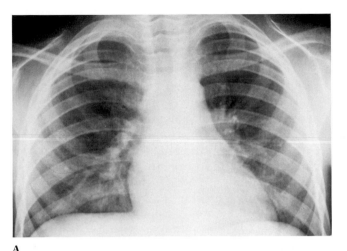
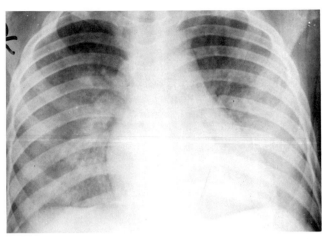

A B

Figure 21-2 *Pneumocystis carinii* **pneumonia.** **A.** Minimal nondescript changes are present in the central lung fields in the very early phase of respiratory distress. Biopsy of the lung established the diagnosis of *P. carinii* infection. **B.** Forty-eight h later, the lungs are diffusely opaque. This pattern represents late disease.

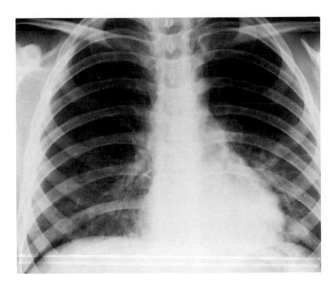

Figure 21-3 *Pneumocystis carinii* **pneumonia—lobar distribution.** A consolidated left lower lobe is present in this patient with biopsy-proven *P. carinii* pneumonia.

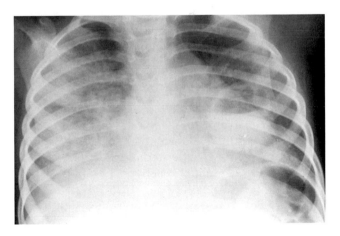

Figure 21-4 **Pneumocystis—cavitation.** There is a cavitary lesion in the left lung in addition to diffuse opacity on the right. While pneumocystis organisms were recovered from the right lung, the exact cause of the left-sided cavitation remained unproved and might have been fungus. The lungs cleared with treatment for both pneumocystis and fungus.

but those techniques that obtain sufficient material for histologic examination are better than ones that produce only fluids. Touch preparations using Bomoni's methanamine silver toluidine blue[7] are often diagnostic within hours for *P. carinii*, the most frequent invader. Biopsy through the thoracoscopy technique is the least traumatic technique for lung biopsy and

usually returns pieces of tissue that are large enough for histologic examination. The procedure can be performed without general anesthesia. However, the techniques employed and their sequence must be selected in accordance with individual clinical parameters and parochial procedures.[33–35]

In spite of the attention that is often focused on

unusual infections such as pneumocystis, cytomegalic inclusion disease, herpes simplex, and fungi, the clinician should be aware that bacterial pneumonias are far and away the most common etiologic agents that invade the lungs, especially in leukemia. Pulmonary changes secondary to leukemia, per se, are extremely uncommon and should not be considered in the differential diagnosis when pulmonary infiltrates develop in these patients.[33,36]

Loeffler's Syndrome (Toxocariasis or Visceral Larval Migrans)

This syndrome is characterized by transitory pulmonary infiltrates and increased numbers of eosinophils in lung tissue and/or peripheral blood, sometimes as high as 70 percent. The terms *Loeffler's syndrome* and *pulmonary infiltrates with eosinophilia* (PIE) are confusing since they represent a wide spectrum of diseases in which the presence or absence of eosinophils is inconstant. These syndromes probably result from an atopic or otherwise unusual allergic response to a variety of stimuli. Among these are drug reactions, collagen-vascular diseases, allergic fungal reactions, helminthic infestations, and probably others.

In children, most cases of Loeffler's syndrome are the result of parasitic infestations, chief of which are the dog roundworm (*Toxocara canis*) and less often the cat roundworm (*Toxocara cati*). Other parasites such as *Ascaris lumbricoides*, *Strongyloides*, and the lung fluke (*Paragonimus*) may be the cause.

The clinical syndrome of visceral larval migrans results when there is extraintestinal invasion by these parasites which travel through the liver, lung, and other organs but do not complete their life cycle. Shifting pulmonary infiltrates, hepatomegaly, and peripheral eosinophilia constitute the clinical manifestations in most cases.[37] The disease affects toddlers most often, especially those who play in dirt contaminated by dogs.

The clinical symptoms derive primarily from the number and location of the granulomatous lesions and from the allergic response of the human host to the larvae.[38] They may range from mild elevation of circulating eosinophils to a fulminant, occasionally fatal disorder with extensive pulmonary and central nervous system involvement.[39] Cough, wheezing, fever, convulsions, and occasional visual impairment are possible complications. Hepatomegaly and hyperglobulinemia are common findings in more serious infestations.[40] Cardiomyopathy may also develop. Examinations for stool ova and parasites are negative.

Clinical signs of pulmonic disease occur in 20 percent of cases; radiographic infiltrates develop in about half. In most cases these represent nondescript alveolar processes (Figure 21-5), but miliary lesions as well as chronic changes are described. The pulmonary opacities shift about as larvae migrate within the pulmonary tissue.

The diagnosis is best confirmed by biopsy of a lesion, usually in the liver, and demonstration of the typical nematode larva within multifocal necrotizing eosinophil-containing granulomas. Capillary tube precipitin tests have been diagnostic in 76 of 80 patients.[41]

Echinococcosis

Echinococcosis (hydatid cyst disease) is caused by infestation with *Echinococcus granulosus*, or *Taenia echinococcus*, the dog tapeworm. The organism lives in dogs, wolves, coyotes, and other Canidae; intermediate hosts include horses, cattle, sheep, and swine. The larval worm is parasitic to humans in regions where it is prevalent among animals. Ova, evacuated in feces, are ingested. Embryos penetrate the intestinal wall and are disseminated by the bloodstream to many parts of the body, especially the liver, where hydatid cysts are produced over a period of many months.

Cardiac and pericardial involvement is an uncommon but reported complication.[42] The lungs are

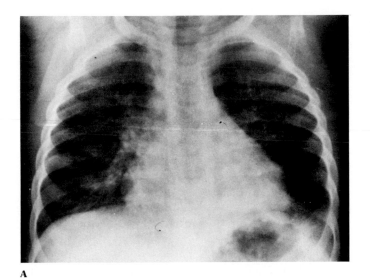

A

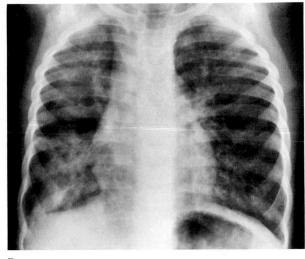

B

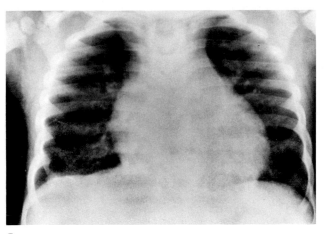

C

Figure 21-5 Visceral larva migrans—Loeffler's pneumonia. This 2½-year-old male had chronic cough; his white blood cell count showed an elevated eosinophil percentage, as high as 57 percent at one time. The lung biopsy revealed eosinophilic pneumonia and remnants of toxocara organisms. **A.** The chest film shows mild cardiomegaly and patchy infiltration, predominantly in the left lower lobe. **B.** One year later, the left lower lobe is clear, but infiltrate has developed in the right lung. **C.** Film taken 1 month later shows remarkable clearing but persistent cardiomegaly.

frequently involved in the pediatric age groups. Hydatidosis is found in all age groups, but it is quite common during childhood and adolescence.[43–46]

Puncture of the cysts is to be avoided because of the danger of anaphylactic shock, hyperpyrexia, pruritis, urticaria, and even death. With the use of computed tomography, this complication should be unlikely. Surgical removal is the treatment of choice, but considerable surrounding lung must be taken along with the cyst.

Radiographic signs depend upon the integrity of the cysts. Intact cysts present a round or ovoid shape with a homogeneous density and smooth outlines. They are often subpleural but may be central or hilar in location (Figure 21-6). The cysts come in all sizes and may be single, multiple, unilateral, or bilateral. Neighboring structures are distorted; bronchi are compressed; but obstruction is not a regular feature.

Pericystic emphysema is a sign of impending cyst rupture.[46,47] Pulmonary complications of ruptured cysts include abscess, cavitation, and residual bronchiectasis. Pneumothorax and hydropneumothorax may result from rupture into the pleural space.

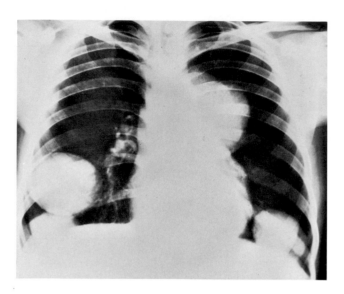

Figure 21-6 Echinococcosis. Multiple, large, rounded, well-marginated densities are present in this native of Turkey. They appear subpleural and hilar in location.

Paragonimiasis

Pulmonary disease attributable to *Paragonimus westermani*, the lung fluke, is endemic in the far east, but also occurs in Africa and South America. With increasing international travel, scattered cases are now being reported in the United States.[48–50] The disease is contracted by ingestion of metacercaria-contaminated water, raw crab, or crayfish. The metacercariae penetrate the wall of the small intestine and eventually penetrate into the lung where they lodge and mature. In the lungs, the fluke may provoke an intense inflammatory response with parenchymal necrosis and cavitation. Migration to the central nervous system and/or skin is a less common but well-known complication.

The most common clinical complaints are cough and hemoptysis, though some patients may remain asymptomatic.[51] Shortness of breath, pleurodynia, and chronic bronchitis or bronchiectasis are frequent.

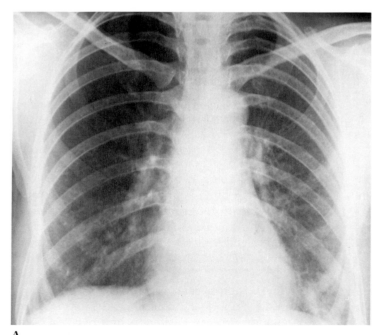

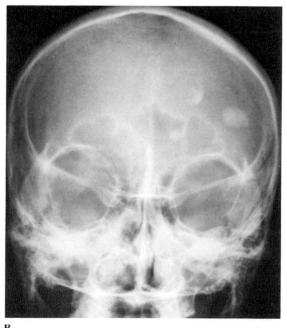

A   B

Figure 21-7 Paragonimiasis. A. The lungs of this Korean native show patchy opacities predominantly located in the central and left lower lung fields. **B.** Intracranial calcifications have developed from central nervous system migration. (Courtesy of Dr. Jae In Ahn, Korea.)

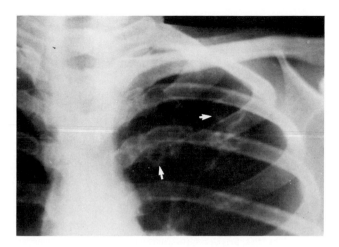

Figure 21-8   Paragonimiasis—signet ring sign. A close-up study of the left upper lung field shows multiple, small, round "cysts" with localized thickened walls (arrows). This configuration resembles a signet ring. (Courtesy of the late Dr. R. John Gould, Philadelphia, Pennsylvania.)

Chest roentgenograms in paragonimiasis are normal in 20 percent of cases, and when positive, the findings are usually inconstant.[52,53] Ill-defined, fluffy, midlung field opacities are seen in the early stages of illness (Figure 21-7A). Cystic, cavitary lesions develop in prolonged, untreated cases. The typical "cysts" are small (1 to 2 cm in diameter) and have a thickened portion of wall in which the parasite is embedded, giving the cyst a "signet ring" configuration (Figure 21-8). Hilar adenopathy, pleural effusions, and lobar consolidations are additional alterations. Rare complications include empyema, abscess formation, and bronchopleural fistula.

Intracranial calcifications result from central nervous involvement.

The pulmonary changes of paragonimiasis, in a patient with chronic cough and hemoptysis, are suggestive of tuberculosis. Melioidosis, an infection also seen in middle and far eastern citizens (Chapter 18), as well as other parasitic and viral diseases, must be considered in the differential diagnosis.

Laboratory tests show mild to moderate eosinophilia in approximately 50 percent of patients.[53] Diagnosis is confirmed by the isolation of characteristic oval eggs in sputum, bronchial washings, and stool.

Treatment with bithionol is effective in 90 percent of cases.[54] Spontaneous resolution of the clinical symptoms and radiographic changes may occur over a period of years.

References

1. Gottlieb MS, Schroff R, Schanker HM, et al: *Pneumocystis carinii* pneumonia and mucosal candidiasis in previously healthy homosexual men. *N Engl J Med* 305:1425, 1981.
2. Cohen BA, Pomeranz S, Rabinowitz JA: Pulmonary complications of AIDS: Radiologic features. *AJR* 143:115, 1984.
3. Epstein DM, Gefter WB, Conard K, et al: Lung disease in homosexual men. *Radiology* 143:7, 1982.
4. Rubinstein A: Acquired immunodeficiency syndrome in infants. *Am J Dis Child* 137:825, 1983.
5. Desposito F, Minnefor A, Oleske J, et al: Acquired immune deficiency syndrome (AIDS): A pediatric perspective. *Pediatr Rev* 5:131, 1983.
6. Stern RG, Gamsu G, Golden JA, et al: Intrathoracic adenopathy: Differential features of AIDS and diffuse lymphadenopathy syndrome. *AJR* 142:689, 1984.
7. Hughes WD: *Pneumocystis carinii* pneumonitis, in Kendig EL Jr, Chernick V (eds): *Disorders of the Respiratory Tract in Children*, 3d ed. Philadelphia, WB Saunders, 1977, p 403.
8. Gajdusek DC: *Pneumocystis carinii*—Etiologic agents of interstitial plasma cell pneumonia of premature and young infants. *Pediatrics* 19:543, 1957.
9. Pass HI, Potter DA, Macher AM, et al: Thoracic manifestations of acquired immune deficiency syndrome. *J Thorac Cardiovasc Surg* 88:654, 1984.
10. Gamsu G, Hecht ST, Birnberg FA, et al: Pneumocystic carinii pneumonia in homosexual men. *AJR* 139:647, 1982.
11. Vanle GT, Heberman R, Lufkin RB: Atypical *Pneumocystis carinii* pneumonia in homosexual men with unusual immunodeficiency. *AJR* 138:1041, 1982.
12. Wollschlager CM, Khan FA, Chitkara RA, et al: Pulmonary manifestations of acquired immune deficiency syndrome (AIDS). *Chest* 85:197, 1984.
13. Forest JV: Radiographic findings of pneumocystis pneumonia. *Radiology* 103:539, 1972.
14. Felman AH, Donnelly WH: Pneumocystic carinii pneumonia in children. *South Med J* 72:1404, 1979.

15. Frazer RG, Paré JAP: *Diagnosis of Diseases of the Chest.* Philadelphia, WB Saunders, 1979, vol. 2, p 856.

16. Hughes WT: Current status of laboratory diagnosis of *Pneumocystis carinii* pneumonitis. *CRC Crit Rev Clin Lab Sci* 6:145, 1975.

17. Lau WK, Young LS, Remington JS: *Pneumocystis carinii* pneumonia: Diagnosis by examination of pulmonary secretions. *JAMA* 236:2399, 1976.

18. Trigg ME, Kohn DB, Sondel DM, et al: Tracheal aspirate examination for *Pneumocystis carinii* cysts as a guide to therapy for pneumocystis pneumonia. *J Pediatr* 102:88, 881, 1983.

19. Hartman B, Koss M, Hui A, et al: *Pneumocystis carinii* pneumonia in acquired immunodeficiency syndrome. Diagnosis in bronchial brushings, biopsy, and bronchoalveolar lavage. *Chest* 87:603, 1985.

20. Pratt JJ, Besson-Leaud M, Lavaud J, Cloup M, et al: Diagnosis of *Pneumocystis carinii* pneumonia using an endobronchial brushing technique. *Eur J Pediatr* 133:41, 1980.

21. Fitzpatrick SB, Stokes DC, Marsh B, et al: Transbronchial lung biopsy in pediatric and adolescent patients. *Am J Dis Child* 139:46, 1985.

22. Feldman NT: An assessment of transbronchial lung biopsy. *N Engl J Med* 293:299, 1975.

23. Nordenstrom B: A new technique for transthoracic biopsy of lung changes. *Br J Radiol* 38:550, 1965.

24. Jareb M, US-Krasovek M: Thin-needle biopsy of chest lesions: Time-saving potential. *Chest* 78:288, 1980.

25. Bandt PD, Blank N, Castellino RA: Needle diagnosis of pneumonitis: Value in high-risk patients. *JAMA* 220:1578, 1972.

26. Ikezoe J, Sone S, Higashihara T, et al: Sonographically guided needle biopsy for diagnosis of thoracic lesions. *AJR* 143:229, 1984.

27. Rodgers BM, Talbert JL: Thoracoscopy for diagnosis of intrathoracic lesions in children. *J Pediatr Surg* 11:703, 1976.

28. Janik JS, Nagaraj HS, Groff DB: Thoracoscopic evaluation of intrathoracic lesions in children. *J Thorac Cardiovasc Surg* 83:408, 1984.

29. Early GL, Williams TE, Kilman JW: Open lung biopsy: Its effect on therapy in the pediatric patient. *Chest* 87:469, 1985.

30. Gaensler EA, Carrington CB: Open biopsy for chronic diffuse infiltrative lung disease: Clinical, roentgenographic, and physiological correlations in 502 patients. *Ann Thorac Surg* 30:411, 1980.

31. Prober CG, Whyte H, Smith CR: Open lung biopsy in immunocompromised children with pulmonary infiltrates. *Am J Dis Child* 138:60, 1984.

32. Imoke E, Dudgeon DL, Colombari P, et al: Open lung biopsy in the immunocompromised pediatric patients. *J Pediatr Surg* 18:816, 1983.

33. Wardman AG, Cooke NJ: Pulmonary infiltrates in acute leukaemia: Empirical treatment or lung biopsy? *Thorax* 39:647, 1984.

34. Tafte JP, et al: Lung biopsy in immunocompromised patients. *Cancer* 48:1144, 1981.

35. Hasleton PS, Curry A: *Pneumocystis carinii:* The continuing enigma. *Thorax* 82:481, 1982.

36. Maile CW, Moore AV, Ulreich S, et al: Chest radiographic-pathologic correlation in adult leukemia patients. *Invest Radiol* 18:495, 1983.

37. Beaver PC, Snyder CH, Carrera GM, et al: Chronic eosinophilia due to visceral larval migrans. Report of three cases. *Pediatrics* 9:7, 1952.

38. Howard WA: Visceral larva migrans, in Kendig EL Jr, Chernick V (eds): *Disorders of the Respiratory Tract in Children* 3d ed. Philadelphia, WB Saunders, 1977, p 1019.

39. Zinkham WH: Visceral larval migrans. A review and reassessment indicating two forms of clinical expression: Visceral and ocular. *Am J Dis Child* 132:627, 1978.

40. Huntley CC, Costas MC, Lyerly A: Visceral larval migrans syndrome: Clinical characteristics and immunologic studies in 51 patients. *Pediatrics* 36:523, 1965.

41. Dafalla AA: The serodiagnosis of human toxocariases by the capillary-tube precipitin test. *Trans R Soc Trop Med Hyg* 69:146, 1975.

42. Hernigou A, Plainfosse MC, Meran S, et al: The value of ultrasonography in the diagnosis of hydatid cysts of the heart. Five cases. *Ann Radiol* 26:648, 1983.

43. Beggs I: The radiology of hydatid disease. *AJR* 145:639, 1985.

44. Lathan WJ: Hydatid disease. *J Fac Radiol* 5:65, 1953.

45. Rakower J: Epidemiology of echinococcus in Israel. *Harefuah* 50:39, 1960.

46. Grünebaum M: Radiological manifestations of lung echinococcus in children. *Pediatr Radiol* 3:65, 1975.

47. Schlanger PM, Schlanger H: Hydatid disease and its roentgen picture. *AJR* 60:331, 1948.

48. Wall MA, McGhee G: Paragonimiasis: Atypical appearances in two adolescent Asian refugees. *Am J Dis Child* 136:828, 1982.

49. Taylor CR, Swett HA: Pulmonary paragonimiasis in Laotian refugees. *Radiology* 143:411, 1982.

50. Burton K, Yogev R, London N, et al: Pulmonary para-

gonimiasis in Laotian refugee children. *Pediatrics* 70:246, 1982.

51. Mayer GJ: Pulmonary paragonimiasis. *J Pediatr* 95:75, 1979.

52. Yang SP, Chang CS, Ghen KM: Chest x-ray findings and some clinical aspects in pulmonary paragonimiasis. *Dis Chest* 27:88, 1955.

53. Ogakwa M, Nwokolo C: Radiologic findings in pulmonary paragonimiasis as seen in Nigeria: A review based on 100 cases. *Br J Radiol* 46:699, 1973.

54. Fischer G, McGrew GL: Pulmonary paragonimiasis in childhood. *JAMA* 243:1360, 1980.

Selected Diseases of the Pulmonary Parenchyma

The diseases covered in this section are difficult to categorize. They are, in fact, grouped together specifically because they share no common denominator.

Chapter 22 is a review of pathophysiologic concepts of diffuse alveolar damage and the "interstitial" disease processes that result. Those (like me) who have never been comfortable using *interstitial* around the view box might find some attraction in this pathophysiologic approach.

The contents of Chapters 23 and 24 are straightforward. Chapter 25 concludes this portion of the book with a group of abnormalities that, for the most part, are rare and esoteric.

Chapter 22

Diffuse Alveolitides (Interstitial Lung Disease)

The matrix or skeleton of the lung consists of the intraalveolar and intralobular tissues that support blood vessels, lymphatics, airways, and intervening tissues. Diseases that affect these interstitial tissues often begin with an inflammatory insult to the alveolar lining cells, the specific cause of which, is often unknown. Over a period of months or years, the inflammatory alveolitis may lead to derangement of alveolar and interstitial structures, loss of functional gas exchange units, and "end-stage lung."[1,2]

Bronchoalveolar lavage, a technique whereby samples of alveolar cellular elements are extracted from the lung and examined histologically, has improved the understanding of the pathogenesis of alveolitis and interstitial lung disease. This procedure also aids in diagnosis and follow-up evaluation of therapy.[1,3,4] Examination of alveolar cellular mixtures is more disease-specific in the early stages of illness; lungs that have reached the end stage manifest remarkably similar lavage characteristics. In certain circumstances, lung biopsy is needed for confirmation of diagnosis. However, bronchoalveolar lavage may be a superior method for assessing the initial intensity and activity of alveolitis, and is a less invasive method for following the course of illness.

Chest radiography remains a standard method for evaluation and follow-up of patients with alveolitis and diffuse interstitial lung disease. However, plain films in adults as well as children are neither sensitive nor specific monitors of the inflammatory alveolar process. In one series, up to 30 percent of patients with biopsy-proven lung disease had chest films interpreted as normal.[5] The alveolar exudation produced by *Pneumocystis carinii* infestation often fails to produce any visible roentgenographic change.[6]

Gallium-67 citrate lung scanning (^{67}Ga index) is another method used to evaluate the presence of alveolitis.[7] Disease activity and therapeutic response can also be followed with this technique. The ^{67}Ga index is not disease-specific, however, since Ga up-take occurs in a variety of pulmonary disorders that produce activated macrophages.[8] Among these are bleomycin toxicity, asbestosis, silicosis, systemic lupus erythematosis, sarcoidosis, usual interstitial pneumonia, Wegener's granulomatosis, histiocytosis X, and other neoplastic and infectious disorders. *Pneumocystis carinii* pneumonia may show in-creased ^{67}Ga in 85 to 98 percent of patients.

The following cryptogenic pulmonary afflictions, characterized by alveolitis, will be considered in this chapter (drug induced alveolitis is covered in Chapter 25):

1. Sarcoidosis
2. Extrinsic allergic alveolitis (hypersensitivity pneumonitis)
3. Intrinsic allergic alveolitis (collagen-vascular disease)
4. Idiopathic interstitial pulmonary fibrosis
5. Histiocytosis X (eosinophilic granuloma)

Sarcoidosis

Mortimer's malady, lupus pernio, uveoparotid fever, lymphogranuloma benignum, and osteitis tuberculosa multiplex cystica were thought of as separate diseases until recognized as a single clinical pathologic entity by Ceasar Boeck, a Norwegian dermatologist, in 1899. The nodular skin lesions are composed of epithelioid cells that resemble sarcoma, hence the term *Boeck's sarcoid*.[9] Sarcoidosis has its major clinical manifestations in the chest; the eyes, skin, and other organs are also involved with variable regularity. The diagnosis is established when clini-coradiographic findings are supported by histologic evidence of widespread noncaseating epithelioid granulomas in more than one organ (Figure 22-1D).[10]

Boeck's sarcoid predominates in adults between 20 and 40 years of age, but also occurs in childhood, mostly between 8 and 15 years.[9,11–19] Sarcoidosis in children commonly produces symptoms, but the clinical manifestations are usually nonspecific.[11,14,15] Malaise, fatigue, and lethargy are the most common initial complaints.[18] Pulmonary disease with hilar ad-enopathy accompanies almost all cases of sarcoidosis in preadolescence and adolescence. Typical laboratory findings consist of hypercalcemia, hyperproteinemia, and eosinophilia.

In young children, initial clinical symptoms of lung disease are less common than in older ages; pulmonary disease is present in less than 22 percent of patients under the age of 4 years. Lung changes often develop later, however.[20] Rash, arthritis, and uveitis are more common in this age group, as are skeletal changes, especially in the hands. Laboratory findings are usually normal.

Sarcoidosis is pathopoietic for many organ systems; chief among these are the lungs and lymph nodes, but skin, bone, and cranial nerves are also affected. Central nervous system disease has been reported in 5 percent of patients with sarcoidosis, but the incidence is 15 percent at autopsy.

Ocular disease is an additional complication of sarcoidosis, often manifesting as uveitis, iritis, or conjunctivitis. Keratitis, retinitis, glaucoma, and eyelid and lacrimal gland involvement are also seen. In some patients, low-grade fever, malaise, and vague gastrointestinal symptoms precede the onset of ocular disease; in others, decreased visual acuity is the initial complaint. Computed tomography (CT) of the anterior pathways is a useful neurodiagnostic study in suspected ocular sarcoid.[21] Magnetic resonance imaging is also well suited to evaluate this region.

Parotid gland swelling is an additional manifestation of sarcoidosis that may lead to permanent induration of the gland. Facial nerve palsy also complicates the disease on rare occasions.

The osseous lesions of sarcoidosis may take several forms. "Lacy" destruction and/or well-defined, "punched-out" patterns are characteristic (Figure 22-1C).[22,23] Localized osteosclerosis also occurs and may simulate metastatic disease.[24] Dense lesions in the terminal phalanges ("bone stones") have been reported in over half of patients with sarcoid lesions of the hands or feet.[25] Other bones of the axillary and appendicular skeleton may be similarly affected.[26] Bone marrow involvement with sarcoidosis may precede the radiographic changes.[27]

Skeletal lesions in children with sarcoidosis primarily affect the small bones of the hands and feet.

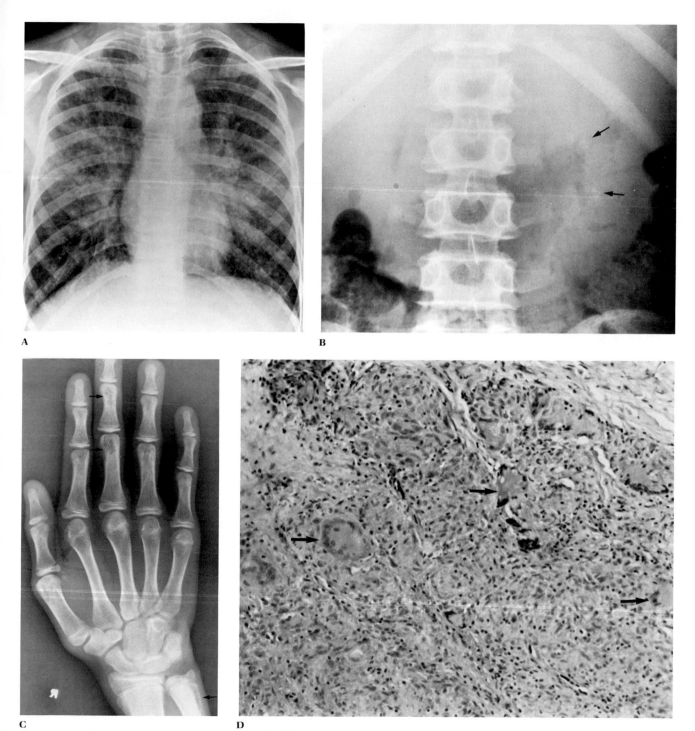

A   B

C   D

Figure 22-1   Sarcoidosis. A. The lungs show diffuse, small, nodular opacities that obscure the normal pulmonary vascular shadows. This nonspecific pattern is produced by lung disease located primarily in the interstitial spaces. Paratracheal adenopathy is also present. **B.** Calcific densities are present in the kidneys (arrows). **C.** Lacelike areas of osseous destruction (arrows) are quite typical of sarcoidosis. **D.** This histologic specimen taken from the conjunctiva shows features of a noncaseating granuloma and large giant cells (arrows) with peripherally located nuclei surrounded by epithelioid histiocytes. There is no necrosis. All stains for acid-fast organisms, fungi, and parasites were negative.

Those children under 4 years of age are more often affected, and half of them develop punched-out lesions of the hands.[22] Arthritic symptoms of sarcoidosis are most often found in young children.[20,28] Boggy effusions and thickened synovial membranes may simulate Still's disease.[29,30]

Skin changes occur in one-third to one-half of patients with sarcoidosis. These consist of small, discrete nodules; large, conglomerate masses; and/or large flat plaques that cover considerable areas of skin. They have a predilection for the face but may occur elsewhere on the body.

Sarcoidosis affects other organ systems less frequently than those mentioned above. Hepatic and splenic abnormalities are often seen at autopsy but usually do not produce clinical symptoms. Glomerulitis, hypercalcemia, nephrolithiasis, and nephrocalcinosis occur when sarcoid granulomas lodge in the renal parenchyma (Figure 22-1B).[31] Cardiac rhythm aberrations result from interference with conduction fibers by sarcoid lesions. Painless, discrete peripheral lymphadenopathy occurs in one-third to three-fourths of children. The nose and paranasal sinuses may also have pathosis.[32]

Pulmonary complications usually develop in childhood sarcoidosis, but in younger children the lungs may be spared during the early course of illness. In most patients, symptoms of pulmonary disease are manifested by dry, hacking cough; wheezing; pleuritic pain, and mild to moderate dyspnea. In rare cases, respiratory symptoms are absent, and the disease resolves spontaneously.[15]

The classic radiographic features of pulmonary sarcoidosis in adults consist of parenchymal infiltrates with or without lymphadenopathy (Figure 22-2).[33,34] Sarcoidosis has been categorized, or staged, in accordance with the various combinations of parenchymal and lymph node involvement.[35]

Stage	Chest Radiograph	Spontaneous Remission
I	Bilateral hilar adenopathy with clear lungs	70 percent
II	Bilateral hilar adenopathy with diffuse parenchymal opacities	31 percent
III	Conglomerate, linear, and/or mixed opacities, evenly distributed throughout the lung (end stage)	10 percent

These stages are not static, and passage from one to the other is to be expected as the disease advances or regresses. The prognosis is, to some extent, based on the roentgenographic stage.[15] Persistent hilar adenopathy is independent of clinical symptoms or parenchymal involvement.[36]

The pulmonary alterations in children with sarcoidosis are similar to those of adults with certain exceptions. Merten et al.[12] found a higher frequency of thoracic lymphadenopathy in children (100 percent) compared with adults (84 percent). The lymph node distribution in their 26 children with sarcoidosis is as follows:

Bilateral hilar	100 percent
Right paratracheal	88 percent
Left paratracheal	75 percent
Subcarinal	10 percent
Posterior mediastinal	8 percent
Anterior mediastinal	8 percent

The occurrence of anterior mediastinal adenopathy in 8 percent of these patients is noteworthy

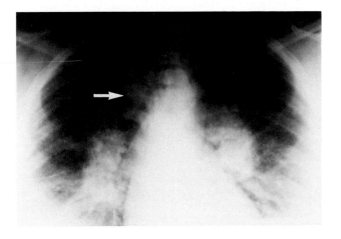

Figure 22-2 Sarcoidosis—lymphadenopathy. Large hilar lymph nodes simulate "potatoes," the classic description of sarcoid lymphadenopathy. The paratracheal lymph nodes are also enlarged (arrow).

since this area has traditionally been thought devoid of adenopathy in sarcoidosis. Other reviews describe subcarinal, anterior, and posterior adenopathy in up to 20 percent of patients.[37,38]

Parenchymal sarcoid involvement in childhood (63 percent) is similar to that found in adults.[12] The most common radiographic pattern consists of an admixture of small, irregular, nodular shadows and fine linear opacities, diffusely scattered about the lung ("reticulonodular pattern") (Figure 22-1A). This appearance may change as the disease advances or regresses. The lymphadenopathy usually does not parallel the parenchymal process.[35] Limited experience with CT of diffuse interstitial lung disease suggests that sarcoidosis produces fine, diffuse nodularity scattered throughout the middle and upper lung zones.[39]

Atypical radiographic chest findings in sarcoidosis are not uncommon.[10] The "alveolar" pattern, occurring in approximately 20 percent of adults with pulmonary involvement, is much less common in children (Figure 22-3). These confluent opacities may represent secondary changes of atelectasis and/or pneumonia rather than actual sarcoid infiltration of the alveoli. On occasion, they occupy the peripheral portions of lung and simulate the pattern of eosinophilic pneumonia.[41] Hilar adenopathy, however, while common in sarcoid, is not a regular feature of eosinophilic pneumonia.

Cavitary lesions develop in adults with sarcoidosis but are usually associated with secondary pyogenic, mycobacterial, or mycotic infections.[42,43] Mycetoma formation is a rare complication of sarcoid cavitation and almost always involves Stage III disease with cystic parenchymal changes.[44,45]

Pleural effusions, mediastinal emphysema, and pneumothorax are additional recognized but uncommon findings of sarcoidosis.[46,47] Fibrosis, bullae, and emphysema are potential sequelae, and cor pulmonale may develop in severe cases.

The incidence of permanent lung damage in children is difficult to evaluate; pulmonary function studies may show variable amounts of lingering restrictive lung disease, even with normal auscultatory findings.[12] Correlation of pulmonary function abnormalities with the radiographic changes is difficult if not impossible in most cases.[14,17,48]

Laboratory studies in sarcoidosis regularly show elevation of serum proteins as well as absolute hyperglobulinemia and reversal of the albumin-globulin ratio. Hypercalcemia in excess of 11 mg/dl serum, as well as eosinophilia and leukopenia, is an additional laboratory change.

Bronchoalveolar lavage is one method used to evaluate the severity of the alveolar inflammation.[8,49,50] A tenfold increase in the number of T-lymphocytes is characteristic of the lavage fluid in patients with sarcoidosis. While little correlation between the cellular content of this fluid and the radiographic pattern can be found, there is a direct relationship between the alveolar lymphocyte count and clinical symptomatology.[2,51] Patients with extrathoracic sarcoidosis also manifest increased numbers of lymphocytes in their bronchoalveolar lavage fluid.[52]

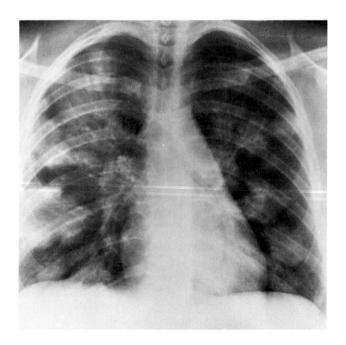

Figure 22-3 Alveolar sarcoidosis. Diffuse alveolar infiltrates are present throughout the lungs in this adult with proven sarcoidosis. (Courtesy of Dr. James Scatliff, Chapel Hill, North Carolina.)

The relationship of lavage fluid content to ultimate prognosis is outlined below:

Alveolitis	Prognosis
High Intensity	
(^{67}Ga index > 50 U; lavage fluid with T-lymphocytes > 28% total cells)	The majority of patients deteriorate in one or more pulmonary function parameters over a 6-month period.
Low Intensity	
(^{67}Ga index < 50 U; lavage fluid with T-lymphocytes ≤ 28% total cells)	Over two-thirds either improve or have no change in pulmonary function.

The systemic immune responses in sarcoidosis are characterized by low numbers of circulating lymphocytes, a low percentage of circulating thymus-processed lymphocytes (T-cells), and hyperglobulinemia, especially levels of immunoglobulin G, immunoglobulin M, and immunoglobulin A.[18] Serum calcium and alkaline phosphatase values may be elevated; eosinophilia and leukopenia are associated findings.

The diagnosis of sarcoidosis is often made by exclusion unless histological material can be obtained. Biopsy of enlarged peripheral lymph nodes or scaline fat pads is most likely to reveal lesions of sarcoidosis. Transbronchial or open lung biopsy is an additional method for obtaining diagnostic material.[53] Epithelioid cell tubercles, with little or no necrosis, are essential to the diagnosis of sarcoidosis.

A positive Kveim-Siltzbach test is helpful but of limited value because of the scarcity of available test material. The serum angiotensin-converting enzyme (ACE) level is increased in patients with active sarcoidosis, but this probably reflects steroid therapy rather than disease activity.[54,55] False-positive elevations of ACE occur in tuberculosis, chronic active hepatitis, berylliosis, and asbestosis.

Gallium-67 scintigraphy, as indicated previously, is useful in the evaluation of pulmonary sarcoidosis as well as other lung diseases, i.e., pneumocystosis, silicosis, pulmonary fibrosis, and drug toxicity reaction.[53,56-59] This test may have greater value in assessing the state of activity rather than in establishing the initial diagnosis.[53,60,61]

Extrinsic Allergic Alveolitis (Hypersensitivity Pneumonitis)

Children and adults are occasionally exposed to substances in the environment that produce a wide spectrum of pulmonary reactions when inhaled. In some circumstances, the lung changes result from local irritation of the respiratory epithelium by the foreign substance; in others, the alterations originate from a hypersensitivity reaction. The diseases produced may be acute, subacute, or chronic.

Farmer's lung, while uncommon in children, is a well-studied hypersensitivity pneumonitis. The disease begins with symptoms of cough, shortness of breath, chills, and fever following exposure to moldy forage. Antigen-antibody reaction to one or more of the thermophilic actinomycetes may account for the symptoms in some patients.

Other inhalant reactions, e.g., pigeon-breeder's disease, allergic aspergillosis, and maple bark disease, are closely related to farmer's lung and produce similar histologic lung changes.[62]

Mushroom-worker's lung is an additional inhalant hypersensitivity. However, this disease is caused by exposure to products in manure and compost.[63] The pulmonary changes in mushroom workers result from inhalation of various fungi during autoclaving and steaming of the plant beds. Most cases are found in and around Chester County, Pennsylvania, where 90 percent of the mushrooms are grown in the United States. A down-wind drive through this countryside on a warm summer day can be quite convincing.

Lycoperdonosis, a form of hypersensitivity pneumonitis, has also been reported in children who inhale the spores of the puffball, a plant related to the mushroom and used topically to stop nosebleeds.[64] The term *lycoperdonosis* was applied to this disease because of the plant's similarity to wolf flatus (from the Greek *lyco* = wolf; *perdesthai* = to break wind). Pituitary snuff sensitivity, pigeon breeding (Figure 22-4), exposure to maple bark, and cave exploring are additional sources of hypersensitivity pneumonitis in childhood.[65-68]

Radiographic patterns of extrinsic allergic alveolitis are usually characterized by disseminated,

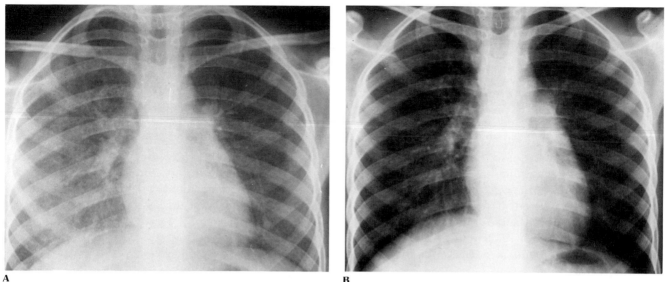

Figure 22-4   Pigeon-breeder's disease. A. The lungs show diffuse opacity that obliterates the normal vascular shadows and lung markings. The right lower lung and left central regions are predominantly involved. **B.** The lungs have returned to normal several weeks after separation from pet birds. (Courtesy of Dr. Mervyn Cohen, Indianapolis, Indiana.)

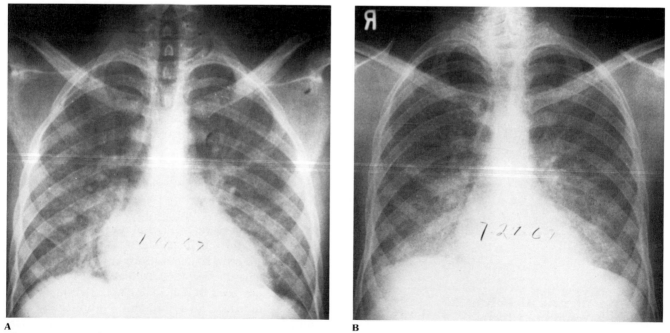

Figure 22-5   Mushroom-worker's lung. A. This film was obtained from an adolescent working on a mushroom farm in Chester County, Pennsylvania. He developed sudden cough, fever, and dyspnea following exposure to fumes in a mushroom barn. The fine, diffuse, predominantly basal densities resemble a sandstorm. **B.** One week later, partial clearing has occurred, but considerable residual radiodensity remains.

small, nondescript opacities that may appear nodular in their early development. While the changes are usually diffuse, they tend to concentrate in the central and lower lung zones (Figure 20-5). Alveolar confluence and hilar adenopathy are inconsistent features of the hypersensitivity pneumonitides. Diffuse fibrosis may result from prolonged exposure to certain substances, especially silica, while mild forms of bronchiolitis fibrosis obliterans are potential sequelae of farmer's-lung disease.

The alveolar lavage characteristics of these inhalant or hypersensitivity pneumonias are similar to other granulomatous diseases, such as sarcoidosis and berylliosis.[69] Increased numbers of macrophages and lymphocytes with relatively expanded proportions of activated T-lymphocytes are the major components.

Gallium scans are also positive during the alveolitis stage of hypersensitivity pneumonitis. The intensity of alveolitis can be gauged by evaluating the ^{67}Ga index and proportion of T-cells in lavage fluid. Prognosis and therapy are based upon these parameters.

As indicated earlier, the diagnosis of most of these conditions depends upon the history of exposure. The following are some additional known hypersensitivity pneumonitides and their precipitating agents (modified from Unger et al.[70]).

Disease	Exposure
Air conditioner or humidifier lung	Contaminated system
Bagassosis	Moldy sugar cane
Cheese-worker's lung	Cheese mold
Malt-worker's lung	Moldy malt
Pituitary snuff-user's lung	Desiccated pituitary snuff
Shower-curtain lung	Moldy shower curtain

Intrinsic Allergic Alveolitis (Collagen-Vascular Disease)

Acute and chronic cardiopulmonary abnormalities may accompany collagen-vascular diseases. The ini-

tial insult causes an alveolitis that typically produces neutrophils as the predominant cell type on bronchoalveolar lavage. However, when neutrophils are numerous, occult inflammatory airway disease must be excluded.

In many cases of collagen-vascular disease, especially scleroderma, pulmonary function tests will become abnormal before any radiographic changes are discernible. In addition, gallium uptake is often positive before the chest films. Nevertheless, radiographic examinations are important in the diagnosis and clinical management of patients with the following collagen-vascular diseases:

1. Rheumatoid arthritis
2. Progressive systemic sclerosis
3. Systemic lupus erythematosus
4. Ankylosing spondylitis

The early radiographic findings of collagen-vascular diseases consist of irregular, connecting, thin lines, sometimes referred to as "reticular." If the condition produces more advanced fibrosis, these lines thicken, become mixed with focal atelectasis and emphysema, and give the lungs a diffuse "honeycomb" appearance.

Although considerable overlap is to be expected, some of these diseases may develop modestly specific radiographic changes. Rheumatoid arthritis causes fibrosis, solitary or multiple necrobiotic nodules, and Caplan's syndrome.[71,72] Pleural effusions may accompany the onset of rheumatoid arthritis or may develop at any time throughout the course of illness. Scleroderma tends to produce a fine, basal pattern of interstitial fibrosis (Figure 22-6). Lupus erythematosus patients more often display a pattern of basal atelectasis, but fibrotic changes are not uncommon (Figure 22-7). Pleural and pericardial effusions are features of all collagen-vascular pulmonary disease, but tend to occur more often with lupus erythematosus (Figure 22-8). Apical pleural disease is occasionally seen in ankylosing spondylitis.

Cardiomegaly is a frequent complication and must be differentiated from pericardial effusion (Figure 22-8B). This distinction is often impossible on plain films; ultrasonography is usually definitive (Figure 22-8C to E).

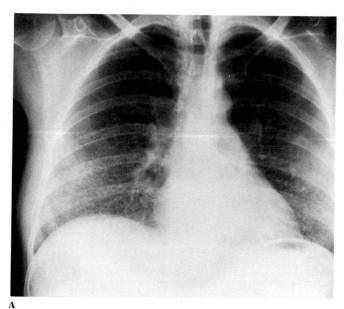

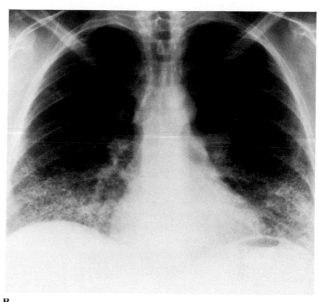

A   B

Figure 22-6   Scleroderma. A. The initial film shows a basal process characterized by fine, randomly oriented ("reticular") shadows. **B.** Three years later, the chest film shows little change; the persistent character of this pattern suggests the development of interstitial fibrosis.

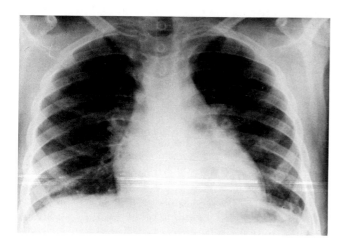

Figure 22-7 Lupus erythematosus—basal atelectasis. This chest film on a young woman shows mild cardiomegaly and bibasilar abnormal lung markings. In the left lower lobe, there is early confluence behind the heart and minimal volume loss.

Spontaneous pneumothorax,[73] pulmonary arteritis,[74] progressive fibrosing alveolitis,[75] and lymphoid interstitial pneumonia[76] are additional pulmonary complications of collagen-vascular disease.

Idiopathic Interstitial Pulmonary Fibrosis

Idiopathic interstitial pulmonary fibrosis (IIPF), also known as usual interstitial pneumonitis, Hamman-Rich syndrome, and cryptogenic fibrosing alveolitis, is a disease of unknown etiology that produces generalized fibrotic changes in the lung. Early cases, described by Hamman and Rich,[77] affect mostly adults; the disease is less common in childhood.[78,79]

As with other types of interstitial lung disease, IIPF probably begins as an alveolitis. The lavage fluid of IIPF is characterized by the presence of neutrophils with normal proportions of lymphocyte subpopulations.[1] The presence of inflammatory tracheobronchial conditions may complicate the diagnosis by falsely increasing the neutrophil population.

Early IIPF is characterized clinically by the insidious onset of dyspnea and tachypnea. As the disease advances, cough, clubbing, and cyanosis are accompanied by cachexia and exertional dyspnea. Lung-function tests are typically abnormal during this phase of the illness.[78]

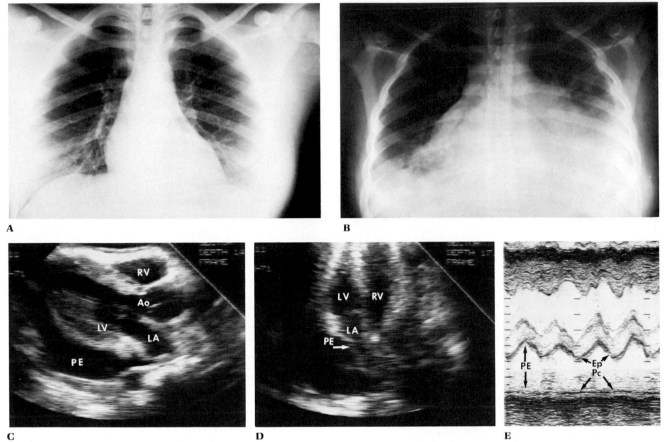

Figure 22-8   Lupus erythematosus—polyserositis. A. During remission, this teenage girl shows an essentially normal chest film; note the extreme obesity from steroid therapy. **B.** Two weeks later, after voluntary cessation of therapy, she has developed marked enlargement of the cardiopericardial silhouette and bilateral pleural effusions. **C.** Two-dimensional echocardiography shows a large pericardial effusion (PE). (LA = left atrium, LV = left ventricle, RV = right ventricle, Ao = aorta.) **D.** The pericardial effusion is large enough to compress the left atrium (arrow) and interfere with diastolic filling. **E.** M-mode echocardiography demonstrates the pleural effusion separating the epicardium (Ep) from the pericardium (Pc).

The radiographic features of IIPF depend upon the degree of activity and the severity of lung involvement. Diffuse, randomly oriented, linear and nodular markings are typical roentgenographic changes of IIPF. Distortion of normal vascular shadows is an additional clue to the presence of interstitial disease. While these changes are the rule, film studies may remain normal even after the development of severely impaired pulmonary functional capacity and significant fibrosis.[79]

Wright and coworkers,[80] using CT in patients with cryptogenic fibrosing alveolitis, demonstrated

subpleural shadowing more commonly seen in the inferior and posterior portions of the lung. The central lung showed three types of change: (1) dense shadowing, sometimes associated with significantly increased gallium uptake, (2) dilated smaller airways with small bullae, suggesting airway disease, and (3) gross bullous change.

After the process of fibrosis has evolved into the so-called end-stage lung, a collection of random linear shadows and focal emphysema produces the radiographic picture of "honeycombing." This honeycomb pattern is not specific and may develop in a large variety of interstitial diseases, including adult respiratory distress syndrome, collagen-vascular diseases, pneumoconioses, and bronchopulmonary dysplasia. When combined with hilar adenopathy, sarcoidosis is a likely diagnosis, while rapidly progressive peripheral lung fibrosis is a feature of chronic eosinophilic pneumonia.

Gallium-67 citrate lung scanning is of value in the diagnosis of IIPF since it is frequently positive before any changes appear on chest films. Moreover, the gallium index is a close reflection of the intensity of underlying alveolitis.[7] In contrast to sarcoidosis, ^{67}Ga does not usually deposit in enlarged lymph nodes.

The histopathologic appearance of IIPF consists of derangement of alveolar walls, replacement of normal epithelium with cuboidal cells, and fibrotic thickening of the interstitium. Areas of focal cystic change with distended emphysematous septa and bullous formation are additional features of advanced disease.

Histiocytosis X

The term *histiocytosis X* is applied to a group of diseases known individually as (1) Letterer-Siwe disease, (2) Hand-Schuller-Christian disease, and (3) eosinophilic granuloma.[81] Their histopathologic features are similar, but they differ in their clinical expression and prognosis. These diseases are also referred to as *nonlipoid reticuloendothelioses* since their pathogenesis is characterized by abnormal reticuloendothelial cells that accumulate normal lipid substances. They differ from the lipoid reticuloendothelioses (Gaucher's disease, Niemann-Pick disease) that are caused by the deposition of abnormal lipids within otherwise normal reticuloendothelial cells.

Histiocytosis X may be localized to the lungs or manifest as a generalized disease.[82,83] The systemic forms produce clinical complexes that are often quite variable. Papular, purpuric, or seborrheic skin rash; hepatosplenomegaly, lymphadenopathy; bone lesions; otitis media; fever; pallor; and growth retar-

dation are among the most common manifestations.[84] When the lungs are involved, an alveolitis develops that is characterized by a predominance of neutrophils.[4] So-called Langerhans cells are also present.

The prognosis depends upon the age of the patient and the patterns of organ involvement. In Lucaya's patients, an overall mortality rate of 33 percent existed, but in neonates it was as high as 77 percent.[84] Onset of disease in older patients is more often characterized by solitary bone involvement. Patients with involvement of several bones have a poorer prognosis than those with solitary lesions. Isolated soft tissue disease carries a mortality of 41 percent; with combined soft tissue and osseous involvement, mortality rises to 50 percent.

Pulmonary histiocytosis X, without evidence of disease elsewhere, is usually referred to as *eosinophilic granuloma of the lung* or *primary pulmonary histiocytosis X*. Eosinophilic granuloma of the lung is analogous to the same pathologic process localized to bone.[82,85]

The precise incidence of pulmonary disease in the generalized malady is difficult to assess. Lucaya[84] found that 12 of 42 children with histiocytosis X had pulmonary involvement. Weber and coworkers[83] reported a 20 percent incidence of lung involvement in patients with generalized histiocytosis X; males were affected five times more commonly than females.

The clinical symptoms of pulmonary histiocytosis X are often absent, nonspecific, or insidious in onset; discovery of the disease is occasionally made on routine chest radiographs in asymptomatic patients. The most common early symptoms are cough and varying degrees of dyspnea.[86] Pneumothorax is a reported complication in 20 to 50 percent of patients. When parenchymal involvement is severe, it can lead to serious disability with chronic respiratory failure, cor pulmonale, and superimposed lung infection.[82,83]

Physical signs of lung pathology are absent or far less evident than might be expected from the radiographic picture. Pulmonary function tests are often abnormal and show restrictive pulmonary mechanics, low diffusion capacity, and occasional changes consistent with airway obstruction. Superimposed pneumonia is a complication found as commonly in patients with generalized histiocytosis X as those with pulmonary involvement.

In nearly one-half of the cases reviewed by Basset et al.,[82] the patient's pulmonary disease stabilized or improved. The remaining cases deteriorated with the appearance of radiographic honeycombing or bullous change, and one-half of these patients died. Poor prognostic features included extremes of age, multiple pneumothoraxes, extensive initial pulmonary radiologic involvement with formation of cysts, and a low CO_2 diffusing capacity.

The radiographic features of pulmonary histio-

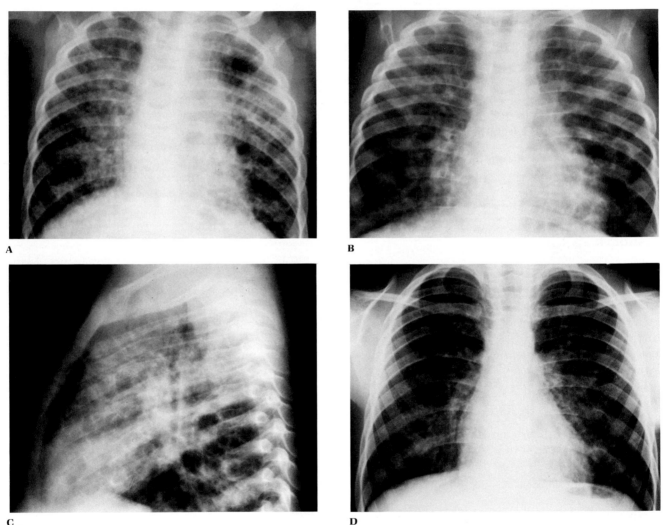

A

B

C   **D**

Figure 22-9   Histiocytosis X.   A. The lungs have a generalized lacy pattern that resembles a honeycomb. All normal lung markings, including the vascular shadows, are completely obscured. **B** and **C.** Five months later the pattern is slightly less evident, but a generalized honeycomb pattern with diffuse overaeration is still apparent. **D.** Three years later the lungs have undergone remarkable clearing with a partial return of the normal parenchymal pattern. Persistent nondescript markings remain, particularly in the left paracardiac region. *Note:* This case represents an unusual resolution of pulmonary histiocytosis X. The lung biopsy following the exposure of the film (part D) revealed interstitial fibrosis.

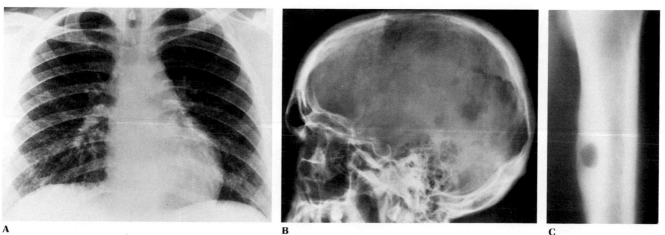

Figure 22-10   Eosinophilic granuloma—lung and bones.   A. The lungs show a diffuse pattern of punctate nodular opacities that were unchanged over several months. **B.** Ill-defined lytic defects are present in the skull of this young adult. **C.** The femoral lesion also represents eosinophilic granuloma.

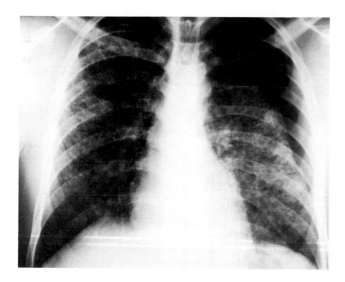

Figure 22-11 Eosinophilic granuloma—spontaneous pneumothorax. This young man developed sudden onset of left chest pain. The frontal chest film shows a diffuse honeycomb pattern with left pneumothorax.

cytosis X are difficult to define since they are characteristically evolutionary and depend upon the type of disease and the age of the patient. Film studies may be normal or slightly overaerated in the early phases of disease. Diffuse nodules of 2 to 3 mm in diameter appear later, with increased markings and occasional thickening of peribronchial tissues. Alveolar infiltrates are uncommon but are difficult to separate from superimposed pneumonia. Hilar and mediastinal adenopathy are inconstant, but conglomerate lymph nodes may cause masses large enough to impinge on adjacent structures. Pleural reactions are rare, but pneumothorax may be the earliest presenting complaint. Gallium-67 citrate is usually concentrated in the lungs of patients in the alveolitis phase of histiocytosis X. As indicated previously, this finding is not specific but may be helpful in a setting of clinical suspicion and normal chest films.

Slow resolution of infiltrates from histiocytosis X usually occurs, and in many cases they are gradually replaced by linear and finely nodular markings suggestive of interstitial disease (Figure 22-9). In some patients, continued progression leads to multiple parenchymal cystic changes, honeycombing, scarring, bullous emphysema, distortion of pulmonary architecture, and end-stage or honeycomb lung.

Primary eosinophilic granuloma of the lung also presents in the above manner, but occasionally it produces solid masses, multiple cystic cavitations, and massive lymphadenopathy. No satisfactory radiographic criteria separate eosinophilic granuloma

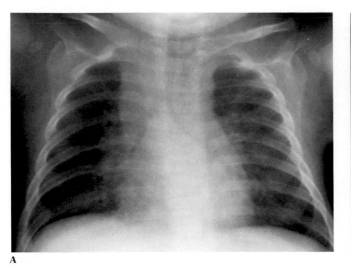
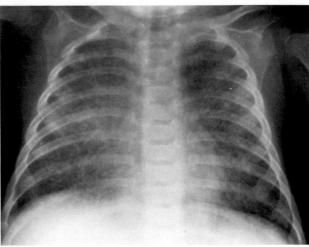

A   B

Figure 22-12   Malignant histiocytosis X.   A. The initial chest film shows minimal central parenchymal opacities and paratracheal lymphadenopathy. **B.** Two months later, the process has worsened significantly with the development of extensive confluent nodular opacities. The child died shortly after this film study.

of the lung from the pulmonary component of generalized reticuloendotheliosis. The presence of bone lesions and/or spontaneous pneumothorax suggests eosinophilic granuloma (Figures 22-10 and 22-11).

Pulmonary histiocytosis X is virtually indistinguishable from other causes of chronic interstitial lung diseases of childhood, i.e., sarcoidosis, bronchopulmonary dysplasia, and idiopathic pulmonary fibrosis. On rare occasions, pulmonary histiocytosis X may undertake a rapid, progressive, malignant course with high mortality (Figure 22-12).

References

1. Crystal RG, Gadek JE, Ferrans VJ, et al: Interstitial lung disease: Current concepts of pathogenesis, staging, and therapy. *Am J Med* 70:542, 1981.
2. Keogh B, Hunninghake G, Line B, et al: Alveolitis parameters as predictors of the natural history of pulmonary sarcoidosis. *Clin Res* 49:171A, 1981.
3. Hunninghake GW, Gadek JE, Kawanami O, et al: Inflammatory and immune processes in the human lung in health and disease: Evaluation by bronchoalveolar lavage. *Am J Pathol* 97:149, 1979.
4. Weinberger SE, Kelman JA, Elson NA, et al: Bronchoalveolar lavage in interstitial lung disease. *Ann Intern Med* 89:459, 1978.
5. Epler GR, McLoud TC, Gaensler EA, et al: Normal chest roentgenograms in chronic diffuse infiltrative lung disease. *N Engl J Med* 298:934, 1978.
6. Felman AH, Donnelly WH: *Pneumocystis carinii* pneumonia in children. *South Med J* 72:1404, 1979.
7. Line BR, Fulmer JD, Reynolds HY, et al: Gallium-67 citrate scanning in the staging of idiopathic pulmonary fibrosis. Correlation with physiological and morphological features and bronchoalveolar lavage. *Am Rev Resp Dis* 118:355, 1978.
8. Hunninghake GW, Line BR, Szapiel SV, et al: Activation of inflammatory cells increases the localization of gallium-67 at sites of disease. *Clin Res* 49:171A, 1981.
9. McGovern JP, Merritt DH: Sarcoidosis in childhood. *Adv Pediatr* 8:97, 1956.
10. James DG, Turiaf J, Hosada Y, et al: Description of sarcoidosis: Report of the Sub-committee on Classification and Definition (Seventh International Conference on Sarcoidosis and Other Granulomatous Disorders). *Ann NY Acad Sci* 278:742, 1976.
11. Cone RB: A review of Boeck's sarcoid with analysis in children. *J Pediatr* 32:629, 1948.
12. Merten DF, Kirks DR, Grossman H: Pulmonary sarcoidosis in childhood. *AJR* 135:673, 1980.

13. Beier FR, Lahey ME: Sarcoidosis among children in Utah and Idaho. *J Pediatr* 65:350, 1964.

14. Jasper PL, Denny FW: Sarcoidosis in children with special emphasis on the natural history and treatment. *J Pediatr* 73:499, 1978.

15. Siltzbach LE, Greenberg GM: Childhood sarcoidosis—A study of 18 patients. *N Engl J Med* 279:1239, 1968.

16. Reed, WG: Sarcoidosis: A review and report of eight cases in children. *J Tenn Med Assoc* 62:27, 1969.

17. Schmitt E, Appelman H, Threatt B: Sarcoidosis in children. *Radiology* 106:621, 1973.

18. Kendig EL: Sarcoidosis. *Am J Dis Child* 136:11, 1982.

19. Schabel SI, Stanley JH, Shelbey BE Jr: Pediatric sarcoidosis. *J SC Med Assoc* 76:419, 1980.

20. Hetherington S: Sarcoidosis in young children. *Am J Dis Child* 136:13, 1982.

21. Beardsley TL, Brown SVL, Sydnor CE, et al: Eleven cases of sarcoidosis of the optic nerve. *Am J Ophthalmol* 97:62, 1984.

22. Holt JF, Owens WI: The osseous lesions of sarcoidosis. *Radiology* 53:11, 1949.

23. Stein GN, Israel HL, Sones M: A roentgenographic study of skeletal lesions in sarcoidosis. *Arch Intern Med* 97:532, 1956.

24. Lin S.-R., Levy W, Go EB, et al: Unusual osteosclerotic changes in sarcoidosis, simulating osteoblastic metastasis. *Radiology* 166:311, 1973.

25. McBrine CS, Fisher MS: Acrosclerosis in sarcoidosis. *Radiology* 115:279, 1975.

26. Stump D, Spack A, Grossman H: Vertebral sarcoidosis in adolescents. *Radiology* 121:153, 1976.

27. Kennedy AC: Boeck's sarcoid: Report of a case with lesions detected in material obtained by sternal puncture. *Glasgow Med J* 31:10, 1950.

28. North AF, Fink CW, Gibson WM, et al: Sarcoid arthritis in children. *Am J Med* 48:449, 1970.

29. Mainley KA, Shulman LE: Joint involvement in sarcoidosis. *Arthritis Rheum* 3:453, 1960.

30. Castellanos A, Galon E: Sarcoidosis: Report of a case in a child simulating Still's disease. *Am J Dis Child* 71:513, 1946.

31. Kogut MD, Neumann LI: Renal involvement in Boeck's sarcoidosis. *Pediatrics* 28:410, 1961.

32. Trachtenberg SB, Wilkinson EE, Jacobson G: Sarcoidosis of the nose and paranasal sinuses. *Radiology* 113:619, 1974.

33. Kirks DR, Greenspan RH: Sarcoid. *Radiol Clin North Am* 11(2):279, 1973.

34. Kirks DR, McCormick VD, Greenspan RH: Pulmonary sarcoidosis: Roentgenologic analysis of 150 patients. *AJR* 177:777, 1973.

35. DeRemu RA: The roentgenographic staging of sarcoidosis: Historic and contemporary perspectives. *Chest* 83:128, 1983.

36. Israel HL, Sperber M, Steiner RM: Course of chronic hilar adenopathy in relation to markers of granulomatous activity. *Invest Radiol* 18:1, 1983.

37. Bein ME, Putman CE, McLoud TC, et al: A reevaluation of intrathoracic lymphadenopathy in sarcoidosis. *AJR* 131:409, 1978.

38. Berman YA, Javors BR: Anterior mediastinal lymphadenopathy in sarcoidosis. *AJR* 127:983, 1976.

39. Bergin CJ, Müller NL: CT in the diagnosis of interstitial lung disease. *AJR* 145:505, 1985.

40. Rockoff SD, Rohatgi PK: Unusual manifestations of thoracic sarcoidosis. *AJR* 144:513, 1985.

41. Glazer HS, Levitt RG, Shackelford GD: Peripheral pulmonary infiltrates in sarcoidosis. *Chest* 85:741, 1984.

42. Rohatgi PK, Schwab LE: Primary acute pulmonary cavitation in sarcoidosis. *AJR* 134:1199, 1980.

43. Tellis CJ, Putman JS: Cavitation in large multinodular pulmonary disease. A rare manifestation of sarcoidosis. *Chest* 71:792, 1977.

44. Gorske KJ, Fleming RJ: Mycetoma formation in cavitary pulmonary sarcoidosis. *Radiology* 95:279, 1970.

45. Wollschlager C, Khan F: Aspergillomas complicating sarcoidosis: A prospective study. *Chest* 86:585, 1984.

46. Freundlich IM, Libshitz HI, Glassman LM, et al: Sarcoidosis: Typical and atypical thoracic manifestations and complications. *Clin Radiol* 21:376, 1970.

47. Amorosa JK, Schaffer RM, Smith PR, et al: Sarcoidosis and mediastinal emphysema. *Radiology* 127:314, 1978.

48. Sillers RD, Siebens AA: The effects of sarcoidosis on pulmonary function, with particular reference to changes in pulmonary compliance. *Am Rev Respir Dis* 9:660, 1965.

49. Hunninghake GW, Crystal RG: Pulmonary sarcoidosis: A disorder mediated by excess helper T lymphocyte activity of sites of disease activity. *N Engl J Med* 305:429, 1981.

50. Hunninghake GW, Kawanami O, Ferrans VJ, et al: Characterization of the inflammatory and immune effector cells in the lung parenchyma of patients with interstitial lung disease. *Am Rev Respir Dis* 123:407, 1981.

51. Arnoux A, Marsac J, Stanislas-Leguern G, et al: Bronchoalveolar lavage in sarcoidosis. *Pathol Res Pract* 175:62, 1982.

52. Davies BH: Sarcoidosis—A gleam of light. *Thorax* 38:165, 1983.

53. Ackart RS, Munzel TL, Rodriguez JJ, et al: Efficacy of 67 Ga-scintigraphy in predicting the diagnostic yield of transbronchial lung biopsy in pulmonary sarcoidosis. *Chest* 82:7, 1982.

54. Lieberman J: Elevation of serum angiotensin-converting enzyme (ACE) level in sarcoidosis. *Am J Med* 59:365, 1975.

55. Parrish RW, Williams JD, Davies BH: Serum beta-2-microglobulin and angiotensin-converting enzyme activity in sarcoidosis. *Thorax* 37:936, 1982.

56. Siemsen JK, Sargent EN, Grebe SF, et al: Pulmonary concentration of ^{67}Ga in pneumoconiosis. *AJR* 120:815, 1974.

57. Niden AH, Mishkin FS, Khurana MML: ^{67}Ga citrate lung scans in interstitial lung disease. *Chest* (suppl), 69:266, 1976.

58. Siemsen JK, Grebe SF, Sargent EN, Wentz D: ^{67}Ga scintigraphy of pulmonary diseases as a complement to radiography. *Radiology* 118:371, 1976.

59. Levenson SM, Warren RD, Richman SD, et al: Abnormal pulmonary gallium accumulation in *P. carinii* pneumonia. *Radiology* 119:395, 1976.

60. Fajman WA, Greenwald LV, Staton G, et al: Assessing the activity of sarcoidosis: Quantitative ^{67}Ga-citrate imaging. *AJR* 142:683, 1984.

61. Schoenberger CI, Line BR, Keogh BA: Lung inflammation in sarcoidosis: Comparison of serum angiotensin-converting enzyme levels with bronchoalveolar lavage and gallium-67 scanning assessment of the T lymphocyte alveolitis. *Thorax* 37:19, 1982.

62. Reyes CN, Wenzel FJ, Lawton BR, et al: The pulmonary pathology of farmer's lung. *Chest* 81:142, 1982.

63. Mindell HJ: Roentgen findings in farmer's lung. *Radiology* 97:341, 1970.

64. Strand RD, Neuhauser EBD, Sornberger CF: Lycoperdonosis. *N Engl J Med* 277:89, 1967.

65. Rankin J, Kobayashi M, Barbee RA, et al: Pulmonary granulomatoses due to inhaled organic antigens. *Med Clin North Am* 51:459, 1957.

66. Dickie HA, Rankin J: The lung's response to inhaled organic dust. *Arch Environ Health* 15:139, 1967.

67. Emanuel DA, Lawton BR, Wenzel FJ: Maple-bark disease. Pneumonitis due to *Coniosporium corticale*. *N Engl J Med* 26:333, 1962.

68. Kadish SP: Long-standing pneumonitis. *JAMA* 211:2004, 1970.

69. Moritz ED, Hunninghake GW, Crystal RG: Activation of lung immune effector cells: A possible precursor to beryllium lung disease. *Am Rev Respir Dis* 123:140, 1981.

70. Unger GF, Scanlon GT, Fink JN, et al: A radiologic approach to hypersensitivity pneumonias. *Radiol Clin North Am* 11:339, 1973.

71. Macfarlane JD, Dieppe PA, Rigden BG, et al: Pulmonary and pleural lesions in rheumatoid disease. *Br J Dis Chest* 72:288, 1978.

72. Spencer-Jones J: An account of pleural effusions, pulmonary nodules and cavities attributable to rheumatoid disease. *Br J Dis Chest* 72:39, 1978.

73. Ayzenerg O, Reiff DB, Levin L: Bilateral pneumothoraces complicating rheumatoid lung disease. *Thorax* 38:159, 1983.

74. Armstrong JG, Steele RH: Localized pulmonary arteritis in rheumatoid disease. *Thorax* 37:313, 1982.

75. Fergusson M, Davidson N, Nuki G, et al: Dermatomyositis and rapidly progressive fibrosing alveolitis. *Thorax* 38:71, 1983.

76. Lovell D, Lindsley C, Langston C: Lymphoid interstitial pneumonia in juvenile rheumatoid arthritis. *J Pediatr* 105:947, 1984.

77. Hamman L, Rich AR: Acute diffuse interstitial fibrosis of the lungs. *Bull Johns Hopkins Hosp* 74:172, 1944.

78. Zapletal A, Houštěk J, Šamánek M, et al: Lung function in children and adolescents with idiopathic interstitial pulmonary fibrosis. *Pediatr Pulmonol* 1:154, 1985.

79. Hewitt CJ, Hull D, Keeling JW: Fibrosing alveolitis in infancy and childhood. *Arch Dis Child* 52:22, 1977.

80. Wright PH, Buxton-Thomas M, Keel L, et al: Cryptogenic fibrosing alveolitis: Pattern of disease in the lung. *Thorax* 39:857, 1984.

81. Lichtenstein L: Histiocytosis X. Integration of eosinophilic granuloma of bone, "Letterer-Siwe disease," and "Hand-Schuller-Christian disease" as related manifestations of a single nosological entity. *Arch Pathol* 56:84, 1953.

82. Basset F, Corrin B, Spencer H, et al: Pulmonary histiocytosis X. *Am Rev Respir Dis* 118:811, 1978.

83. Weber WN, Margolin FR, Nielson SL: Pulmonary histiocytosis X. A review of 18 patients with report of 6 cases. *AJR* 107:280, 1969.

84. Lucaya J: Histiocytosis X. *Am J Dis Child* 121:289, 1971.

85. Auld D: Pathology of eosinophilic granuloma of lung. *Arch Pathol* 63:113, 1959.

86. Lewis JG: Eosinophilic granuloma and its variants with special reference to lung involvement: Report of 12 patients. *Q J Med* 33:337, 1964.

Chapter 23

Tumors and Tumor-Like Conditions

Primary pulmonary tumors are uncommon in childhood and most that occur are benign. Pulmonary metastases have assumed increasing importance with the availability of therapeutic modalities such as radiation, chemotherapy, and surgery.

Hamartoma

Pulmonary hamartomas are bulky, circumscribed mass lesions composed of pulmonary, bronchial, and cartilaginous elements. While their etiology is unknown, they probably arise from poorly organized embryologic rests. Most are discovered on chest films taken for other reasons in patients between the ages of 14 and 76 years.[1]

Hamartoma of the lung and congenital adenomatoid malformation are sometimes considered as the same neoplasm; the presence of cartilage tissue in hamartomas is used as a differential criterion. In the newborn, an unusual and distinctive hamartoma may present as a large, bulky, poorly encapsulated mass.[2] Teratomas, rarely found in the lung, are easily differentiated histologically.

Most hamartomas occur in the parenchyma of the lung, more often in the right lower lobe, but endobronchial and chest wall involvement is possible (Figure 23-1). Atypical radiographic appearance of a well-circumscribed, solitary, lobulated, nodular lesion smaller than 4 cm in diameter with popcorn calcification permits confident diagnosis. More often, however, hamartomas produce nonspecific nodular opacities that cannot be differentiated from primary or metastatic malignant neoplasm. Calcification occurs with variable frequency. Differentiation from bronchogenic carcinoma is important in adults, but less so in children. Enlargement on serial roentgenograms has been reported.[3] Additional evi-

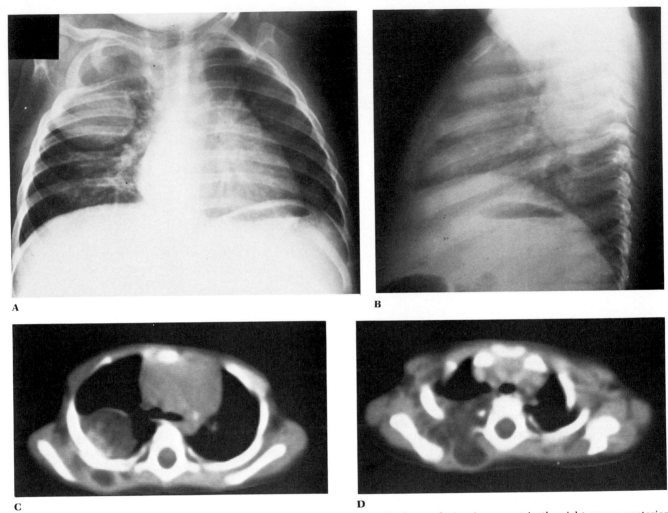

Figure 23-1   Fibrolipomatous hamartoma. A and **B.** A well-circumscribed mass lesion is present in the right upper posterior thorax. The second intercostal space is widened, and the adjacent ribs are deformed. **C** and **D.** Computed tomography confirms the presence of a posterior thoracic chest lesion protruding through the rib cage and into the prescapular and paraspinous region. The lucent areas represent fatty tissue. (From Hoffman AD: Pediatric case of the day. *AJR* 142:1072, 1984. Copyright © by American Roentgen Ray Society. With permission.)

dence for the dynamic potential of this tumor is derived from reports of cystic change over time.[4] Multiple hamartomas are reported in adults, but these are extremely rare.[5]

Fine-needle aspiration is an accepted diagnostic technique for lung tumors, but there is little experience in the pediatric age group. Repeat attempts are often needed in order to obtain sufficient tissue.[6]

Pulmonary Choristoma

Choristoma, or "heterotopic rest," is a rare developmental anomaly that closely resembles hamartoma. However, hamartomas contain only lung tissue, while choristomas have nonpulmonary elements. They occur most often in the gastrointestinal tract

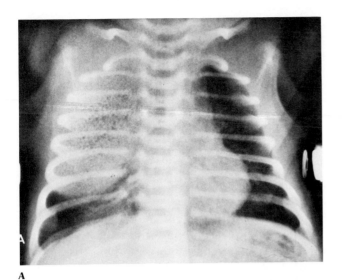

A

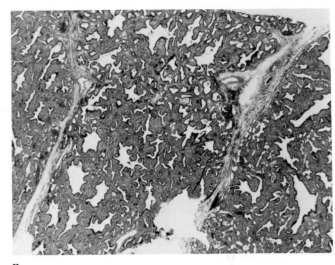

B

C

Figure 23-2 Pulmonary choristoma. A. This frontal film, taken at 10 days of age, reveals a large right upper lobe expansile process of "mixed air" and solid texture. *Note:* There is a depressed, bulging right middle lobe fissure and minimal tracheal deviation to the left. **B** and **C.** Well-differentiated striated muscle fibers enclose irregular cystic spaces lined by well-differentiated, pseudostratified, ciliated columnar epithelium. The presence of striated muscle, not normally found in the lung, distinguishes choristoma from hamartoma (see the text). Scattered throughout are well-formed bronchi containing smooth muscle and cartilage in their walls. (From Wat K, Toomoy F, Wat BY, et al.: Pulmonary choristoma in a neonate. *AJR* 139:377, 1982. Copyright © by American Roentgen Ray Society. With permission. Courtesy of Dr. Frances Toomey, Loma Linda, California.)

and heart, but have been reported in the lung as well.

Unlike hamartomas, choristomas have no known growth potential. However, the lesion reported by Wat and coworkers occupied the entire right upper lobe in a neonate (Figure 23-2).[7]

Intrathoracic Lipoma

...mas account for less than 2 per-
...rs in adults.[8,9] They are

usually discovered during removal of overlying superficial lipomas, but are occasionally seen as mass lesions on incidental chest films.[10] Massive enlargement and encroachment on vital structures may produce clinical symptoms. The majority are benign, and surgical removal is usually curative.

Most intrathoracic lipomas are situated in the mediastinum;[11,12] subpleural and endobronchial locations are much less common.[13,14] Chest wall and subpleural lipomas may contain both intrathoracic and extrathoracic components, thus producing an hourglass configuration. The external mass may extend into the neck, to the suprasternal notch, or through an intercostal space.[15] Lipomas of the thorax may also involve the thymus (thymolipomas).[16,17] (See Chapter 8.)

The radiographic features of intrathoracic lipomas depend mostly upon their location and size. Mediastinal lesions present as well-defined masses but may alter shape with changes in bodily attitude. Although soft and malleable, they may displace the trachea and esophagus (Figure 23-3). The lipomatous nature of these tumors is not usually evident on plain films, but computed tomography (CT) will disclose their characteristic fatty tissue elements. Endobronchial lipomas often present with findings of pulmonary collapse; the obstructing mass may be visible on plain films or tomograms of the bronchus.

Thoracic wall and subpleural lipomas present as mass lesions along the inner chest wall or above the diaphragm. Adjacent rib erosion and widened intercostal spaces are accompanying radiographic signs that suggest extension of tumor through the chest wall. (Figures 23-1 and 23-3).[18] These findings are not specific for chest wall lipomas; they may also be seen in neurogenic tumors as well as chest wall infections, i.e., empyema necessitans. (See Chapter 20.)

Pulmonary Blastoma (Carcinosarcoma, Mixed Malignant Tumor)

Pulmonary blastoma is a malignant tumor of the lung, initially reported by Barnard[19] as a "lung embryoma." Spencer[20] described four such tumors under the label of "pulmonary blastoma," because of their histologic similarity to nephroblastoma. Additional cases have since been observed, approximately one-fourth in children.[21,22]

Pulmonary blastomas rarely produce symptoms and are discovered most often on routine chest films. Like many other pulmonary tumors, they have few, if any, distinguishing clinical or radiologic features. Pulmonary blastomas are usually small, well-

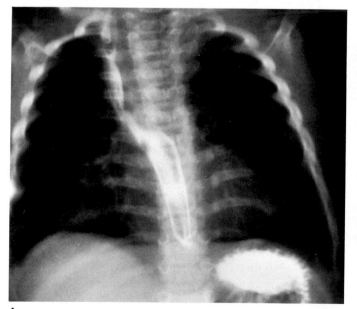

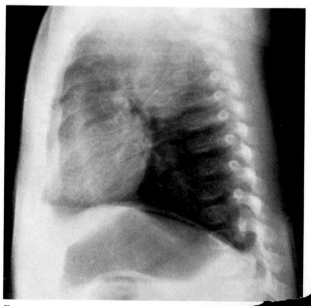

A

B

Figure 23-3 Subpleural lipoma. A. A posterior mediastinal mass is displacing the barium-filled esophagus widening of the right second-third and third-fourth intercostal spaces. **B.** The lateral film demonstrates ment by the posterior mass.

defined, unilateral, peripheral masses, with a predilection for upper lung fields (Figure 23-4).[23,24] Large masses may exist and occupy an entire lobe; hilar nodes are not usually enlarged.[25,26] Calcification within a tumor has been reported with CT.[24] Sumner et al.[27] have reported a case arising within a cystic lesion in the lung. Others have observed similar findings, but true cavitation is infrequent.[25,28]

Histologically, pulmonary blastoma consists of a spindle cell stroma containing glandular elements (Figure 23-4C and D). The small number of cases makes realistic prognosis impossible; four of the pa-

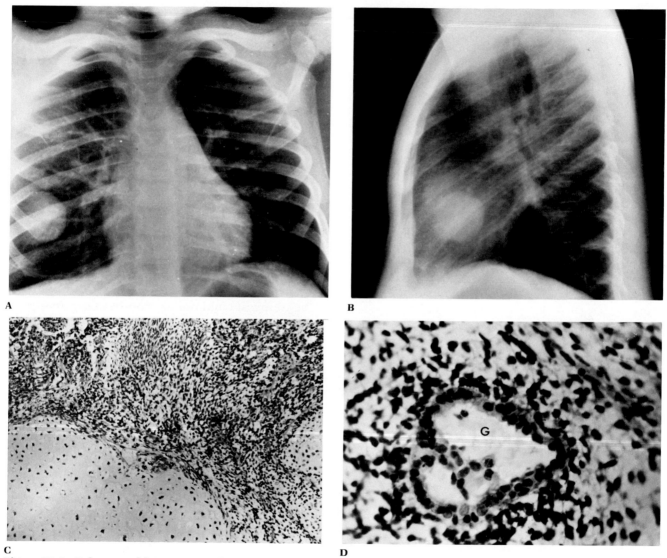

Figure 23-4   Pulmonary blastoma. A and **B.** A solitary, round, masslike lesion is present in the right lung base. **C.** The histologic section shows the mesenchymal portion of the tumor with chondrosarcomatous and smooth muscle differentiation. **D.** The epithelial component consists of glandlike spaces (G) lined by poorly differentiated epithelium and surrounding undifferentiated tumor cells. (From Sumner TE, Phelps CE, Crowe JE, et al: Pulmonary blastoma in a child. *AJR* 133:147, 1979. Copyright © by American Roentgen Ray Society. With permission.)

tients with pulmonary blastoma died within 1 year of operation.[29]

Treatment consists of surgical removal by wedge resection or pneumonectomy. Radiation therapy and chemotherapy have been used but are of unknown value.

Askin Tumor (Malignant Thoracopulmonary Small Cell Tumor)

The Askin tumor is a rare, malignant, small cell neuroepithelioma that originates in the soft tissues of the chest wall or lung.[30] Histologically, the tumor simulates Ewing's sarcoma, rhabdomyosarcoma, neuroblastoma, and malignant lymphoma, a group that composes the bulk of chest wall neoplasms in the pediatric age group.[31,32] Specific immunocytochemical and electron microscopic features distinguish Askin tumors from other lesions with similar appearance on light microscopy. These patients may present with symptoms of chest wall invasion or spontaneous pneumothorax, but occasional lesions are discovered on incidental chest films.

Radiographic demonstration of a mass in the chest wall or back is the most common feature of Askin tumor. Additional findings include pleural involvement with effusions and/or rib destruction (Figure 23-5). Radionuclide bone scan may also disclose local rib involvement. Calcifications within the tumor occur uncommonly.

Local recurrence and direct invasion of pleura and lung are consequences of most lesions. Distant metastases to liver, adrenal, skeleton, and sympathetic chain are also reported.[32]

Infections and Other Masslike Lesions

Plasma Cell Granuloma

The term *plasma cell granuloma* was first used by Bahadori and Liebow[33] to describe a lesion of the lung previously classified as *postinflammatory pseudotumor, xanthoma, fibroxanthoma, xanthogranuloma,* and *plasmacytoma.*[34] Immunohistochemical techniques are available to identify various immunoglobulins within these lesions that confirm their inflammatory origin.[35] Monzon and coworkers[35] reported 3 children with plasma cell granuloma and reviewed 41 previously reported cases in children. The youngest child was 12 months of age. In 41 percent of patients, the process was detected on incidental chest films in asymptomatic patients.

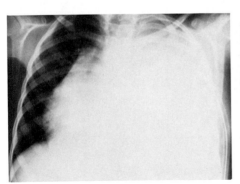
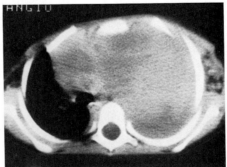
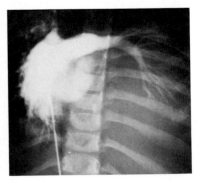

A   B   C

Figure 23-5   Askin (malignant thoracopulmonary small cell) tumor. A. This 5-year-old girl presented with respiratory distress and was found to have a large pleural effusion and left chest mass. **B.** Computed tomography discloses anterior chest wall involvement, cardiac displacement to the right, and complete occupation of the left hemithorax by mass and fluid. **C.** The pulmonary arteriogram shows substantial stretching of the left pulmonary artery around the lesion and associated destruction of the left, fifth anterior rib. (Courtesy of Dr. Barry D. Fletcher, Cleveland, Ohio.)

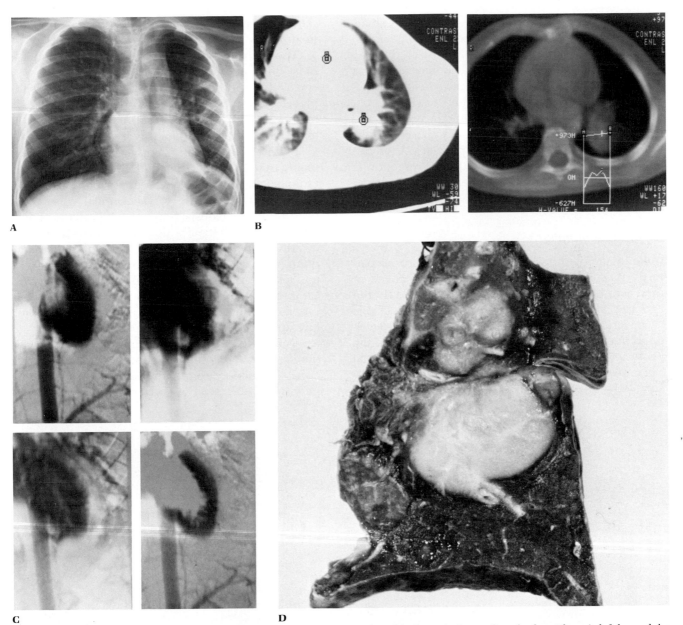

Figure 23-6   Plasma cell granuloma. A. A left lower lobe ovoid mass is visible through the cardiac shadow. There is left lower lobe volume loss and compensatory overaeration of the right lung. **B.** Computed tomography shows the mass adjacent to the left hilum and surrounded by aerated lung. **C.** Digital subtraction angiography shows no aberrant vessel to the lower lobe or to the mass. **D.** The gross specimen shows the lesion surrounding and compressing the left lower lobe bronchus.

Plasma cell granulomas may range from small, well-circumscribed, coinlike lesions to large intrapulmonary masses (Figure 23-6). In isolated cases, calcification is encountered on plain films as well as on CT. Most plasma cell granulomas are located peripherally; esophageal obstruction has been observed with central lesions.[36] Pulmonary artery and mediastinal invasions are additional rare complications.[37,38] The clinical course of plasma cell granuloma is almost always benign; surgical resection is usually curative, but radiation therapy has also been used.

Round Pneumonia

Inflammatory lesions of the lung may assume patterns that simulate tumors of the parenchyma or mediastinum.[39–41] Rose and Ward[42] reported that in 21 cases of round pneumonia clinical signs of disease were inconstant. Their patients had well-developed radiopacities located predominantly in the posterior lung fields (Figure 23-7). Unlike the usual inflammatory pattern, air bronchograms were absent. Polymorphonuclear lymphocytosis was universal, and patients responded rapidly to antibiotic treatment.

Though difficult to prove, round pneumonia is most often caused by the pneumococcus. Clinical correlation is of utmost importance to establish the presence of infection and exclude the possibility of neoplasm. Complete radiographic clearing is to be expected after appropriate therapy.

Round pneumonia is another pulmonary abnormality that illustrates the need for close clinical and radiologic follow-up. The frequency of filming must be individually tailored to the clinical course and presumptive diagnosis; however, all patients should be followed until their radiograph returns to normal. In adult patients, the fear that an underlying carcinoma as a cause for "pneumonia" is ever present, and follow-up chest films are always recommended. Children have different causes for incomplete resolution of pulmonary disease, but no less need for follow-up until complete clearing has occurred.

Numerous conditions may interfere with the resolution of pneumonia. Chief among these is bronchial obstruction from (1) foreign body, (2) mucous plug with atelectasis, (3) congenital stenosis or atre-

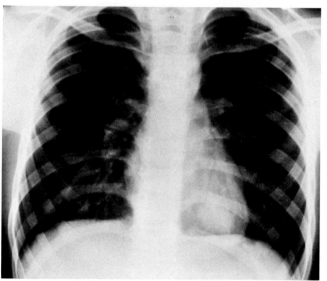 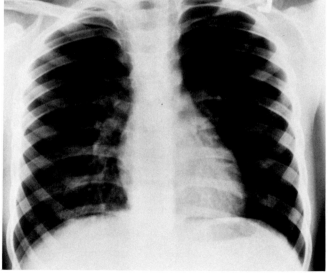

A   B

Figure 23-7 Round pneumonia (possible pneumococcus). A. A round, well-defined, left lower lobe opacity is visible through the cardiac shadow. **B.** Two weeks later, following antibiotic treatment, the film is normal.

sia, (4) adenopathy or mass, and (5) vascular anomaly. Other pulmonary lesions may simulate pneumonia or recurrent pneumonia: (1) sequestration, (2) adenomatoid malformation, (3) tumors, and (4) preexisting acquired lung lesion. Vertebral infections and neoplasms may also simulate parenchymal infection.

The right middle lobe is especially prone to atelectasis. This volume loss may be overlooked unless films are taken in the lateral as well as the usual frontal projection. In confusing or unclear circumstances, lordotic projection will help. After all, one cannot always judge everyone from the front. A judicious side peek is often more convincing, but be careful with the lordotic.

Nodular Residua of Atypical Measles

Rounded, well-defined pulmonary parenchymal opacities occur in children previously immunized with inactivated measles virus vaccine who subsequently develop measles and measles pneumonia. In the future, this should become less common although sporadic outbreaks of measles continue to occur. Once these nodules develop, they may remain into adulthood.[43,44] Calcification occurs in rare cases.

Pulmonary Varix

Most pulmonary varices are discovered in adults, but cases have been reported in newborns and infants (see Chapter 12). In contrast to arteriovenous fistulas, pulmonary varix produces no symptoms. The diagnosis may be confirmed by pulmonary angiography or contrast-enhanced CT. Reports in children are isolated.[45,46]

References

1. Blair TC, McElvein RB: Hamartoma of the lung. A clinical study of 25 cases. *Dis Chest* 44:296, 1963.
2. Jones CJ: Unusual hamartoma of the lung in a newborn infant. *Arch Pathol* 48:150, 1949.
3. Weisel W, Glicklich M, Landis FB: Pulmonary hamartoma, an enlarging neoplasm. *Arch Surg* 71:128, 1955.
4. Doppman J, Wilson G: Cystic pulmonary hamartoma. *Br J Radiol* 38:629, 1965.
5. Sargent EN, Bares RA, Schwinn CP: Multiple pulmonary fibroleiomyomatous hamartomas. *AJR* 110:694, 1970.
6. Sinner WN: Fine-needle biopsy of hamartomas of the lung. *AJR* 138:65, 1982.
7. Wat K, Toomey F, Wat BY, et al: Pulmonary choristoma in a neonate. *AJR* 139:377, 1982.
8. Arrigoni MG, Woolner LB, Bernatz PE, et al: Benign tumors of lung. A ten year experience. *J Thorac Cardiovasc Surg* 60:589, 1970.
9. Peleg H, Pauzner Y: Benign tumors of lung. *Dis Chest* 47:179, 1965.
10. Kauffman SL, Stout AP: Lipoblastic tumors in children. *Cancer* 12:912, 1959.
11. Heuer GJ: The thoracic lipomas. *Ann Surg* 98:801, 1933.
12. Keeley JL, Vana AJ: Lipomas of the mediastinum. *Surg Gynecol Obstet* 103:313, 1956.
13. Schraufnagel DE, Morin JE, Wang NS: Endobronchial lipoma. *Chest* 75:97, 1979.
14. Smart J: Intra-thoracic and intra-bronchial lipomata. *Br J Tuberc* 47:16, 1953.
15. Saini VK, Wahi PL: Hourglass transmural type of intra-thoracic lipoma. *J Thorac Cardiovasc Surg* 47:600, 1964.
16. Bigelow NH, Ehler AA: Lipothymoma: Unusual benign tumor of thymus gland. *J Thorac Cardiovasc Surg* 23:528, 1952.
17. Falor WH, Ferro FE: Lipothymoma. *Surgery* 39:291, 1956.
18. Ten Eycke EA: Subpleural lipoma. *Radiology* 74:295, 1960.
19. Barnard WG: Embryoma of the lung. *Thorax* 7:299, 1952.
20. Spencer H: Pulmonary blastomas. *J Pathol* 82:161, 1961.
21. Fung CH, Lo JW, Yonan TN, et al: Pulmonary blastoma. *Cancer* 39:153, 1977.
22. Kodaira Y, Okiyama H, Morikawa M, et al: Pulmonary blastoma in a child. *J Pediatr Surg* 11:239, 1976.
23. Greene R, McLoud TC, Stark P: Other malignant tumors of the lung. *Semin Roentgenol* 12:225, 1977.
24. Solomon A, Rubinstein ZJ, Rogoff M, et al: Pulmonary blastoma. *Pediatr Radiol* 12:148, 1982.
25. Han SS, Wills JS, Allen OS: Pulmonary blastoma: Case report and literature review. *AJR* 127:1048, 1976.

26. Peacock MJ, Whitwell F: Pulmonary blastoma. *Thorax* 31:197, 1976.

27. Sumner TE, Phelps CE, Crowe JE, et al: Pulmonary blastoma in a child. *AJR* 133:147, 1979.

28. Martinez JC, Pecero FC, Gutierrez de la Pana C, et al: Pulmonary blastoma: Report of a case. *J Pediatr Surg* 13:93, 1978.

29. Valderrama E, Saluja G, Shende A, et al: Pulmonary blastoma: Report of two cases in children. *Am J Surg Pathol* 2:415, 1978.

30. Askin FB, Rosai J, Sibley RK, et al: Malignant small cell tumor of the thoracopulmonary region in childhood. A distinctive clinicopathologic entity of uncertain histogenesis. *Cancer* 43:2438, 1979.

31. Kumar APM, Green A, Smith JW, et al: Combined therapy for malignant tumor of the chest wall in children. *J Pediatr Surg* 12:991, 1977.

32. Fink IJ, Kurtz DW, Cazenave L, et al: Malignant thoracopulmonary small-cell ("Askin") tumor. *AJR* 145:517, 1985.

33. Bahadori M, Liebow AA: Plasma cell granulomas of lung. *Cancer* 31:191, 1973.

34. McCall IW, Woo-Ming M: The radiological appearance of plasma cell granuloma of the lung. *Clin Radiol* 29:145, 1978.

35. Monzon CM, Gilchrist GS, Burgert EO Jr, et al: Plasma cell granuloma of the lung in children. *Pediatrics* 70:268, 1982.

36. Hutchins GM, Eggleston JC: Unusual presentation of pulmonary inflammatory pseudotumor (plasma cell granuloma) as esophageal obstruction. *Am J Gastroenterol* 71:501, 1979.

37. Berdon W: Personal communication, 1983.

38. Wagner M: Progressive plasma cell granuloma. *Proceedings of the John Caffey Society*, Carmel, California, 1981.

39. Greenfield H, Gyepes MT: Oval-shaped consolidations simulating new growth of the lung. *AJR* 91:125, 1964.

40. Talner LB: Pleuropulmonary pseudotumors in childhood. *AJR* 100:208, 1967.

41. Swenson PC, Leaming RH: Chest lesions often confused roentgenographically with primary cancer of the lung. *AJR* 63:629, 1950.

42. Rose RW, Ward BN: Spherical pneumonias in children simulating pulmonary and mediastinal masses. *Radiology* 106:179, 1973.

43. Mitnick J, Becker MH, Rothberg M, et al: Nodular residua of atypical measles pneumonia. *AJR* 134:257, 1980.

44. Young LW, Smith DI, Glasgow LA: Pneumonia of atypical measles. Residual nodular lesions. *AJR* 110:439, 1970.

45. Chilton SJ, Campbell JB: Pulmonary varix in early infancy: Case report with 8 year follow up. *Radiology* 129:400, 1978.

46. Bartram C, Strickland B: Pulmonary varices. *Proc R Soc Med* 64:839, 1971.

Chapter 24

Chest Trauma

Despite preventive efforts (seat belt laws, packaging laws, and other safety regulations), accidents remain the most common cause of death in childhood. This chapter will review two major categories of chest trauma: (1) external chest trauma and (2) iatrogenic trauma.

External Chest Trauma

The causes of thoracic trauma depend heavily upon geographic area and socioeconomic conditions. Blunt injuries (automobile accidents) account for over one-half of patient trauma in nonurban areas.[1-3] Meller and coworkers,[4] reporting on patients in the inner-city area, found blunt trauma most often in younger ages, but penetrating injuries more common in older ages (Figure 24-1). Knives and

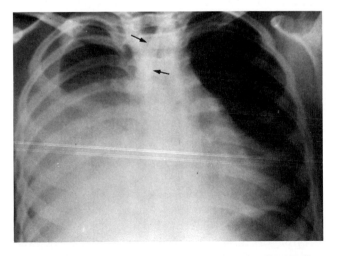

Figure 24-1 Penetrating injury—glass. While playing games with his father, this child ran through a plate glass door. A large pleural effusion is present in the right hemithorax. The sharp, pointed object overlying the trachea (arrows) proved to be a piece of glass impaled in the chest wall. *Note:* All glass is radiopaque.

bullets are the most frequent causes of penetrating injuries. Thoracic perforations also result from fractured ribs and clavicles and from insertion of tubes and needles. In addition to the initial trauma, aspiration of foreign bodies, especially teeth, large quantities of blood, or gastric contents may complicate the lung injury.[5]

Serious damage to thoracic contents may exist with mild or absent symptoms.[6] Physical findings are also lacking in approximately 20 percent of children with trauma-induced radiographic changes.[7]

Thoracic Cage Injuries

Rib fractures are the most common sequela of chest trauma. However, the presence or absence of rib fractures is not a good indicator of the extent of injury.[4] When rib fractures occur in children, flail chest or ventilatory difficulty rarely follows.[4,5] Paraspinous rib fractures, especially in different stages of healing, should raise the suspicion of child abuse. Additional fractures may be evident on the humeri when included on the chest film.

The identification of underlying great vessel injury is of critical importance in the initial evaluation of patients with chest trauma. While deceleration injuries are most often responsible, ascending aortic laceration may result from other mechanisms, including traction-torsion forces.[8] The significance of fractures of the first two or three ribs and their relation to underlying vascular injury has been a cause of concern in the adult patient suffering from blunt chest trauma.[6] Subsequent reviews regarding the relationship of rib fractures to vascular injuries suggest more of a coincidental than causative connection.[7-12] Data on vascular injuries in children are less complete, but Meller and coworkers reported only one great vessel injury in 68 cases.

Other roentgenographic signs of aortic injury include widening of the mediastinum, deviation of an esophageal tube to the right, loss of the aortic knob silhouette, depression of the left stem bronchus, widening of the paratracheal stripe, and development of an apical cap or pleural effusion.[13-16] Burney and coworkers,[15] in a comparison of seven radiographic signs, found "widening of the mediastinum

and obscuration of the aortic knob" the most reliable findings of traumatic rupture of the aorta. Others have suggested that deviation of the esophagus is the most reliable plain-film finding.[17] It is apparent from the above that several radiographic signs point to vascular injury; the importance of each may vary from patient to patient. Careful clinicoradiologic correlation is essential when making the decision to perform angiography.

Extensive, elaborate positioning and filming of the severely traumatized patient to ascertain the presence of insignificant, occult rib fractures should be avoided since their presence or absence is of little importance to the immediate management of the patient.[18] Follow-up films are often better indicators of rib fractures, as the healing process renders them more visible.

Fractures of the eleventh and twelfth ribs are more often associated with ruptures of subphrenic organs, specifically the liver or spleen.

Tracheobronchial Tree Injury

Ruptured bronchus is a serious complication of chest trauma. In one series of adult patients with ruptured bronchus, 53 percent showed a fracture of one or more of the first three ribs. In children and young adults, however, major injuries and ruptures of the bronchi occurred in the absence of rib fractures.[19,20]

Most traumatic airway lacerations occur through stem bronchi within 2 or 3 cm of the carina, but occasional tears involve the trachea or peripheral bronchi. A fracture through the bronchus may be complete or partial. The immediate diagnosis is often extremely difficult and frequently compounded by additional injuries that produce similar clinical and radiographic findings.[21] Approximately 10 percent of patients with fractured bronchus will have no radiographic or physical findings, presumably because of preservation of the integrity of the bronchial sheath.[6]

Pneumomediastinum, pneumothorax, and/or subcutaneous emphysema, especially in the deep cervical fascia, suggest the presence of bronchial rupture (Figure 24-2).[21-24] The pneumothorax that accompanies this injury may or may not develop

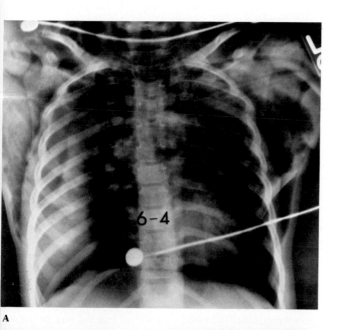

A

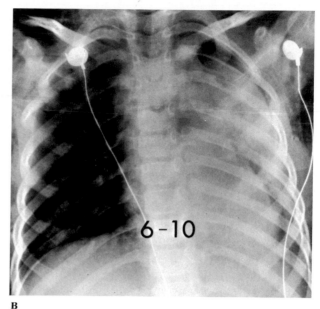

B

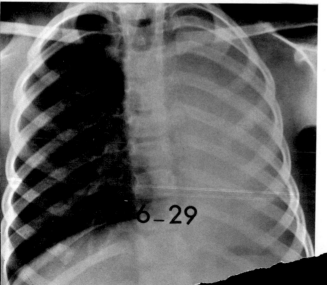

C

Figure 24-2   Fractured bronchus. A girl riding in front of her father on a motorcycle at night was struck across the chest by a low-hanging steel cable. **A.**
emphys

though the damage may not be recognized for months or years after the original insult, complete repair and reconstruction is possible in some cases.[25-27] On occasion, resection of a diseased lung is necessary.

Parenchymal Injury

Significant lung damage may occur from external blunt trauma with few clinical signs or symptoms of pulmonary injury.[1,28] Simultaneous trauma to the abdomen, urinary tract, central nervous system, and other organs often produces symptoms that overshadow the thoracic injury. For example, pulmonary contusion may be confused with edema caused by central nervous system injury (neurogenic) or by aspirated blood and/or gastric contents.

Lung contusion is the most common parenchymal injury following blunt chest trauma.[29] Transmission of forces through the thoracic cage is responsible for the pathologic changes that are characterized by exudation of fluid and erythrocytes into the alveoli. Arteriolar and capillary dilatation, as well as lacerations and hematomas, are additional sequelae.

Lung contusion is usually evident radiographically on arrival in the emergency facility; late changes may develop in some cases. Wiot[6] has emphasized the importance of the time sequence in separating lung contusion from fat embolism, a condition that produces similar, but delayed, roentgenographic features.

The roentgenographic changes of lung contusion vary from irregular, patchy, scattered infiltrates to _____ (Figure 24-3). Lin-

the lungs clear. They simulate mass lesions, but on occasion may cavitate and develop air-fluid levels. These lesions are generally self-limited, and slow resolution without sequelae is the rule (Figure 24-3B). Conservative treatment is recommended even though complete resolution may be delayed for several months or years. Superimposed bacterial infection should be suspected when there is progressive infiltration associated with clinical symptoms of systemic toxicity.

Traumatic Wet Lung

This complication of pulmonary injury, first described by Burford and Burbank,[34] apparently results from a combination of excess tracheobronchial secretions, hemorrhage, depressed cough from pain, and difficulty eliminating accumulated material in the lung. Clinical symptoms that herald the onset of traumatic wet lung include increasing dyspnea, cyanosis, apprehension, and labored respiratory movement. Wheezes and rales occur along with copious amounts of mucus, serum, and frank blood in the tracheobronchial tree. A similar clinical complex occasionally follows open heart surgery and/or periods of shock.[35,36]

The lungs are characterized by focal parenchymal opacities and areas of regional atelectasis, or by a disseminated alveolar pattern, secondary to pulmonary hemorrhage or edema (Figure 24-4A). Adult respiratory distress syndrome may supervene either as a part of the underlying disease or from the administration of oxygen and baropressure or both. (See Chapter 25.)

___ic Air Leak

___ural space and medias-
___ thoracopul-
___ into

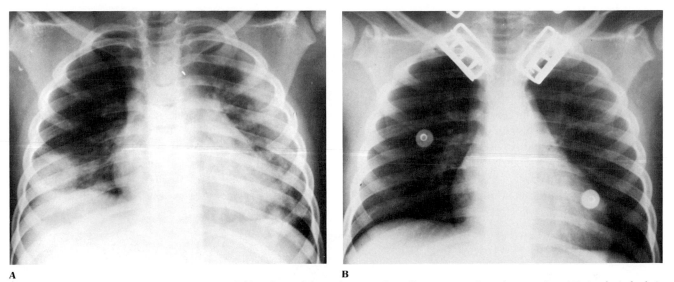

A   B

Figure 24-3   Lung contusion. A. The initial film shows bilateral areas of confluent parenchymal contusion. Minimal air leak is present on the left. No thoracic fractures are present. **B.** A follow-up study shows normal lungs.

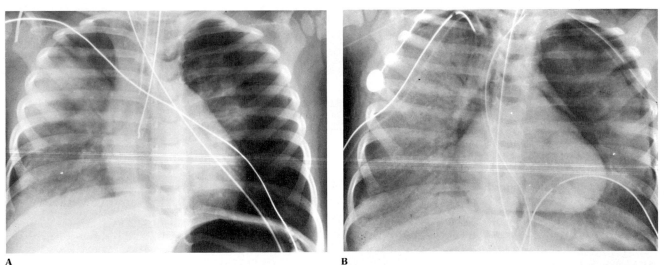

A   B

Figure 24-4   Traumatic wet lung. This child was left alone in an automobile with the motor running. She accidentally engaged the gear shift, and the car drove about in a circle. Repeated attempts to enter the vehicle were unsuccessful, and it was stopped by shooting out the tires. **A.** The initial film shows edema and contusion of the right lung. A pneumothorax is present on the left. **B.** In the ensuing 24 h, all attempts to ventilate and oxygenate the child were futile. The lungs are totally opaque, presumably from an outpouring of edema and blood. Left pneumothorax, pneumomediastinum, and pneumopericardium are also present. The child died shortly after this film.

from mechanical-assisted ventilation or anesthesia may ensue. Wall and coworkers[37] have called attention to the discovery of previously unrecognized pneumothorax during computed tomography (CT) of the abdomen in traumatized patients.

Spontaneous pneumothorax, particularly ones less than 20 percent, may be treated by simple aspiration.[38] Sequential films are of greater help than the actual size when deciding on thoracotomy.

Pleural air may collect in unusual locations, depending upon the characteristics of the underlying lung, nature of the disease process, or condition of the pleural space. A localized pneumothorax anterior to collapsed lung is a well-known finding.[39,40] Air may become trapped within the pulmonary ligament, especially in neonates, and present as a loculated pneumatocele or pneumothorax.[32,41,42] In older patients, this air collection probably represents loculated pneumothorax behind, rather than within, the pulmonary ligament (Figure 24-5).[43,44] Watchful waiting is the treatment of choice, as these collections almost invariably disappear spontaneously once the air leak is controlled.

Considerable controversy exists within the com-

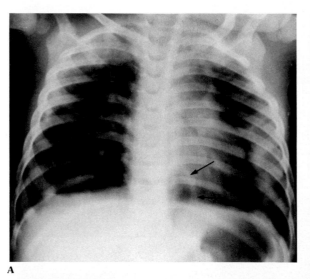

A

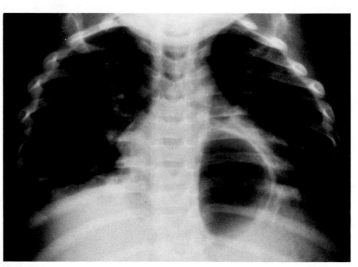

B

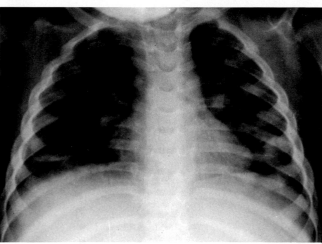

C

Figure 24-5 Traumatic pneumatocele in pulmonary ligament. A. This film study taken shortly after chest trauma shows bilateral pneumothorax, lung contusion, and a small left-sided paraspinous air collection (arrows). **B.** Seventeen days later, the air collection has enlarged and appears under tension. Several attempts at needle aspiration failed to drain this air. **C.** A film taken 1 month after injury shows spontaneous disappearance of the pneumatocele. The possibility exists that this collection is loculated in the pleural space behind the pulmonary ligament (see the text). *Note:* There is healing in the left anterior rib fractures. (From Felman, Rodgers, Talbert, et al,[41] with permission.)

munity of chest surgeons regarding the most efficacious treatment for pneumothorax. Tube thoracostomy and various drainage hookups are recommended for traumatic pneumothorax and spontaneous pneumothorax where underlying lung disease inhibits normal lung expansion. Hamilton and Archer[38] have treated spontaneous pneumothorax successfully by simple aspiration (single or multiple) with an intravenous catheter.

Pneumomediastinum may accompany traumatic pneumothorax. Most often, this complication requires no specific treatment, although administration of 100% oxygen might relieve symptoms in some cases.[45]

Spontaneous pneumomediastinum, originally described by Hamman,[46] has several clinical features:

1. It may occur with little effort.
2. Pain may be severe and radiate to the back, neck, and shoulders.
3. Constitutional symptoms are absent.
4. A distinctive sound (Hamman's crunch) may be heard over the chest wall.
5. Subcutaneous emphysema (crepitus) in the neck and supraclavicular area is diagnostic.

A variety of events may precipitate pneumomediastinum. Among these are sudden pulling or pushing,[47] laughing, coughing, yelling,[48] vomiting, and other activities that vigorously increase intrathoracic pressure. The radiographic findings of mediastinal emphysema vary from a minimal collection of air along the left heart border and over the aortic knob, to large, irregular air collections along the entire mediastinum extending into the neck and supraclavicular soft tissues. Small amounts of free air are often seen to best advantage behind the sternum in the lateral projection (see Figure 14-9). As with small pneumothoraxes, expiratory films may reveal a small pneumomediastinum that is otherwise not apparent.

Posttraumatic Diaphragmatic Hernia

This complication of chest trauma occurs in children as well as adults. Ball and coworkers[49] reported a series of 42 patients aged 18 to 69 years. In their cases the correct diagnosis was made when (1) the injury was recent, (2) the tear was left-sided and large, with readily identifiable structures herniated, and (3) the chest film, upper gastrointestinal examination, barium enema, nuclear liver scan, and CT scan were performed. Right-sided hernias containing liver or other water density organs were more often missed.

Iatrogenic Pulmonary Trauma

Tube Thoracotomy

The widespread use of ventilatory assistance in the management of respiratory failure in the newborn has resulted in a dramatic increase in the incidence of pneumothoraxes requiring chest tube drainage. While tube thoracotomy is performed readily and safely in the majority of patients, complications may accompany this procedure. The least common is hemorrhage from a puncture made along the interior border of the superior rib. Traumatic arteriovenous fistula between the chest wall and lung is an additional uncommon complication of intercostal catheter placement.[50] A more frequent and serious problem of chest tube insertion is perforation of the lung by the chest tube.[51–54] This complication occurs more commonly with hyaline membrane disease, wherein the lung is stiff and less able to recoil from the chest wall. Banagale et al.[53] suggest that the perforation is produced by a trocar inserted through the chest wall before the placement of a catheter, while others have shown the lung perforated by the chest tube.[51,54]

Lung perforation is not easily recognized radiographically but should be suspected when a pneumothorax fails to resolve, especially if the catheter tip appears to be well positioned in relation to the free air. Changes of atelectasis and/or infiltration near the tip of the chest tube are indirect evidence for lung perforation. Two additional signs that suggest lung perforation are hemorrhage into the pleural space and blood return from the endotracheal tube.

Chest tubes may cause damage to other structures including the phrenic nerve, leading to the development of diaphragmatic paralysis (Figure 24-6).

A tube positioned within a fissure may render it ineffective.[55]

The use of central venous catheters creates an additional danger of thrombosis, perforation, and extravasation (Figure 24-7).[56] The rapid opacification of the thorax in the presence of an indwelling vascular catheter suggests extravasation of fluid. Thoracentesis will usually confirm the diagnosis; catheter injection with contrast material is also helpful in selected cases.

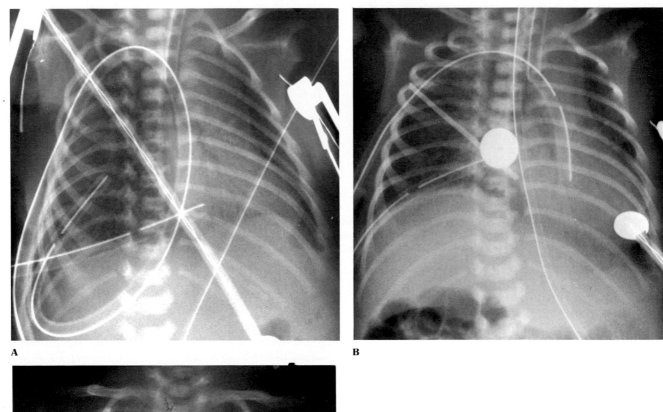

A   B

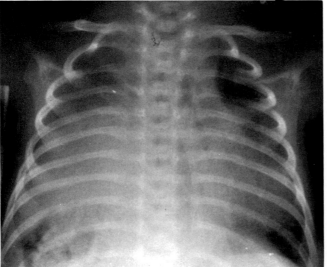

C

Figure 24-6   Traumatic diaphragmatic paralysis. A. Chest tubes were inserted for pneumothorax in this newborn with hyaline membrane disease. The tube is coiled against the mediastinal structures. **B.** One week later, the tube is seen extending across the midline; the right hemidiaphragm is elevated. **C.** One month later, the right hemidiaphragm is more elevated and immobile on fluoroscopic examination.

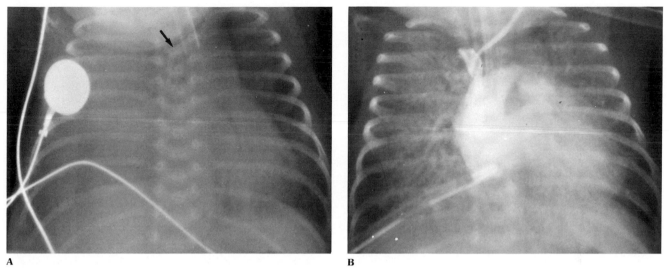

Figure 24-7   Catheter fluid extravasation. A. The right hemithorax is opaque with mediastinal shift to the left. *Note:* catheter in the innominate vein (arrow). **B.** Intravenous fluid was drained from the right chest. Contrast injection several days later shows no extravasation. The perforation of the vein had apparently sealed.

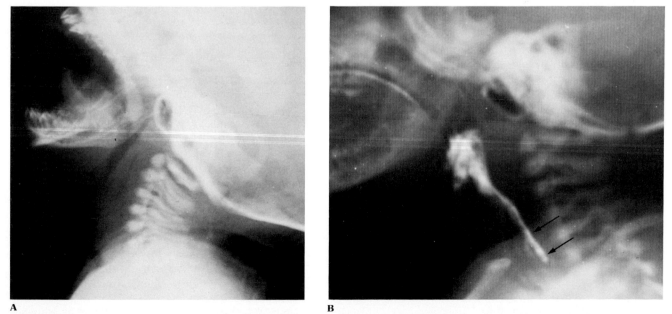

Figure 24-8   Traumatic pharyngeal perforation. A. The air collection in the thickened prevertebral soft tissue suggests a retropharyngeal perforation following oropharyngeal suction. **B.** A barium-water swallow outlines the traumatic diverticulum (arrows).

Tracheal Perforation

Tracheal perforation is a rare complication of endotracheal intubation.[57,58] Onset of severe pneumomediastinum, pneumothorax, and respiratory distress suggests the presence of this complication. The trachea may be punctured with minimal pressure.

Pharyngeal Perforation and Mediastinitis

Perforation of the pharynx may occur during resuscitation efforts of newborn infants. Return of blood during oropharyngeal suction should suggest the possibility of a perforation. Occasionally, the resulting pseudodiverticulum may be confused with esophageal atresia and tracheoesophageal fistula.[59,60] Swallowed foreign bodies that lodge in the esophagus may also cause perforation. Objects in the mouths of children are additional sources of injury.

When the inflammatory process is localized to the mediastinum, chronic infection with formation of a mass lesion usually requires surgical drainage. When perforations extend into the pleural space, the use of antibiotics and external chest drainage is often sufficient.[61]

Radiographs of the injured area will frequently show air within the prevertebral soft tissues or in the anterior mediastinum. Contrast study of the esophagus may help delineate these problems (Figure 24-8). Additional discussion of mediastinitis is covered in Chapter 13.

References

1. Kilman JW, Charnock E: Thoracic trauma in infancy and childhood. *J Trauma* 9:863, 1969.
2. Bellinger SB: Penetrating chest injuries in children. *Ann Thorac Surg* 14:635, 1972.
3. Smyth BT: Chest trauma in children. *J Pediatr Surg* 14:41, 1979.
4. Meller JL, Little AG, Shermeta DW: Thoracic trauma in infants. *Pediatrics* 74:813, 1984
5. Haller JA Jr, Shermeta DW: Major thoracic trauma in children. *Pediatr Clin North Am* 22:341, 1975.
6. Wiot JF: The radiologic manifestations of blunt trauma. *JAMA* 231:500, 1975.
7. Poole GV, Myers RT: Morbidity and mortality rates in major blunt trauma to the upper chest. *Ann Surg* 193:70, 1981.
8. Lundell C, Quinn M, Finck E: Traumatic laceration of the ascending aorta: Angiographic assessment. *AJR* 145:715, 1985.
9. Livoni JP, Barcia TC: Fracture of the first and second rib: Incidence of vascular injury relative to type of fracture. *Radiology* 145:31, 1982.
10. Fisher RG, Ward RE, Ben-Menachem Y, et al: Arteriography and the fractured first rib: Too much for too little? *AJR* 138:1059, 1982.
11. Woodring JH, Fried AM, Hatfield DR, et al: Fractures of the first and second ribs: Predictive value for arterial and bronchial injury. *AJR* 138:211, 1982.
12. Lazrove S, Harley DP, Grinnell VS, et al: Should all patients with first rib fracture undergo arteriography? *J Thorac Cardiovasc Surg* 83:532, 1982.
13. Sefczek DM, Sefczek RJ, Deeb ZL: Radiographic signs of acute rupture of the thoracic aorta. *AJR* 141:1259, 1983.
14. Brandt B III, Cram AE, Chow KC: Esophageal displacement secondary to blunt chest trauma. *Chest* 81:99, 1982.
15. Burney RE, Gundry SR, Mackenzie JR, et al: Chest roentgenograms in diagnosis of traumatic rupture of the aorta. Observer variation in interpretation. *Chest* 85:5, 1984.
16. Woodring JH, Pulmano EM, Stevens RK: Right paratracheal stripe in blunt chest trauma. *Radiology* 143:605, 1982.
17. Marnocha KE, Maglinte DDT, Wood J, et al: Mediastinal-width/chest-width ratio in blunt chest trauma: A reappraisal. *AJR* 142:275, 1984.
18. De Luca SA, Rhea JT, O'Malley T: Radiographic evaluation of rib fractures. *AJR* 138:91, 1982.
19. Chesterman JT, Satsangi PN: Rupture of the trachea and bronchi by closed injury. *Thorax* 21:21, 1966.
20. Larizadele R: Rupture of the bronchus. *Thorax* 21:28, 1966.
21. Mills SA, Johnston FR, Hudspeth AS, et al: Clinical spectrum of blunt tracheobronchial disruption illustrated by seven cases. *J Thorac Cardiovasc Surg* 84:49 1982.
22. Lotz PR, Martell W, Rohwedder JJ, et al: Significance of pneumomediastinum in blunt trauma to the thorax. *AJR* 132:819, 1979.
23. Kirsh MM, Orringer MB, Behrendt DM, et al: Management of tracheobronchial disruption secondary to non-penetrating trauma. *Ann Thorac Surg* 22:93, 1976.

24. Guest JL Jr: Major airway injury in closed chest trauma. *Chest* 72:63, 1977.

25. Hood RM, Sloan HE: Injuries to the trachea and major bronchi. *J Thorac Cardiovasc Surg* 38:458, 1959.

26. Silberger ML, Kushner LN: Tracheobronchial perforation: Its diagnosis and treatment. *Radiology* 85:242, 1965.

27. Mahaffey DE, Creech O Jr, Boren HG, et al: Traumatic rupture of the left main bronchus successfully repaired 11 years after injury. *J Thorac Surg* 32:312, 1956.

28. Stevens E, Templeton AW: Traumatic nonpenetrating lung contusion. *Radiology* 85:247, 1965.

29. Shulman HS, Samuels TH: The radiology of blunt trauma. *J Assoc Can Radiol* 34:204, 1985.

30. Sorsdahl OA, Powell JW: Cavitary pulmonary lesions following non-penetrating chest trauma in children. *AJR* 95:118, 1965.

31. Fagan CJ: Traumatic lung cyst. *AJR* 97:186, 1966.

32. Fagan CJ, Swischuk LE: Traumatic lung and paramediastinal pneumatoceles. *Radiology* 120:11, 1976.

33. Cochlin DL, Shaw MRP: Traumatic lung cysts following minor blunt chest trauma. *Clin Radiol* 29:151, 1978.

34. Burford TN, Burbank B: Traumatic wet lung. *J Thorac Surg* 14:415, 1945.

35. Neville WE, Kontaxis A, Gavin T, et al: Post-perfusion pulmonary vasculitis. *Arch Surg* 86:126, 1963.

36. Ostendorf P, Birzle H, Vogel W, et al: Pulmonary radiographic abnormalities in shock. *Radiology* 115:257, 1975.

37. Wall SD, Federle MP, Jefrey RB, et al: CT diagnosis of unsuspected pneumothorax after blunt abdominal trauma. *AJR* 141:915, 1983.

38. Hamilton AAD, Archer GJ: Treatment of pneumothorax by simple aspiration. *Thorax* 38:934, 1983.

39. Berdon W, Abramson S, Dee G, et al: Localized pneumothorax adjacent to a collapsed lobe: A sign of bronchial obstruction. *Radiology* 150:691, 1984.

40. Lams P, Jolles H: The effect of lobar collapse on the distribution of free intrapleural air. *Radiology* 142:309, 1982.

41. Felman AH, Rodgers BM, Talbert JL: Traumatic paramediastinal air cyst: A case report. *Pediatr Radiol* 4:120, 1976.

42. Volberg FM Jr, Everett CJ, Brill PW: Radiologic features of inferior pulmonary ligament air collections in neonates with respiratory distress. *Radiology* 130:357, 1979.

43. Friedman PJ: Adult pulmonary ligament pneumatocele: A loculated pneumothorax. *Radiology* 155:575, 1985.

44. Godwin JD, Merten D: Paramediastinal pneumatocele: Alternative explanations to gas in the pulmonary ligament. *AJR* 145:525, 1985.

45. Munsell WP: Pneumomediastinum. *JAMA* 202:689, 1967.

46. Hamman L: Spontaneous mediastinal emphysema. *Bull Johns Hopkins Hosp* 64:1, 1939.

47. Sturtz GS: Spontaneous mediastinal emphysema. *Pediatrics* 74:432, 1984.

48. Feldtman RW, Oram-Smith JC, Manning LG, et al: Spontaneous mediastinal emphysema. *J Pediatr Surg* 15:648, 1980.

49. Ball T, McCrory R, Smith JO, et al: Traumatic diaphragmatic hernia: Errors in diagnosis. *AJR* 138:633, 1982.

50. Cox PS, Keshishian JM, Blades BB: Traumatic arteriovenous fistula of the chest wall and lung. *J Thorac Cardiovasc Surg* 54:109, 1976.

51. Wilson AJ, Kraus HF: Lung perforation during chest tube placement in the stiff lung syndrome. *J Pediatr Surg* 9:213, 1974.

52. Moessinger AC, Driscoll JM, Wigger HJ: High incidence of lung perforation by chest tube in neonatal pneumothorax. *J Pediatr* 92:635, 1978.

53. Banagale RC, Outerbridge EW, Aranda JV: Lung perforation: A complication of chest tube insertion in neonatal pneumothorax. *J Pediatr* 94:973, 1979.

54. Strife JL, Smith P, Dunbar JS, et al: Chest tube perforation of the lung in premature infants: Radiographic recognition. *AJR* 141:73, 1983.

55. Webb WR, LaBerge JM: Radiographic recognition of chest tube malposition in the major fissures. *Chest* 85:81, 1984.

56. Dhande V, Kattwinkel J, Alford B: Recurrent bilateral pleural effusions secondary to superior vena cava obstruction as a complication of central venous catheterization. *Pediatrics* 72:109, 1983.

57. Schild JP, Wuilloud A, Kollberg H, et al: Tracheal perforation as a complication of nasotracheal intubation in the neonate. *J Pediatr* 86:596, 1975.

58. Serlin SP, Daily WJR: Tracheal perforation in the neonate: A complication of endotracheal intubation. *J Pediatr* 86:596, 1975.

59. Wells SD, Leonidas JC, Conkle D, et al: Traumatic prevertebral pharyngoesophageal pseudodiverticulum in the newborn infant. *J Pediatr Surg* 9:217, 1974.

60. Girdany BR, Sieber WK, Osman MZ: Traumatic pseudodiverticulum of the pharynx in newborn infants. *N Engl J Med* 280:237, 1969.

61. Johnson DE, Foker J, Munson DP, et al: Management of esophageal and pharyngeal perforation in the newborn infant. *Pediatrics* 70:592, 1982.

Chapter 25

Miscellaneous Diseases

Something old, something new, something borrowed, something blue.

This chapter covers pulmonary conditions that have unknown or obscure causes and diverse pathogeneses. They are difficult to classify and are therefore included as a miscellaneous group. The following diseases are covered in this chapter:

1. Diffuse pulmonary hemorrhage and pulmonary hemosiderosis
2. Adult respiratory distress syndrome
3. Smoke inhalation
4. Drug-induced pulmonary disease
5. Lymphocytic (lymphoid) interstitial pneumonitis
6. Gaucher's disease
7. Pulmonary veno-occlusive disease
8. Pulmonary alveolar proteinosis
9. Pulmonary calcification and/or ossification
10. Pulmonary vasculitides
    a. Wegener's granulomatosis
    b. Lymphomatoid granulomatosis
    c. Allergic granulomatous angiitis (Churg-Strauss syndrome)

Diffuse Pulmonary Hemorrhage and Pulmonary Hemosiderosis

Pulmonary hemorrhage has been classified by Albelda and coworkers[1] into the following six groups:

1. Pulmonary hemorrhage associated with glomerulonephritis and anti-glomerular basement membrane (anti-GBM) antibodies (Goodpasture's syndrome)
2. Diffuse pulmonary hemorrhage associated with renal disease without demonstrable immunologic abnormalities
3. Pulmonary hemorrhage associated with glomerulonephritis and immune complex disease (systemic lupus erythematosus)
4. Pulmonary hemorrhage and immune complex disease without renal disease
5. Pulmonary hemorrhage and anti-GBM antibodies without renal disease
6. Pulmonary hemorrhage without demonstrable immunologic associations or renal disease

The conditions listed in the first five groups are primarily seen in adults; group 6 includes several complexes that afflict children as well. Those with known etiology are bleeding disorders, acute lung injury, foreign body ingestion, drug reactions, pulmonary venous hypertension, and chronic infections.

Idiopathic pulmonary hemosiderosis (Ceelem's disease) is a disease of unknown etiology that is also included in this group. Children and young adults are mostly affected and characteristically present with cough, fever, tachypnea, and abdominal pain associated with pulmonary hemorrhage. These symptoms are often accompanied by leukocytosis, elevated erythrocyte sedimentation rate, and occasional hemoptysis. Additional features of this syndrome include pallor, dyspnea, wheezing, hepatosplenomegaly, recurrent iron-deficiency anemia, and growth retardation. Hypochromic, microcytic anemia and low serum iron concentrations occur in spite of excessive accumulation of iron sequestered in the macrophages of the lung.

The diagnosis is often delayed because the clinical signs and symptoms simulate acute pulmonary infection, and improvement often follows antibiotic treatment. The recurrence of similar episodes should lead to consideration of this entity, however, and trigger the appropriate diagnostic studies. Recovery of iron-laden macrophages (siderophages) from the stomach in the presence of otherwise unexplained pulmonary disease is presumptive evidence of pulmonary hemosiderosis.[2] Stools may be positive for blood during exacerbations. Lung biopsy will usually show degeneration and hyperplasia of alveolar epithelium with excessive shedding of cells, siderocytes, interstitial fibrosis, and sclerotic vascular changes.[3] Injection of [51]Cr- or [59]Fl-labeled red blood cells will show a decrease in plasma radioactivity along with increased radioactivity in the lungs.[4,5] Pulmonary function tests may show impaired diffusion, decreased compliance, airway obstruction, and other reduced functions.

If the child is radiographed during the acute hemorrhagic episode, the lungs assume a generalized, filmlike, "hazy" quality that is scattered throughout the lungs and not confined to the borders of lobes (Figure 25-1B).[6] As the illness abates, the lungs gradually return to their prehemorrhagic appearance and remain normal during remission (Figure 25-1A and C). However, after repeated episodes of hemorrhage, a mottled, finely nodular persistent pattern remains and is obscured only by the hemorrhagic episodes. In time, the repeated pulmonary insults leave permanent fibrotic residua.

In some patients, lobar or segmental infiltrates appear, disappear, and surface in other regions. These opacities represent more intense focal hemorrhage and may be misinterpreted as pneumonia. However, recognition of recurrent patterns of alveolar opacities and progressive, persistent, nodular, parenchymal changes over weeks and months should suggest the diagnosis within the proper clinical setting. These patients frequently accumulate heavy film envelopes; the diagnosis of pulmonary hemosiderosis lies not on the view box but in those envelopes.

Lung scintigraphy following the injection of ^{51}Cr-labeled red blood cells or ^{99m}Tc pertechnetate may show abnormal uptake in patients with several varieties of pulmonary hemorrhage including idiopathic pulmonary hemosiderosis.[7,8]

The etiology of primary pulmonary hemosiderosis remains obscure. Heiner and coworkers[9] have demonstrated antibodies to cow's milk in the serum of 7 of 14 children with pulmonary hemosiderosis, but milk precipitins have not been consistently present in other subjects with this disorder. Others have cast doubt on this theory since they found milk precipitins in children with a variety of recurrent pulmonary inflammatory disorders not associated with bleeding.[10]

Electron microscopy studies of biopsied lung tissue show breaks in the continuity of basement membranes of alveolar capillaries, but attempts to implicate an autoimmune reaction as the cause of the basement membrane lysis have been unsuccessful.[11] Nevertheless, the favorable response of patients with idiopathic pulmonary hemorrhage to immunosuppressive therapy suggests an underlying immunopathologic mechanism.[1] Before making the diagnosis of primary or idiopathic pulmonary hemosiderosis, it is necessary to exclude other causes for pulmo-

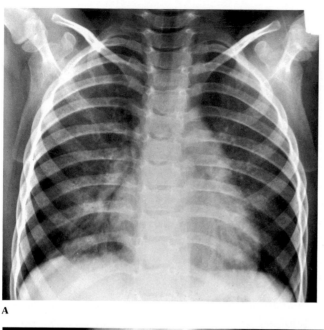

A

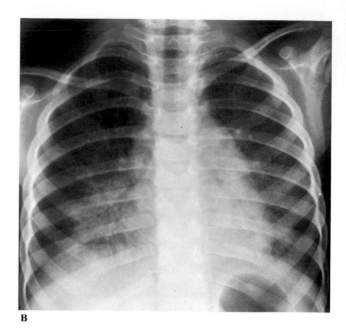

B

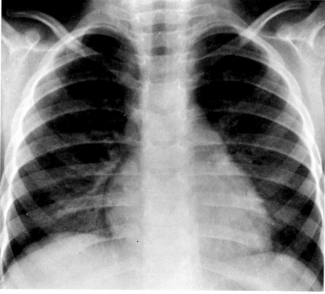

C

Figure 25-1 Idiopathic pulmonary hemorrhage (hemosiderosis). This child suffered from repeated bouts of pulmonary hemorrhage. Three examples of chest studies taken at different stages of illness are illustrated. **A.** This film shows diffuse, subtle radiopacities in the central basal lung segments during a recovery phase. **B.** Six months later, there are well-defined alveolar opacities in both lower lung fields. The child was acutely ill with tachypnea, tachycardia, and anemia on this occasion. **C.** A representative film, 1 year later, during relatively good health shows return to the baseline conditions. The lungs have poorly defined central and basal vessels. The parenchyma contains finely nodular densities, often difficult to appreciate and even harder to photograph. *Note:* More than any other disease, this entity requires careful scrutiny of all old films. The clinician should find a large bank of view boxes and a grease pencil to date each film and put them all up in sequence; then the physician will have a good chance at the diagnosis.

nary hemorrhage, including renal disease, with or without autoimmune abnormalities, and chronic elevation of pulmonary venous pressure.[12] Systemic lupus erythematosus (SLE) is another cause for pulmonary hemorrhage to be excluded.[13] This may present difficulty in selected patients since recurrent pulmonary hemorrhage may precede the more typical clinical manifestations of SLE.

Adult Respiratory Distress Syndrome

Although the word *adult* suggests an older age for patients with this syndrome, considerable experience with adult respiratory distress syndrome (ARDS) has been accumulated in children.[14–17] The clinical, radiologic, and pathologic abnormalities of this syndrome, also known as *shock lung*, are summarized as follows:

1. Clinical
   a. Tachypnea (> 20 breaths per minute)
   b. Pulmonary insufficiency (hypoxemia)
   c. Increased alveolar-arterial oxygen gradient
   d. Decreased lung compliance and capacity
   e. Left ventricular wedge pressure < 12 cmH$_2$O
2. Radiologic
   a. Diffuse alveolar infiltrates (early, 24 to 72 h)
   b. Pulmonary edema (early, 24 h)
   c. Chronic, slowly changing opacities suggesting "interstitial" disease (later, 3 to 10 days)
   d. Air leak (in some cases)
   e. Gradual return to "normal" (in some cases)
3. Pathologic
   a. Hyaline membranes
   b. Atelectasis
   c. Pulmonary edema
   d. Type II pneumocyte proliferation
   e. Alveolar macrophages
   f. Increased septal cellularity

The pathophysiology of ARDS begins with injury to the alveolar-capillary basement membrane leading to pulmonary edema, atelectasis, intrapulmonary shunting, and hypoxemia.

The following is a list of some precipitating causes for this syndrome:[18]

1. Shock (septic, hemorrhagic, cardiogenic, anaphylactic)
2. Trauma (direct contusion of the lung or nonpulmonary injury)
3. Infection (bacterial, viral, miliary tuberculosis, legionella)
4. Near-drowning
5. Emboli (fat, amniotic fluid)
6. Toxic inhalation (smoke, phosgene, oxides of nitrogen)
7. Oxygen toxicity
8. Drugs (heroin, methadone, salicylates)
9. Postradiation

Radiographic findings, invariably present, depend largely upon the nature of the original insult. Generalized air space opacities resembling and often representing pulmonary edema are characteristic (Figures 25-2A and C and 25-3B). After therapy is initiated, the pattern gradually alters, depending upon the patient's response and the type of treatment being administered. Therapy of ARDS is based upon the delivery of oxygen under positive end expiratory pressure (PEEP) between 5 and 15 cm of water. This mechanical ventilation is designed to open collapsed alveoli and may give the lung a relatively "clear" appearance by distending the air space and dissipating the edema fluid. Air leak phenomena are natural consequences from this therapy and often complicate the radiographic picture (Figure 25-2B). As chronicity develops, however, a pattern resembling interstitial fibrosis or honeycombing may ensue (Figure 25-4). The onset of superimposed pneumonia is difficult to assess under these circumstances. Careful examination from sequential films is important in this regard. Multiple cavitary processes are rare but significant indicators of infection. Failure of resolution of the pulmonary infiltrates also suggests superimposed pneumonia.

Since ARDS may be precipitated by a wide spectrum of insults, the prognosis will frequently depend upon the character and severity of the initial annoyance. Even with successful treatment, mortality from ARDS may approach 20 to 50 percent in children (Figure 25-5); significant morbidity in adults may reach 40 percent.[15]

Long-term sequelae are more common in children than adults and consist primarily of abnormal gas exchange.[19] The ultimate effect of ARDS on the growing lung is still to be determined.

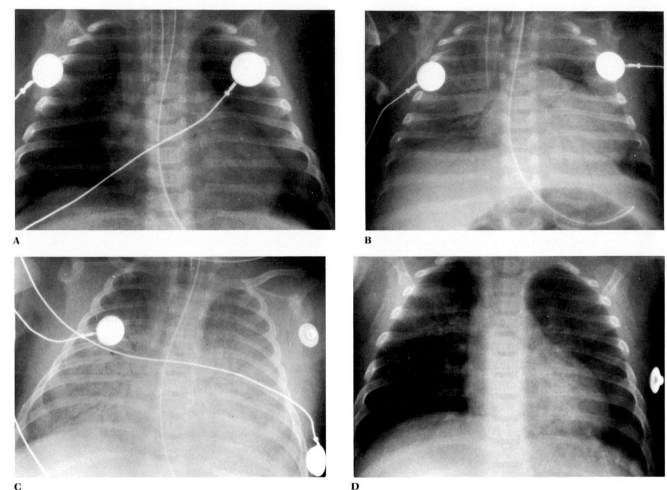

Figure 25-2   Adult respiratory distress syndrome—septic shock. This patient presented with systemic signs of overwhelming sepsis and hypotension. **A.** The initial film study is normal. **B.** A disseminated alveolar pattern has developed during the ensuing 48 h of mechanical ventilation therapy. Minimal air leak is present in the central lung field. **C.** At the height of this patient's illness the lungs are almost completely opacified. **D.** Approximately 2 weeks later (1 month after the onset of illness) the lungs have returned to near normal.

Smoke Inhalation

Two general areas of smoke inhalation are considered: (1) acute and (2) passive.

Acute Smoke Inhalation

The consequences of acute smoke inhalation depend upon the duration of exposure to smoke and the chemical constituents of the burning substance. Irritant aldehydes are produced from burning wood; oxides of sulfur, nitrogen, and other elements are formed when synthetic substances (plastics) are consumed by fire.[20,21]

Two major anatomic areas of the tracheobronchial tree are injured from acute smoke inhalation: (1) the trachea and stem bronchi and (2) the peripheral bronchioles and alveoli. In most cases the damage is reversible, but central and peripheral airway

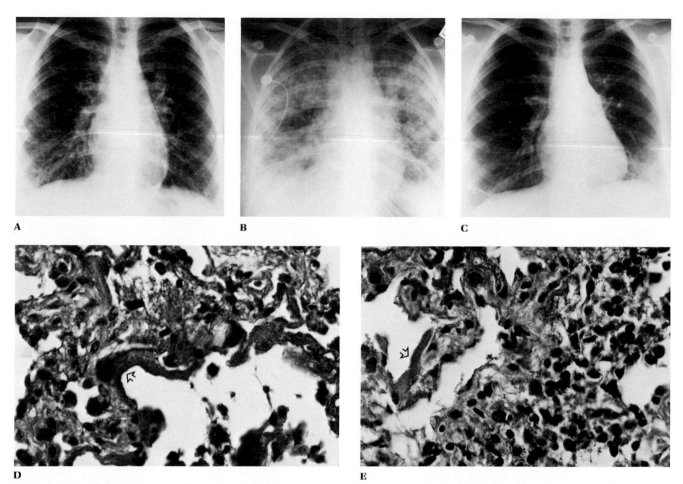

Figure 25-3 Adult respiratory distress syndrome—overwhelming pneumonia (psittacosis). This adolescent girl presented with extremely severe pulmonary symptoms and toxicity. **A.** The admission film shows diffuse interstitial disease. **B.** After 48 h the lung fields are opacified by a diffuse alveolar process. **C.** Following 1 month of therapy, the lungs have returned to near normal. **D** and **E.** Histologic sections of lung biopsy show an inflammatory reaction consisting of both mononuclear cells and granulocytes that are thickening the interstitial septa. The dark-staining homogeneous material lining the pulmonary alveoli are hyaline membranes (arrows).

obstruction are potential long-term complications of smoke-induced tracheobronchitis.[22]

Damage to the pulmonary parenchyma does not always accompany tracheobronchitis. However, injury to the alveolar epithelium leads to increased capillary permeability, pulmonary edema, and altered gas exchange.[22,23] Heart failure, fluid overload,[22,23] and adult respiratory distress may begin at any time after original injury.

Teixidor and coworkers[21] found radiographic evidence of acute smoke inhalation in all but 4 of 35

patients with chest films taken within 24 h of exposure. These consisted predominantly of vascular unsharpness, peribronchial cuffing, and mixed alveolar and interstitial edema. A predilection for the central lung and upper lobes was noted. Little data exist that relate the radiographic findings to the patients' prognosis.

Passive Smoking

The association of chronic smoke inhalation with symptoms of cough, wheezing, recurrent pneu-

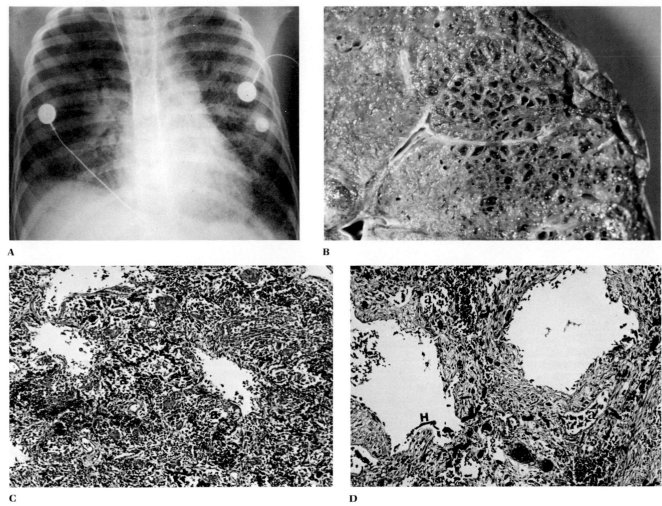

Figure 25-4   Adult respiratory distress syndrome—end-stage lung. This 4-year-old child developed septic shock from a ruptured appendix. He died after 2 weeks of oxygen and ventilator therapy. **A.** This film, the last study obtained during life, demonstrates a pattern of generalized honeycombing. **B.** The cut surface of the gross lung specimen shows an array of small, cystic spaces of variable sizes and shapes. These correspond to the radiographic and histologic pattern. **C** and **D.** Low- and high-power photomicrographs illustrate marked thickening of the interalveolar septa with extensive fibrosis and cellular infiltration. Many alveoli (a) are collapsed, and others are filled with macrophages. The large, "cystic" air spaces are lined by fragmenting hyaline membranes (H).

monia, bronchitis, and unspecified lower respiratory illness is now recognized.[24–26] Evidence suggests that the greatest danger to the child is in the first year or two of life and that maternal rather than paternal smoking is a more significant threat.[27]

There is controversy over the magnitude of the health risk for children exposed to parents who smoke cigarettes. Obstructive lung disease in later life may well result from exposure to parental smoking. Greater incidence of smoking by children of smoking parents threatens to perpetuate this problem.

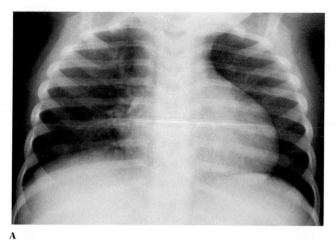

A

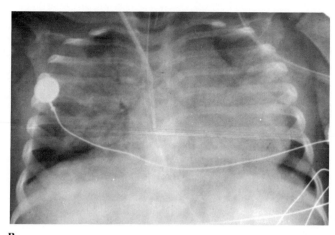

B

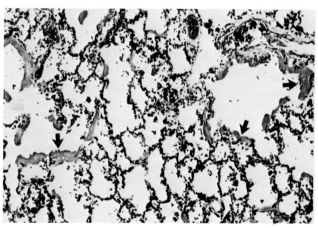

C

Figure 25-5 Adult respiratory distress syndrome—early changes. This 13-month-old boy developed flulike symptoms and systemic toxicity. **A.** The initial film shows minimal early right-sided infiltration. By 24 h, infiltration had progressed to involve most of the lung. **B.** At 48 h, just before death, this film study retains a diffuse alveolar pattern. **C.** The histologic specimen shows severe congestion, diffuse alveolar damage, and focal bronchopneumonia. The gray material represents early hyaline membrane formation (arrows).

Drug Induced Pulmonary Disease

The relationship between drug intake and lung disease is a well-established but extremely complex and poorly understood phenomenon. A wide variety of drugs may cause pulmonary injury that is characterized by diffuse damage to the alveolar lining cells.[28] Continued exposure to these agents causes progressive alterations within the supporting lung structures, leading to interstitial pneumonia, fibrosis, and possible ARDS. These alveolar injuries and fibrotic sequelae are not limited to drug ingestion but may follow a variety of other insults, including (1) infectious agents, (2) inhalants, (3) systemic shock, (4) lung irradiation, and (5) other known and unknown causes (see Chapter 22).

Clinical symptoms of cough, dyspnea, respiratory distress, and occasional fever accompany the onset of drug-induced hypersensitivity pneumonitis. Unfortunately, these symptoms often simulate those of the underlying disease process under therapy. Peripheral eosinophilia frequently accompanies these complications, and when present, the condition is often referred to as *Loeffler's syndrome*. This syndrome, however, is not limited to drug sensitivity, but is associated with a variety of other reactions, frequently atopic in nature (see Chapter 21).

The radiographic patterns produced by drug ingestion are nonspecific. In acute reactions, especially with drug overdose, an exudative process predominates with the production of a pulmonary edema-like, or disseminated alveolar, radiographic pattern (Figure 25-6; also see Chapter 16.) With continued exposure, an indolent picture of proliferative organization ensues, producing subtle, diffuse nodular and occasionally fibrotic opacities. Almost any composite of radiographic features may develop, especially in the presence of preexisting lung disease or superimposed infection. With some drugs (e.g., bleomycin) the reaction is dose-related, while in others it is idiosyncratic. Synergistic reactions may alter the clinical and radiographic response since many of these patients are receiving multiple drugs and/or pulmonary irradiation.

Antibiotics

Penicillin

The lung reaction caused by penicillin sensitivity is often characterized by pulmonary infiltrates with

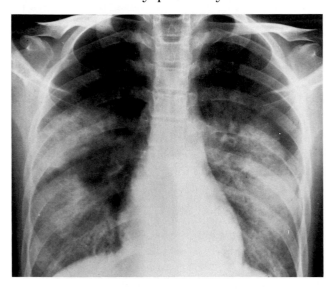

Figure 25-6   Methotrexate lung disease. The lungs have developed generalized alveolar infiltration after treatment with methotrexate. The pattern regressed following cessation of the drug. This radiograph is nonspecific. It is compatible with virtually any cause for the diffuse alveolar pattern.

eosinophilia (Loeffler's syndrome). The radiographic features may range from "accentuated" lung markings to diffuse patchy infiltration that may be evanescent or persistent. The lung lesions often regress when the peripheral eosinophilia reaches its maximum.[29]

Clinical symptoms usually accompany the pulmonary changes of penicillin sensitivity. The plasma lupus erythematosus (LE) factor has been demonstrated in patients manifesting hypersensitivity to penicillin, but pulmonary infiltrates in these individuals are uncommon.[30]

Tetracycline

Hypersensitivity to tetracycline has been implicated in the genesis of SLE; untoward reaction to the drug may be the first clue to the presence of this disease. Ingestion of tetracyclines may also cause accelerated systemic spread of discoid lupus or precipitate a disastrous exacerbation in the clinical course of patients with SLE. Domz and coworkers[31] reported three cases of SLE felt to be secondary to the administration of tetracycline. Hydralazine (Apresoline) is another drug that apparently has the capacity to initiate systemic syndromes that simulate collagen diseases such as SLE and rheumatoid arthritis.[32,33]

Chemotherapeutic Agents

Nitrofurantoin

Numerous reports have documented the occurrence of pulmonary pathology in patients receiving nitrofurantoin.[34–41] Pulmonary infiltrates with eosinophils are characteristic histologic findings. Most often, the drug reaction is acute with sudden onset of cough, dyspnea, and fever; symptoms regress rapidly following drug withdrawal.

In some patients, the pulmonary reaction to nitrofurantoin has a gradual, insidious onset of dyspnea without fever.[34,41] This complication may follow long periods of therapy—6 months to as long as 6 years.[42]

In the acute reaction to nitrofurantoin, the pulmonary infiltrates usually affect the lower lobes.

Pleural effusions are occasionally seen.[34,37,43] As with other lung reactions, acute inflammatory disease cannot always be excluded from the initial chest films, especially in the presence of pleural effusions. The radiologic pattern in the more chronic, insidious variety consists of diffuse, nonspecific, linear opacities. Cessation of drug therapy and treatment with steroids will clear most cases, but irreversible fibrosis may result.

Bleomycin

Bleomycin, an antibiotic used in the treatment of Hodgkin's disease, may cause pulmonary toxicity, but a direct relationship is often difficult to prove. Abnormal pulmonary function tests, present in about one-third of patients receiving the drug, do not appear dose-related.[44] However, significant increase in pulmonary toxicity at total doses greater than 450 mg has been reported.[45,46] Lung reaction also occurs with lower doses of bleomycin, possibly because of synergistic action with concomitantly administered irradiation or other chemotherapeutic agents.[47]

The histologic alterations of bleomycin toxicity are those of interstitial fibrosis, alveolar squamous metaplasia, and hyalinization.

Radiographic features consist mostly of fine, nodular, bilateral opacities. Lymphadenopathy and/or pleural effusions are not usually observed. Elevated diaphragm and decreased lung volume have been reported.[48]

Methotrexate

Methotrexate, used in long-term therapy for a host of diseases including leukemia, psoriasis, Wegener's granulomatosis, and multiple solid tumors, is occasionally associated with pulmonary complications.[49-53] Typically, methotrexate toxicity causes acute symptoms of cough, fever, and dyspnea about 1 or 2 weeks to several months after administration of the drug. In an unusual instance a patient received the drug for 5 years before onset of symptoms.[52] Others may have a more chronic and indolent course resembling that seen in nitrofurantoin toxicity. Peripheral eosinophilia is an additional finding.

Although many drugs produce reactions that progress inexorably to irreversible interstitial fibrosis with high mortality, the lung reaction of methotrexate toxicity is frequently reversible and may be responsive to corticosteroid therapy. This response may be explained by the development of granulomatous lesions in this condition rather than the diffuse alveolar damage so often noted with other drug reactions.

The radiographic appearance of methotrexate toxicity varies from linear streaky shadows to confluent opacities (Figure 25-6). Hilar and paratracheal lymphadenopathy are rare but have been reported.[53] The roentgenographic abnormalities clear with interruption of the medication or following treatment with steroids.

Cyclophosphamide

Cyclophosphamide (Cytoxan) is an alkylating agent used in the treatment of a wide variety of tumors. Rare cases of associated pulmonary complications following the administration of this drug are reported. Topilow and coworkers[54] reported a patient under therapy for Hodgkin's disease who developed widespread interstitial pneumonia with bilateral confluent infiltrates. In another report, diffuse opacification and extensive histologic changes were observed in a 3-year-old child receiving the drug.[55] It is not clear from these two cases whether the pulmonary findings resulted from the cyclophosphamide or from other drugs also administered at some course in the disease. Nevertheless, it seems reasonable to assume that cyclophosphamide may contribute to permanent pulmonary injury including fibrosis and restrictive lung disease.

Sulfonamides

Sulfa drugs are used less frequently than in the past and rarely cause pulmonary complications. Migratory pneumonia with eosinophils has been observed in a patient taking oral sulfadimethoxyine (Madribon).[56] In sensitive individuals, SLE may be precipitated or exacerbated by the administration of sulfa drugs.[57]

Diphenylhydantoin

The cause-and-effect relationship between pulmonary disease and diphenylhydantoin (Dilantin) intake is not clear. In 1959, Moore[58] reported "accentuated" markings and fibrosis in patients taking diphenylhydantoin; Livingston and coworkers[59] found no lung changes. Hilar lymphadenopathy is reported in association with diphenylhydantoin ingestion,[60] and osseous changes of rickets may develop in growing children taking the drug.

Narcotics

Heroin

Four types of pulmonary complications may occur as a result of heroin abuse: (1) edema, (2) embolic pneumonia and/or lung abscess, (3) upper respiratory tract infection and superimposed bacterial pneumonia, and (4) pulmonary fibrosis and/or granulomatosis. Heroin overdose usually leads to pulmonary edema, but the relationship is not clear. If the patient survives the initial overdose, the pulmonary edema resolves rapidly. Adult respiratory distress syndrome with chronic fibrosis is not an uncommon sequela of heroin overdose in patients who require treatment with ventilators, oxygen, and other life-support methods.

The radiographic appearance of heroin-induced pulmonary edema is nonspecific. Pulmonary emboli, frequent complications of heroin abuse, are usually associated with infection. Superimposed pneumonia, as evidenced by prolonged infiltration, apparently relates to duration of drug use rather than to dosage.[61] The development of pulmonary fibrosis may be associated with intravenous injection of cotton fibers used to remove impurities.

Drug overdose should be considered in a child or adult with acute pulmonary edema and no antecedent disease.[62]

Methadone

Methadone hydrochloride is a synthetic narcotic used for the detoxification and maintenance of drug addicts. When taken in abusive amounts, this drug may cause pulmonary edema.[63–65] The underlying mechanism is thought to be similar to edema caused by other narcotic overdoses.

Codeine and propoxyphene hydrochloride (Darvon) are other narcotics capable of causing pulmonary changes of edema, fibrosis, and acute and chronic lung disease.[62–68]

Anti-Inflammatory Agents

Acetylsalicylic Acid (Aspirin)

Salicylate ingestion is a rare cause for pulmonary edema.[69–71] The lung changes may occur with therapeutic administration or overdose.[72] The pathophysiologic explanation for salicylate-induced edema appears related to increased pulmonary vascular permeability and escape of fluid and protein into the interstitial-alveolar space.[73] The radiographic findings of salicylate-induced edema are not specific.

Endocrine

Corticosteroids

Pulmonary changes from cortisone ingestion are limited to widening of the mediastinum from fat accumulation, a phenomenon that has been reported from exogenous steroids and Cushing's syndrome.[74,75] The development of secondary lymphoma in patients on long-term immunotherapy, including steroids, might occasionally lead to mediastinal lymphadenopathy. Computed tomography (CT) and magnetic resonance imaging are useful for distinguishing between mediastinal fat and adenopathy.

The thymus regresses in young children on steroid therapy. High doses of steroids may cause diminished bone mineral, collapsed vertebrae, aseptic necrosis of the proximal humeral epiphysis, and excess fat accumulation in the soft tissues.

Lymphocytic (Lymphoid) Interstitial Pneumonitis

Lymphocytic interstitial pneumonitis (LIP) is one of the interstitial pneumonic processes Liebow and Carrington[76] described in 1969. It occurs primarily in adults but has been reported in infants and children.[76-78] Patients present with cough, fatigue, dyspnea, and, on occasion, systemic symptoms.

This disease may occur in association with conditions that manifest abnormal immunoglobulins, especially immunoglobulin M, i.e., Sjögren's syndrome and Waldenstrom's macroglobulinemia. Juvenile rheumatoid arthritis is also complicated by LIP on rare occasions.[79,80] The prognosis of LIP is unpredictable. Some patients survive for variable lengths of time, while others develop a progressive illness with high mortality.[78]

The radiologic features of LIP overlap many other diseases. The presence of the term *interstitial* should not be taken as necessarily descriptive of the radiographic findings. Unfortunately, many diseases are named for their histologic appearance. To be sure, LIP often produces a coarse, honeycomb, "interstitial" pattern, but fluffy, cloudlike alveolar or air space shadows with air bronchograms also occur. Heitzman and coworkers[81] have described coarse, flame-like shadows along with alveolar air space opacities in LIP. Adding to the confusion is the fact that air bronchograms and other characteristic criteria of alveolar-air space disease are occasionally produced by lung processes having mostly interstitial changes on histologic examination.[82]

Gaucher's Disease

Gaucher's disease is a relatively uncommon abnormality of enzyme B-betaglucosidase activity that results in the accumulation of glucosyleramide in reticuloendothelial cells. These altered reticuloendothelial cells (Gaucher's cells) appear swollen and foamy on histologic examination. Accumulation of Gaucher's cells in the liver, spleen, and lymph nodes causes marked enlargement of these organs. Deposition of abnormal cells in bones may alter their shape, cause fractures, and lead to periosteal cloaking and aseptic necrosis, especially of the hip.

Gaucher's disease exists in two major forms: infantile and adult. Infantile Gaucher's disease is characterized by severe neurologic deterioration. The onset is usually in the first 6 months of age, with rapid clinical progression and pulmonary infection. The adult form of Gaucher's disease may begin in childhood but progresses slowly into older age with the development of hypersplenism, bone pain, pathologic fractures, and hematologic aberrations. The central nervous system is usually spared. An intermediate or juvenile variation resembles the infantile form of Gaucher's disease with central nervous system involvement but has an indolent clinical progression.

Pulmonary involvement in Gaucher's disease is uncommon but well documented. Wolson[83] reported 3 patients (1 adult) and reviewed 10 previously described examples in children. In most patients with Gaucher's disease the radiographs show diffuse, irregular densities throughout the lungs (Figure 25-7). A predominantly miliary pattern also occurs.[84-86] The lung changes are produced by the accumulation of Gaucher's cells in alveolar walls and sacs. Both hilar and mediastinal lymphadenopathy result from similar deposition in the lymph nodes.[86,87] Obstruction to pulmonary capillaries is a rare complication that may lead to pulmonary hypertension.[88] Recurrent pulmonary infections and occasional severe pulmonary hemorrhage may supervene.

Pulmonary Veno-Occlusive Disease

Pulmonary veno-occlusive disease results from primary obliterative obstruction of pulmonary veins and venules resulting in pulmonary hypertension.

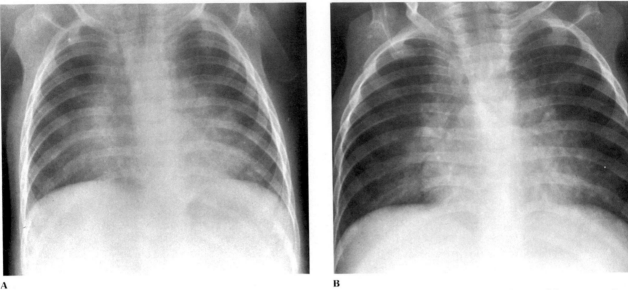

A   B

Figure 25-7   Gaucher's disease. A. The cardiac borders and pulmonary markings are completely obscured by a generalized parenchymal infiltrate. **B.** Six months later, the lungs are little changed and continue to demonstrate central opacities. The unchanging process probably represents the pulmonary manifestation of Gaucher's disease.

The disease affects males and females equally. Patients from 39 days to 48 years of age have been reported, with a little over one-half 16 years of age or younger.[89,90]

Patients present clinically with signs and symptoms of pulmonary arterial hypertension, most commonly dyspnea on exertion. Syncopal and cyanotic attacks, hemoptysis, and fever occur less frequently. Right ventricular hypertrophy and failure are eventual sequelae.

The etiology of veno-occlusive disease is unknown. Infections, hematologic clotting disorders, and immune complex reactions have been suspected, but to date there is no clear-cut answer. Isolated examples of veno-occlusive disease are reported in association with Hodgkin's disease,[91] following bone marrow transplant,[92] and after chemotherapy (bleomycin, mitomycin, and cisplatin).[93] Familial factors are occasionally operative, and isolated examples of the disease in siblings have been reported.[94-96]

Histologic examination of the lungs usually shows extensive constriction or occlusion of venous channels. These often contain multiple thrombi, many of which are partially recanalized. Fibrous intimal proliferation of the preacinar arteries may also develop, probably as a secondary phenomenon.[94]

Prognosis is poor regardless of treatment; most patients die within 2 years of onset. Occasional transient improvement with heparin therapy has been reported.[97,98]

Plain chest films often provide clues to the diagnosis. Radiographic findings are characterized by signs of right-sided cardiac enlargement and dilatation of the pulmonary arteries. Swollen interlobular septae, pulmonary edema, and pleural effusions are helpful when present (Figures 25-8 and 25-9). Mitral stenosis must be considered in the differential diagnosis but can usually be excluded by normal left atrial size, absent left atrial appendage enlargement, and negative history of rheumatic fever. Primary pulmonary hypertension may produce a radiographic picture of enlarged pulmonary arteries but should not cause the pattern of swollen interlobular septae associated with veno-occlusive disease.

Combined echocardiography, CT, and pulmo-

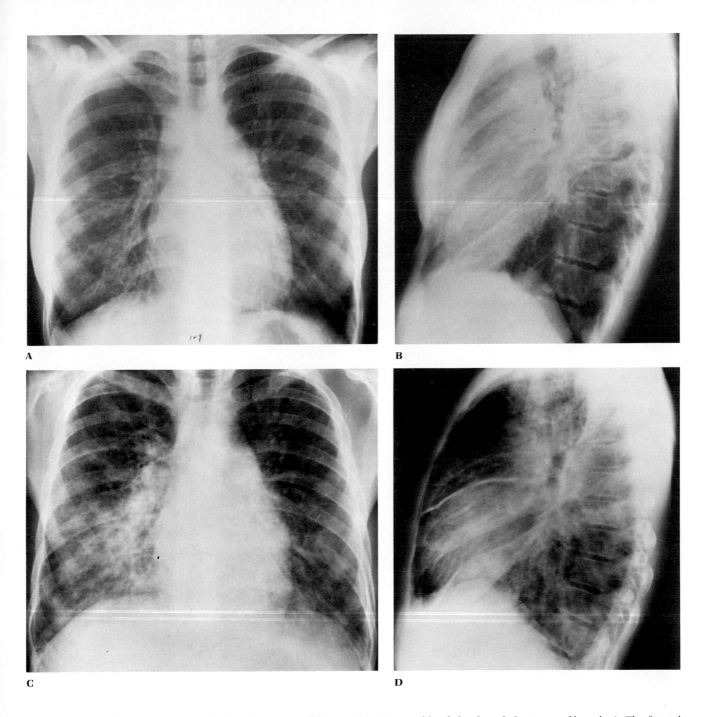

Figure 25-8 Pulmonary veno-occlusive disease in siblings. This 12-year-old girl developed shortness of breath. **A.** The frontal film shows a prominent main pulmonary artery and numerous fine, linear, irregular markings, mostly in the basal segments. **B.** The hila are ill-defined, fissures are thickened, and there are Kerley C lines (fine linear white shadows behind the sternum). **C.** This 14-year-old male sibling has more advanced disease. The lungs show diffuse linear shadows that are confluent centrally and discrete peripherally. Kerley lines and pleural edema are evident. The pulmonary artery segment is prominent. **D.** The lateral film shows more striking evidence of thickened fissures, ill-defined hila, and vascular unsharpness. *Note:* Differentiation from pulmonary edema of mitral stenosis or left heart failure is difficult, but the normal-sized heart and absence of left atrial enlargement are helpful clues. (Courtesy of Dr. Eugene Blank, Portland, Oregon.)

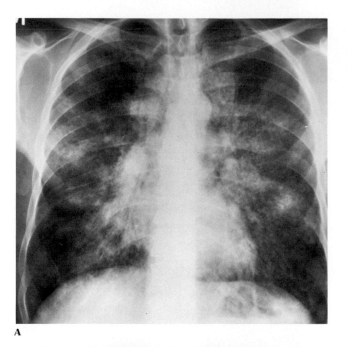

A

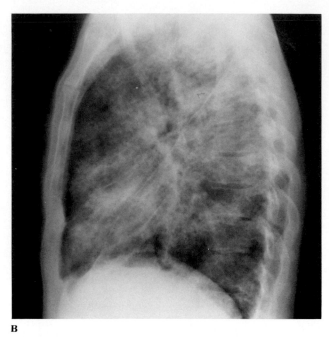

B

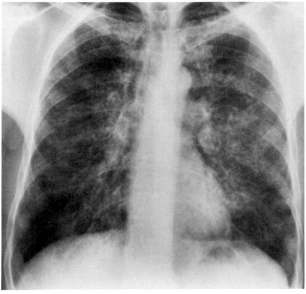

C

Figure 25-9 Pulmonary alveolar proteinosis—no associated disease. A and **B.** A disseminated alveolar pattern is evident in this young adult. The heart is normal, and there are no signs of interstitial fluid. **C.** Gradual improvement occurred without specific therapy. The lungs retain a nonspecific pattern of irregular markings, but some normal vascular shadows have reappeared.

nary angiography may be used to exclude other causes of pulmonary arterial and/or venous hypertension, i.e., thromboembolic disease, mediastinal fibrosis, congenital stenosis of pulmonary veins, left atrial myxoma, and cor triatriatum.[99] Enlarged central pulmonary arteries and slow flow through the lungs are the salient features of pulmonary angiography. The left atrium is not enlarged, and the pulmonary wedge pressure is normal in this condition.

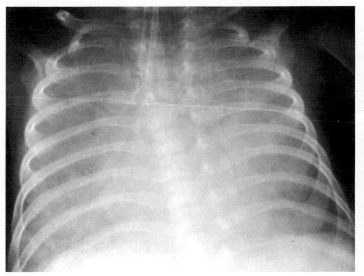

A

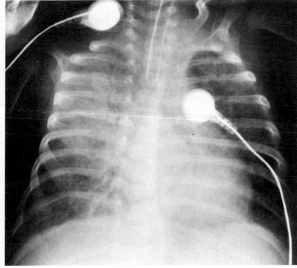

B

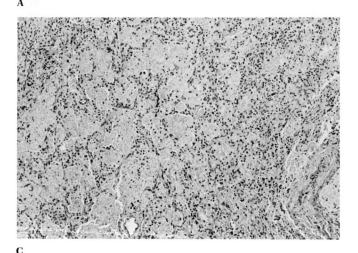

C

Figure 25-10 Pulmonary alveolar proteinosis—lavage therapy. A. A 3-month-old boy with a chronic pulmonary process that began at 1 month of age. The lungs are completely opacified. **B.** Film taken 6 h following bronchoalveolar lavage shows partial clearing, but there is residual opacity in the right mid and upper lung. **C.** The histologic section of lung shows all alveoli filled with homogeneous, granular, pink-staining, proteinaceous material. Tests for *Pneumocystis carinii* were negative. (See Chapter 21, Figure 21-1C, and Chapter 26, Figure 26-60.) (Courtesy of Dr. Jon Williams, Gainesville, Florida.)

Pulmonary Alveolar Proteinosis

The original description of pulmonary alveolar proteinosis was based upon 27 cases collected from autopsy or biopsy specimens.[100] It is a disease of unknown etiology characterized by the accumulation of protein, phospholipids, cholesterol, and free fatty acids within the alveolar spaces. The diagnosis is confirmed by typical electron-microscopic findings in sputum, lung washings, or lung biopsy. Most cases occur in adults, but occasional pediatric pa-

tients have been reported.[101,102] Males are affected twice as often as females.

Clinical symptoms are nonspecific, but pulmonary disability and hypoxemia are regular features; however, occasional patients are asymptomatic. The diagnosis should be considered in patients with tuberculosis, hematologic malignancy, or immunologic incompetence who develop diffuse alveolar pulmonary infiltrates that fail to resolve.[103,104]

The radiographic appearance of pulmonary alveolar proteinosis may assume almost any configuration but is typically characterized by a disseminated alveolar pattern (Figures 25-9 and 25-10). The infiltrates are often diffuse, perihilar, and butterfly-like in distribution. Bibasilar location is also common, and lobar consolidation may mimic pneumonia. Pleural effusions and cavitations are unusual and suggest the presence of superimposed infection. The pattern may simulate pulmonary edema, but pleural effusions and swollen interlobular septa are usually absent. A normal-sized heart and a stable or slowly changing pattern of radiopacities also tend to exclude pulmonary edema.

Histologic examination reveals the deposition of homogeneous-appearing eosinophilic material in the alveolar spaces (Figure 25-10C). The picture is not unlike that produced by *Pneumocystis carinii* infestation. Poor clinicoradiologic correlation is common; the lung biopsy may show extensive alveolar filling in the face of a normal chest radiograph.[105]

Superimposition of infections and fungal disease may complicate the course of this illness.[106] Inappropriate therapy with corticosteroids potentiates these dangers.

Whole lung lavage is a recognized treatment and may be effective when begun early in the illness.[107] This procedure may be curative in some cases, but occasionally patients need repeat lavage.

Pulmonary Calcification and/or Ossification

The deposition of calcified mineral in the lung may take the form of bone or calcium. Idiopathic pulmonary ossification, as the name implies, has no known etiology. It may be superimposed upon calcified deposits or occur without previous calcification. Ossification also develops through osteoid metaplasia of preexisting interstitial fibrosis and intraalveolar proteinaceous material.[108]

The radiographic lesions of pulmonary ossification appear as fine linear shadows, 1 to 4 mm thick, arranged in a branching or netlike configuration and located predominantly in the lower lobes.[109] Punctate, miliary, or small nodular opacities are occasion-

ally seen.[110] The disease is usually progressive but may remain indolent; regression never occurs.

Metastatic calcification is most commonly associated with chronic renal failure, destructive diseases of bone, and primary hyperparathyroidism (Figure 25-11).[111] Other causes include calcified metastatic tumors, chronic pulmonary venous hypertension (mitral stenosis), congenital heart lesions, calcified thrombi, healed infection, granulomatous disease (impotent white blood cells), and chronic lung disease. The calcification is usually confined to the interstitium, particularly the alveolar walls.[111–113]

Beerman and coworkers[111] described three subgroups of patients with pulmonary calcification. In the first, the patients had no roentgenographic abnormalities despite pulmonary calcification at autopsy. The second group of patients developed pulmonary infiltrates indistinguishable from opportunistic pneumonia or pulmonary edema. The opacities did not appear calcified and remained stable in contrast to the rapidly changing pattern of pulmonary edema or pneumonia. The third and smallest group developed infiltrates whose calcific nature was apparent without resorting to other imaging techniques or open lung biopsy.

Pulmonary Vasculitides

The pulmonary vasculitides constitute a heterogeneous group of rare disorders characterized by inflammation of blood vessel walls. Three varieties that occur in children and primarily affect the lungs are (1) Wegener's and limited Wegener's granulomatosis, (2) lymphomatoid granulomatosis, and (3) allergic granulomatous angiitis (Churg-Strauss syndrome). Other generalized diseases, in which pulmonary vasculitis may play a part, include collagen-vascular disorders, eosinophilic pneumonias, sarcoidosis, organic dust diseases (hypersensitivity pneumonitis, extrinsic allergic alveolitis), and others.

Considerable overlap in the radiographic presentation is the rule in this group of afflictions. Definitive diagnosis, in most patients, can only be made from histologic examination of lung tissue.[114]

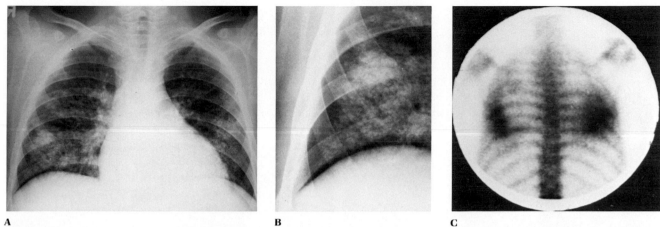

A   B   C

Figure 25-11   Pulmonary calcification/ossification. A 16-year-old boy with chronic renal failure. **A.** The chest film shows diffuse parenchymal infiltrates that spare apices and peripheral lungs. **B.** On closer examination, pulmonary parenchymal shadows are of greater density than expected for pneumonia. They represent diffuse pulmonary calcification. **C.** Technetium-99m diphosphonate scintigraphy shows radionuclide uptake within the lung corresponding to pulmonary parenchymal infiltrates. (From Beerman PJ, Crome JE, Sumner TE, et al: Radiological case of the month. *Am J Dis Child.* 137:1119, 1983. Copyright 1983, American Medical Association. With permission. Courtesy of Dr. Thomas E. Sumner, Winston-Salem, North Carolina.)

Wegener's Granulomatosis

Wegener's granulomatosis is a necrotizing granulomatous angiitis, most often found in adults but also reported in children.[115,116] The disease may be generalized or limited. The generalized form is characterized by a triad of diagnostic findings: (1) granulomatous vasculitis of the upper and lower respiratory tract, (2) a generalized, systemic small vessel vasculitis, and (3) focal glomerulonephritis. The kidneys, skin, and central nervous system may be involved, and segmental necrotizing glomerulitis may lead to hematuria and renal failure. The segmental arteritis is frequent and indistinguishable from polyarteritis nodosa.[117]

The limited form of Wegener's granulomatosis, sometimes referred to as *midline lethal granuloma,* is confined primarily to the sinuses and respiratory tract.[118,119] Submucosal granulomas and ulcerations of the upper respiratory passages and paranasal sinuses characterize this variety.

The systemic and pulmonary signs and symptoms in limited Wegener's are similar to the disseminated form of the disease, and the radiologic and pathologic changes in the lung are identical.[120] Early

differentiation between the generalized and limited forms is difficult, and may only be accomplished as the disease progresses.[121]

Midline lethal granuloma usually starts with persistent rhinorrhea, epistaxis, and sinusitis. Obstruction and ulceration of the nose and nasopharynx, perforation of the nasal septum, and further destruction of midfacial structures are unhappy consequences.

Radiographic changes of the lung are seen in almost all patients, even those with only minimal symptoms (Figure 25-12). Multiple pulmonary nodular opacities ranging in size from 1 to 10 cm are characteristic (Figure 25-12B). These nodules may be single or multiple, and cavitation is a frequent feature.[122] Constantly changing patterns with clearing in some areas and progression in others are typical.[123] Infiltrates may be fleeting and transient. Cavitations are common and usually have irregular, thick walls; pleural reactions are also reported.[124] The course of pulmonary radiographic changes cannot give any estimate of disease severity or prognosis.[125]

Treatment with cyclophosphamide has improved the outcome of this disease, but prognosis should remain guarded.[126 – 128] In isolated cases, surgical re-

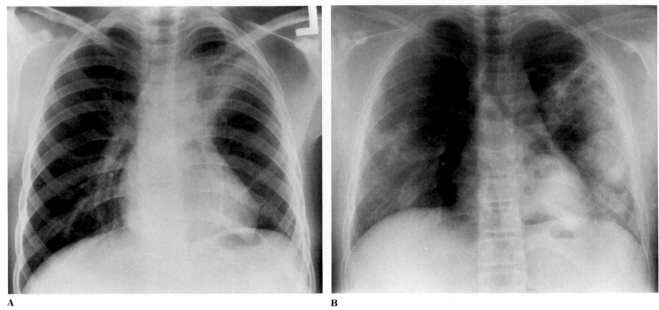

A   B

Figure 25-12   Wegener's granulomatosis. A 12-year-old boy with chronic cough. **A.** The initial film shows a left upper lobe opacity radiating to the hila. The lesion was biopsied and found to be compatible with Wegener's granulomatosis. **B.** Steroid therapy caused regression of the original left upper lobe process, but 6 months later there are round, homogeneous opacities in the left lung and irregular, patchy infiltrates on the right. Apparent cavitation has occurred in one or two of the larger lesions. The child also suffered from a skin rash and recurrent hematuria.

moval of solitary lesions may be curative. Fulminating pulmonary hemorrhage is an uncommon but dreaded complication.[129]

Lymphomatoid Granulomatosis

Originally described by Liebow and coworkers,[130] lymphomatoid granulomatosis primarily attacks the lungs, but other organs such as the kidneys, skin, central nervous system, and adrenal glands are frequently involved. It may well be the most common form of pulmonary angiitis and granulomatosis.[131–133]

The precise relationship of this disorder to pulmonary lymphoma is not definitively established. Considerable overlap exists in their clinicopathologic picture. Lymphomatoid granulomatosis has been reported to progress into a picture indistinguishable from pulmonary lymphoma in 10 percent of cases.[134] As with lymphoma, the mortality rate is high.

In contrast to lymphomatoid granulomatosis, lymphoma more often involves lymph nodes, spleen, and bone marrow and has fewer complications of the skin and central nervous system.

Lymphomatoid granulomatosis predominates in middle age but occurs in childhood as well. Although the lungs are almost always affected early in the course of illness, rare examples of delayed pulmonary changes are reported.[135] Onset and progression of clinical symptoms are generally rapid; cough, dyspnea, malaise, fever, and arthralgia with occasional hemoptysis are characteristic.[130,134]

The chest radiographs of lymphomatoid granulomatosis are characterized by multiple, often poorly marginated nodules that coalesce and occasionally cavitate (Figure 25-13A and B). Unilateral or bilateral lobar consolidations and pleural-based lesions are commonplace. The disease has a predilection for the lower lobes, but the lesions are characteristically evanescent and may shift about the lung. "Reticulo-

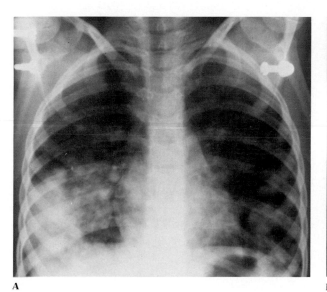
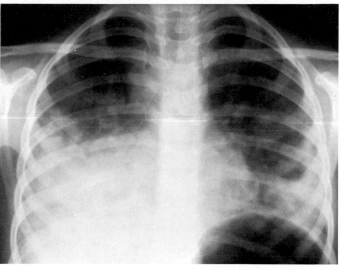

A   B

Figure 25-13   Lymphomatoid granulomatosis. A. Diffuse, fluffy, nodular opacities are present throughout both lower lung fields. Early coalescence is evident in the right lower lobe. Adenopathy is absent. **B.** This process has advanced and now appears more confluent. The child died shortly after this film study.

nodular" infiltrates have also been described. The development of pulmonary infarctions may explain many of the pulmonary opacities observed in this disease and also account for the transient nature of the infiltrates.[136]

Differential diagnosis of the nodular form of lymphomatoid granulomatosis includes primary and secondary neoplasms, pulmonary infarcts, rheumatoid nodules, pulmonary lymphoma, classical and limited Wegener's granulomatosis, and sarcoidosis. Although the diagnosis of such a rare disease is unlikely from chest films alone, the proper radiographic patterns in patients with a systemic process involving the skin and central nervous system should suggest the diagnosis of lymphomatoid granulomatosis.

Treatment of lymphomatoid granulomatosis is very discouraging; cytotoxic agents have been tried with little success.[118] Sustained remissions have been produced with high doses of prednisone.[131,133] The prognosis is worse for patients under 25 years of age who have elevated white blood cell counts and neurologic and hepatic involvement. Katzenstein et al.[134]

reported a mortality of 63.5 percent and a median survival of 14 months. Death is usually the result of pulmonary insufficiency.

Allergic Granulomatous Angiitis (Churg-Strauss Syndrome)

Several types of idiopathic angiitis have been recognized; among these are periarteritis nodosa and its variants, and hypersensitivity angiitis. Another distinct type, allergic granulomatous angiitis, was described by Churg and Strauss.[137] This is a multisystem disease characterized by severe asthma, fever, and hypereosinophilia, together with symptoms of vascular embarrassment in organ systems such as the liver, kidney, and gastrointestinal tract.

Of the original 13 cases reported by Churg and Strauss, 11 had pulmonary disease, a finding in marked contrast to periarteritis nodosa.[137] The parenchyma is involved with more or less extensive pneumonic processes that involve the interstitial septa as well as alveoli. Eosinophils predominate in the acute stage with typical granulomatous nodules in the septa, similar to those found in Loeffler's syndrome. Histologic evidence of asthma (hyalinization of the basement membrane, increased mucous secretion, eosinophilic infiltration of bronchial walls) is also present.

The paucity of cases reported precludes any definitive statement regarding the radiographic appearance of the lungs.

References

1. Albelda SM, Gefter WB, Epstein DM, et al: Diffuse pulmonary hemorrhage: A review and classification. *Radiology* 154:289, 1985.

2. Heiner DC: Pulmonary hemosiderosis, in Kendig EL Jr, Chernick V (eds): *Disorders of the Respiratory Tract in Children*, 3d ed. Philadelphia, WB Saunders, 1977, p 538.

3. Soergel KH, Sommers SC: The alveolar epithelial lesions of idiopathic pulmonary hemosiderosis. *Am Rev Respir Dis* 85:540, 1962.

4. Dutau G, Ghisolfi J, Rochiccioli P, et al: Idiopathic pulmonary hemosiderosis in the child: 7 cases. *Rev Tuberc (Paris)* 36:19, 1972.

5. Faulon E, Nagues C, Joron F, et al: Idiopathic pulmonary hemosiderosis in children: Two cases. *Ann Pediatr (Paris)* 21:145, 1974.

6. Elgenmark O, Kjellberg SR: Hemosiderosis of the lungs—Typical roentgenological findings. *Acta Radiol* 29:32, 1947.

7. Miller T, Tanaka T: Nuclear scan of pulmonary hemorrhage in idiopathic pulmonary hemosiderosis. *AJR* 132:120, 1979.

8. Kurzwell PR, Miller DR, Freeman JE, et al: Use of sodium Cr 51 in diagnosing childhood idiopathic pulmonary hemosiderosis. *Am J Dis Child* 138:746, 1984.

9. Heiner D, Sears J, Kniker W: Multiple precipitins to cow's milk in chronic respiratory disease. *Am J Dis Child* 103:634, 1962.

10. Holland N, Hong R, Davis N, et al: Significance of precipitating antibodies to milk proteins in the serum of infants and children. *J Pediatr* 61:181, 1962.

11. Hyatt RW, Adelstein ER, Halazun JF, et al: Ultrastructure of the lung in idiopathic pulmonary hemosiderosis. *Am J Med* 52:822, 1972.

12. Thomas HM, Irwin RS: Classification of diffuse intrapulmonary hemorrhage. *Chest* 64:483, 1975.

13. Ramirez RE, Glasier C, Kirks D, et al: Pulmonary hemorrhage associated with systemic lupus erythematosus in children. *Radiology* 152:409, 1984.

14. Nussbaum E: Adult-type respiratory distress syndrome. *Clin Pediatr* 22:401, 1983.

15. Lyrene, RK, Truog WE: Adult respiratory distress syndrome in a pediatric intensive care unit: Predisposing conditions, clinical course and outcome. *Pediatrics* 64:790, 1981.

16. Pfenninger J, Gerber A, Tschaddeler H, et al: Adult respiratory distress syndrome in children. *J Pediatr* 101:352, 1982.

17. Effman EL, Merten DF, Kirks DR, et al: Adult respiratory distress syndrome. *Radiology* 157:69, 1985.

18. Petty TL, Fowler AH: Another look at ARDS. *Chest* 82:98, 1982.

19. Fanconi S, Kraemer R, Weber J, et al: Long-term sequelae in children surviving adult respiratory distress syndrome. *J Pediatr* 106:218, 1985.

20. Fein A, Leff A, Hopewell PC: Pathophysiology and management of the complications resulting from fire and the inhaled products of combustion. *Crit Care Med* 8:94, 1980.

21. Teixidor HS, Rubin E, Novick GS, et al: Smoke inhalation: Radiologic manifestations. *Radiology* 149:383, 1983.

22. Mellins RB, Park S: Respiratory complications of smoke inhalation in victims of fires. *J Pediatr* 87:1, 1975.

23. Moylan JA: Supportive therapy in burn care. Smoke inhalation. Diagnostic techniques and steroids. *J Trauma* 19:917, 1979.

24. Colley JRT, Holland WW, Corkhill RT: Influence of passive smoking and parental phlegm on pneumonia and bronchitis in early childhood. *Lancet* 2:1031, 1974.

25. Weiss ST, Tager IB, Speizer FE, et al: Persistent wheeze; its relationship to respiratory illness, cigarette smoking and level of pulmonary function in a population sample of children. *Am Rev Resp Dis* 122:696, 1980.

26. Fergusson DM, Horwood LJ, Shannon FT, et al: Parental smoking and lower respiratory illness in the first three years of life. *J Epidemiol Community Health* 35:180, 1981.

27. Weiss ST, Tager IB, Speizer FE: Passive smoking: Its relationship to respiratory symptoms, pulmonary

function and nonspecific bronchial responsiveness. *Chest* 84:651, 1983.

28. Katzenstein AA, Askin FB: *Surgical Pathology of Non-Neoplastic Lung Disease.* Philadelphia, WB Saunders, 1982, p 34.

29. Reichlin S, Loveless MH, Kane EG: Loeffler's syndrome following penicillin therapy. *Ann Intern Med* 38:112, 1953.

30. Walsh JR, Zimmerman HJ: The demonstration of the "L.E." phenomenon in patients with penicillin hypersensitivity. *Blood* 6:65, 1953.

31. Domz CA, McNamara DE, Holzapfel HF: Tetracycline provocation in lupus erythematosus. *Ann Intern Med* 50:1217, 1959.

32. Perry JM Jr, Schroeder HA: Syndrome simulating collagen disease caused by hydralazine (Apresoline). *JAMA* 154:670, 1954.

33. Dustan HD, Taylor RD, Corcoran AC, et al: Rheumatic and febrile syndromes during prolonged hydralazine treatment. *JAMA* 154:23, 1954.

34. Israel HL, Diamond P: Recurrent pulmonary infiltration and pleural effusion due to nitrofurantoin sensitivity. *N Engl J Med* 266:1024, 1962.

35. Hailey FJ, Glascock HW Jr, Hewitt WF: Pleuropneumonic reactions to nitrofurantoin. *N Engl J Med* 281:1087, 1969.

36. Murray MJ, Kronenberg R: Pulmonary reactions simulating cardiac pulmonary edema caused by nitrofurantoin. *N Engl J Med* 273, 1185, 1965.

37. Rosenow EC, De Remee RA, Dines DE: Chronic nitrofurantoin pulmonary reaction. Report of five cases. *N Engl J Med* 279, 1258, 1968.

38. Strauss WG, Griffin LM: Nitrofurantoin pneumonia. *JAMA* 199:175, 1967.

39. Geller M, Dickie H, Kass D: The histopathology of acute nitrofurantoin-associated pneumonitis. *Ann Allergy* 37:275, 1976.

40. Holonberg L, Boman G, Böttiger L, et al: Adverse reactions to nitrofurantoin. Analysis of 921 reports. *Am J. Med* 69:733, 1980.

41. Bone R, Wolfe J, Sobonya R, et al: Desquamative interstitial pneumonia following long-term nitrofurantoin therapy. *Am J Med* 60:697, 1976.

42. Katzenstein AA, Askin FB: *Surgical Pathology of Non-Neoplastic Lung Disease.* Philadelphia, WB Saunders, 1982, p 9.

43. Robinson BR: Pleuropulmonary reaction to nitrofurantoin. *JAMA* 189:239, 1964.

44. Yagoda A, Mickherji B, Young C, et al: Bleomycin, an anti-tumor antibiotic. Clinical experience in 274 patients. *Ann Intern Med* 77:861, 1972.

45. Luna M, Bedrossian C, Lichtiger B, Salem P: Interstitial pneumonitis associated with bleomycin therapy. *Am J Clin Pathol* 58:501, 1972.

46. Blum RH, Carter SK, Agri K: A clinical review of bleomycin—A new antineoplastic agent. *Cancer* 31:903, 1973.

47. Iacovino J, Leitner J, Abbas A, et al: Fatal pulmonary reaction from low doses of bleomycin. An idiosyncratic tissue response. *JAMA* 235:1253, 1976.

48. Horowitz AL, Friedman M, Smith J, et al: The pulmonary changes of bleomycin toxicity. *Radiology* 106:65, 1973.

49. Clarysse AM, Cathey WJ, Cartwright GE, et al: Pulmonary disease complicating intermittent therapy with methotrexate. *JAMA* 209:1861, 1969.

50. Robertson JH: Pneumonia and methotrexate. *Br Med J* 2:156, 1970.

51. Whitcomb ME, Schwarz MI, Tormey DC: Methotrexate pneumonitis: Case report and review of the literature. *Thorax* 27:636, 1972.

52. Filip DJ, Logue GL, Harle TS, et al: Pulmonary and hepatic complications of methotrexate therapy for psoriasis. *JAMA* 216:881, 1971.

53. Goldman GC, Moschella SL: Severe pneumonitis occurring during methotrexate therapy. *Arch Dermatol* 103:194, 1971.

54. Topilow AA, Rothenberg SP, Cottrell TS: Interstitial pneumonia after prolonged treatment with cyclophosphamide. *Am Rev Respir Dis* 108:114, 1973.

55. Rodin AE, Haggard ME, Travis LB: Lung changes and chemotherapeutic agents in childhood: Report of a case associated with cyclophosphamide therapy. *Am J. Dis Child* 120:337, 1970.

56. Feigenberg DS, Weiss C, Kirshman H: Migratory pneumonia with eosinophilia associated with sulfonamide administration. *Arch Intern Med* 120:85, 1967.

57. Honey M: Systemic lupus erythematosus presenting with sulphonamide hypersensitivity reaction. *Br Med J* 1:1272, 1956.

58. Moore MT: Pulmonary changes in hydantoin therapy. *JAMA* 171:1328, 1959.

59. Livingston S, Whitehouse D, Pauli LL: Study of effects of diphenylhydantoin sodium on the lungs. *N Engl J Med* 264:648, 1961.

60. Heitzman ER: Lymphadenopathy related to anticonvulsant therapy. Roentgen findings simulating lymphoma. *Radiology* 89:311, 1967

61. Lauria DB, Hensle T, Rose J: The major medical complications of heroin addiction. *Ann Intern Med* 67:1, 1967.

62. Lynch K, Grunbaum E, O'Loughlin BJ: Pulmonary edema in heroin overdose. *Radiology* 94:377, 1970.

63. Wilen SB, Ulreich S, Rabinowitz JG: Roentgenographic manifestations of methadone-induced pulmonary edema. *Radiology* 114:51, 1975.

64. Frand UI, Shim CS, Williams MH Jr: Methadone-induced pulmonary edema. *Ann Intern Med* 76:975, 1972.

65. Fraser DW: Methadone overdose. Illicit use of pharmaceutically prepared parenteral narcotics. *JAMA* 217:1387, 1971.

66. Sklar J, Timms RM: Codeine-induced pulmonary edema. *Chest* 72:230, 1972.

67. Katz S, Aberman A, Frank UI, et al: Heroin pulmonary edema: Evidence for increased pulmonary capillary permeability. *Am Rev Respir Dis* 106:472, 1972.

68. Bogartz LJ, Miller WC: Pulmonary edema associated with propoxyphene intoxication. *JAMA* 215:259, 1971.

69. Davis PR, Burch RE: Pulmonary edema and salicylate intoxication. *Am Intern Med* 80:553, 1974.

70. Tashima CK, Rose M: Pulmonary edema and salicylates. *Ann Intern Med* 81:274, 1974.

71. Hrnicek G. Shelton J, Miller WC: Pulmonary edema and salicylate intoxication. *JAMA* 230:866, 1974.

72. Broderick TW, Reinke RT, Goldman E: Salicylate-induced pulmonary edema. *AJR* 127:865, 1976.

73. Bowers RE, Brigham KL, Owen PJ: Salicylate pulmonary edema: The mechanism in sheep and review of the clinical literature. *Am Rev Respir Dis* 115:261, 1977.

74. Price JE, Rigler LG: Widening of the mediastinum resulting from fat accumulation. *Radiology* 96:497, 1970.

75. Teates CD: Steroid-induced mediastinal lipomatosis. *Radiology* 96:501, 1970.

76. Liebow AA, Carrington CB: The interstitial pneumonias, in Simon M, Potchen EJ, LeMay M (eds): *Frontiers of Pulmonary Radiology*, New York, Grune & Stratton, 1969, p 102.

77. Halprin GM, Famirez RJ, Pratt, PC: Lymphoid interstitial pneumonia. *Chest* 62:418, 1972.

78. O'Brodovich HM, Moser MM, Lu L: Familial lymphoid interstitial pneumonia. A long-term follow-up. *Pediatrics* 65:523, 1980.

79. Talal N, Sokoloff L, Barth WF: Extrasalivary lymphoid abnormalities in Sjögren's syndrome (reticulum cell sarcoma, "Pseudolymphoma," macroglobulinemia). *Am J Med* 43:50, 1967.

80. Liebow AA, Carrington CB: Diffuse pulmonary reticular infiltrations associated with dysproteinemia. *Med Clin North Am* 57:809, 1973.

81. Heitzman ER, Markarian B, DeLise CT: Lymphoproliferative disorders of the thorax. *Semin Roentgenol* 10:73, 1975.

82. Reed JC, Madewell JE: The air bronchogram in interstitial disease of the lung. A radiological-pathological correlation. *Radiology* 116:1, 1975.

83. Wolson AH: Pulmonary findings in Gaucher's disease. *AJR* 123:712, 1975.

84. Kauser A: Morbus Gaucher-spezifische Lungeninfiltration unter dem Bilde einer Miliartbc. *Monatsschr Kinderheilkd* 98:252, 1950.

85. Levin B: Gaucher's disease: Clinical and roentgenologic manifestations. *AJR* 85:685, 1961.

86. Jackson DC, Simon G: Unusual bone and lung changes in a case of Gaucher's disease. *Br J Radiol* 38:698, 1965.

87. Myers B: Gaucher's disease of the lungs. *Br Med J* 2:8, 1937.

88. Roberts WC, Frederickson DS: Gaucher's disease of the lung causing severe pulmonary hypertension with associated acute recurrent pericarditis. *Circulation* 35:783, 1967.

89. Wagenvoort CA, Losekoot G, Mulder E: Pulmonary veno-occlusive disease of presumably intrauterine origin. *Thorax* 26:429, 1971.

90. Hora J: Zur Histologie der klinischen "Primaren Pulmonalsklerose." *Frankf 2 Pathol* 47:100, 1934.

91. Capewell SJ, Wright AJ, Ellis DA: Pulmonary veno-occlusive disease in association with Hodgkin's disease. *Thorax* 39:554, 1984.

92. Troussard X, Bernaudin JF, Cordonnier C, et al: Pulmonary veno-occlusive disease after bone-marrow transplantation. *Thorax* 39:956, 1984.

93. Joselson R, Warnock M: Pulmonary veno-occlusive disease after chemotherapy. *Hum Pathol* 14:88, 1983.

94. Davies P, Reid L: Pulmonary veno-occlusive disease in siblings: Case report and morphometric study. *Hum Pathol* 13:911, 1982.

95. Rosenthal A, Vawter G, Wagenvoort CA: Intra-pulmonary veno-occlusive disease. *Am J Cardiol* 31:78, 1973.

96. Wagenvoort CA, Wagenvoort N: The pathology of pulmonary veno-occlusive disease. *Virchows Arch [Pathol Anat]* 364:69, 1974.

97. Brown CH, Harrison CV: Pulmonary veno-occlusive disease. *Lancet* 2:61, 1966.

98. Liu L, Sackler JP: A case of pulmonary veno-occlusive disease. *Angiology* 23:299, 1972.

99. Shackelford GD, Sacks EJ, Mullin JD, et al: Pulmonary

veno-occlusive disease: Case report and review of the literature. *AJR* 128:643, 1977.

100. Rosen SH, Castleman B, Liebow AA: Pulmonary alveolar proteinosis: The nature and origin of alveolar lipid. *Am J Med* 45:502, 1958.

101. Sunderland WA, Campbell RA, Edwards MJ: Pulmonary alveolar proteinosis and pulmonary cryptococcosis in an adolescent boy. *J Pediatr* 80:450, 1972.

102. Wilkinson RH, Blanc WA, Hagstrom JWC: Pulmonary alveolar proteinosis in 3 infants. *Pediatrics* 41:510, 1968.

103. Bala RM, Snidal D: Pulmonary alveolar proteinosis: A case report and a review of the literature. *Dis Chest* 49:643, 1966.

104. Carnovale R, Zornoza J, Goldman AM, et al: Pulmonary alveolar proteinosis: Its association with hematologic malignancy and lymphoma. *Radiology* 122:303, 1977.

105. Larson RK, Gordinier R: Pulmonary alveolar proteinosis: Report of six cases, review of the literature and formulation of a new theory. *Ann Intern Med* 62:292, 1965.

106. Davidson JM, Macleod WM: Pulmonary alveolar proteinosis. *Br J Dis Chest* 63:13, 1969.

107. DuBois RM, McAllister WAC, Branthwaite MA: Alveolar proteinosis: Diagnosis and treatment over a 10 year period. *Thorax* 38:360, 1983.

108. Pear BL: Idiopathic disseminated pulmonary ossification. *Radiology* 91:746, 1968.

109. Felson B, Schwarz J, Lukin RR, et al: Idiopathic pulmonary ossification. *Radiology* 153:303, 1984.

110. Hughes WP: Roentgenogram of the month. *Dis Chest* 47:441, 1965.

111. Beerman PJ, Crowe JE, Sumner TE, et al: Radiological case of the month. *Am J Dis Child* 137:1119, 1983.

112. Conger JD, Hammond WS, Alfrey AC, et al: Pulmonary calcification in chronic dialysis patients: Clinical and pathological studies. *Ann Intern Med* 83:330, 1975.

113. Phelan MS, Lams P: Massive pulmonary complications in two infants with congenital cardiac lesions. *Clin Radiol* 34:381, 1983.

114. Fulmer JD, Kaltreider HB: The pulmonary vasculitides. *Chest* 82:615, 1982.

115. Roback SA, Herdman RC, Hoyer J, et al: Wegener's granulomatosis in a child: Observations of pathogenesis and treatment. *Am J Dis Child* 118:608, 1969.

116. McSweeney W: *Proceedings of the John Caffey Society,* Carmel, California, 1981.

117. Askin FB: in Kissane JM (ed): *Pathology of Infancy and Childhood.* St. Louis, CV Mosby, 1975, p 108.

118. DeRemee RA, McDonald TJ, Harrison EG Jr, et al: Wegener's granulomatosis: Anatomic correlates, a proposed classification. *Mayo Clin Proc* 51:777, 1976.

119. Carrington CB , Liebow AA: Limited forms of angiitis and granulomatosis of Wegener's type. *Am J Med* 41:497, 1966.

120. Edwards CW: Vasculitis and granulomatosis of the respiratory tract. *Thorax* 37:81, 1982.

121. Neumann G, Benz-Bohm G, Rister M: Wegener's granulomatosis in childhood: Review of the literature and case report. *Pediatr Radiol* 14:267, 1984.

122. Israel HL, Patchefsky AS, Saldana MJ: Wegener's granulomatosis, lymphoid granulomatosis, and benign lymphocytic angiitis and granulomatosis of lung. Recognition and treatment. *Ann Intern Med* 87:691, 1977.

123. Gohal VK, Dalinka MC, Israel HK, et al: The radiological manifestations of Wegener's granulomatosis. *Br J Radiol* 46:427, 1973.

124. Epstein DM, Gefter WB, Miller WT, et al: Spontaneous pneumothorax: An uncommon manifestation of Wegener's granulomatosis. *Radiology* 135:327, 1980.

125. Fauci AS, Wolff SM: Wegener's granulomatosis: Studies in eighteen patients and a review of the literature. *Medicine* 52:535, 1973.

126. Singsen BS, Platzker ACG: Pulmonary involvement in the rheumatic disorders (so-called collagen diseases) of childhood, in Kendig EL Jr, Chernick V (eds): *Disorders of the Respiratory Tract in Children,* 3d ed. Philadelphia, WB Saunders, 1977, p 1052.

127. Novack SN, Pearson CM: Cyclophosphamide therapy in Wegener's granulomatosis. *N Engl J Med* 284:938, 1971.

128. Reza MJ, Dornfeld L, Goldberg LS, et al: Wegener's granulomatosis. Long term follow-up of patients treated with cyclophosphamide. *Arthritis Rheum* 18:501, 1975.

129. Stokes TC, McCann BG, Rees RT, et al: Acute fulminating intrapulmonary hemorrhage in Wegener's granulomatosis. *Thorax* 37:315, 1982.

130. Liebow AA, Carrington CRB, Friedman PJ: Lymphomatoid granulomatosis. *Hum Pathol* 3:457, 1972.

131. Wechsler RJ, Steiner RM, Israel HL, et al: Chest radiograph in lymphomatoid granulomatosis: Comparison with Wegener's granulomatosis. *AJR* 142:79, 1984.

132. Fauci AS, Haynes BF, Costa J, et al: Lymphomatoid granulomatosis, prospective clinical and therapeutic experience over ten years. *N Engl J Med* 306:68, 1982.

133. Israel HL: Pulmonary angiitis and granulomatosis, in Fishman AP (ed): *Update: Pulmonary Diseases and Disorders.* New York, McGraw-Hill, 1982, 243–255.

134. Katzenstein AL, Carrington CB, Liebow AA: Lymphomatoid granulomatosis. A clinicopathological study of 152 cases. *Cancer* 43:360, 1979.

135. Yockey CC, Leichter SB, Hampton JR: Lymphomatoid granulomatosis presenting as fever of unknown origin. *JAMA* 237:2633, 1977.

136. Dee PM, Arora NS, Innes DJ Jr: The pulmonary manifestations of lymphomatoid granulomatosis. *Radiology* 143:613, 1982.

137. Churg J, Strauss L: Allergic granulomatosis, allergic angiitis, and periarteritis nodosa. *Am J Pathol* 27:277, 1951.

Chest Imaging

While plain-film radiography and fluoroscopy remain the most important tools in the radiologic diagnosis of thoracopulmonary disease, the utilization of ultrasonography, computed tomography, and magnetic resonance imaging is now commonplace and indispensable. Examples of these techniques are detailed in selected cases in this section and should improve the understanding of these most important modalities.

Chapter 26

Computed Tomography of the Chest

Mervyn D. Cohen, M.B., Ch.B.

Techniques for Chest Computed Tomography Scanning in Children

Computed tomography (CT) scanning of the chest is extremely well tolerated by children of all ages. Children are not merely small adults, and there are many differences in the techniques utilized for CT scanning of the chest of children when compared with adults. Careful attention to preparing the child and to details in performing the scans will result in excellent images.

Patient Preparation

Since many children who are to undergo chest CT scanning will be given intravenous contrast during the scanning procedure, children should have nothing to eat or drink for about 3 to 4 h before the study.

It is desirable for the children to have an empty stomach at the start of the study because the contrast may induce vomiting. The scanning procedure should be explained in detail to children older than 3 to 4 years of age. They should be told that there is no discomfort (apart from an intravenous injection); in addition, if breath holding is to be utilized, this should be explained to the child, and the breath-holding methods should be practiced. A small, important, but often neglected, point is to have all children, old enough to understand, empty their bladders before starting the study.

Sedation

Almost all children under the age of 1 year or over the age of 4 years can be scanned successfully without the utilization of any sedative. Although some workers would advocate the routine use of sedation for children aged 1, 2, or 3 years, it is preferable to evaluate each child individually. Although the risks of sedation are small, there is no reason to take any risk unless absolutely necessary. Discussion with the parents and observation of the child on arrival at the CT unit will often identify those children who do require sedation.

The choice of sedative is wide. Intramuscular sedatives may have a more predictable response than oral sedatives, and some workers would advocate the use of intramuscular sedatives in all patients.[1] Others have found very little difference in the failure rate between the use of intramuscular and oral sedatives.[2] Because many of the intramuscular sedatives will depress respiration, they should not be utilized unless a nurse is available to monitor the patients continuously while they lie within the scanner.[3] Chloral hydrate is a good choice of sedative. In most children, providing an adequate dose is given, it will produce effective sedation within 15 to 30 min following oral administration. A dose of between 50 to 100 mg per kilogram of body weight given by mouth is appropriate. Contraindications to the use of chloral hydrate are renal failure and impaired pulmonary function.

Study Planning

Before starting the chest CT scanning, the patient's chart and other radiographs must be reviewed. It is only by obtaining a thorough knowledge of the patient that specific objectives for the chest CT scan can be formulated. These will influence the manner in which the study is performed. It is desirable for the pediatric radiologist to monitor the study and review the CT images before the patient is allowed off the table.

Imaging Parameters

Patients are imaged using between 120 and 140 kV and usually 100 to 300 mA. If children are to be successfully imaged, it is extremely important to use a rapid scan time. Scan times of longer than 2 s will usually produce inferior images. This is more crucial with children than with adults because children are less able to hold their breath for more than 2 s. For most patients, 1-cm-thick contiguous slices should be taken from the apices of the lungs down to a level below the costophrenic recesses. Occasionally, thinner slices through focal regions of abnormality may be needed for better anatomic resolution. In general, most patients should be scanned in the supine position. In the evaluation of fluid collections, repeat scans with the patient in a side position or in a prone position may sometimes be helpful.[4] The patient's arms should be positioned above the head to reduce artifacts produced by the bones in the arms adjacent to the side of the chest. A scout view of the chest should be initially obtained to identify the start and finish levels of the scan sequence and also to assist in accurate localization of any particular image slice (Figure 26-1).

Breath Holding

Most children under the age of 5 cannot cooperate with breath holding, and so these children should be scanned during quiet respiration. For some older children this method is desirable as well. For those children who can hold their breath, the easiest and

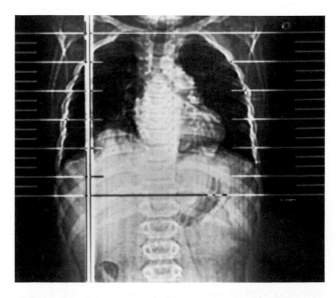

Figure 26-1   Normal scanogram. This scan view of the chest is performed at the start of the study. It identifies the levels of the first, last, and intermediate slices.

most reproducible level in which to suspend respiration is at the end of quiet respiration. Forced inspiration or maximal expiration varies greatly from effort to effort and is not nearly as reproducible. The patient should be instructed to breathe in quietly, let the breath out, and then hold it.

Intravenous Contrast Material

Intravenous contrast material should be utilized for all studies of suspected mediastinal disease. For some studies directed primarily at the lung parenchyma, e.g., lung evaluation for metastases, it is quite reasonable to omit routine use of intravenous contrast material. The contrast agent used should have an iodine concentration of between 50 and 60 percent and should be administered in a dose of 1 to 2 ml per kilogram of body weight. For most studies of the chest, contrast is used principally to opacify and identify blood vessels rather than to cause enhancement of a region of pathology. For this reason it is usually best to administer the contrast material in a bolus given fairly rapidly over a 30- to 60-s period. The images should be acquired as rapidly as possible following the administration of contrast material. The maximal effect of a bolus of injected intravenous contrast material is only seen for about 1 min.[4] Older children can be injected on the table. For young children in whom the injections might induce crying, it may often be advisable to start an intravenous infusion about 15 to 30 min before starting the CT study.

Parents

The question of whether or not to permit the parent into the scan room should be judged separately for each case. Some children will settle better with their parents in the room; some will become more agitated if they can see but not be held by their parents.

Window Levels

Completely different window settings are required to visualize the lungs and the soft tissues. If the bones are to be optimally visualized, a third set of window settings is required. A window level is the midpoint of the gray scale display. As a general guideline it is best to set the window level at the level of the tissue of interest (either air, soft tissue, or bone). The window width is the range of CT numbers included in the display. A narrow window width gives a small range of display with very high contrast between different tissues. A wide width gives a better latitude with more structures being seen on a single display but less contrast between different individual structures. In general, very wide window widths (greater than 1500) should be utilized for lung images, and narrower window widths (100 to 200) should be utilized for soft tissue or bone display. Keep in mind that the apparent size of an object changes as the window level is altered. Studies with phantoms have shown that an accurate depiction of the structure size will be obtained when the window level is set halfway between the intensity of the structure and the adjacent background intensity.

Radiation Dose

It is difficult to give an accurate dose from a CT scan of the chest because the dose will vary significantly between different CT scanners and also between different-sized patients. A study in 1982 suggested a mean dose of seven different CT scanners for children was in the order of 1.5 rad. Some scanners were significantly lower than this.[5] The dose for chest CT is lower than that for head or abdomen CT.[6]

Normal Computed Tomography Appearance of the Chest

Computed tomography shows the thickness of the soft tissues overlying the chest wall. The bones of the thoracic cage are well visualized. The thymus can be identified in all normal children (Figure 26-2).[4] The normal gland is about 15 g in weight and increases to a maximum of about 35 g at puberty.[7] Below the age of puberty the thymus is of very homogenous soft tissue intensity[7] and shows little or no enhancement following the administration of intravenous contrast material.[8] After puberty the appearance of the thymus becomes nonhomogenous due to the deposition of fat within the gland.[9] The thymus is variable in its appearance.[10] The right and left lobes

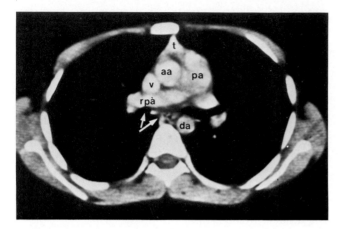

Figure 26-2   Normal anatomy at the level of the right pulmonary artery. The thymus (t) is small and triangular. It is seen in the anterior mediastinum. The right pulmonary artery (rpa) lies behind the superior vena cava (v) and in front of the bronchus intermedius (small arrow). The azygoesophageal recess is clearly identified (large arrow). The ascending aorta (aa) lies in front of the right pulmonary artery, and the descending aorta (da) lies just to the left of the spine. (pa = main pulmonary artery.)

can usually be distinguished. The lateral margins of the lobes are well seen, contrasted against the adjacent air in the lungs.[11] The posterior margins are poorly identified as they are molded to the adjacent heart and great vessels of the mediastinum.[11] Normal thymus can extend between the superior vena cava and the aorta[7] and can also extend into the posterior mediastinum (Figure 26-3).[7] Posterior extension of the normal thymus is recognized by a smooth, continuous lateral margin joining the anterior and posterior parts of the thymus and by a uniform intensity of the entire thymus. The normal thymus can occasionally displace normal mediastinal vessels, the trachea,[11] and the esophagus (Figure 26-4).

Small normal lymph nodes can frequently be identified in the mediastinum. In adults, nodes of up to 1 cm in diameter are considered to be normal.[12] The upper limit for normal-size lymph nodes in children is not known. Many normal structures identified on the CT scan may mimic enlarged lymph nodes. It is important to be aware of these. Some of these structures are an aberrant right subclavian artery, a right aortic arch, and partial volume averaging of the top of the left pulmonary artery. The right superior intercostal vein lies adjacent to the right side of spine as it runs to join the azygos vein. It may be mistaken for a lymph node. Similarly, the left superior intercostal vein lies lateral to the aortic arch on

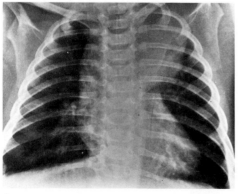

A

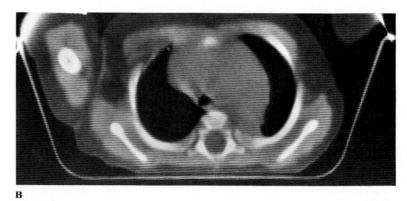

B

Figure 26-3   Posterior mediastinal extension of the normal thymus. A. The chest radiograph shows a large left superior mediastinal mass lesion with moderately well defined lateral margins. **B.** The CT scan shows that the abnormality extends from the anterior to the posterior mediastinum. A smooth lateral margin extends all the way from front to back. The intensity of the lesion is homogeneous. At surgery the entire mass was found to be normal thymus.

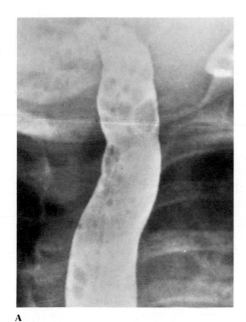
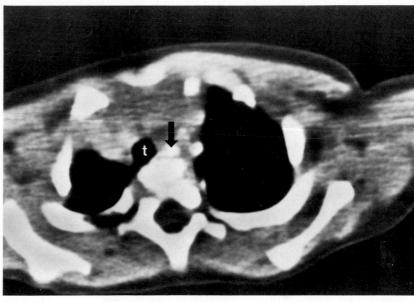

A   **B**

Figure 26-4   Esophageal displacement by normal thymus. A. The esophogram shows displacement of the esophagus to the left at the level of the thoracic inlet. **B.** The CT scan shows a prominent but normal thymus. No other mass lesion can be identified. The thymus extends between the trachea (t) and the esophagus (black arrow). The esophagus is identified by the presence of an intraluminal nasogastric tube.

its way to the left innominate vein. A left superior vena cava is a fairly common normal variant. This vessel passes lateral to the aortic arch and anterior to the left hilum to enter the coronary sinus. An azygos vein, particularly if enlarged (as with azygos continuation of the inferior vena cava, may mimic an enlarged lymph node. The azygos vein may also mimic an enlarged lymph node if only part of it is captured in an image slice. The pericardial recesses, especially if a pericardial effusion is present, can mimic enlarged lymph nodes. The right atrial appendage normally extends anterior to the ascending aorta and superior vena cava and may simulate an enlarged anterior mediastinal lymph node. Internal mammary vessels may mimic anterior mediastinal nodes. The junction of the right superior pulmonary vein anteriorly and the right interlobar pulmonary artery posteriorly may cause a lobular appearance to the right hilum which resembles node enlargement. A similar appearance may be seen on the left side.[13,14]

The trachea is well seen on CT images. The trachea cross-sectional area can be accurately mea-

sured by tracing around the margins of the trachea with a region-of-interest cursor. Two methods can be used to make corrections for window settings. The first is to make the measurements with a window width of -1000 Hounsfield units and a level of -500 Hounsfield units.[15] Alternatively, one can measure with a window level of 100 Hounsfield units and a width of 20 Hounsfield units. A correction factor is then applied in which the actual tracheal cross-sectional area equals the measured area multiplied by the mean CT number of the air in the trachea divided by 1000.[16] Tables for normal tracheal dimensions corrected for height, weight, age, and body surface area are available.[16] The angle of obliquity of the trachea is measured from the lateral scanogram and a correction made for the measured tracheal cross-sectional area.[15] The error due to tracheal obliquity is believed to be less than 6 percent.[16] The paraspinal lines can be well seen on CT images.[17] The pericardium forms several recesses where it reflects off adjacent mediastinal structures. Knowledge of the location of these normal recesses is important if they are not to be confused with disease.[18] Large recesses include the transverse recess behind the ascending aorta and pulmonary artery, the oblique recess behind the left atrium, and the left pulmonic recess between the left pulmonary artery and the left superior pulmonary vein. Smaller recesses are found between the superior and inferior pulmonary veins, posterolateral to the superior vena cava, and between the inferior vena cava and coronary sinus.[18] These re-

cesses fill with fluid when pericardial effusion is present and may be confused with lymph nodes, cysts, or other tumors.[18]

The normal anatomy of the hilar and mediastinal vessels can be appreciated by dividing the chest into a number of anatomic levels as follows:[4]

1. *Sternoclavicular junction.* At this level the brachiocephalic veins run obliquely in the anterior mediastinum. The brachiocephalic artery, left carotid, and left subclavian arteries are seen as transverse densities (Figure 26-5), posterior to the veins.
2. *Aortic arch.* At the level of the superior part of the aortic arch, the arch appears as an oblique structure. The superior vena cava lies to the right (Figure 26-6).
3. *Level of left pulmonary artery.* At this level the ascending aorta and descending aorta appear as circular structures (Figure 26-7). The superior vena cava lies to the right of the ascending aorta. The left pulmonary artery is seen in the left hilum. On the right side the right upper lobe bronchus is identified (Figure 26-8). It divides into an anterior and posterior branch. The right superior pulmonary vein lies in the angle between these two divisions (Figure 26-7).

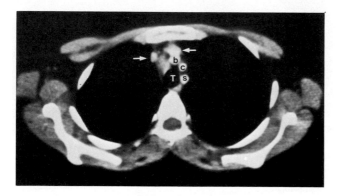

Figure 26-5   Normal anatomy at the level of the sternoclavicular junction. The trachea (T) appears as a round or slightly oval lucency. The brachiocephalic veins (arrows) lie anterior to the great vessels. The brachiocephalic artery (b), left carotid artery (c), and left subclavian artery (s) are seen as transverse densities just superior to the origin from the aortic arch.

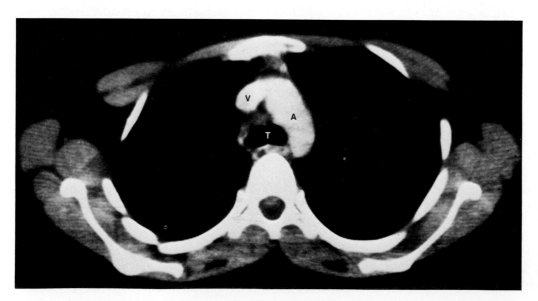

Figure 26-6 Normal anatomy. The CT scan at the level of the aortic arch shows the aortic arch (A) and the superior vena cava (V). The image is obtained at the level of the tracheal (T) bifurcation.

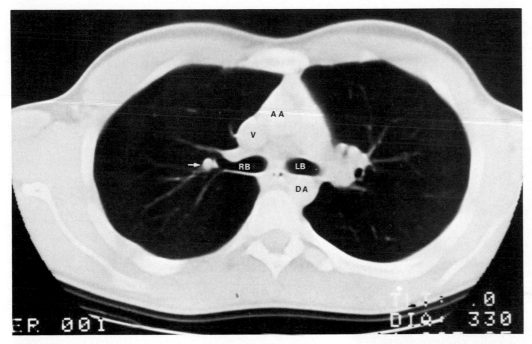

Figure 26-7 Normal anatomy. This image at the level of the left pulmonary artery shows the ascending aorta (AA), descending aorta (DA), and superior vena cava (V). The main pulmonary artery and left pulmonary artery are present. The left bronchus (LB) and right bronchus (RB) are also seen. The right bronchus divides into anterior and posterior segments. The right superior pulmonary vein (arrow) lies in the angle of this bifurcation.

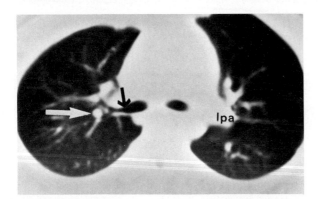

Figure 26-8 Normal anatomy at the level of the left pulmonary artery. The left pulmonary artery (lpa) is seen in the left hilum. The right upper lobe bronchus (black arrow) divides into anterior and posterior branches. The superior pulmonary vein (white arrow) lies in the angle between the anterior and posterior divisions.

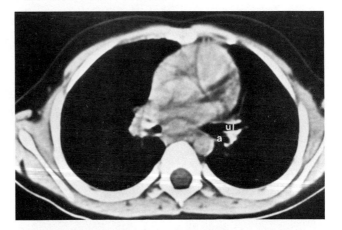

Figure 26-9 Normal anatomy. This study shows the left upper lobe bronchus (ul) and the origin of the bronchus to the apical segment of the left lower lobe (a).

4. *Level of right pulmonary artery* (Figure 26-2). The right pulmonary artery is identified. It runs from the main pulmonary artery posteriorly and to the right, passing behind the superior vena cava and in front of the bronchus intermedius. At this level

the left lower lobe pulmonary artery is seen lying behind the left main stem bronchus. On the right side, lung tissue may be seen behind the bronchus intermedius in the azygoesophageal recess. This recess is less well developed in children than in adults. One centimeter inferiorly, the origin of the bronchus to the apical segment of the left lower lobe can be identified (Figure 26-9).

5. *Level of left atrium* (Figure 26-10). At this level the left atrium and right atrium are well seen. The

aorta and main pulmonary artery appear as circular densities. The pulmonary artery lies anterior to the proximal aorta. To the left and anterior to the spine lies the descending aorta. A smaller structure identified in a similar position on the

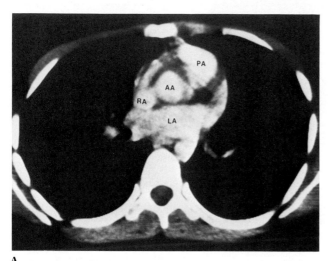

A

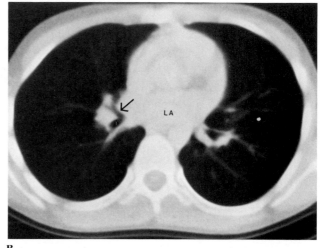

B

Figure 26-10   Normal anatomy at the level of the left atrium. A and **B.** These images are obtained at the same level. They show the left atrium (LA), right atrium (RA), ascending aorta (AA), main pulmonary artery (PA), and origin of the middle lobe bronchus (black arrow) from the bronchus intermedius (i). The division of the middle lobe bronchus into medial and lateral segmental bronchi can also be identified.

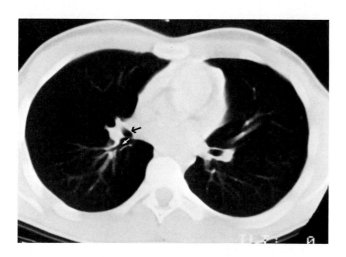

Figure 26-11   Normal anatomy at the level of the left atrium. This image shows the origin of the bronchus to the apical segment of the right lower lobe (white arrow). It arises at the same level as the middle lobe bronchus (black arrow).

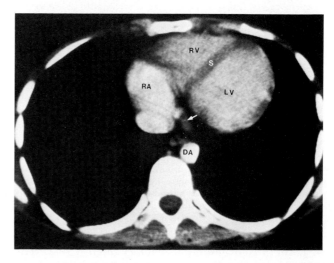

Figure 26-12 Normal anatomy at the ventricular level. The interventricular septum (S) appears as an oblique band lying between the left ventricle (LV) and the right ventricle (RV). The coronary sinus (white arrow) drains into the right atrium (RA). The descending aorta (DA) can also be identified.

right side is the azygos vein. The pulmonary veins can be seen entering the left atrium. Also at this level the right middle lobe bronchus arises from the bronchus intermedius. The medial and lateral segments of the middle lobe bronchus can be identified in many cases. The origin of the bronchus to the apical segment of the right lower lobe is apparent (Figure 26-11).

6. *Level of ventricles* (Figure 26-12). Both the ventricles are evident. The septum lies obliquely between the ventricles. The coronary sinus can be identified between the right ventricle and the inferior vena cava.

The presence of an azygos lobe causes characteristic changes on the CT scan. The azygos vein lies in a more cephalad position than normal, the axis of the superior vena cava is tilted, and the lung may extend into the pretracheal and posttracheal mediastinal spaces.[19]

In the lung, the pulmonary arteries (Figure 26-13) and veins are well seen. The arteries radiate from the hilum, and the veins converge on the left atrium. On thin slices the fissures can be identified as thin lines with adjacent lucent areas.[20] The lucency results from normal tapering of peripheral vessels on each side of the fissure. On images with a slice thickness of 1 cm or greater, the fissures will often not be identifiable, although their location can be inferred by identification of zones of lucency (Figure 26-14).

Indications for Computed Tomography

The indications for performing a CT scan of the chest are as follows:

1. Screening for pathology when the chest radiograph is negative. The most common indication for this is a search for pulmonary metastasis from a known "lung-seeking" neoplasm.
2. Evaluating an area of suspicious abnormality (e.g., suspected widened mediastinum) apparent on the chest radiograph.
3. Further evaluating a definite abnormality identified on a chest radiograph. The CT scan would be performed to help define the extent of the abnormality, its tissue of origin, and its internal structure.
4. Monitoring the response of a known abnormality to therapy.

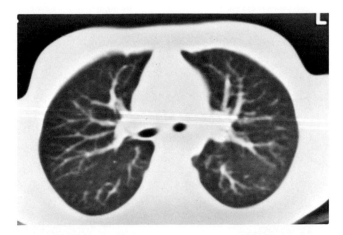

Figure 26-13 Normal peripheral pulmonary arteries. This CT scan obtained just below the level of the bifurcation of the trachea shows normal branching pulmonary arteries in both lung fields. Both lungs are fairly symmetrical. The vessels radiate outward from the hila and have a fairly regular branching pattern with a decrease in size toward the lung periphery.

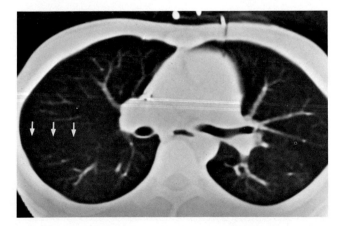

Figure 26-14 Normal right oblique fissure. Although the oblique fissure cannot be identified separately on this 1-cm-thick CT image, the position of the fissure can be inferred by a band of lucency (arrows). The lucency is due to the relatively small size of the blood vessels on either side of the fissure.

Advantages of Computed Tomography for Chest Imaging

Computed tomography displays images in cross section and has excellent soft tissue contrast resolution. It is more sensitive than chest radiograph for evaluating mediastinal lesions,[21] for defining the extent and tissue of origin of chest masses,[22] for differentiating vascular from nonvascular abnormalities,[4] for evaluating widening of the paraspinal lines,[7] and for identifying lung metastases.[22,23] Computed tomography may diagnose certain vascular malformations without the need of angiography.[24] With mediastinal masses it may often identify secondary effects of the mass lesion such as tracheal compression.[23] Computed tomography is also superior to chest radiograph for identification of lesions in the pleura.[24] It also complements the chest radiograph when differentiating abscess from empyema.[22] Computed tomography identifies areas of the lung hidden on chest radiograph.[22]

Computed tomography may permit guided needle biopsy of lesions that were previously thought to be too dangerous to approach or that were poorly localized on fluoroscopy.[24]

Although CT is expensive, it is cost-effective in many situations since it replaces other imaging modalities, e.g., lung tomograms, esophograms, angiograms, and isotope scans.[24]

Problems and Pitfalls with Computed Tomography Imaging of the Chest in Children

1. Because of their size, each individual structure appears smaller in children than in adults.[23,25] Children are not as capable as adults of suspending respiration.[1]
2. Children have much less fat than adults. When present, fat acts as a natural contrast agent separating out the individual mediastinal structures.[4,23,25]
3. Computed tomography is relatively expensive and has a higher radiation dose than chest radiograph.[20,25]
4. The thymus is large in children, and it may be difficult to distinguish normal gland from diffuse infiltrating disease of the thymus or an adjacent

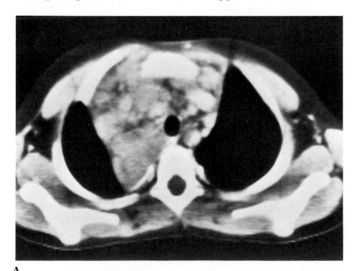
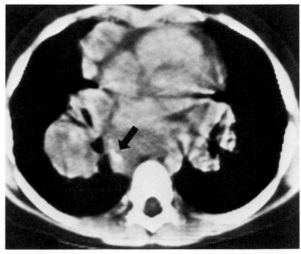

A
B

Figure 26-15 Hodgkin's disease. A. The CT scan at the level of the midtrachea identifies massively enlarged lymph nodes, mainly on the right side. The enlarged lymph nodes involve the anterior mediastinum and paratracheal area and also extend into the posterior mediastinum. The tracheal lumen is not decreased. **B.** The CT scan taken below the level of the tracheal bifurcation identifies enlarged lymph nodes in the anterior mediastinum, in the subcarinal area, and in both pulmonary hila. *Note:* The presence of calcification in the enlarged lymph nodes in the azygoesophageal recess (arrow). This may represent old histoplasma infection.

soft tissue mass (Figure 26-15).[4,23,25]

5. Computed tomography numbers do not completely characterize tissue. They vary from patient to patient and machine to machine.[20]

6. If the wrong window settings are chosen to display the image, pathology may be missed. For example, unless the trachea is viewed with lung window settings, foreign bodies or tumors in the lumen of the trachea will be overlooked.[14]

7. Apposition of the walls of the esophagus may cause the esophagus to appear as two separate air-containing cavities.[14]

8. Focal pulmonary nodules may escape detection for the following reasons:

    a. If they are of the same size as adjacent pulmonary vessels sliced transversely, they may be mistaken for the vessels.

    b. If sequential slices are obtained in markedly different phases of respiration, a small nod-

ule might move out of the plane of interest on each image slice and therefore not be visualized.

9. The anterior end of the rib may be partial-volume-averaged into an image slice and mimic a pulmonary parenchymal nodule (Figure 26-16).[26]

10. Pulmonary nodules may be confused with adjacent vessels (Figure 26-17). Several factors help in differentiating a nodule from a vessel. Vessels will be identified as being contiguous on adjacent slices, they will alter in size if a patient's position is changed, they will enhance with contrast, and they may show a "twinkling star" appearance of radiolinear artifacts due to pulsation.[27] This is usually only seen with scan times longer than 2½ s.

11. Metallic clips or radiopaque catheters in or on the patient will cause streak artifacts which may obscure pathology (Figures 26-18 and 26-19).

12. In the mediastinum many normal structures may be mistaken for enlarged lymph nodes (Figure 26-20).

13. Patchy densities due to gravity pooling of fluid in the posterior aspects of the lungs might be confused with pulmonary infiltrates.

14. The superior aspect of the diaphragm may mimic a lung mass (Figure 26-21).

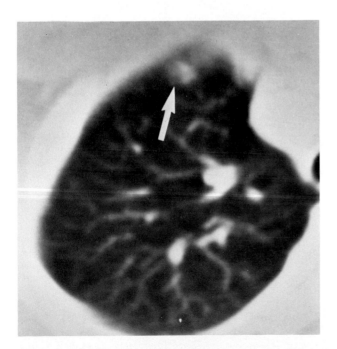

Figure 26-16 Rib simulates pulmonary lung nodule. The anterior end of the first rib (arrow) is partially visualized on the CT image. It simulates the presence of a pulmonary lung nodule.

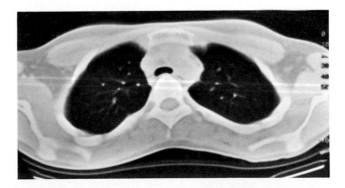

Figure 26-17 Pulmonary vessels mimic metastatic nodules. This CT scan shows multiple nodular densities in both lung fields. They are of fairly uniform size. Almost all of them are continuous with an adjacent vessel. They are therefore much more likely to be vessels imaged transversely, rather than metastatic nodules. *Note:* A nodule and vessel of similar size cannot be accurately differentiated.

Congenital Anomalies

Computed tomography can identify a wide variety of congenital anomalies of the thorax. Many of these anomalies may be adequately diagnosed without the use of CT. In some cases, however, CT provides unique information, helpful in diagnosis and therapy.

Bronchogenic Cyst

Computed tomography can accurately identify bronchogenic cysts (Figures 26-22 to 26-24). The sharply defined smooth margins of the cyst are well seen. While in some cases the contents of the cyst appear to have the intensity of fluid, the contents can sometimes appear to have the same intensity as that of soft tissue (Figure 26-23). In these situations the cor-

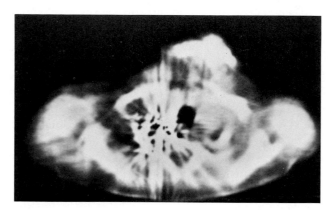

Figure 26-18   Streak artifacts from metallic clips. This patient previously had a large neuroblastoma resected. Metallic clips were left in the tumor bed. A small soft tissue recurrence was clearly identified on chest radiograph. Because of the large streak artifacts caused by the presence of the clips, the recurrence cannot be diagnosed on the CT scan.

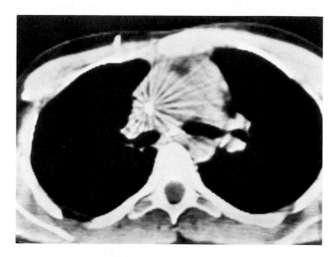

Figure 26-19   Artifacts from a venous catheter. The distal end of a radiopaque subclavian venous catheter lies in the superior vena cava. It is causing significant radial streak artifacts.

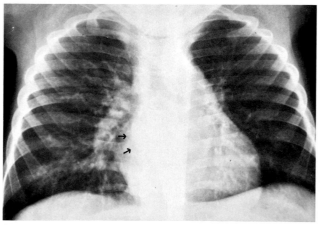

A

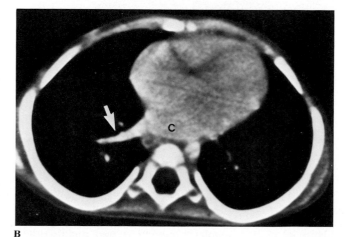

B

Figure 26-20   Normal confluence of the pulmonary veins mimics enlarged lymph nodes. A. The chest radiograph shows a soft tissue density (arrows) through the right atrium. **B.** The CT scan shows this confluence (C) to be the same intensity as the adjacent heart. The right inferior pulmonary vein (arrow) enters this confluence.

rect diagnosis may be missed. The reason for the high-intensity appearance is that bronchogenic cysts are sometimes filled with a thick proteinaceous material.[28] This material has a high CT Hounsfield number. Computed tomography can accurately identify the effects of bronchogenic cysts on adjacent structures. There may be compression of adjacent pulmonary veins or heart. There may also be compression of either the trachea or the left or right main stem bronchi. If one bronchus is compressed, secondary collapse (Figure 26-24) or emphysema of the ipsilateral lung may result (Figure 26-22).

Cystic Adenomatoid Malformation

In the first few hours of life these malformations appear as mixed areas of fluid and soft tissue density.[29] Some of the fluid later is replaced by air,[29] and the lesions then appear as irregular abnormalities containing soft tissue, fluid, and air (Figure 26-25). Usually only a single lobe is involved; however, the lobe may be so expanded as to give the impression that more than one lobe is involved. Sometimes the lesions can also be bilateral, and they may also appear as giant cysts (Figure 26-25).

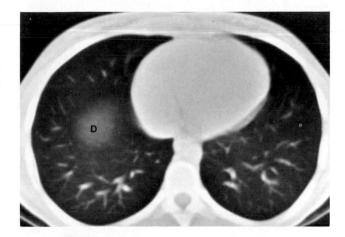

Figure 26-21 Normal diaphragm simulates a lung nodule. This scan is obtained through the superior portion of the dome of the right hemidiaphragm (D). The rest of the diaphragm lies inferior to the plane of this image. The small segment of diaphragm that has been imaged mimics the presence of a round mass lesion in the right lung.

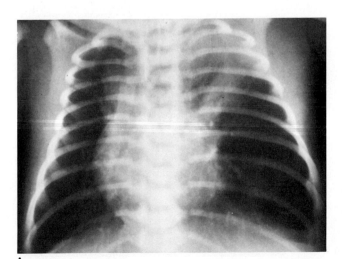

A

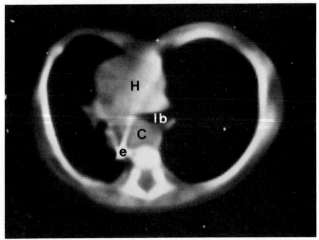

B

Figure 26-22 Bronchogenic cyst. A. The chest radiograph shows hyperlucency of the left lower lung field with some ill-defined hazy opacification of the upper lung field. **B.** The CT scan shows a low-intensity bronchogenic cyst (C). It lies behind the left bronchus (lb), which it partially compresses. This causes emphysema of most of the left lung with displacement of the heart (H) and mediastinum from the left to the right. The esophagus (e) is identified by the presence of a nasogastric tube within it. It is displaced posteriorly by the cyst which lies between the bronchi and the esophagus.

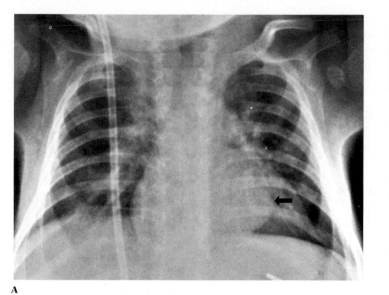

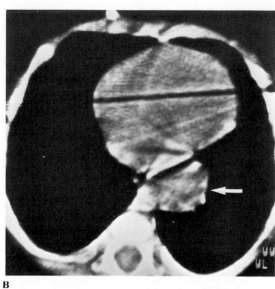

A   B

Figure 26-23   Bronchogenic cyst. A. The chest radiograph shows a mass lesion lying behind the heart (arrow). **B.** The CT scan shows the same lesion (arrow). It has fairly well defined, smooth margins. Some edge enhancement artifacts are seen in the periphery of the lesion. The overall intensity of the cyst is similar to that of the paraspinal muscle. The cyst contains mucoid material which caused the relatively high signal intensity from the cyst.

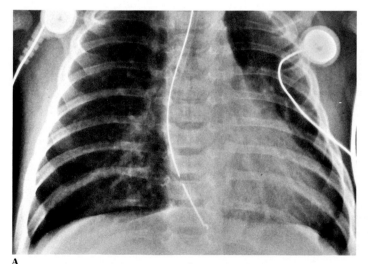

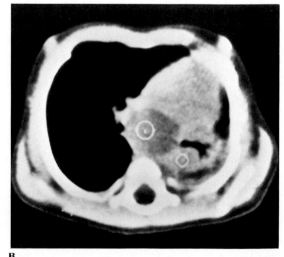

A   B

Figure 26-24   Bronchogenic cyst causing a partial collapse and emphysema. A. A chest radiograph shows displacement of the esophagus to the right. The margins of the cyst cannot be identified. The esophagus is indicated by a nasogastric tube. **B.** The CT scan shows a very low intensity, well-defined cystic lesion (large circle) lying in front of the spine and just below the carina. Compression of the left main stem bronchus by the cyst is causing partial collapse of the left lung (small circle), compression of the right main stem bronchus, and emphysema of the right lung, with a shift of the heart and mediastinum from the right to the left.

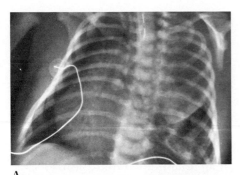
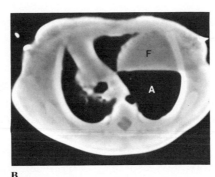
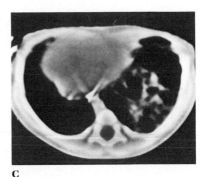

A   B   C

Figure 26-25   Cystic adenomatoid malformation with a giant cyst. A. The chest radiograph features an ill-defined, hazy opacification of the left upper lung field. Patchy densities are seen in the left lower lung field. The changes are due to a giant cystic adenomatoid malformation of the left lower lobe. This diagnosis, however, cannot be made from the chest radiograph. **B.** The CT scan at the level of the midtrachea shows a gigantic cyst. There is an air-fluid level between the fluid (F) and air (A) within the cyst. The study was performed with the patient prone. **C.** The CT scan taken at the level of the heart shows patchy areas of soft tissue abnormality interspersed with regions containing air. Pathology showed a cystic adenomatoid malformation involving the left lower lobe. The lobe was markedly expanded. The superior segment contained a single gigantic cyst. The inferior segment contained mixed areas of soft tissue tumor and cyst.

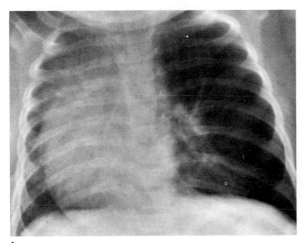
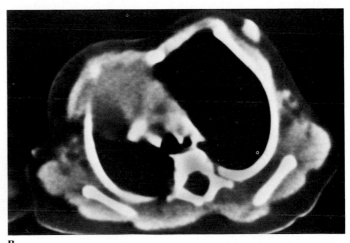

A   B

Figure 26-26   Congenital lobar emphysema (left upper lobe). A. The chest radiograph shows emphysema of the left upper lobe. The ribs are separated. The mediastinal structures are displaced to the right. The partially collapsed left lower lobe appears as a region of streaky density in the inferior medial aspect of the left hemithorax. **B.** The CT scan shows marked overexpansion of the left hemithorax with displacement of the mediastinal structures to the right. No underlying cause for the emphysema (such as a bronchogenic cyst compressing the bronchus) could be identified. The appearance is compatible with congenital lobar emphysema.

Lobar Emphysema

In most patients, lobar emphysema is idiopathic. If a CT scan is performed, it will show the hyperinflation of the affected upper or middle lobe (Figure 26-26). However, CT is not usually employed, as the diagnosis can be made effectively from a plain-chest radiograph.

Sequestration

The diagnosis of sequestration is usually suspected by the presence of a persistent abnormality in the lower lung fields on chest radiograph. Although CT will not always give a specific diagnosis, it may be helpful by excluding other conditions such as a simple lobar collapse, abscess, or tumor. Utilizing a bolus injection of contrast material, CT may occasionally identify anomalous vessels to and from the sequestration.

Vascular Anomalies

Computed tomography can identify arteriovenous malformations[30] and may show more lesions than the chest radiograph. In addition, enlarged vessels leading to and from a malformation may also be identified. Bolus injection of contrast material will result in marked enhancement of many vascular malformations in the lungs. Although not the major method for evaluation of abnormalities of the great vessels, CT can effectively demonstrate a large number of malformations, including the position of the great vessels in transposition. Right aortic arch and anomalous right and left subclavian arteries are well seen. In children with pulmonary atresia, a CT scan can be utilized to identify the size of the pulmonary arteries.[31,32] Computed tomography can also accurately diagnose the presence of a double aortic arch, left superior vena cava, anomalous left pulmonary artery, and azygos continuation of the inferior vena cava.[24]

Mechanical Disorders

Trauma

Although not routinely utilized in the evaluation of children with chest trauma, CT can sometimes yield information not obtained from other studies.[33] It can identify the extent of soft tissue abnormality in the chest wall, and rib fractures can be seen. Also, it is more accurate than plain-film radiograph in estimating the volume of blood in the pleural space. In the lung, CT can identify the extent of lung contusion. Great vessel tears following chest trauma are extremely rare in children.

Lobar Collapse

Lobar collapse can be accurately diagnosed from plain-film radiograph. Computed tomography can also accurately diagnose collapse (Figures 26-27 and 26-28). In addition, it may frequently identify the underlying cause of the collapse. Such pathology will include lesions within the lumen or wall of the bronchi or compression by an extrinsic mass.

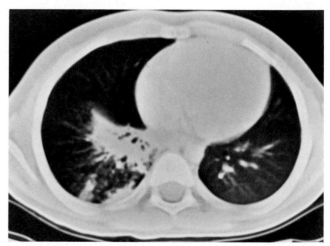

A   **B**

Figure 26-27   Partial collapse of the right lower lobe. A. The chest radiograph shows patchy densities in the medial aspect of the right lower lobe. Infection cannot be clearly differentiated from patchy collapse. **B.** The CT scan shows patchy opacification of the medial aspect of the right lower lobe. The right oblique fissure provides a sharp anterior margin to the abnormality. The presence of volume loss in the medial aspect of the right lower lobe is indicated by the posterior displacement of the oblique fissure and by the compensatory emphysema of the middle lobe. The middle lobe is seen as an area of increased lucency.

Tracheal Size

The size of the trachea can be accurately seen on CT images. Marked tracheal dilatation due to high ventilation pressures is illustrated in Figure 26-29.

Foreign Bodies

Computed tomography is extremely accurate in localizing metallic foreign bodies anywhere within the thorax. In many situations CT is not required, however, as the location of the foreign body can be made from plain-film radiographs and/or barium studies, in selected cases it is helpful.[34] Soft tissue foreign bodies are frequently aspirated into the trachea and bronchi by children. The diagnosis is usually made from the history, plain-film radiographs, and observation of mediastinal movement under fluoroscopy. It can accurately identify soft tissue foreign bodies in the lungs, trachea, and main bronchi (Figure 26-30).[35]

Scoliosis

Computed tomography can define the spinal angles and the amount of vertebral rotation.[36]

Other

A pneumatocele is seen on CT scans as a low-intensity region with no blood vessels in it and no significant wall (Figure 26-31).

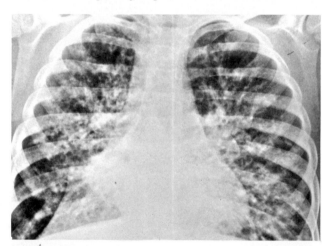

A

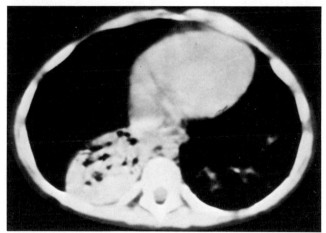

B

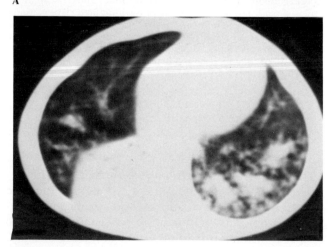

C

Figure 26-28 Cystic fibrosis—collapsed right lower lobe. A. The chest radiograph shows extensive bilateral densities consistent with the known diagnosis of cystic fibrosis. Collapse of the right lower lobe is identified. **B** and **C.** The CT scan was taken at the level of the right lower lobe collapse. Part B was obtained with soft tissue window settings and part C with lung window settings. In the left lung the severe extensive abnormality due to the cystic fibrosis is easily identified as patchy nodular and streaky densities. The amount of disease is even more than one would suspect from the chest radiograph. On the right side the collapsed right lower lobe is seen. The sharply defined margin is due to the interface between the collapsed lower lobe and the fully expanded adjacent middle and upper lobes. Multiple lucent regions are seen within the collapsed lobe. These are presumably due to foci of emphysema or bronchiectasis which have not collapsed together with the rest of the lobe. The middle lobe, in part C, is much more hyperlucent than the left lung. This is due to compensatory overinflation.

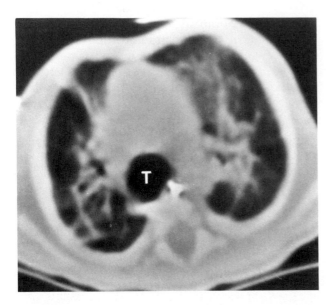

Figure 26-29   Tracheomegaly. This CT scan in a 3-month-old infant shows massive distension of the trachea (T). The trachea was a normal size in the first few weeks of life. The dilatation is believed to be due to mechanical distension from high ventilator pressure. Note too the diffuse patchy changes in both lung fields due to bronchopulmonary dysplasia (see Figure 1-15).

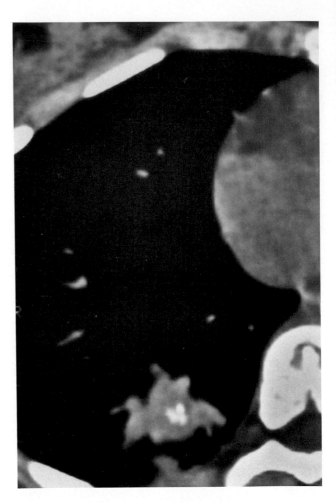

Figure 26-30   Timothy grass granuloma. The CT scan identifies a mass lesion in the right lower lung field. The margins are very irregular. The main mass of the lesion is of soft tissue intensity. Several areas of calcification are present as well. At surgery this was found to be a foreign body granuloma due to the presence of inhaled timothy grass (see Figure 17-13).

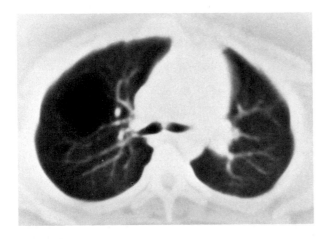

Figure 26-31   Pneumatocele. The CT scan identifies a large pneumatocele in the right upper lobe. The pneumatocele is displacing adjacent vessels. No normal vessels are seen within it. The margins are fairly well defined, but no definite wall is present.

Tumors

The major role that CT plays in imaging of the pediatric chest is in the evaluation of benign thoracic tumors and primary and secondary malignant tumors. Computed tomography consistently provides more information than other imaging modalities.

Mediastinal Masses

The differential diagnosis of mediastinal masses has already been discussed in Chapter 9. Computed tomography is much better than plain-film radiographs at identifying and characterizing mediastinal masses (Figures 26-22, 26-23, and 26-24),[17,37] at defining the extent of the mass,[17,37] and in localizing the mass.[4,24] Accurate localization of a mediastinal mass is most important as this information greatly assists in formulating a differential diagnosis. Masses in the anterior mediastinum include the normal thymus, abnormal thymus, metastases, teratoma, germ cell neoplasms,[38] soft tissue component of osteomyelitis of the sternum,[39] enlarged lymph nodes, lymphoma, and tuberculosis.[39] Midmediastinal masses include enlarged lymph nodes, vascular malformations, and enteric and bronchogenic cysts.[4] One of the commonest posterior mediastinal masses is neuroblastoma. Less common posterior mediastinal masses include posterior extension of the thymus,[40] teratoma,[41] mediastinal extension of spinal lipomas,[42] hematomas, abscess, paraspinal Ewing's sarcoma,[43] and loculated effusions.[17]

Computed tomography is superior to chest radiograph for the identification of lymph nodes particularly in the subcarinal area.[44]

In addition to identifying and locating mediastinal masses, CT can often characterize the tissues in the mass, and this may in many cases suggest the correct diagnosis. For example, CT can accurately identify calcification, fat, or fluid within mass lesions.[4] The fact that bronchogenic cysts can occasionally appear as solid lesions on CT scan has been discussed already.

Computed tomography can also accurately demonstrate secondary effects of mass lesions in the mediastinum. Tracheal compression is an important secondary effect (Figures 26-32 and 26-33). It may be seen with bronchogenic cysts, neurofibromas, lymphomas, and other disorders. It is important, as it may occur in as many as 55 percent of patients with Hodgkin's disease on initial presentation.[45] The level of the tracheal narrowing and the amount of reduction in the cross-sectional area can be accurately identified.[24,45]

Computed tomography can identify partial or complete obstruction of major vessels in the mediastinum due to compression from adjacent mass lesions.[24,39] Dilated collateral vessels can also be seen.[24]

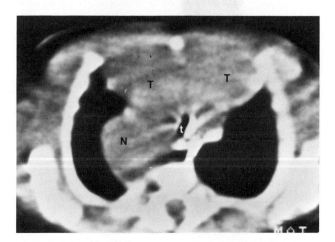

Figure 26-32 Neuroblastoma. This patient has a well-defined posterior mediastinal mass lesion on the right side. This is a neuroblastoma (N). No calcification is identified in the mass. The mass is causing significant compression of the trachea (t). There are no specific features to characterize the lesion as a neuroblastoma—many posterior mediastinal lesions could have a similar appearance. In addition to the neuroblastoma, note the large, but normal, thymus (T) in the anterior mediastinum.

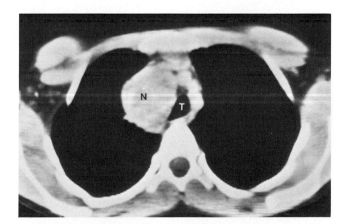

Figure 26-33 Compression of the trachea by Hodgkin's disease. The CT scan identifies right paratracheal lymph nodes (N) that are markedly enlarged. These are causing slight displacement of the trachea (T) to the left and moderate indentation of the right wall of the trachea.

Although CT is very accurate in identifying mass lesions in the mediastinum, lungs, and chest wall, it may not always be possible to differentiate benign from malignant lesions or tumors from infections or other diseases.[24] Most cystic lesions, particularly if well defined, are benign.[24] However, cystic degeneration of tumors may sometimes cause confusion, and it may be impossible to differentiate a necrotic tumor either from a cyst into which hemorrhage has occurred or from an abscess. With intravenous contrast injection, the walls of an abscess will frequently show more enhancement than will a tumor or hemorrhagic cyst.[4] An abscess will usually have a much more irregular rim than will a hemorrhagic cyst.

Widening of the mediastinum is a not infrequent finding on a chest radiograph. This may be due to

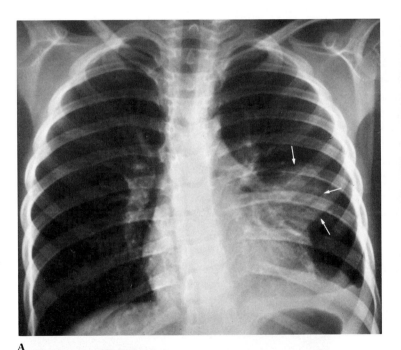

A

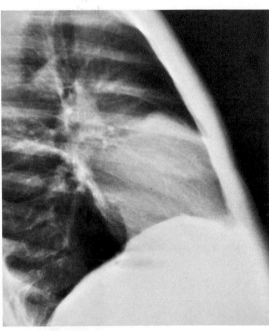

B

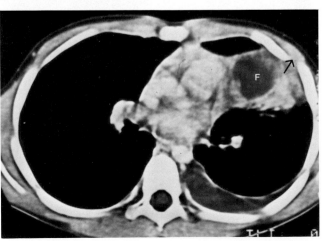

C

Figure 26-34   Mediastinal teratoma. A. The frontal chest radiograph shows an ill-defined region of opacification in the left midlung (arrows). It obscures part of the heart border, suggesting an anterior location. **B.** The lateral chest radiograph shows the anterior location of the abnormality seen on the frontal radiograph. **C.** The CT scan shows a large mass lesion arising from the anterior mediastinum. Involvement of the chest wall can be identified (arrow). The mass has fairly sharply defined margins, suggesting a mediastinal rather than a pulmonary origin. A large central area of low intensity is due to fluid (F) within the lesion as well as pleural effusion. No calcium is seen within the mass. The sharp margins, chest wall involvement, and fluid suggest the diagnosis of mediastinal teratoma. The differential diagnosis includes an abscess or necrosis within the enlarged lymph nodes.

disease or to normal tissue.[4] Computed tomography can often help differentiate normal from abnormal mediastinal widening.

Teratoma

Mediastinal teratomas usually are located in the anterior mediastinum but may occur elsewhere (Figure 26-34).[41] The classic teratoma has regions of fluid, fat,

calcium, and soft tissue, and in these cases an accurate diagnosis can be made from the CT scan. In some cases, particularly when calcium and fat are not present, it may not be possible on the CT scan to differentiate teratomas from other mediastinal mass lesions.

Neuroblastoma

Neuroblastomas are one of the commonest mediastinal mass lesions. They are almost always found in the posterior mediastinum (Figure 26-35) but extend into the midmediastinum and even cause tracheal compression (Figure 26-32). In many cases they are calcified, and the identification of calcium in a posterior mediastinal mass strongly suggests the diagnosis of neuroblastoma. These lesions may cause displacement or even erosion of the adjacent ribs, and this can be accurately seen on CT scans. Mediastinal neuroblastomas will sometimes extend into the spinal canal. The routine CT scan may suggest this diagnosis, but to identify the true extent of the tumor in the spinal canal, the region should be rescanned using thin-sliced sections and following the injection of metrizamide into the subarachnoid space.

Posterior mediastinal neuroblastomas always have a smooth, sharp interface between the tumor

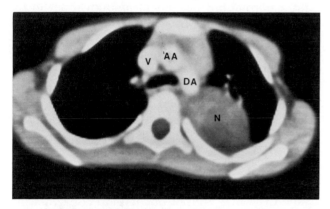

Figure 26-35   Neuroblastoma. There is a large, left-sided posterior neuroblastoma (N). The margins of the mass are relatively well defined. No rib destruction can be identified. The tumor does not extend into the spinal canal. The superior vena cava (V), ascending aorta (AA), and descending aorta (DA) are all well identified.

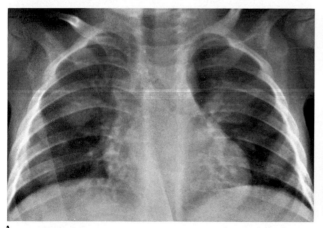
A

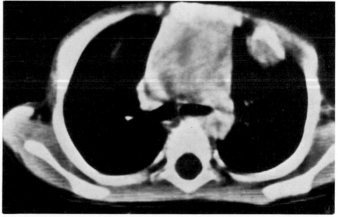
B

Figure 26-36   Rib metastases from neuroblastoma. A. The chest radiograph identifies three large nodular soft tissue densities. Two overlie the right lung, and one overlies the left midlung. The chest radiograph cannot distinguish pulmonary metastases from chest wall nodules. **B.** The CT scan taken through the superior part of the left nodule shows that the nodule arises from the anterior end of the left rib.

and the adjacent lung tissue. The interface with adjacent mediastinal structures may be less well defined. On occasion, a tumor can infiltrate around the adjacent descending aorta or azygos vein.

Metastases from neuroblastoma to the ribs may be associated with adjacent soft tissue masses[36] which mimic lung nodules on chest radiograph. The origin from the ribs is clearly shown by CT (Figure 26-36).

Thymic Tumors

Fifteen percent of adult patients with myasthenia gravis have a thymoma.[24] Thymomas can be accurately identified by CT. They are seen as focal soft tissue nodules in the thymus. They may or may not cause a bulge in the contour of the thymus.

Cysts in the thymus are rare but can occasionally be seen in patients with Hodgkin's disease who have had radiation therapy.[46] They are identified as fluid intensity, well-defined lesions in the thymus. The thymus is not infrequently involved with lymphoma. Diffuse enlargement of the thymus with lymphoma can be very difficult to distinguish from a normal but prominent thymus. After therapy for lymphoma, it is not uncommon to see a marked rebound increase in thymic size,[4] and this may be difficult to differentiate from a recurrent tumor in the thymus (Figure 26-37).

Fatty Tumors

The demonstration of fat within abnormalities of the mediastinum is relatively easy. Fat is of very low intensity on the CT image and has a CT number well below that of fluid. The demonstrated fat may be normal fat, a lipoma, or fat in a teratoma.[4,24] Patients with a normal but prominent amount of fat in the mediastinum usually have a large amount of subcutaneous fat present as well. Lipomas show a homogenous intensity and are well defined. Occasionally a spinal lipoma can be seen extending into the posterior mediastinum.[42] If fat is identified in a teratoma, the correct diagnosis can usually be made, especially if there is associated calcium (see Figures 9-4 and 9-5).

Cystic Hygroma

Cystic hygromas are not uncommon congenital tumors in the newborn. While they occur predominantly in the neck, they may extend into the thorax. In planning surgery, it is important to accurately de-

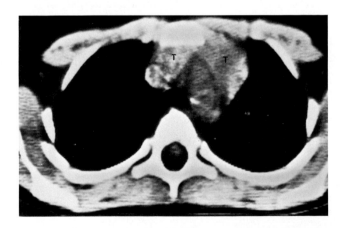

Figure 26-37 Rebound enlargement of the thymus. The CT scan shows an enlarged thymus (T). The patient had just completed therapy for non-Hodgkin's lymphoma. Previous CT studies had shown a much smaller thymus. The CT scan cannot differentiate a normal thymus from a recurrent lymphoma involving the thymus. At surgery this patient was found to have a normal thymus.

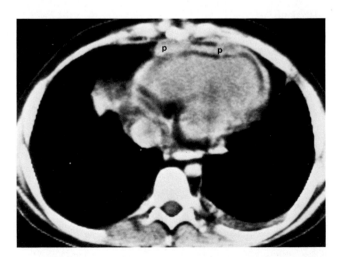

Figure 26-38 Non-Hodgkin's lymphoma with pericardial involvement. The CT scan shows marked thickening of the pericardium (p) due to infiltration by non-Hodgkin's lymphoma.

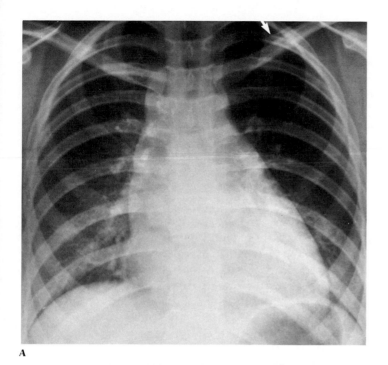

Figure 26-39 Hodgkin's disease of lymph nodes, sternum, and chest wall. A. The chest radiograph shows mild widening of the anterior mediastinum. There is indentation of the right side of the trachea by enlarged lymph nodes. A normal soft tissue companion shadow (arrow) was identified on the left side. No shadow is seen in the right supraclavicular area because of the presence of enlarged lymph nodes in this region. The CT scan shows the extent of the abnormality far better than the chest radiograph. **B.** This CT scan, taken at the level of the thoracic inlet, shows enlarged supraclavicular lymph nodes (N). **C.** On this CT scan, taken at the level of the trachea, the enlarged lymph nodes extend down into the right parasternal region. Enlarged right paratracheal nodes are identified. Note the heavy calcification (C) lying just to the right of the trachea. **D** and **E.** These scans were obtained with soft tissue and bone window settings at the level of the tracheal bifurcation. There is extensive patchy destruction of the sternum. A large soft tissue mass surrounds the sternum. This is contiguous with the massively enlarged mediastinal lymph nodes. Again, note the heavy calcification around the right main stem bronchus. **F.** This CT scan, taken 2 cm lower than the previous two scans, shows extensive abnormality involving the entire sternum, chest wall, and anterior mediastinum. The calcification is believed to be due to old histoplasmosis rather than to Hodgkin's disease.

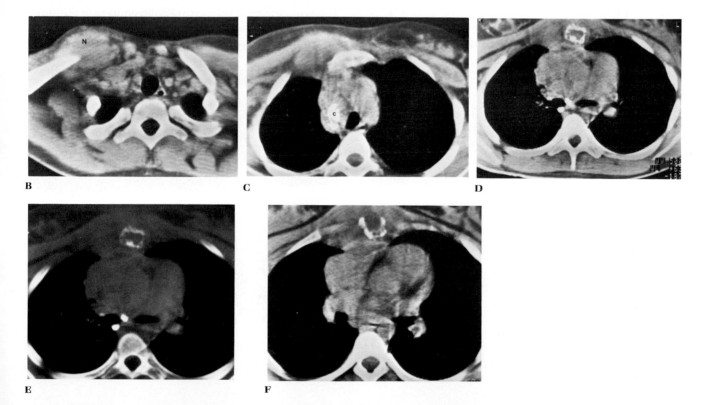

fine the intrathoracic extension of these tumors. They appear as well-defined mass lesions with a large number of cystic spaces separated by bands of soft tissue of varying thickness. Computed tomography defines the neck component and the intrathoracic extension of these tumors extremely well. In the thorax they may extend anterior or posterior to the lung and into the mediastinum. In this situation they usually cause minimal displacement of the mediastinal structures but may infiltrate between the great vessels and trachea.

Mesenchymoma

Mesenchymomas[47] are rare tumors occurring in the newborn. They arise from the chest wall and may be very large, often filling an entire hemithorax. Computed tomography will identify these tumors, define their extent, and also show associated rib displacement and erosion. Many of these tumors regress spontaneously.

Lymphoma

Computed tomography plays a major role in the management of children with Hodgkin's and non-

Hodgkin's lymphoma (Figures 26-15, 26-33, and 26-37 to 26-39). It can identify disease not seen on chest radiograph (Figure 26-40).[4] The CT findings are important in differential diagnosis, staging the tumor, and monitoring the response to therapy. They are also utilized in planning the field for radiation therapy.[48] The major findings in the chest in lymphoma are the presence of enlarged lymph nodes in the anterior mediastinum, the midmediastinum, and the hila. Node enlargement can be identified in any or all of these sites. The differential diagnosis includes infection, particularly histoplasmosis. The presence of calcification in the lymph nodes does not exclude the diagnosis of lymphoma (Figures 26-15 and 26-39), because in geographic regions where histoplasma is endemic, patients with old histoplasma infection may also subsequently develop lymphoma. The enlarged mediastinal lymph nodes may compress mediastinal vessels and/or the trachea (Figure 26-33). The nature of such compression is accurately identified by CT.

Lymphoma also may involve the lung (Figure 26-41). The abnormality may be seen as ill-defined infiltrates or as nodular densities. The demonstration of pulmonary disease in lymphoma does alter staging

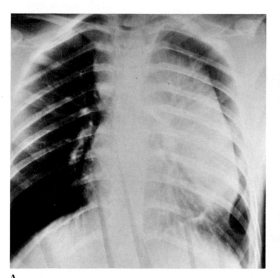
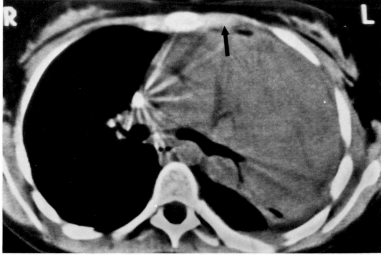

A   B

Figure 26-40   Mediastinal Hodgkin's disease. A. The chest radiograph shows a large left-sided mass. **B.** The CT scan shows an extensive soft tissue mass lesion involving the anterior mediastinum and extending around the side of the chest to the posterior mediastinum. The mass is of soft tissue density. No calcium or cysts can be identified within it. Subtle involvement of the anterior chest wall can be identified (arrow). At biopsy this was Hodgkin's disease.

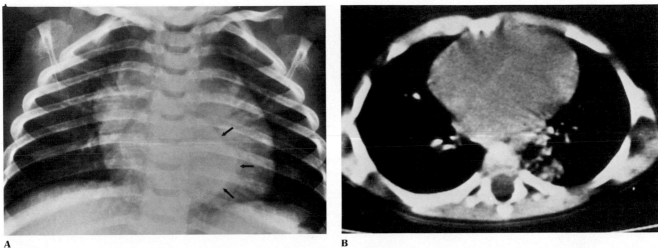

A   B

Figure 26-41   Pneumonia mimics a mediastinal mass. This child presented with fever. **A.** The chest radiograph shows a density through the cardiac silhouette. The margins are moderately well defined laterally (arrows), suggesting a mediastinal tumor rather than pneumonia. **B.** The CT scan shows patchy, ill-defined densities in the medial aspect of the left lower lobe consistent with infection rather than tumor. A repeat radiograph after 2 weeks of antibiotic therapy showed complete resolution of the lesion (see Figure 23-7).

and is an important finding. Malignant effusions are not uncommon findings in children with lymphoma. Computed tomography will identify the amount of fluid present. In some patients, solid tumor plaques can also be identified in the pleura. Involvement of the chest wall occurs in up to 10 percent of patients with lymphoma (Figure 26-39).[48,49] This finding is far better demonstrated on CT than on chest radiograph,[48,49] and its presence will alter tumor staging.[49] Chest wall lymphoma can be identified even without the presence of mediastinal or lung tumor.[48] Lymphoma may also involve the pericardium (Figure 26-38).

Lung Metastases

Computed tomography is extremely accurate in the identification of lung metastases (Figures 26-42 to 26-44)[22] and is an excellent modality for screening the lungs for metastases in children with known remote primary tumors.[4] Computed tomography has consistently been shown to identify more pulmonary nodules than either chest radiograph or whole-lung tomography.[4] It is also more accurate than chest radiograph for identifying pleural metastases[50] (Fig-

ures 26-43 and 26-44). Occasionally, especially with osteogenic sarcoma, spontaneous pneumothorax can occur with lung metastases (Figure 26-44). Most thoracic metastases are in the lung, but they may involve the chest wall and spinal canal (Figure 26-45).

There are a number of problems in the CT evaluation of the lungs for metastases:

1. Computed tomography may miss nodules, either because a small nodule has moved with respiration out of the imaging plane or because a nodule is of similar size to adjacent vessels imaged transversely.

2. Computed tomography cannot always accurately differentiate benign from malignant nodules.[4] One study of lung nodules in children with known primary malignancies elsewhere reported that as many as one-third of such nodules were benign.[51] Such benign nodules may be due to histoplasma, pseudotumors, radiation, hamartoma, round pneumonia, fibrosis, or round atelectasis.[10,51–53]

3. Calcification in a lung nodule usually indicates the presence of previous infection such as histoplasmosis (Figure 26-46). With histoplasma, calci-

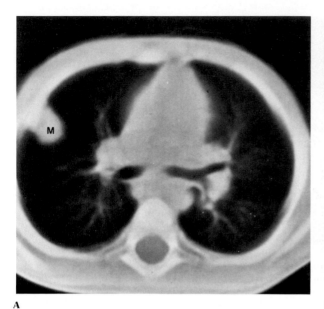

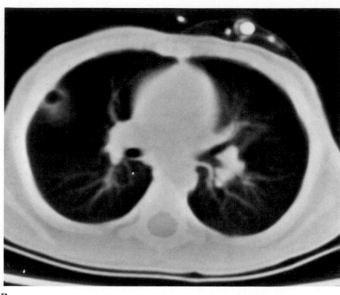

A   **B**

Figure 26-42   Metastasis from Wilms's tumor. A. A large nodular metastasis (M) is seen in the periphery of the right lung field. Scans at other levels showed multiple metastases in this patient with a known Wilms's tumor. **B.** This CT scan taken after 3 months of chemotherapy shows a residual abnormality at the site of the metastasis. A cavitating lesion is now present. This is an unusual feature in Wilms's tumor. In most patients metastases respond to therapy by disappearing completely.

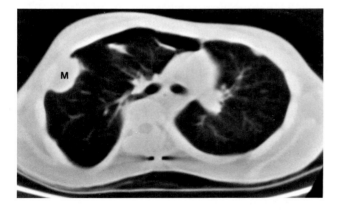

Figure 26-43   Metastasis from an osteogenic sarcoma. A large metastatic mass (M) is located adjacent to the pleura in the right midlung field. The asymmetry of the two lungs in this patient is due to moderately severe congenital scoliosis.

4. Although CT is the most sensitive imaging modality for identifying lung nodules, there are limitations to its resolution. Many reports indicate that more nodules are found during planned surgical resection than were demonstrated on the CT scan.

5. The appearance of the lung metastases is relatively nonspecific, and metastases from a variety of tumors may all look similar (Figures 26-42 and 26-48). In addition, benign lesions such as inflammatory pseudotumors or histoplasma granulomas may mimic metastases. Primary lung tumors, although rare, may also look similar (Figure 26-49).

fied lymph nodes may be seen as well. With some primary tumors, such as osteogenic sarcoma, calcification can occur in pulmonary metastases (Figure 26-47). This would be an extremely rare finding in metastases from tumors other than those arising in bone.

Other Tumors

Many other unusual tumors can occur in the thorax. The CT appearance of several such tumors is illustrated in Figures 26-50 to 26-56.

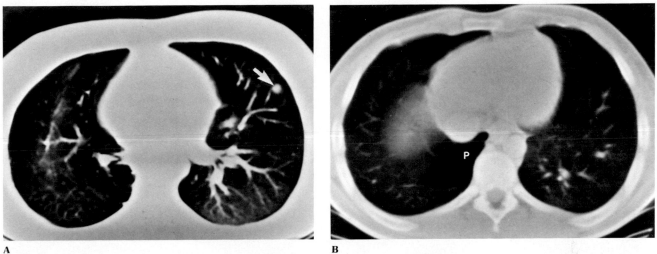

A   B

Figure 26-44   Metastasis from an osteogenic sarcoma with a spontaneous pneumothorax. A. A small metastasis (arrow) is seen in the left upper lobe. Multiple metastases were present at other levels. **B.** The CT scan at a lower level in the same patient shows a small pneumothorax (P).

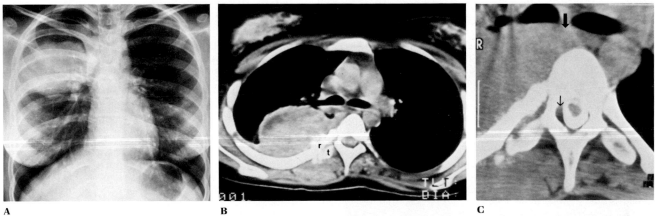

A   B   C

Figure 26-45   Metastasis from an osteogenic sarcoma with involvement of the chest wall, rib, and spinal canal. A. This patient had a primary osteogenic sarcoma of the right leg. The chest radiograph shows a large mass lesion in the right hemithorax. The posterior ribs are separated, but rib destruction cannot be clearly identified. **B.** The CT scan localizes the lesion to the posterior chest wall. It shows a large soft tissue mass lesion extending into the thoracic cage, extensive involvement of the medial aspect of the adjacent rib (r), involvement of the transverse process (t) of the vertebra, and extension into the soft tissues behind the rib. **C.** This thin-section CT image, obtained at the same level as part B following injection of subarachnoid metrizamide, again shows a large soft tissue mass with bone destruction. Extension of the tumor into the spinal canal is clearly identified (small arrow). Extension of the tumor into the subcarinal region is also evident (large arrow). Both of these findings indicate that the tumor metastasis cannot be resected.

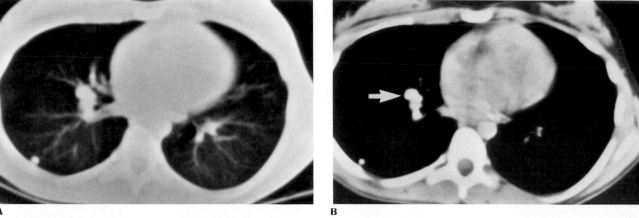

A   B

Figure 26-46 Chronic histoplasmosis. The lung window (**A**) and soft tissue window (**B**) CT scans both show a calcified nodule in the posterior aspect of the right lower lobe. The calcification involves almost the entire aspect of the nodule, with no significant surrounding soft tissue mass identifiable. Heavy calcification is also identified in the hilar lymph nodes (arrow).

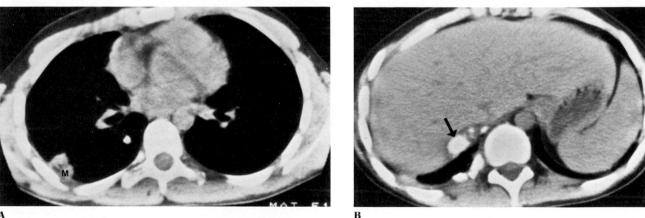

A   B

Figure 26-47 Calcified metastasis from an osteogenic sarcoma. A. A pleural-based metastasis (M) is present in the posterior right chest. **B.** Another pleural-based metastasis is identified (arrow). This lesion lies posteriorly in the inferior aspect of the pleura. Because of this location it could be difficult to differentiate this chest metastasis from a neuroblastoma or from a primary liver mass. At surgery the thoracic origin was confirmed.

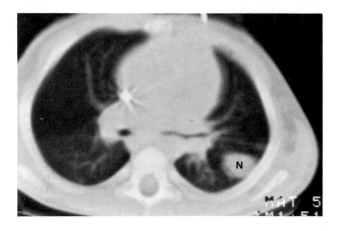

Figure 26-48 Lung metastasis from a hepatocellular carcinoma. A large, well-defined nodular density (N) appears in the left lower lung field posteriorly. This was a metastasis from a patient's known liver tumor. The appearance of the metastasis is nonspecific, with no specific feature to indicate the organ of origin.

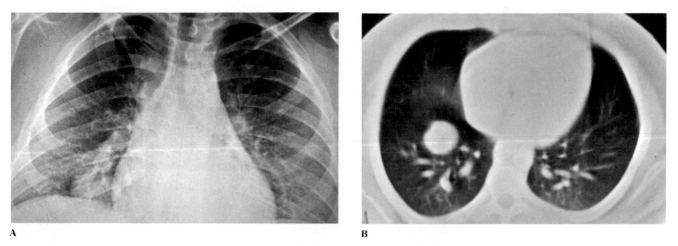

A   B

Figure 26-49   Malignant schwannoma. A. The chest radiograph in this patient with known neurofibromatosis shows an ill-defined nodular density in the right lower lung field. **B.** The CT scan shows this to be a well-localized soft tissue nodule without calcification in the right lower lobe. The lesion was completely resected and found to be a malignant schwannoma.

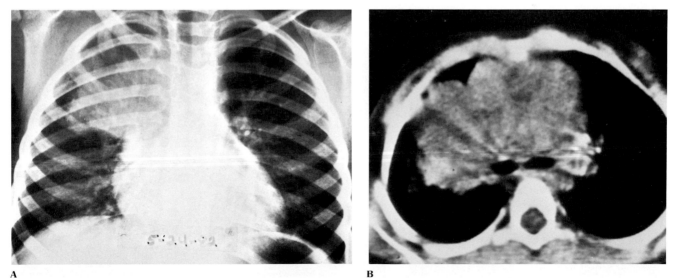

A   B

Figure 26-50   Mucoid epidermoid carcinoma of the lung. A. The chest radiograph shows an opacification in the right upper lung field. The slight elevation of the horizontal fissure indicates some volume loss of the right upper lobe. Infection, with mild superimposed collapse is suggested from the chest film. **B.** The CT scan identifies a large mass lesion in the right upper lung field. The margins are moderately well defined and lobulated, suggesting the presence of a tumor rather than pneumonia or collapse. The lesion was completely resected and found to be a malignant tumor.

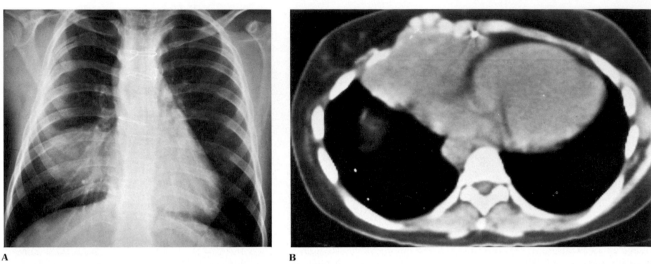

A   B

Figure 26-51   Mesenchymal tumor of the right lung and chest wall. The patient had a ventricular septal defect repaired 3 years before the present study. **A.** The chest radiograph identifies an area of homogenized opacification in the right lower lung field. The margins are poorly defined. The appearance is nonspecific. Involvement of the chest wall cannot be identified. **B.** The CT scan shows a large right anterior mass lesion causing displacement of the heart to the left. The lesion is invading the chest wall. The margins are moderately well defined. The lesion is of fairly uniform homogeneous soft tissue density. The relatively sharp margins and the involvement of the chest wall exclude infection or collapse and suggest the correct diagnosis of tumor. The lesion was completely resected.

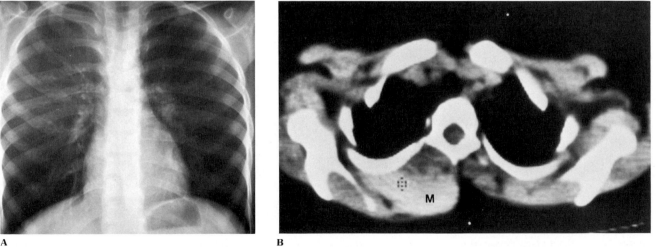

A   B

Figure 26-52   Benign fibrous desmoid. A. The chest radiograph shows an increased density in the right upper lung field. No boundaries to the abnormality can be identified. It is not possible to distinguish a chest wall abnormality from lung disease. **B.** The CT scan shows a moderately well defined mass (M) in the right posterior chest wall. The lesion is of relatively high intensity due to its dense fibrous nature. It was completely resected.

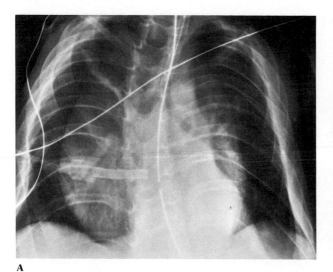
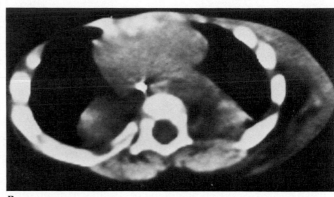

A

B

Figure 26-53   Massive lymphangiomatosis. A. The chest radiograph shows large mass lesions in both sides of the chest. **B.** The CT scan shows large posterior mediastinal mass lesions on both the right and left sides. In addition to this, an ill-defined mass is seen in the left chest wall. The appearance of these lesions is relatively nonspecific. The patient had diffuse lymphangiomas affecting many regions of the body. (See Figures 12-1 and 12-2.)

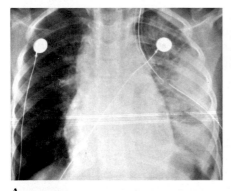
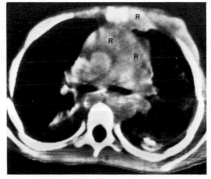
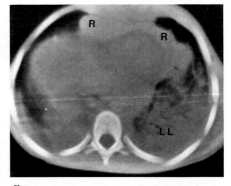

A   **B**   **C**

Figure 26-54   Rhabdomyosarcoma with pleural effusion and secondary collapse of the left lower lobe. A. The chest radiograph shows a large density in the left lung. It is moderately confluent laterally and more patchy closer to the midline. The outline of the left hemidiaphragm is lost. The gas in the bowel indicates elevation of the left hemidiaphragm. On the chest radiograph, tumor, collapse, and effusion cannot be differentiated. Chest wall involvement is not identified. **B.** The CT scan shows a large rhabdomyosarcoma (R) involving the anterior mediastinum and the left anterior chest wall. The mediastinal margins of the tumor are poorly defined. **C.** A CT scan taken more inferiorly than part B again shows tumor (R) involving the anterior chest wall and the anterior mediastinum. The collapsed left lower lobe (LL) is differentiated from tumor by the presence of air bronchograms within the collapsed lung tissue.

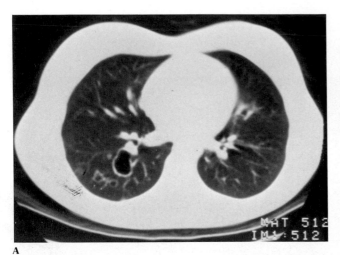
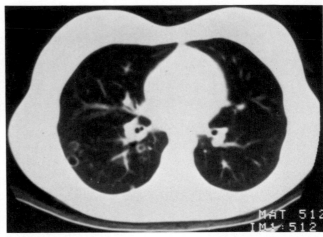

A   **B**

Figure 26-55   Laryngeal papillomatosis with extension into the lungs. A and **B.** The CT images show multiple cavitating nodules of varying size. The nodules have well-defined walls. No air-fluid levels are identified within the nodules. This appearance is fairly typical of pulmonary involvement with laryngeal papillomas. (See Figures 17-14 and 17-15.)

Infections

For most children with thoracic infection, chest radiograph is the only imaging modality required to manage their cases. The chest radiograph will identify the infection and can be utilized to monitor response to therapy. In selected patients, however, CT is of great benefit. Some of the uses of CT are as follows:

1. *Persistence of suspected pneumonia in the lungs following therapy.* For patients who are suspected of having pneumonia, with or without collapse, but who fail to respond to adequate therapy, CT scan might yield additional information. The failure to respond to therapy might be due to obstruction of the draining bronchus from either enlarged lymph nodes or a tumor (Figure 26-56). Both can be identified by CT. Another reason for the failure of infection to respond to therapy is that the infection may have occurred in an underlying pulmonary abnormality such as pulmonary sequestration or a cystic adenomatoid malformation. Again CT might demonstrate specific features suggesting the correct underlying diagnosis. In sequestration it might demonstrate feed-

ing vessels. In cystic adenomatoid malformation it might demonstrate areas of cystic change.

2. *Management of abscesses.* Computed tomography is more sensitive than chest radiograph in the diagnosis of a suspected pulmonary abscess (Figure 26-57). The abscess will usually appear as a mass lesion with irregular margins and a poorly defined interface with the adjacent lung.[22] The walls of the abscess may show significant enhancement following an injection of intravenous contrast material. The amount of fluid in the abscess cavity can be identified with CT. Computed tomography may also be successfully utilized to guide the placement of drainage needles and catheters into the abscess.[54]

3. *Unusual infections.* With some unusual infections, CT will accurately define the extent of the abnormality and suggest the underlying cause. For example, a number of infections will involve the chest wall, the pleura and lung, and sometimes the adjacent ribs. Demonstration of such an extensive abnormality would suggest the diagnosis of fungal infection, tuberculosis, staphylococcal infection, or occasionally lymphoma.[55]

4. *Empyema.* Computed tomography has several roles to play in the evaluation of empyema. It will

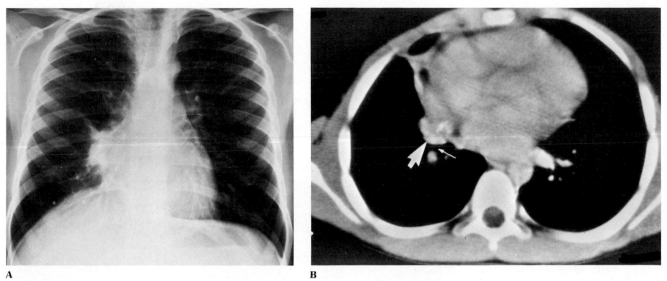

A   B

Figure 26-56   Inflammatory pseudotumor. A. The chest radiograph shows loss of the right heart border, suggesting the presence of collapse in the middle lobe. No definite focal mass lesion can be identified. **B.** The CT scan shows a mass lesion (large arrow) at the origin of the middle lobe bronchus (small arrow). Patchy collapse is seen in the middle lobe.

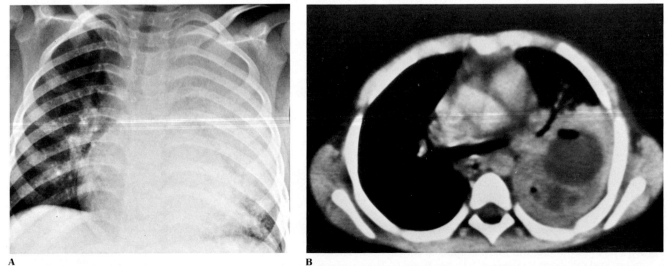

A   B

Figure 26-57   Cavitating pneumonia. A. This chest radiograph in a 12-year-old girl with fever shows extensive consolidation of the left upper lobe. **B.** The CT scan shows that the central regions of the lesion have liquefied. Small air collections show the early development of a cavity.

demonstrate the extent of the abnormal fluid collection. Following drainage, CT will evaluate the adequacy of the drainage procedure and identify loculated areas of fluid collection remote from the catheter position. It will also help differentiate empyema from underlying adjacent inflammation or abscess formation in the lungs.

5. *Evaluation of pneumonia that mimics a mass lesion.* Areas of pneumonia may occasionally mimic mass lesions on chest radiograph. By identifying air bronchograms in the abnormal areas, CT can give the correct diagnosis (Figures 26-41 and 26-58).

6. *Cystic fibrosis.* In patients with cystic fibrosis, CT may show even more extensive and severe disease than the chest radiograph (Figure 26-28).

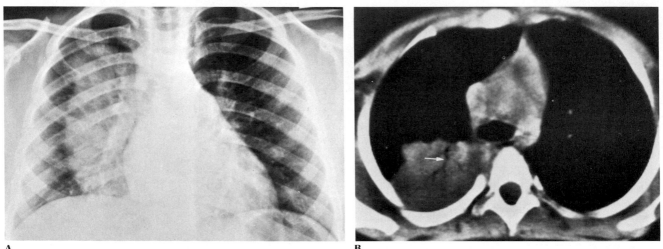

A   **B**

Figure 26-58   Pneumonia mimics a tumor. This patient presented with a fever of 104° for 3 days. **A.** The chest radiograph shows a large right-sided abnormality with fairly well defined lateral margins. The appearance suggests a mediastinal mass lesion. **B.** The chest CT shows extensive consolidation of the right lower lobe (arrow). An air bronchogram is clearly identified within the abnormal region, indicating the correct diagnosis of pneumonia.

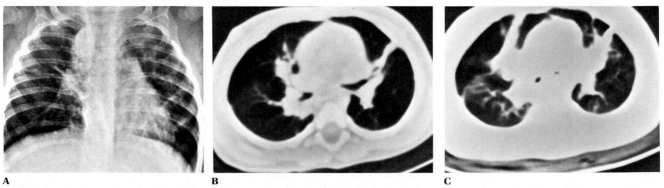

A   **B**   **C**

Figure 26-59   Bronchopulmonary dysplasia. A. The chest radiograph shows diffuse abnormality in both lung fields. Patchy areas of lucency and increased density can be seen. **B** and **C.** The CT scans show much more severe abnormality than can be appreciated from the chest radiograph. Broad bands of soft tissue density probably represent regions of collapse and/or fibrosis. The very severe nonuniform distribution of air throughout the lungs is also clearly identified, with multiple areas of emphysema seen as patchy regions of very low intensity.

Diffuse Lung Disease

There is little experience of CT scanning of diffuse lung disease.[24] Computed tomography has been reported to show abnormality in bullae, interstitial fibrosis, and diffuse granulomas.[56] Many of the disorders such as emphysema, fibrosis, or edema will look different on CT images.[24] The clinical utility of these findings is, however, not well established.

In bronchopulmonary dysplasia (Figure 26-59), CT will identify diffuse abnormality. The severity of the abnormality is more readily appreciated on the

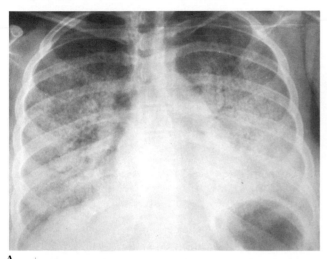
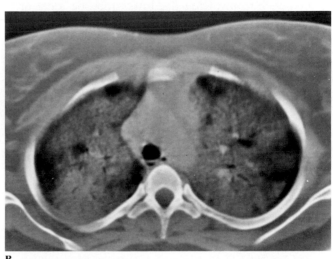

A **B**
Figure 26-60 Alveolar proteinosis. A. The chest radiograph shows diffuse, hazy, granular opacification of both lung fields, with relative sparing of the apices. **B.** The CT scan shows a moderately uniform, diffuse soft tissue infiltrate throughout the lung fields. (See Figures 25-9 and 25-10.)

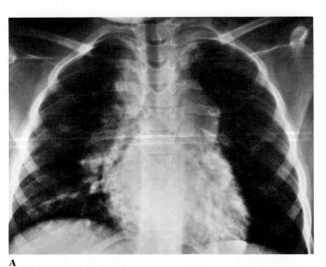
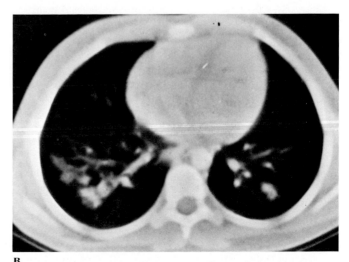

A **B**
Figure 26-61 Hodgkin's disease of the mediastinum and lung. A. This overpenetrated chest radiograph shows widespread mediastinal lymph node enlargement. The trachea and bronchi are not significantly compressed. **B.** The CT scan, taken at the level of the midheart, shows patchy densities in both lower lobes. The densities are more extensive on the right side. These were due to pulmonary involvement with tumor.

CT scan than on the chest radiograph. Computed tomography can demonstrate areas of collapse, areas of infection, and focal areas of emphysema. Bands of fibrous tissue are also identified.

Alveolar proteinosis appears as a very uniform, hazy, diffuse abnormality seen throughout the lung fields (Figure 26-60).

Lymphoma involving the lungs may be focal or widespread (Figure 26-61).

References

1. Kirks DR, Korobkin M: Computed tomography of the chest in infants and children: Techniques and mediastinal evaluation. *Radiol Clin North Am* 19:409, 1981.
2. Thompson JR, Schneider S, Ashwal S, et al: The choice of sedation for computed tomography in children: A prospective evaluation. *Radiology* 143:475, 1982.
3. Mitchell AA, Louik C, Lacouture P, et al: Risks to children from computed tomographic scan premedication. *JAMA* 247:2835, 1982.
4. Lee J, Sagel S, Stanley R (eds): *Computed Body Tomography*. New York, Raven Press, 1983, pp 55–131.
5. Brasch RC, Cann CE: Computed tomographic scanning in children: II. An updated comparison of radiation dose and resolving power of commercial scanners. *AJR* 138:127, 1982.
6. Fearon T, Vucich H: Pediatric patient exposures from CT examinations: GE CT/T 9800 scanner. *AJR* 144:805, 1985.
7. Francis IR, Glazer GM, Bookstein FL, et al: The thymus: Re-examination of age-related changes in size and shape. *AJR* 145:249, 1985.
8. Salonen OLM, Kivisaari ML, Somer JK: Computed tomography of the thymus of children under 10 years. *Pediatr Radiol* 14:373, 1984.
9. Dixon AK, Hilton CJ, Williams GT: Computed tomography and histological correlation of the thymic remnant. *Clin Radiol* 32:255, 1981.
10. Hidalgo H, Korobkin M, Kinney TR, et al: The problem of benign pulmonary nodules in children receiving cytotoxic chemotherapy. *AJR* 140:21, 1983.
11. Salonen OLM, Kivisaari ML, Somer JK: Computed tomography of the thymus of children under 10 years. *Pediatr Radiol* 14:373, 1984.
12. Glazer GM, Cross BH, Quint LE, et al: Normal mediastinal lymph nodes: Number and size according to American Thoracic Society mapping. *AJR* 144:261, 1985.
13. Glazer HS, Aronberg DJ, Sagel SS: Pitfalls in CT recognition of mediastinal lymphadenopathy. *AJR* 144:267, 1985.
14. Proto AV, Rost RC Jr: CT of the thorax: Pitfalls in interpretation. *RadioGraphics* 5:693, 1985.
15. Griscom NT: Computed tomographic determination of tracheal dimensions in children and adolescents. *Radiology* 145:361, 1982.
16. Effman EL, Fram EK, Vock P, et al: Tracheal cross-sectional area in children: CT determination. *Radiology* 149:137, 1983.
17. Gaisie G, Oh KS: Paraspinal interfaces in the lower thoracic area in children: Evaluation by CT. *Radiology* 149:133, 1983.
18. Levy-Raveth M, Auh YH, Rubenstein WA, et al: CT of the pericardial recesses. *AJR* 144:707, 1985.
19. Speckman JM, Gamsu G, Webb WR: Alterations in CT mediastinal anatomy produced by an azygos lobe. *AJR* 137:47, 1981.
20. Godwin JD: *Computed Tomography of the Chest*. Philadelphia, JB Lippincott Company, 1980.
21. Shurin SS, Haaga JR, Wood RE, et al: Computed tomography for the evaluation of thoracic masses in children. *JAMA* 246:65, 1981.
22. Kirks DR, Korobkin M: Computed tomography of the chest wall, pleura, and pulmonary parenchyma in infants and children. *Radiol Clin North Am* 19:421, 1981.
23. Kirks DR, Korobkin M: Chest computed tomography in infants and children. An analysis of 50 patients. *Pediatr Radiol* 10:75, 1980.
24. Webb WR: Advances in computed tomography of the thorax. *Radiol Clin North Am* 21:723, 1983.
25. Kirks DR, Korobkin M: Computed tomography of the chest in infants and children: Techniques and mediastinal evaluation. *Radiol Clin North Am* 19:409, 1981.
26. Paling MR, Dwyer A: The first rib as the cause of a "pulmonary nodule" on chest computed tomography. *J Comput Assist Tomogr* 4:847, 1980.
27. Kuhns LR, Borlaza G: The "Twinkling Star" sign. An aid in differentiating pulmonary vessels from pulmonary nodules on computed tomograms. *Radiology* 135:763, 1980.
28. Marvasti MA, Mitchell GE, Burke WA, et al: Misleading density of mediastinal cysts on computerized tomography. *Ann Thorac Surg* 31:167, 1981.

29. Tucker TT, Smith WL, Smith JA: Fluid-filled cystic adenomatoid malformation. *AJR* 129:323, 1977.

30. Rankin S, Faling LJ, Pugatch RD: CT diagnosis of pulmonary arteriovenous malformations. *J Comput Assist Tomogr* 6:746, 1982.

31. Sondheimer H, Oliphant M, Schneider B, et al: Computerized axial tomography of the chest for visualization of "absent" pulmonary arteries. *Circulation* 65:1020, 1982.

32. Day DL: Aortic arch in neonates with esophageal atresia: Preoperative assessment using CT. *Radiology* 155:99, 1985.

33. Davis SJ, Bryson BL, Thompson JS, et al: The role of computed tomography in blunt trauma. *Nebraska Med J* 70:3, 1985.

34. Adler OB, Rosenberger A: Localization of metallic foreign bodies in the chest by computed tomography. *J Comput Assist Tomogr* 6:955, 1982.

35. Berger PE, Kuhn JP, Kuhns LR: Computed tomography and the occult tracheobronchial foreign body. *Radiology* 134:133, 1980.

36. Edelstein G, Levitt RG, Slaker DP, et al: CT observation of rib abnormalities: Spectrum of findings. *J Comput Assist Tomogr* 9:65, 1985.

37. Sones PJ Jr, Torres WE, Colvin RS, et al: Effectiveness of CT in evaluating intrathoracic masses. *AJR* 139:469, 1982.

38. Levitt RG, Husband JE, Glazer HS: CT of primary germ-cell tumors of the mediastinum. *AJR* 142:73, 1984.

39. Rana SR, Saxena SB, Gumbs RV: Tuberculous mediastinal lymphadenitis with a chest wall mass. *Pediatr Radiol* 15:127, 1985.

40. Cohen MD, Weber TR, Sequeira FW, et al: The diagnostic dilemma of the posterior mediastinal thymus: CT manifestations. *Radiology* 146:691, 1983.

41. Weinberg B, Rose JS, Efremidis SC, et al: Posterior mediastinal teratoma (cystic dermoid): Diagnosis by computerized tomography. *Chest* 77:694, 1980.

42. Quinn SF, Monson M, Paling M: Spinal lipoma presenting as a mediastinal mass: Diagnosis by CT. *J Comput Assist Tomogr* 7:1087, 1983.

43. Weinstein JB, Siegel MJ, Griffith RC: Spinal Ewing sarcoma: Misleading appearances. *Skeletal Radiol* 11:262, 1984.

44. Muller NL, Webb WR, Gamsu G: Subcarinal lymph node enlargement: Radiographic findings and CT correlation. *AJR* 145:15, 1985.

45. Kirks DR, Fram EK, Vock P, et al: Tracheal compression by mediastinal masses in children: CT evaluation. *AJR* 141:647, 1983.

46. Baron RL, Lee JKT, Sagel SS, et al: Computed tomography of the abnormal thymus. *Radiology* 142:127, 1982.

47. Campbell AN, Wagget J, Mott MG: Benign mesenchymoma of the chest wall in infancy. *J Surg Oncol* 21:267, 1982.

48. Cho CS, Blank N, Castellino RA: Computerized tomography evaluation of chest wall involvement in lymphoma. *Cancer* 55:1892, 1985.

49. Press GA, Glazer HS, Wasserman TH, et al: Thoracic wall involvement by Hodgkin disease and Non-Hodgkin lymphoma: CT evaluation. *Radiology* 157:195, 1985.

50. Cohen M, Grosfeld J, Baehner R, et al: Lung CT for detection of metastases: Solid tissue neoplasms in children. *AJR* 139:895, 1982.

51. Cohen M, Smith WL, Weetman R, et al: Pulmonary pseudometastases in children with malignant tumors. *Radiology* 141:371, 1981.

52. Cohen MD, Mirkin DL, Provisor A, et al: Lung nodules after whole lung radiation. *Am J Pediatr Hematol/Oncol* 5:283, 1983.

53. Cohen M, Slabaugh R, Smith JA: Unusual non-metastatic nodules in the lungs of children with cancer. *Clin Radiol* 33:57, 1982.

54. Gobien RP, Stanley JH, Gobien BS, et al: Percutaneous catheter aspiration and drainage of suspected mediastinal abscesses. *Radiology* 151:69, 1984.

55. Webb WR, Sagel SS: Actinomycosis involving the chest wall: CT findings. *AJR* 139:1007, 1982.

56. Nakata H, Kimoto T, Nakayama T, et al: Diffuse peripheral lung disease: Evaluation by high-resolution computed tomography. *Radiology* 157:181, 1985.

Chapter 27

Magnetic Resonance Imaging of the Chest

Mervyn D. Cohen, M.B., Ch.B.

Background Physics and Principles of Image Interpretation

Magnetic resonance (MR) images are produced by utilizing a strong magnetic field to align the hydrogen atoms in the body along the vertical axis of the body, parallel to the magnetic field. The magnet looks rather like a computed tomography (CT) machine, and the patient lies on a table within the center of the magnet. Short bursts of radio waves are aimed into the patient. These bursts are a fraction of a second in duration. The radio waves cause the hydrogen atoms to tip away from their alignment with the magnetic field. As the atoms rotate, they absorb energy from the radio waves. When the radio wave pulse is turned off, the hydrogen atoms return to their resting position. As they do so, they release the absorbed energy back into the environment, again in the form of radio waves. These radio waves are de-

tected by an aerial which is either wrapped around the patient or placed on the body surface. From the pattern of strength and distribution of the returned radio waves, an image of the body tissues can be formed. The computer manipulations involved in this image construction are similar to those used in CT scanning. In CT (and other radiography) the image intensity depends on a single parameter, namely differential attenuation of the x-ray beam by different tissues. In MR images, however, the intensity of signal in any particular spot in the image depends on three independent factors: the local concentration of hydrogen atoms and the T_1 and T_2 relaxation times of the hydrogen atoms. The T_1 and T_2 relaxation times refer to the speed with which the hydrogen atoms return the radio wave signals to the environment. They are two independent properties of the hydrogen atoms and depend entirely on the micro-local environment in which the atoms are located. It is because of these local differences in environment that various body organs and tissues appear different and can be distinguished on the MR image. By altering the rate and number of radio waves which are aimed into the patient, one can generate MR images that emphasize either the concentration of hydrogen atoms or their T_1 or T_2 relaxation times. These images will all appear very different. In conventional radiography the final image depends only on the degree of absorption of x-rays by tissues. Thus on a conventional chest radiograph or on a CT scan, the bones always appear white, the soft tissues gray, the lungs black, and fat as an intensity between that of air and soft tissue. On the MR image this gray scale relationship between the tissues is not constant and will vary depending on the pulse sequence that has been chosen to create the image.

The whiteness seen on the image depends on the intensity of signal received from the body. The stronger the intensity signal received from a particular region, the whiter it will appear on the final image.

On MR images a strong signal (and hence a strong intensity on the image) is obtained from tissues with:

1. A high concentration of hydrogen
2. A short T_1 relaxation time
3. A long T_2 relaxation time

Weak signals (and therefore regions of low intensity) are obtained from tissues with:

1. A low concentration of hydrogen atoms
2. A long T_1 relaxation time
3. A short T_2 relaxation time
4. Flowing blood

The reason that flowing blood produces no signal is that the hydrogen atoms which have absorbed energy from the radio waves will have flowed out of the imaging plane by the time they return the signal to the environment.

The different tissues of the body have the following appearance in MR images:

1. *Fat.* Fat has a high concentration of hydrogen, a short T_1 relaxation time, and a long T_2 relaxation time. Because of this it will appear of strong intensity irrespective of the imaging pulse sequence chosen.
2. *Air.* Air in the lungs has a very low concentration of hydrogen and will therefore appear black irrespective of the pulse sequence chosen.
3. *Flowing blood.* In almost all situations, flowing blood will produce very little signal, so that the lumen of the blood vessels or the heart appears black and is strongly contrasted against the stronger signal received from the wall of the vessel. Exceptions to this occur if the flow of blood is extremely slow or if a paradoxically enhanced signal is obtained from the blood. Paradoxical enhancement of signal from the blood occurs in the first few slices, into which blood is flowing, when a series of multiple body slices is obtained simultaneously.
4. *Bone marrow.* The bone marrow gives a relatively strong signal because of the fat within it. The signal from the ribs and vertebra is not quite as strong as that obtained from the bone marrow of the humerus because the marrow in the flat bones does not lie in a central bone cavity.
5. *Bone cortex.* The cortex of bone produces little or no signal because it has an extremely short T_2 relaxation time and a very long T_1 relaxation time.
6. *Soft tissues.* The soft tissues of the chest wall and mediastinum produce signals of varying intensity which will alter depending on the pulse sequence that has been chosen to generate image.
7. *Diseased tissues.* Like soft tissues, diseased tissues will produce signals of varying intensity depending on the nature of the disease process, and also on the pulse sequence chosen to create the image.

Normal Anatomy

The chest wall tissues and structures can be seen fairly well. The subcutaneous fat of the chest wall produces a very strong uniform signal. It is clearly differentiated from the underlying muscle of the chest wall, which has a lower signal. The ribs and vertebra are identified by the strong signal received from the marrow within them and from the lack of signal from the bone cortex.

In the mediastinum the soft tissues are clearly distinguished from blood vessels and trachea. No signal is obtained from the blood vessels or trachea, and this contrasts well with the intermediate signal obtained from the mediastinal soft tissues. The thymus is seen as a soft tissue organ of intermediate signal strength. On the coronal images, the right and left lobes are clearly identified by their characteristic triangular shape. The trachea is also well-defined because of the lack of signal from the air within its lumen. The lungs on the MR image appear very different from those on a chest radiograph. They appear as a featureless, uniform black region, because no signal is obtained from the air in the lungs or the flowing blood in the pulmonary vessels. The soft tissues of the alveolar walls provide a very fine, hazy background of very low signal to the lung fields. The fissures are not usually identifiable in the normal individual.

Advantages and Disadvantages of Magnetic Resonance Imaging in the Chest

The advantages of MR imaging are

1. It uses no ionizing radiation.[1]
2. It is very safe.[2]
3. It is well tolerated by patients. There is no discomfort, and the study is noninvasive.
4. It is able to scan in any plane.[3,4] Hence, many of the thoracic structures can be seen along their long axis on a single image.
5. Magnetic resonance images have a very high soft tissue contrast.
6. Mediastinal vessels are clearly seen without the need for injection of contrast agents.

The disadvantages of MR imaging are

1. The cost is high.

2. The scan time is long. It takes between 30 and 60 min to image a single patient. However, technology improvements are rapidly decreasing the scan time.
3. It is poor for identifying small areas of calcification.
4. Cardiac and respiratory motion degrade images. However, this can be overcome by the use of gating techniques.

Focal Lung Disorders

A wide variety of different focal disorders of the lung can be identified by MR. Magnetic resonance is very sensitive for the identification of disease in the lungs, and it is probably true to say that almost every abnormality seen on a chest radiograph or CT scan can be identified by MR as well. The exact role of MR, however, is still to be defined.

Congenital Anomalies

Cystic adenomatoid malformations (Figure 27-1) appear as lesions with relatively poorly defined margins. There is marked variation of signal intensity on both T_1- and T_2-weighted images. This reflects the mixed pathology of the malformation, which includes air, fluid-filled cysts, and soft tissue masses.

A small right lung and a secondary small right hemithorax have been identified in a patient with agenesis of the right pulmonary artery.[5]

Areas of emphysema in the lungs appear as regions of diminished intensity on all pulse sequences because of the increased volume of air relative to the amount of interstitial soft tissue. Lobar emphysema is identified as a large homogeneous area of decreased intensity, corresponding in position to either the left or right upper lobe or the middle lobe on the right or lingular on the left (Figures 27-2 and 27-3). The margins of the abnormality are well-defined, and varying degrees of mediastinal shift may be identified.

Sequestration appears as a moderately well defined abnormality in the lower lung fields (Figure 27-

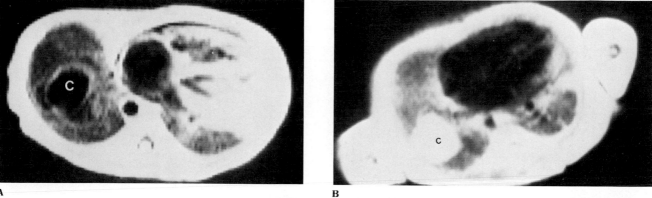

Figure 27-1 Cystic adenomatoid malformation. A. In this T_1-weighted image [spin echo (SE) = 30 and repetition time (TR) = 500], the margins of the lesions are not defined. The center of the abnormality has a very low intensity due to the presence of fluid within a cystic area (C) of the malformation. The heart is seen on the left. **B.** The T_2-weighted image shows a very strong signal from the cystic component (C) of the malformation. There has been much less change of signal intensity from the rest of the abnormality.

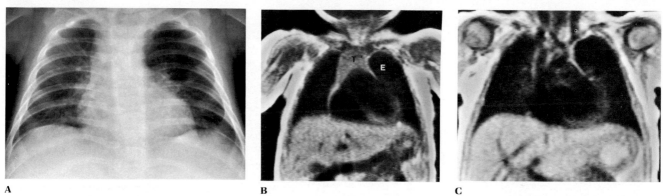

Figure 27-2 Lobar emphysema—left upper lobe. A. The chest radiograph shows mild hyperinflation of the left upper lobe with a slight shift of the mediastinum from left to right. **B.** The coronal T_1-weighted MR image shows expansion of the left upper lobe. There is a slight shift of the mediastinum to the right, and there is a slight reduction of signal intensity from the emphysematous lobe (E). *Note:* There is excellent visualization of both the right and left lobes of the thymus (T). **C.** This T_1 MR image was obtained more posteriorly. This again shows an expansion of the left upper lobe with a slight displacement of the mediastinal structures to the right.

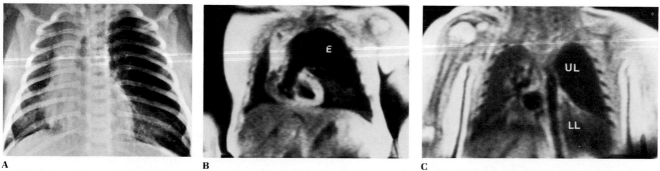

Figure 27-3 Lobar emphysema—left upper lobe. A. The chest radiograph shows marked hyperinflation of the left upper lung field with separation of the ribs and displacement of the mediastinal structures to the right. **B.** The T_1-weighted coronal MR image shows similar findings to those on the chest radiograph. There is marked hyperinflation of the left upper lobe (E) with significant displacement of the heart and mediastinal structures to the right. **C.** The T_1-weighted image was obtained more posteriorly. There is hyperinflation of the left upper lobe. *Note:* There is significant reduction in signal intensity from the emphysematous left upper lobe (UL), and there is a clear demarcation between the abnormal upper lobe and the slightly compressed lower lobe (LL).

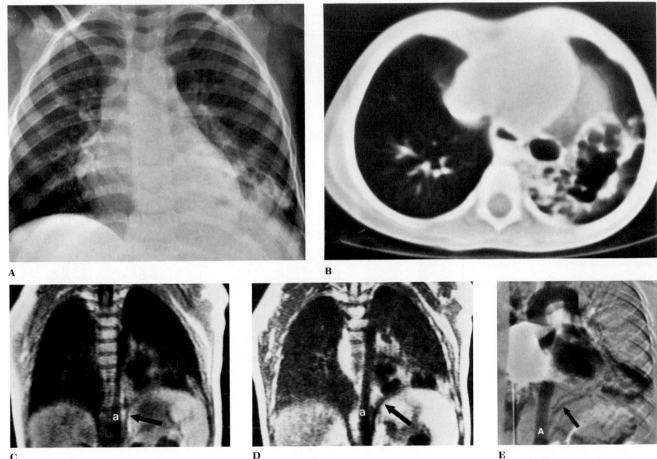

Figure 27-4   Pulmonary sequestration. A. This child presented with recurrent episodes of fever and persistent abnormality on chest radiograph. The chest radiograph shows patchy densities in the left lower lung field. The outline of the left hemidiaphragm cannot be defined. Some ill-defined areas of increased lucency are also seen in the left lower lung field. **B.** The CT scan shows a complex lesion in the left lower lung field. There are abnormal areas of soft tissue density. Fluid and air-filled cystic areas are also identified. **C** and **D.** These are coronal T_1- and T_2-weighted MR images. Both images show a complex lesion in the left lower lung field. The soft tissue components of the abnormality have a moderate intensity on the T_1-weighted image and demonstrate increased signal intensity on the T_2-weighted image. Both images show the descending aorta (a). An abnormal vessel (arrow) is seen running from the descending aorta to the pulmonary sequestration. **E.** This digital vascular angiogram also shows the abnormal vessel (arrow) running from the descending aorta (A) to the sequestration.

4). The internal structure varies considerably on both T_1- and T_2-weighted pulse sequences. Magnetic resonance can identify feeding vessels from the aorta to the region of sequestration (Figure 27-4). When these vessels are identified, the diagnosis of sequestration can be confidently made.

Trauma and Mechanical Disorders

Areas of contusion in the lungs can be identified following blunt trauma to the chest wall (Figure 27-5). The appearance of blood on MR images is complex and varies depending on its age. In the acute phase, blood has a relatively long T_1 and long T_2 relaxation

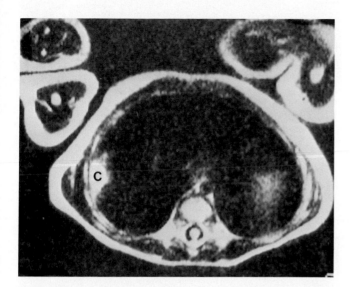

Figure 27-5 Pulmonary contusion. This T_2-weighted image was obtained several days after direct trauma to the lower right side of the chest wall. A moderately well defined region of high intensity is seen adjacent to the pleural surface. This is believed to be a region of pulmonary contusion (C).

time. Over a period of a few days the T_1 relaxation time shortens significantly. Blood thus appears of relatively strong signal intensity on T_2-weighted images, irrespective of age. On the T_1-weighted images, the intensity is low initially and increases with time. The appearance of a contusion in the lung will be very similar to that of a pulmonary infarct on MR imaging.

Lobar collapse (Figures 27-6 and 27-7) is readily identified by MR imaging. There is a sharp interface between the collapsed lobe and the adjacent normal lung (Figure 27-7). The ability to image in multiple planes allows excellent anatomic delineation of collapsed lobes or segments of lung. Total lung collapse can also be seen (Figure 27-8). Collapsed lung appears to show less change in signal intensity (Figure 27-7) between T_1- and T_2-weighted images than acute inflammation or tumor in the lung. In difficult cases, this finding might help in distinguishing focal areas of collapse from infection. Air bronchograms with crowding of bronchi may be seen in collapsed lung

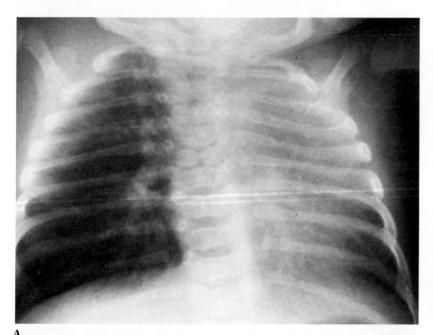

A

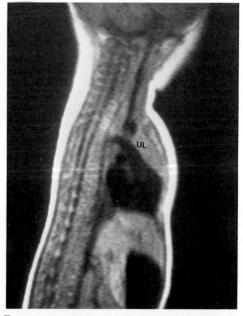

B

Figure 27-6 Collapsed left upper lobe. A. The chest radiograph shows opacification of the left upper lung field with a shift of the mediastinal structures to the left. **B.** The sagittal T_1-weighted MR image shows a collapsed left upper lobe (UL). There is sharp demarcation between the upper and lower lobes.

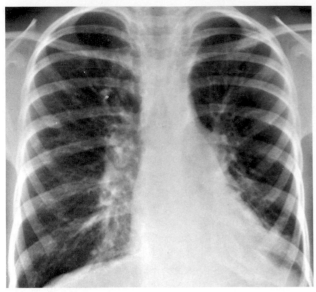

A

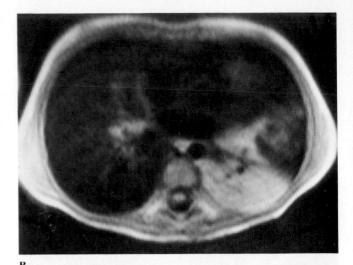

B

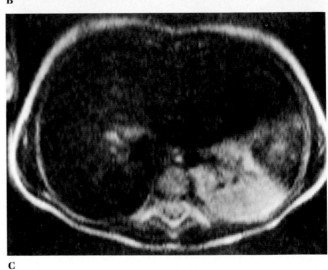

C

Figure 27-7 Collapsed left lower lobe. A. The chest radiograph shows a collapsed left lower lobe. **B.** The T_1-weighted image shows a moderate signal from the left lower lobe. There is crowding of the bronchi. The volume of the lobe is small. **C.** On this strongly T_2-weighted image [echo time (TE) = 150 and TR = 1000], the abnormality of the left lower lobe is again seen. The extent appears similar to that seen on the T_1-weighted image. There has been a very slight change in the signal intensity between the T_1- and T_2-weighted images. This finding suggests the absence of any acute inflammatory process.

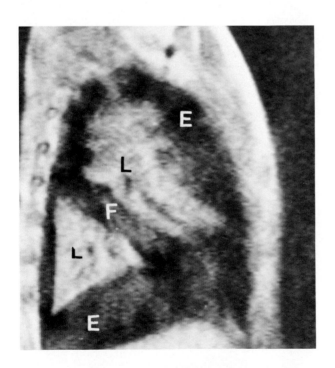

Figure 27-8 Massive pleural effusion with secondary collapse of the underlying lung. The coronal T_1-weighted MR image clearly distinguishes collapsed lung from pleural effusion. The collapsed lung (L) has a moderately strong signal. The surrounding effusion (E) is of very low intensity. Fluid in the oblique fissure (F) is nicely demonstrated.

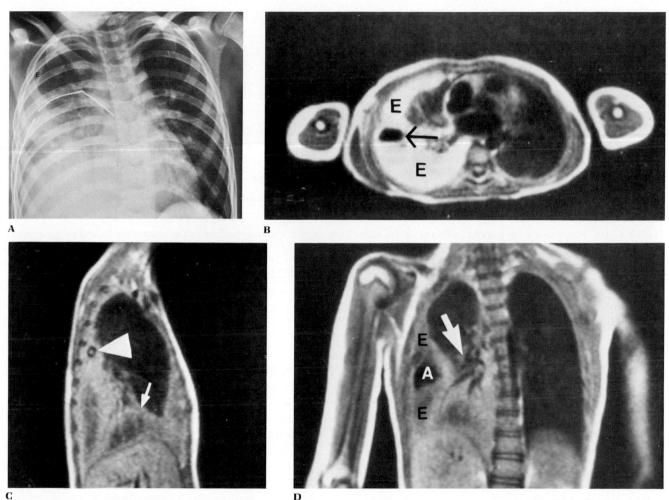

Figure 27-9   Staphylococcal empyema. A. This chest radiograph, taken several days after the insertion of a chest drainage tube, shows a large opacification of the right lower lung field. The chest radiograph cannot distinguish residual empyema from collapsed right lower lung or pneumonic consolidation of the right lower lung. **B, C,** and **D.** These three MR images, taken in the transverse, sagittal, and coronal planes, respectively show the presence of a very large residual empyema (E). Some collapsed right lower lobe is identified because of visualization of an air bronchogram. In part B, a T_2-weighted gated image (TE = 60), the empyema (E) is seen as a thick band of very high intensity. A small amount of air (arrow) is seen in the pleural space. In part C, a sagittal T_1-weighted gated image (TE = 30), the signal from the empyema fluid is much lower than that seen on the T_2-weighted image. Collapse in the right lower lobe is identified by the presence of an air bronchogram, with crowding of the bronchi (arrow). The pleural drainage tube (arrowhead) is identified in the superior aspect of the oblique fissure. It lies away from the main mass of the empyema and is thus ineffective in draining the empyema. In part D, a coronal T_1-weighted gated image (TE = 30), shows the empyema (E), air (A) in the pleural space, and air bronchogram in the collapsed right lower lobe (arrow).

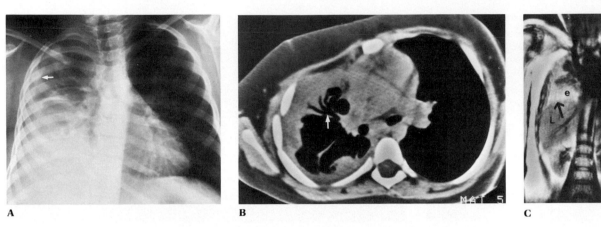

A   B   C

Figure 27-10   Empyema with partial collapse of the right lung. A. The chest radiograph shows opacification of the right lower lung field with pleural fluid seen superiorly (arrow). There is overinflation of the left lung. **B.** The CT scan shows irregular thickening of the pleura due to the presence of empyema. An air bronchogram, with crowding of bronchi, is seen anteriorly (arrow). This indicates the presence of collapsed lung tissue. There is no sharp demarcation between the lung and the empyema. *Note:* There is marked asymmetry of the hemithorax due to overinflation of the left lung and collapse on the right. **C.** This coronal T_1-weighted MR image (TE = 30, TR = 500) shows extensive abnormality in the right lung but does not clearly differentiate empyema from lung collapse or inflammation. The elevated hemidiaphragm (arrow) is well seen. The liver (L) is of much lower intensity than the empyema fluid (e). The overexpansion of the left hemithorax and the reduction in size of the right hemithorax are easily identified.

segments (Figure 27-9) with significant volume loss in one side of the chest. Coronal MR images clearly show the reduction in size of the affected hemithorax, the elevation of the hemidiaphragm, the mediastinal shift, and opposite compensatory emphysema (Figure 27-10).

Inflammatory Disorders

Magnetic resonance can identify areas of pneumonia (Figures 27-11 to 27-13), abscesses, and pseudotumors. In patients with pneumonia the extent of abnormality seen on MR corresponds fairly well with that of chest radiographs (Figures 27-11 and 27-12). The margins of abnormal lung are sharp when the pneumonia is adjacent to a fissure (Figure 27-12), but ill-defined and irregular where no such contact exists. Areas of pneumonia show significant change in signal intensity between T_1- and T_2-weighted images (Figures 27-13 and 27-14). Compared with the intensity of the muscles of the chest wall, the areas of pneumonia have a relatively low intensity on T_1-weighted images and a very high intensity on T_2-

weighted images. Air bronchograms can usually be identified within the pneumonic areas. Except for the air bronchograms, the regions of pneumonia usually appear fairly homogeneous on both T_1- and T_2-weighted images (Figure 27-11). Abscesses can be clearly identified in most cases (Figures 27-15 to 27-17). The cavity of the abscess may or may not contain air. When inflammatory fluid is present, it usually has a very strong signal intensity on T_2-weighted images, similar to that of fat. On T_1-weighted images the signal intensity will vary, depending significantly on the nature of the fluid in the cavity. When it is very liquid, the signal will often be low. When the fluid is more viscous, a stronger signal may be obtained. The wall of the abscess, presumably because of the presence of less inflammatory edema, shows less change in signal intensity between T_1- and T_2-weighted images (Figure 27-16) than does the abscess cavity or surrounding pneumonia. The amount of pneumonic consolidation around the abscess will vary considerably between patients (Figures 27-16 and 27-17). Inflammatory pseudotumors (Figure 27-18) in the lung show less change in signal intensity between T_1- and T_2-weighted images than do areas of pneumonia.

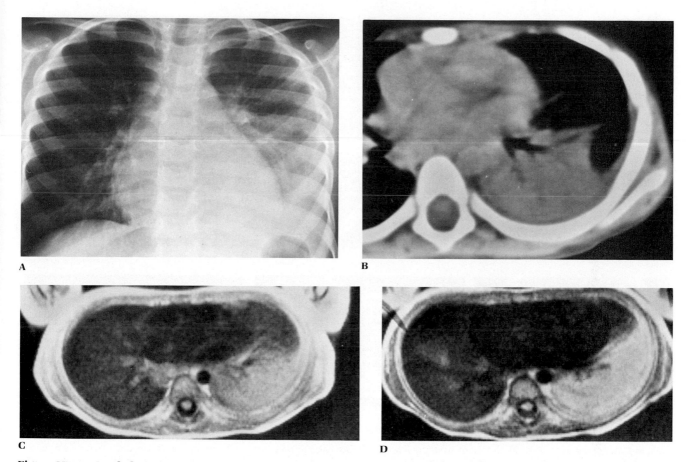

Figure 27-11   Staphylococcal pneumonia. A. The chest radiograph shows consolidation of the left lower lobe. A small associated pleural effusion is seen. **B.** The CT scan shows opacification of the left lower lung consistent with pneumonia. **C.** On the T_1-weighted MR image (TE = 30, TR = 500), an extensive, moderately homogeneous, increased signal can be seen in the left lower lobe. No significant volume loss is appreciated. **D.** On the T_2-weighted MR image (TE = 60, TR = 1000), there is a moderate increase in signal intensity from the pneumonia in the left lower lobe. The extent of the consolidation is again well shown.

They may cause compression of the airway and associated peripheral collapse.

Magnetic resonance may be more sensitive than chest radiographs for monitoring the response of infections to therapy (Figure 27-14).

Tumors

Lung metastases are visualized as well-defined focal areas of increased intensity seen in the lung parenchyma (Figure 27-19). Magnetic resonance imaging has not yet proved to be as sensitive as CT for

identifying small lung metastases (Figure 27-20),[6] nor has it been found to be specific for distinguishing metastases from other causes of lung nodules (Figure 27-21). In most regions of the lung, CT can identify smaller lung nodules than can be identified by MR. Magnetic resonance is better than CT only for identifying some small nodules lying close to vessels of similar diameter. On the CT scan the nodules appear of similar intensity to vessels, but on MR the vessels are of very low intensity. Primary tumors of the lung are rare, but they can be identified by MR imaging (Figure 27-22). No specific features distin-

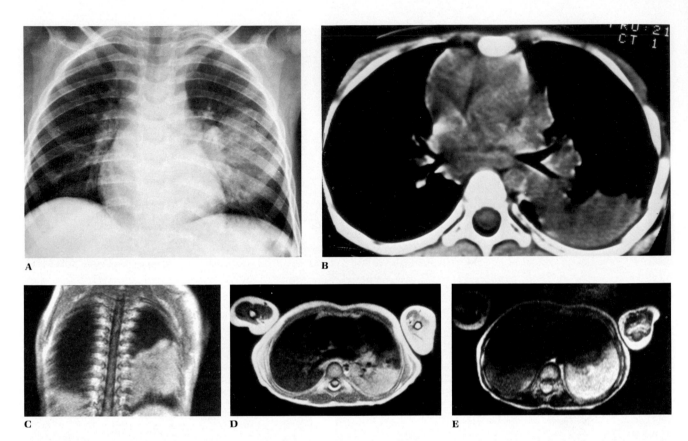

Figure 27-12 Chronic suppurative pneumonia. This patient had persistent episodes of infection of the left lower lobe. **A.** The chest radiograph shows consolidation of most of the left lower lobe with sparing of the inferior aspect. **B.** On the CT scan, a nonspecific soft tissue opacification appears in the region of the left lower lobe. **C.** The coronal T_1-weighted MR image (TE = 30, TR = 500), taken through the posterior aspect of the chest, shows the extent of abnormality in the left lower lobe extremely well. There is a homogeneous increased signal from almost the entire lower lobe. The inferior segment is spared. **D.** On the transverse T_1-weighted MR image (TE = 30, TR = 500), an increased signal is seen from the left lower lobe. There is no significant volume loss. **E.** On the strongly T_2-weighted transverse image (TE = 90, TR = 1000), a very strong signal is obtained from the pneumonia in the left lower lobe. There is a moderately sharp demarcation between the diseased lobe and the adjacent normal lung.

Figure 27-13 Histoplasma pneumonia of the left upper lobe with extension into the mediastinal lymph nodes. A and B. The posteroanterior and lateral chest radiographs show opacification of the left upper lobe. A slight displacement of the proximal part of the left main stem bronchus (arrow) suggests the presence of adjacent enlarged hilar lymph nodes. **C.** The CT scan shows homogeneous opacification of the left upper lobe. It is clearly distinguished from the thymus (T) and the contrast-opacified mediastinal vessels (arrows). An enlarged lymph node (N) can be seen adjacent to the trachea. **D.** The transverse T_1-weighted MR image (TE = 30, TR = 500) shows a homogeneous abnormality of the left upper lobe. The signal intensity is just above that of muscle. Without the use of contrast agents the superior vena cava (s) and the aortic arch (a) are easily seen. An enlarged lymph node (n) is identified. **E and F.** These are T_1-weighted (TE = 30, TR = 500) and T_2-weighted (TE = 120, TR = 2000) coronal images. Both show the pneumonia (P) in the left upper lobe. *Note:* There is a very marked change in signal intensity between the T_1- and T_2-weighted images. This suggests an acute inflammatory process. These coronal images show extensive paratracheal lymph node enlargement (arrows). The coronal images also show the extent of the lymph node disease to a greater degree than the chest radiograph or CT scan. *Note:* The signal intensity of the lymph nodes changes to the same extent as that of the inflamed lung.

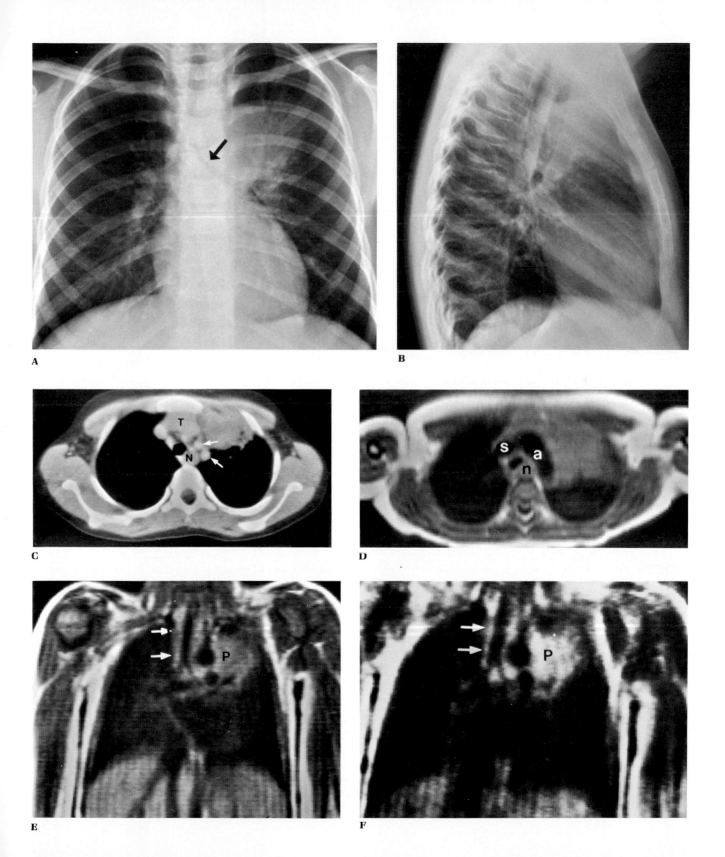

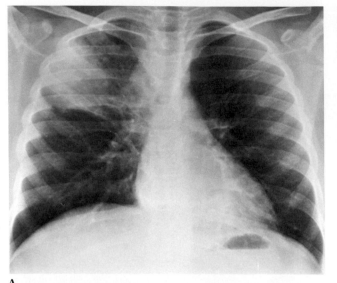

A

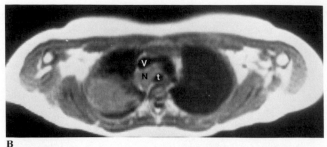

B

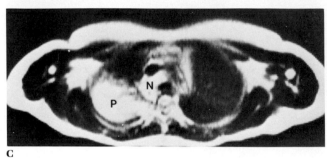

C

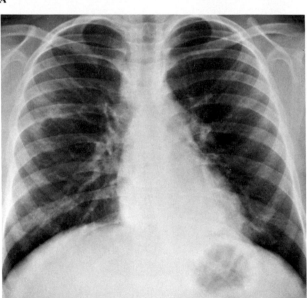

D

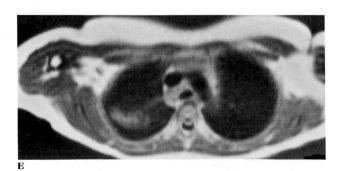

E

Figure 27-14 Right upper lobe pneumonia—pretherapy and posttherapy images. An 8-year-old girl with cystic fibrosis developed fever. **A.** The chest radiograph reveals a density in the right upper lobe. **B.** The T_1-weighted transverse MR image (TE = 30, TR = 500) shows an increased signal from the posterior segment of the right upper lobe. *Note:* There is a sharp posterior interface where the fissure demarcates the diseased upper lobe from the normal apical segment of the lower lobe. The anterior margins of the pneumonia are poorly defined because there is no sharp anatomic interface between the anterior and posterior segments of the upper lobe. An enlarged lymph node (N) is seen between the superior vena cava (V) and the trachea (t). It is of similar intensity to the pneumonia. **C.** The T_2-weighted transverse image (TE = 90, TR = 1000) also shows the pneumonia (P) in the right upper lobe and disease in the mediastinal lymph nodes (N). There has been marked increase in the signal intensity of both the pneumonia and the lymph node compared with the T_1-weighted image (part B). This is compatible with an acute rather than a chronic inflammatory process or collapse. **D.** On the chest radiograph taken after 3 weeks of antibiotics, there is an ill-defined hazy opacification in the right upper lobe. **E.** The MR scan taken on the same day as the chest radiograph (part D) shows more clearly the residual abnormality in the right upper lobe and in the paratracheal lymph nodes. The extent of disease is significantly less than it was before antibiotic therapy.

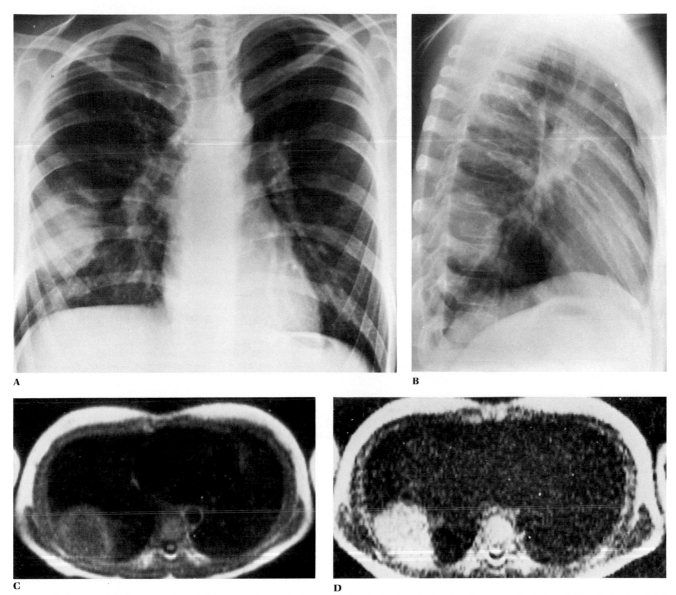

Figure 27-15   Lung abscess.   A and **B.** The posteroanterior and lateral chest radiographs show a well-defined density in the right lower lobe. On the frontal radiograph, a small amount of air can be seen in the superior aspect of the abscess. **C.** The T_1-weighted MR image identifies the abscess clearly. The abscess has a well-defined wall of slightly higher intensity than the central content. Very little surrounding inflammation in the lung parenchyma can be identified. **D.** The transverse, strongly T_2-weighted image shows a marked change in signal intensity from both the wall and central region of the abscess. The wall and central region can no longer be differentiated. Again note the absence of significant inflammation in the surrounding lung tissues. The change in signal intensity between the T_1- and T_2-weighted images is consistent with an acute inflammatory process.

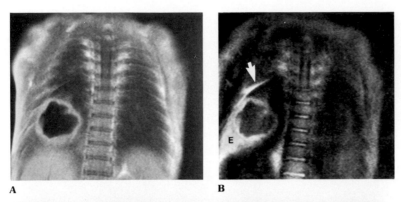

A

B

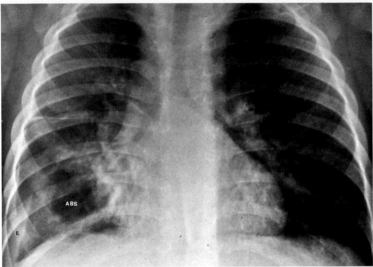

C

Figure 27-16 Abscess—right lower lobe. A.
On the T_1-weighted image (T = 30, TR = 500), the
abscess in the right lower lobe is clearly seen. The
abscess contains air which appears black. The abscess wall is well defined. It is of moderate thickness and moderate intensity. **B.** On the strongly T_2-
weighted image (TE = 60, TR = 2000), a very
strong intensity signal is obtained from a pleural
effusion (E). Some fluid is seen extending into the
horizontal fissure (arrow). There has been very little change in the signal intensity from the abscess
wall. Little inflammation is seen in the surrounding lung. **C.** The chest radiograph shows an ill-defined cavity in the right lower lung field. There is
a pleural effusion (E). Another density lies between
the lateral effusion and the abscess cavity (ABS).
On chest radiograph one cannot distinguish between lung consolidation and posteriorly placed
effusion fluid. The MR image suggests that the entire abnormality is due to the pleural effusion,
which lies lateral and posterior to the lung.

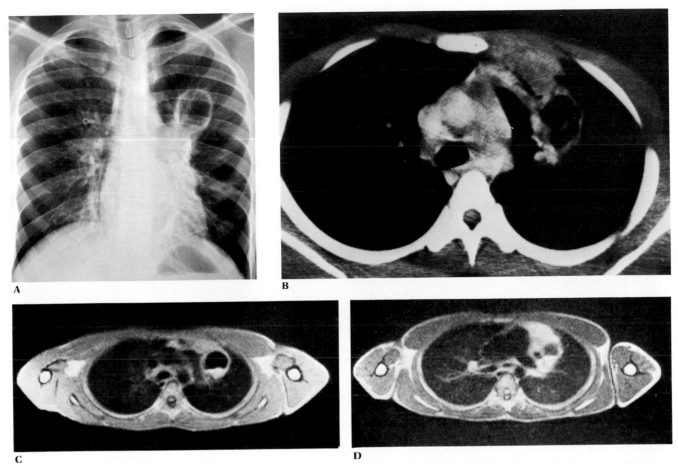

Figure 27-17   Lung abscess. A. On the chest radiograph, a cavity appears in the left upper lung field. It has a thin but well-defined margin. A more homogeneous density overlies the left hilum. **B.** The CT scan shows the cavity in the left upper lobe. The density seen overlying the hilum on the chest radiograph is shown to lie anteriorly. Computed tomography cannot distinguish collapsed lung tissue from infection. **C** and **D.** These are transverse MR images. Part C is a T_1 weighted image (TE = 30, TR = 500) and part D is a T_2-weighted image (TE = 60, TR = 1000). Image C is obtained at a slightly higher level than D. Both images, however, show the cavitation in the left upper lobe. On the T_1-weighted image the wall has a moderately strong signal, slightly greater than that of muscle. The adjacent soft tissue abnormality has a lower signal. On the T_2-weighted image there has been a significant enhancement of signal from the lung parenchyma around the abscess cavity. This strongly suggests the presence of pneumonic consolidation rather than collapse.

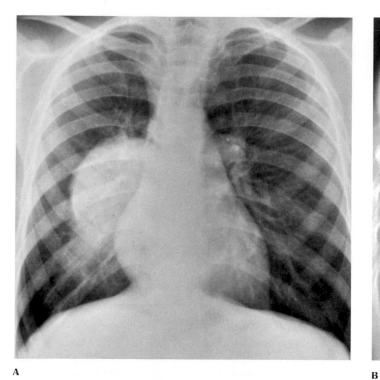

A

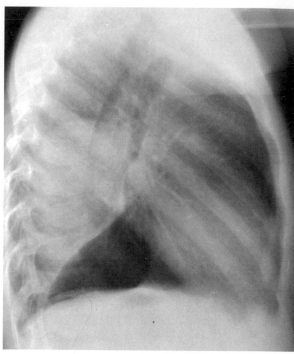

B

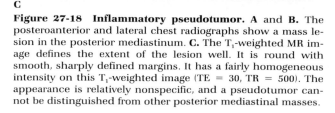

C

Figure 27-18 Inflammatory pseudotumor. A and **B.** The posteroanterior and lateral chest radiographs show a mass lesion in the posterior mediastinum. **C.** The T_1-weighted MR image defines the extent of the lesion well. It is round with smooth, sharply defined margins. It has a fairly homogeneous intensity on this T_1-weighted image (TE = 30, TR = 500). The appearance is relatively nonspecific, and a pseudotumor cannot be distinguished from other posterior mediastinal masses.

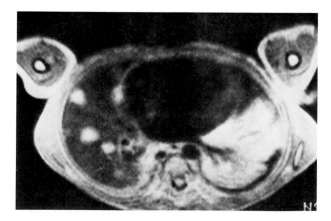

Figure 27-19 Pulmonary metastasis from Wilms's tumor. This transverse MR image (TE = 30, TR = 2000) shows multiple nodules in the right lower lung field. These are of moderately strong intensity. They are metastases from the patient's known Wilms's tumor.

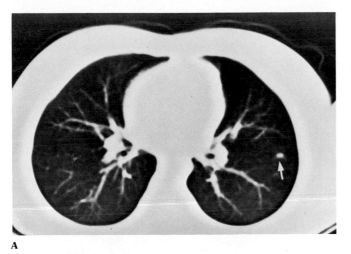

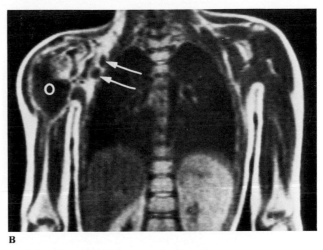

A

B

Figure 27-20 Osteogenic sarcoma metastases. A. The CT scan shows a metastasis in the left midlung field (arrow). **B.** The T_1-weighted MR image (TE = 30, TR = 500) fails to demonstrate the lung metastasis. The primary osteogenic sarcoma (O) is seen in the right proximal humerus. Calcified metastases are seen in the axillary lymph nodes (arrows).

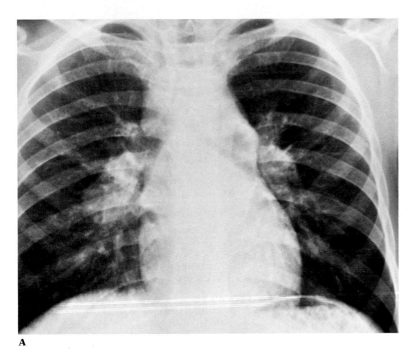

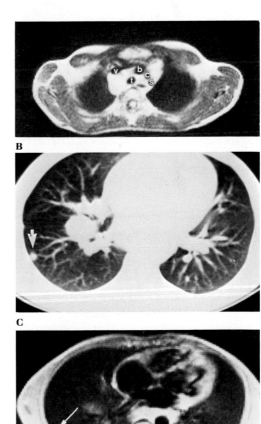

A

B

C

D

Figure 27-21 Hodgkin's disease of the mediastinum and lung. A. The chest radiograph shows enlargement of mediastinal and hilar lymph nodes. **B.** The transverse T_2-weighted image (TE = 60, TR = 1000) is taken through the level of the upper mediastinum. Massive lymph node enlargement is identified. The lymph nodes all appear white. The superior vena cava (v), brachiocephalic artery (b), left common carotid artery (c), and left subclavian artery (s) are well identified. The trachea (t) is surrounded by nodes. **C.** The CT scan through the lower chest shows a metastatic nodule in the right lower lung field (arrow). **D.** The T_1-weighted MR image (TE = 30, TR = 500) also shows the lung nodule (arrow).

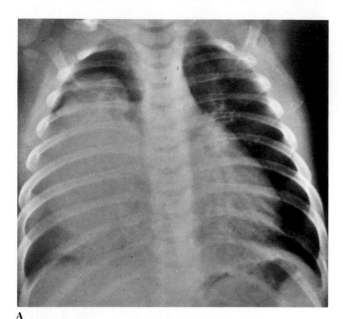

A

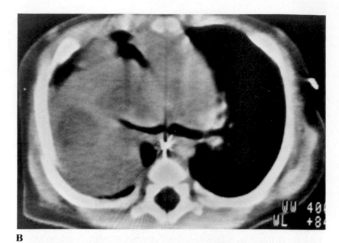

B

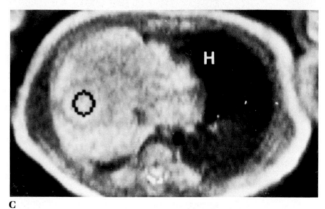

C

Figure 27-22 Rhabdomyosarcoma of the lung. A. The chest radiograph shows a large mass lesion in the right hemithorax. It is of soft tissue intensity. **B.** The CT scan also shows a large right-sided mass lesion of varying intensity. The tumor cannot be distinguished from the adjacent mediastinal structures, and it is not possible to determine whether it arises from the mediastinum, lung, or pleura. **C.** The transverse spin density MR image shows a large tumor mass. The margins are much better defined than on the CT scan. The tumor appears of very high intensity. The heart (H) is displaced toward the left.

guish benign lesions from malignant ones. Chronic inflammatory nodules can also be identified. Small areas of calcification which frequently appear on CT are not seen on MR. This is a significant disadvantage of MR, except for calcification in osteogenic metastases, as almost all calcified nodules in the lung are benign. There is a suggestion, however, that because of their fibrous nature, benign nodules such as old histoplasmosis will show little change in signal intensity between T_1- and T_2-weighted images. It is believed that this finding will help to distinguish such nodules from metastases, which typically are of much greater intensity on T_2- than on T_1-weighted images. It must be remembered, however, that in areas where histoplasma is endemic, patients with tumors may have both metastases and histoplasma nodules in their lungs.

Diffuse Lung Disorders

Many diffuse lung disorders appear similar on chest radiographs, and in many cases a biopsy is required to obtain a definitive diagnosis. Initial studies with MR evaluation of diffuse lung disease indicate that some disorders, indistinguishable on chest radiographs, appear different on MR images. The exact specificity and sensitivity of MR for the evaluation of diffuse lung disease are, however, not yet known.

On MR images, miliary tuberculosis (Figure 27-23) has moderately well-defined nodules distributed throughout both lungs. The intensity of the nodules is similar to that of muscle on T_1-weighted images, but becomes very strong, similar to the intensity of fat, on T_2-weighted images. In addition to the lung

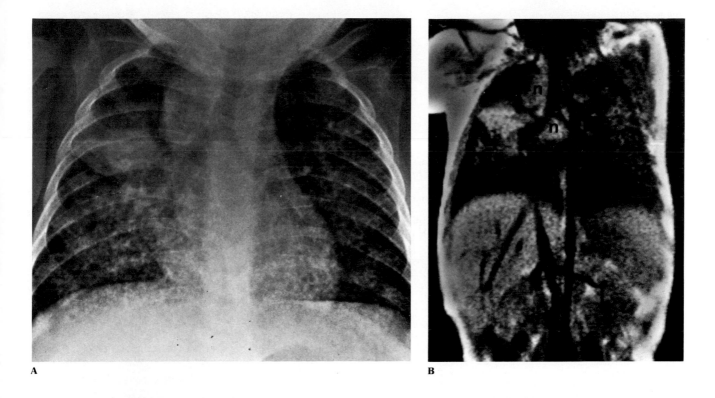

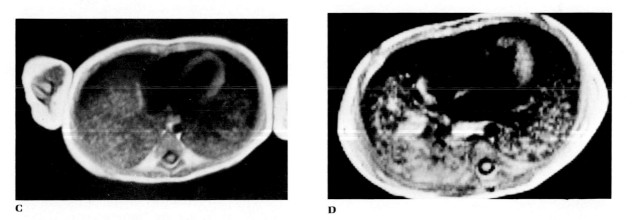

Figure 27-23   Miliary tuberculosis. A. The chest radiograph shows diffuse nodules throughout both lung fields. There is an area of more confluent consolidation in the right upper lobe. Enlarged right paratracheal lymph nodes are also identified. **B** and **C.** The transverse and coronal T_1-weighted MR images (TE = 30, TR = 500) show a diffuse, granular abnormality throughout both lung fields. The coronal image shows the confluent pneumonia in the right upper lobe. The right paratracheal lymph nodes (n) are clearly seen. In addition the MR identifies diseased lymph nodes (n) in the subcarinal area. **D.** The T_2-weighted MR image (TE = 60, TR = 1000) shows a significant increase in signal intensity from the nodules. The nodules are more discrete with this pulse sequence. The change in image intensity compared with that of the T_1 image suggests an acute inflammatory process.

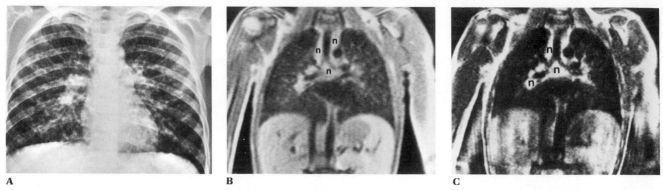

Figure 27-24   Disseminated pulmonary histoplasmosis with mediastinal lymph node involvement. A. The chest radiograph shows ill-defined nodular abnormality of both lung fields. **B.** The coronal MR image (TE = 30, TR = 1000) shows a hazy, ill-defined abnormality in both lung fields. Enlarged lymph nodes (n) are seen in the paratracheal, subcarinal, and hilar regions. **C.** The T_2-weighted MR image (TE = 60, TR = 1000) shows a significant increase in signal from the mediastinal lymph nodes (n). The nodes are easily identified and distinguished from the trachea and mediastinal vessels. The pulmonary disease is much less readily appreciated on this pulse sequence. This is very different from the patient with tuberculosis (Figure 27-23).

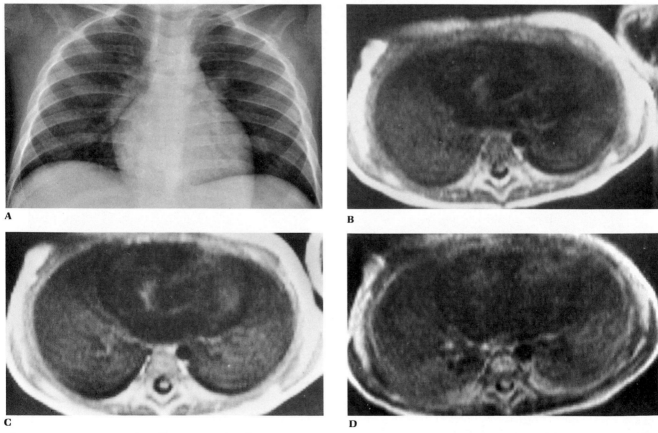

Figure 27-25   Letterer-Siwe disease. A. The abnormality is difficult to identify on this chest radiograph. There is a subtle, hazy, nodular pattern in the lung fields. **B, C,** and **D.** These images are transverse inversion recovery (TI = 450, TR = 500), T_1-weighted (TE = 30, TR = 500), and T_2-weighted (TE = 60, TR = 2000) images. All show a definite, hazy, uniform granularity distributed throughout both lung fields. Much more abnormality is seen on the MR images than on the chest radiograph. The signal intensity from the diseased lungs is fairly similar on all three pulse sequences. This is very different from the appearance seen in miliary tuberculosis.

disease, enlarged lymph nodes in the hila and mediastinum can also be identified. With diffuse histoplasmosis, enlarged lymph nodes, similar to those in tuberculosis, can be identified. The diffuse nodular densities seen on chest radiographs with diffuse histoplasmosis are much less well visualized and much less sharply defined on MR images than are tuberculosis nodules (Figure 27-24). They show much less change in signal intensity between T_1- and T_2-weighted images.

With Letterer-Siwe disease (Figure 27-25), MR shows more abnormality than is evident on chest radiographs. On the MR image, the diseased area takes on a hazy, granular, ground-glass appearance with much less definition of the lung nodules than with tuberculosis. No individual nodules can be identified. The appearance in allergic alveolitis is somewhat similar to that seen with Letterer-Siwe disease, but allergic alveolitis responds far more quickly to therapy.

Pulmonary edema (Figure 27-26) appears as a hazy granularity varying in texture from fine to coarse. On the coronal images the perihilar distribution of the edema can be well-identified (Figure 27-26). When the pulmonary edema is cardiogenic in origin, an enlarged heart can usually be identified as well (Figure 27-26). Associated pleural effusions are also often present.

In patients with cystic fibrosis it is hoped that MR might be able to resolve some of the problems that are encountered on the chest radiograph. The findings on chest radiographs will often not correlate with the clinical status of the patients. A clinical relapse may occur with little change in the chest radiograph. It is also often difficult on the chest radiograph to distinguish areas of collapse caused by mucous plugs or pneumonia. In patients with cystic fibrosis the blood vessels produce linear branching structures of very low intensity, whereas mucoid-impacted bronchi are seen as linear branching structures of intermediate or moderate intensity. Peribronchial inflammation causes curved branching areas of increased intensity outlining the lumina of the adjacent bronchi.[7]

Diffuse pulmonary vascular malformations (Figure 27-27) may be difficult to identify if the flow of blood is fast and the malformations have little soft tissue component. Where blood flow is slow, paradoxical enhancement of the signal from the flowing blood will be seen.

Pulmonary lymphangiectasia (Figure 27-28) has a coarse, patchy abnormality with a mild increase in signal on T_2-weighted images. Magnetic resonance shows more abnormality than chest radiograph.

Pleural Effusions

Magnetic resonance may accurately identify pleural effusion (Figure 27-29). The signal intensity will de-

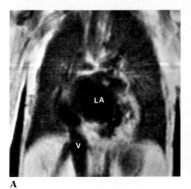 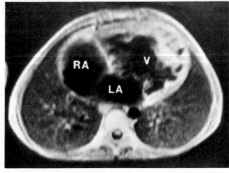 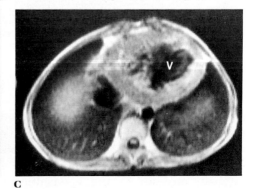

A   B   C

Figure 27-26   Pulmonary edema. Complex congenital heart disease. All images have a TE of 30 ms and are gated. **A.** The coronal image shows pulmonary edema. There is an increased perihilar signal intensity from the lung. The left atrium (LA) is enlarged, and the inferior vena cava (V) is also significantly enlarged. **B** and **C.** These transverse images are taken in diastole and systole. They show an enlarged heart. There is a single ventricle (V), and the right atrium (RA) and left atrium (LA) can be distinguished. The hazy abnormality in the lung fields is consistent with edema.

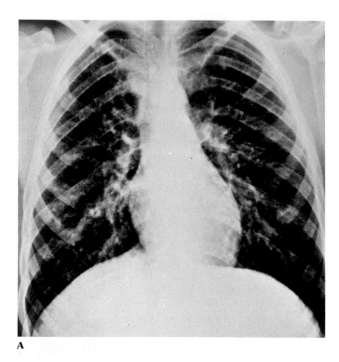

A

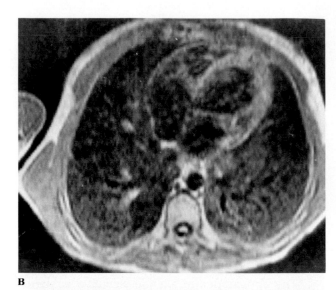

B

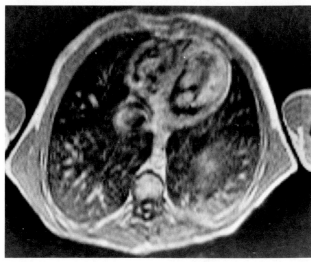

C

Figure 27-27 Pulmonary arteriovenous malformations. Diffuse, small pulmonary arteriovenous vascular malformations are present in this cyanotic child (proved by angiography and isotope studies). **A.** The chest radiograph shows a normal-sized heart. No focal vascular malformations can be seen in the lung fields, but diffusely irregular vessels are present. **B** and **C.** These are T_1-gated MR images with a TE of 30 ms. Part B is obtained in diastole, and part C, in systole. The diastolic image shows a fairly uniform, hazy granularity in both lung fields. On the systolic image, branching structures of high intensity are seen toward the lung periphery. These are believed to be prominent vessels, with the strong signal due to paradoxical enhancement from altered flow rates. The MR images show much more abnormality than the chest radiograph.

pend on the nature of the liquid. There is a correlation between the protein content of the effusion and the T_1 relaxation time.[8] Because of the presence of fat in chylous effusions, this type will have a very strong intensity on both T_1- and T_2-weighted images. Empyema (Figure 27-10) will have margins that are not as smooth as simple effusions, and more often produce loculation. Massive effusions can collapse the underlying lung (Figure 27-8).

Mediastinum

Magnetic resonance is excellent for evaluating the mediastinum. The ability to image in the coronal plane frequently yields additional information, and there is excellent natural contrast between the blood vessels and the adjacent structures (Figures 27-13 and 27-30).

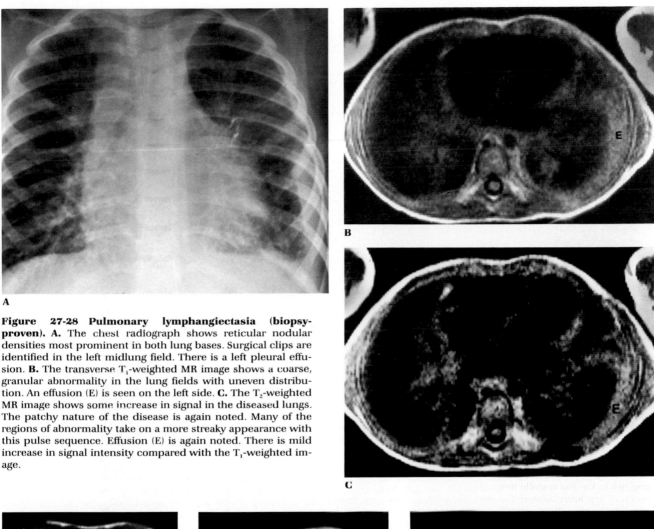

Figure 27-28 Pulmonary lymphangiectasia (biopsy-proven). A. The chest radiograph shows reticular nodular densities most prominent in both lung bases. Surgical clips are identified in the left midlung field. There is a left pleural effusion. **B.** The transverse T_1-weighted MR image shows a coarse, granular abnormality in the lung fields with uneven distribution. An effusion (E) is seen on the left side. **C.** The T_2-weighted MR image shows some increase in signal in the diseased lungs. The patchy nature of the disease is again noted. Many of the regions of abnormality take on a more streaky appearance with this pulse sequence. Effusion (E) is again noted. There is mild increase in signal intensity compared with the T_1-weighted image.

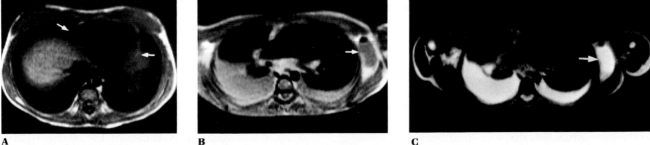

Figure 27-29 Pleural and pericardial effusions due to non-Hodgkin's lymphoma. A. The transverse image (TE = 30, TR = 2000) shows a moderate signal from a small pericardial effusion (arrows). **B** and **C.** On these transverse images (TE = 30, TR = 2000; TE = 150, TR = 2000, respectively), pleural effusions are identified on both sides. The images were taken following percutaneous partial drainage of the left effusion. Following needle withdrawal, some fluid has leaked from the pleural space into the soft tissues (arrow). The effusion is of moderate intensity on the mildly T_2-weighted image (part B) and of very high intensity on the strongly T_2-weighted image (part C). On these images, simple effusion cannot be distinguished from malignant effusion.

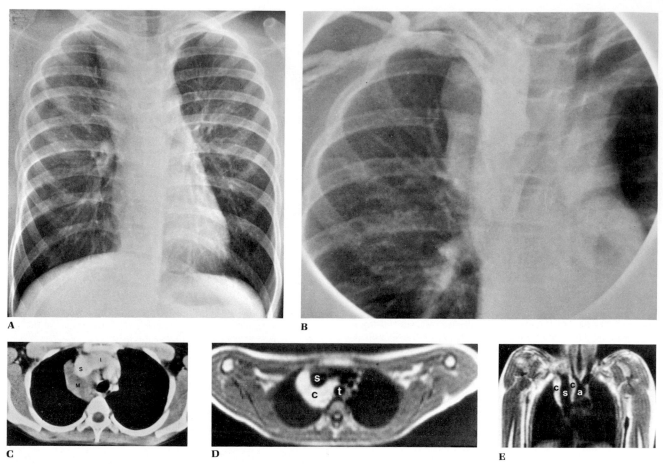

Figure 27-30 Mediastinal extension of cystic hygroma. This 9-year-old child had a cervical cystic hygroma excised in infancy. She presented with a mediastinal mass. **A.** The chest radiograph shows widening of the right superior mediastinum with displacement of the trachea to the left. **B.** The venogram shows a patent, but slightly widened, superior vena cava. **C.** The CT scan shows a moderately well defined soft tissue mass (M) of intensity slightly below that of muscle. The innominate vein (I) and superior vena cava (S) are well identified following bolus contrast injection. **D** and **E.** The transverse and coronal T_1-weighted MR images (TE = 30, TR = 500) clearly identify a well-defined mediastinal mass lesion of high intensity. This was cystic hygroma (c). It is clearly distinguishable from the superior vena cava (s), the trachea (t), and the aorta (a). *Note:* The lesion extends between the superior vena cava and the trachea and aorta. For this reason it is not surgically resectable. The high signal from the fluid in the cystic hygroma is believed to be due to a very high protein content of the fluid.

Magnetic resonance can identify a wide range of mediastinal abnormalities, localize the lesions, and in many cases categorize the disease. Congenital mass lesions that may be identified include bronchogenic cysts and extension of cystic hygroma into the thorax (Figure 27-30). Bronchogenic cysts appear as well-defined cystic lesions with low intensity on T_1-weighted images and with very high intensity on T_2-weighted images. Although fluid in nature, cystic hygromas will often give a very strong signal on T_1-weighted images. This is presumed to be due to lipid contained within the fluid of the cyst.

On a chest radiograph the thymus is often very difficult to distinguish from abnormal mediastinal mass lesions. The coronal MR images show the classical triangular shape of the lobes of the thymus and in many cases will accurately distinguish the thymus from other mass lesions in the anterior mediastinum.

Many anomalies of the great vessels can be readily identified by MR imaging. The position of the aortic arch in right aortic arch anomaly or in transposition of the great vessels is easily appreciated. Aberrant vessels, such as an aberrant subclavian artery, can also be readily seen.

In patients with infection or lymphoma, MR can identify enlarged lymph nodes in the anterior mediastinum and midmediastinum (Figures 27-21 and 27-24). Magnetic resonance has no difficulty in identifying nodes in the paratracheal, hilar, or subcarinal regions. The nodes contrast strongly with the adjacent vessels, trachea, and lung (Figures 27-13 and 27-14). They appear of intermediate intensity on T_1-weighted images and strong intensity on T_2-weighted images. Although MR can accurately define the number, size, and location of enlarged lymph nodes, it is not always able to separate inflammation from tumor (Figures 27-13 and 27-14). In patients with lymphoma, MR cannot distinguish Hodgkin's from non-Hodgkin's disease.

Displacement of the trachea due to lung disease or to mediastinal masses is readily appreciated. Tracheal narrowing by compression from adjacent mass lesions can also be identified and evaluated.

References

1. Zeitler E, Schittenhelm R: Nuclear magnetic resonance tomography (NMR tomography) and its clinical application possibilities. *Electromedica* 3:134, 1981.
2. Alfidi RJ, Haaga JR, El Yousef SJ, et al: Preliminary experimental results in humans and animals with a superconducting, whole-body, nuclear magnetic resonance scanner. *Radiology* 143:175, 1982.
3. Lufkin RB, Larsson SG, Hanafee WN: Work in progress: NMR anatomy of the larynx and tongue base. *Radiology* 148:173, 1983.
4. Hriack H, Williams RD, Spring DB, et al: Anatomy and pathology of the male pelvis by magnetic resonance imaging. *AJR* 141:1101, 1983.
5. Ross JS, O'Donovan PB, Novoa R, et al: Magnetic resonance of the chest: Initial experience with imaging and in vivo T_1 and T_2 calculations. *Radiology* 152:95, 1984.
6. Muller NL, Gamsu G, Webb WR: Pulmonary nodules: Detection using magnetic resonance and computed tomography. *Radiology* 155:687, 1985.
7. Gooding CA, Lallemand DP, Brasch RC, et al: Magnetic resonance imaging in cystic fibrosis. *J Pediatr* 105:384, 1984.
8. Revel D, Terrier F, Hricak H, et al: Determination of the nature of pleural effusions with MR imaging. RSNA Scientific Program, Washington, DC, Radiological Society of North America, 1984.

Chapter 28

Ultrasound of the Chest

Mervyn D. Cohen, M.B., Ch.B.

Technique

It is technically possible to obtain good ultrasound images of many of the thoracic structures. It is often helpful to scan the patient in different positions. The only limiting technical factor is that one must have an access window to the region of suspected disease.[1] Lesions of the chest wall are easily scanned without any problem; for the intrathoracic structures, the bony thorax does provide some problem. In young children, however, it is frequently possible to obtain satisfactory scans through the ribs. In older children, scans must be performed either through the intercostal spaces or by angling up from the abdomen or down through the suprasternal and supraclavicular regions. For this reason a sector scanner is almost always to be preferred over a linear array. In children, the thymus usually provides an adequate window to most of the mediastinum. The

thymus has a fine very homogeneous echo pattern.[2] Pulmonary parenchymal lesions can only be identified if they lie in the lung periphery adjacent to the pleura.[3] More centrally placed lung lesions cannot be identified because they are obscured by the overlying air in the lung. The actual technique of performing the ultrasound scans is the same as that used for the chest and for other sites in the body. The transducer should have the highest frequency that will give the desired depth penetration. A 5-MHz transducer is most often used.

Other problems are encountered in ultrasound scanning of the thorax. In many areas there are no clearly identifiable anatomic landmarks, and for this reason some lesions may be difficult to localize anatomically.[1] All lesions in the lung or adjacent to the lung will demonstrate strong posterior echoes irrespective of whether they are solid or cystic. This is because of the strong reflection of echoes from the air in the adjacent lung.[1,3]

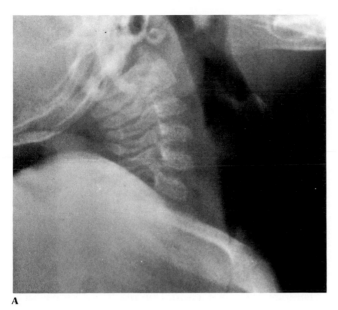

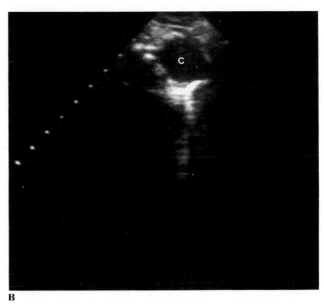

A   B

Figure 28-1   Enteric duplication cyst. A. The lateral neck radiograph shows a mass lesion of soft tissue density lying behind the trachea. The trachea is displaced forward. The lumen is markedly narrowed. The differential diagnosis is extensive. **B.** The cervical ultrasound clearly identifies the abnormality as a cyst (C). The margins are sharply defined. No echoes are obtained from the lesion. There is good through transmission of the sound waves with posterior enhancement. This appearance is due to either a bronchogenic or enteric duplication cyst. No additional studies were done. The lesion was successfully removed at surgery.

Indications

The use of ultrasound of the chest is indicated for evaluating the pleura, diaphragm, and mediastinum. Ultrasound is extremely useful in defining whether a lesion is cystic or solid (Figure 28-1),[4] although occasionally a bronchogenic or other cyst will be encountered which appears solid (Figure 28-2).[5] This is due to the presence of fatty or viscous material within the cysts, causing a return of echoes. In addition to identifying lesions as solid or fluid, ultrasound is very useful for localizing small fluid collections, particularly in the pleura, for needle aspiration.[1] The differentiation of solid from cystic lesion will often determine which studies are to be performed in the future. If a lesion is shown by ultrasound to be cystic, then CT should not be performed, as this will rarely add additional information.[6] In many cases, particularly in the

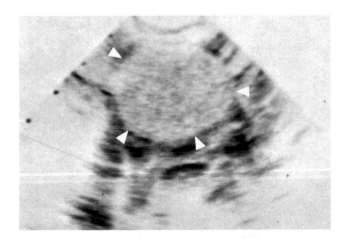

Figure 28-2   Cystic teratoma. The ultrasound scan of an anterior mediastinal mass shows a well-defined, large mass lesion (arrowheads). Uniform echoes of moderately low intensity were obtained from the lesion. This suggests that the lesion is solid and not cystic. At surgery, almost all the mass was found to be a large cyst. There were several small adjacent soft tissue components of this tumor. The reason that the cyst appeared solid on the ultrasound is that it was filled with thick, milky, mucoid material.

mediastinum, demonstration of a cystic lesion will result in surgery being performed without any further imaging studies. In the newborn presenting with an opaque hemithorax, ultrasound can distinguish cystic lesions from solid tumors. Another area where ultrasound has a major role to play is in the evaluation of the diaphragm. The diaphragm is seen as a strongly echogenic curvilinear structure. Ultrasound can very accurately determine the degree of excursion of the diaphragm and diagnose diaphragm paralysis. With diaphragmatic hernias (Figure 28-3) or eventration, particularly if the kidney or liver is involved, ultrasound can identify the abnormality and the herniated tissue.[1] (See Figures 12-18 and 12-19.) Visualization of the left diaphragm can sometimes be difficult if there is a large amount of gas in the stomach or splenic flexure.[3]

Cystic Hygroma

Cystic hygromas arise in the neck and may extend into the thorax. They are identified by ultrasound as multiple septate anechoic cysts of varying sizes.[7] Ul-

trasound can accurately define the margins and extent of most of these lesions. Hemorrhage into the cysts may produce internal echoes. Secondary inflammation and fibrosis may cause significant thickening of the cyst walls. Occasionally, cystic hygromas may occur in the mediastinum alone, and in these cases they can be impossible to differentiate from other mediastinal tumors, such as teratoma.[8]

Tumors

Ultrasound can identify a wide range of tumors of the chest wall, mediastinum, pleura, and adjacent lung. Most of these tumors appear as solid mass lesions (Figure 28-4). In many cases, ultrasound can accurately define the extent of the abnormality. The appearance in most cases is fairly nonspecific, and a histologic diagnosis cannot be made. Lesions which have been demonstrated include hemangiomas,[7] rhabdomyosarcoma, Ewing's tumor, neuroblastoma, lymphomas, and metastases from abdominal tumors.[7]

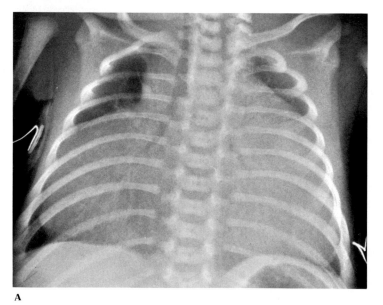

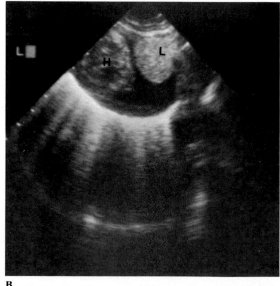

A   B

Figure 28-3   Diaphragmatic hernia. The liver herniated into the pericardial sac. **A.** The chest radiograph of this newborn infant shows a very large opacity involving right and left sides of the lower thorax. The medial border of the heart cannot be defined. **B.** Longitudinal oblique ultrasound shows the heart (H). There is a moderate amount of fluid (F) in the pericardial sac. The liver (L) is herniated into the pericardial sac.

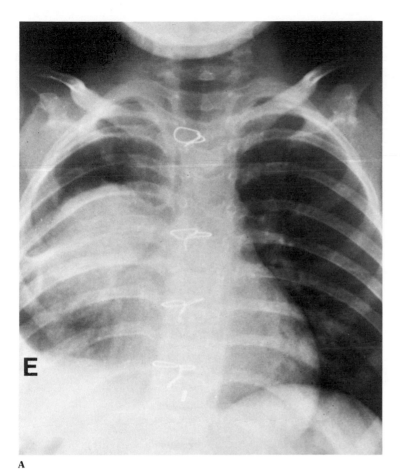

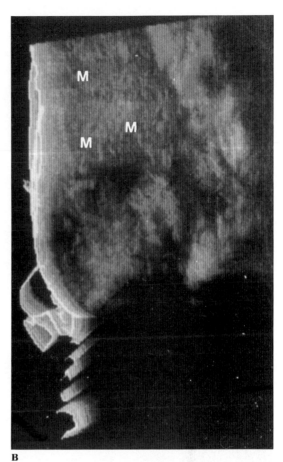

A   B

Figure 28-4   Pleural metastasis from Wilms's tumor. A. The chest radiograph shows a moderately well defined, round density in the right middle lung field. There is a large, right-sided pleural effusion (E). Differential diagnosis for the midlung lesion included a tumor or effusion loculated in the transverse fissure. **B.** An ultrasound study of the midlung lesion shows it to be solid and not cystic. It was in fact a metastasis (M) from the patient's known Wilms's tumor.

Cystic Adenomatoid Malformation

Cystic adenomatoid malformation is seen as a complex mass in the lung,[7] with cysts and solid tissue components (see Figure 3-10).[9] The cysts vary in size.[10] In type III cystic adenomatoid malformation, there are multiple, very small cysts with marked expansion of the lung. This type appears as a predominantly solid tumor mass.[11] Cystic adenomatoid malformation can be diagnosed in utero;[10,11] with type III malformation there may be associated fetal hydrops and hydramnios.[11] Differential diagnosis of cystic mass lesions seen in the lungs in utero or shortly after birth includes cystic adenomatoid malformation, sequestration, fluid-filled congenital lobar emphysema, and fluid-filled bowel loops with diaphragmatic hernia.

Parenchymal Lung Disease

Tumors, metastases, collapse, and infection all appear in the lung as echogenic abnormalities. The appearance is moderately nonspecific. Lung abscesses will have varying echoes, and may be almost echo-

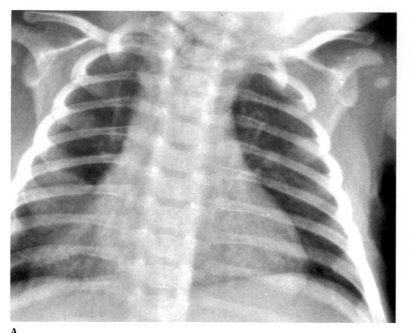

A

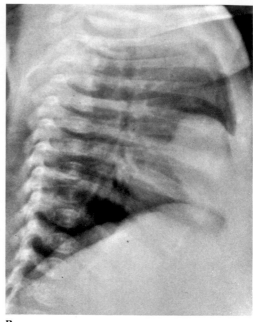

B

C

Figure 28-5   Right middle lobe abscess in a 3-week-old. A and **B.** The frontal and lateral radiographs show a moderately well defined opacity in the anterior aspect of the lower right lung field. A mediastinal lesion cannot be differentiated from a lung lesion. **C.** The longitudinal ultrasound identifies the liver (L) and diaphragm (D). Just above the diaphragm a moderately well defined cystic mass lesion (M) is seen. At surgery this was found to be an abscess of the middle lobe. The imaging studies could not differentiate this lesion from a pericardial cyst.

free if the pus is very liquid (Figure 28-5). The clinical utility of these findings is probably low because the lesions cannot be identified unless they are adjacent to the pleural surface.

Pleural Effusions

Ultrasound may identify pleural effusion in utero[12] or after birth. Simple effusions are anechoic and usually triangular.[3] Empyema appears as a complex pleural abnormality with solid and cystic lesions (Figure 28-6).[7] Ultrasound can distinguish effusion from fibrosis or other pleural masses,[13] define the extent of the abnormality, identify focal loculations, and guide needle aspiration.

Mediastinal Masses

Most mediastinal masses may be identified by ultrasound and characterized as solid (Figure 28-7) or cystic (Figure 28-1). As mentioned above, bronchogenic cysts can occasionally appear solid rather than cystic. Enteric duplication cysts can also be seen as well-defined cystic masses (Figure 28-1).

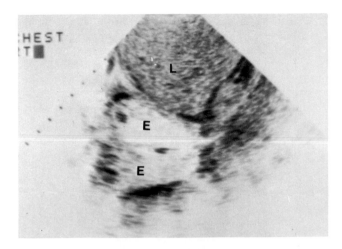

Figure 28-6   Empyema. A longitudinal ultrasound study on the right side shows a fairly homogeneous echo pattern from the normal liver (L). The diaphragm is seen as a strongly echogenic curvilinear structure between the liver and the adjacent empyema. The empyema (E) appears as a predominantly echo-free region just above the diaphragm. Patchy internal echoes are seen, due either to regions of very thick pus or to nonliquefied inflammation (see Figure 16-19).

References

1. Haller J, Schneider M, Kassner G, et al: Sonographic evaluation of the chest in infants and children. *AJR* 134:1091, 1980.
2. Parker LA, Gaisie G, Scatliff JH: Computerized tomography and ultrasonographic findings in massive thymic hyperplasia. *Clin Pediatr* 24:90, 1985.
3. Matalon TA, Neiman HL, Mintzer RA: Noncardiac chest sonography. The state of the art. *Chest* 4:675, 1983.
4. Jaffe C: Sonograms, radiographs and the mediastinum. *AJR* 137:422, 1981.
5. Ries T, Carrarino G, Nikaidoh M, et al: Real time ultrasonography of subcarinal bronchogenic cysts in two children. *Radiology* 145:121, 1982.
6. Cohen MD, Smith JA, Greenman GF: Ultrasound diagnosis of liquid-filled lesions in children. *Br J Radiol* 56:527, 1983.
7. Miller J, Reid BS, Kemberling CR: Water bath ultrasound of the chest in childhood. *Radiology* 152:401, 1984.

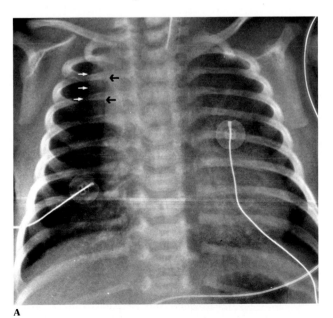

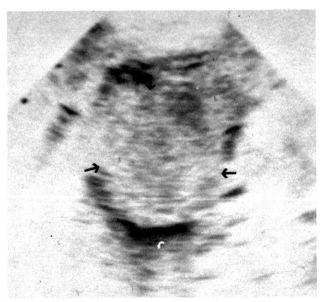

A   B

Figure 28-7   Neuroblastoma. A. This chest radiograph of a 3-week-old infant identifies a large mass lesion in the right upper mediastinum. The lateral margin of the lesion is outlined by white arrows. The lateral margin of the thymus (black arrows) is seen to lie more medially. Fluoroscopy showed some displacement of the trachea to the left together with tracheal narrowing. This caused respiratory difficulty, and the patient required intubation. **B.** An ultrasound examination shows the lesion to be moderately well defined (arrows) and to be completely solid. No cystic components are identified. This made the diagnosis of an enteric duplication cyst most unlikely.

8. Sumner TE, Volberg FM, Kiser PE, et al: Mediastinal cystic hygroma in children. *Pediatr Radiol* 11:160, 1981.

9. Hartenberg MA, Brewer WH: Cystic adenomatoid malformation of the lung: Identification by sonography. *AJR* 140:693, 1983.

10. Pezzati R, Isler R: Antenatal ultrasound diagnosis of cystic adenomatoid malformation of the lung. *JCU* 11:342, 1983.

11. Diwan RV, Brennan JN, Philipson EH, et al: Ultrasonic prenatal diagnosis of type III congenital cystic adenomatoid malformation of lung. *JCU* 11:218, 1983.

12. Canty T, Leopold G, Wolf D: *Ultrasonography of Pediatric Surgical Disorders.* New York, Grune & Stratton, 1982, pp 14–15, 37–60.

13. Phillips G, Baron MG: Use of 5.0 MHz transducer in the evaluation of pleural masses. *AJR* 137:1085, 1981.

Index

Page numbers in *italic* indicate illustrations.